MANUAL *of* VETERINARY ECHOCARDIOGRAPHY

MANUAL
of VETERINARY
ECHOCARDIOGRAPHY

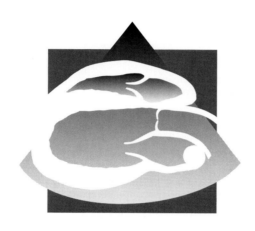

June A. Boon, MS
College of Veterinary Medicine and Biomedical Sciences
Department of Clinical Sciences
Colorado State University
Ft. Collins, Colorado

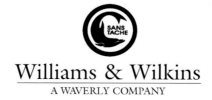

Williams & Wilkins
A WAVERLY COMPANY

BALTIMORE • PHILADELPHIA • LONDON • PARIS • BANGKOK
BUENOS AIRES • HONG KONG • MUNICH • SYDNEY • TOKYO • WROCLAW

Editor: Carroll C. Cann
Managing Editor: Paula Brown
Marketing Manager: Diane M. Harnish
Design Coordinator: Mario Fernandez

Copyright © 1998 Williams & Wilkins

351 West Camden Street
Baltimore, Maryland 21201-2436 USA

Rose Tree Corporate Center
1400 North Providence Road
Building II, Suite 5025
Media, Pennsylvania 19063-2043 USA

Printed in the United States of America

Library of Congress Cataloging-in-Publication Data

Boon, June A.
    Manual of veterinary echocardiography / author, June A. Boon.—1st
  ed.
      p.   cm.
    Includes index.
    ISBN 0-683-00938-9
    1. Veterinary echocardiography.   I. Title.
  SF811.B66 1998
  636.089′61207543—dc21

97-43333
CIP

The publishers have made every effort to trace the copyright holders for borrowed material. If they have inadvertently overlooked any, they will be pleased to make the necessary arrangements at the first opportunity.

To purchase additional copies of this book, call our customer service department at (800) **638-0672** or fax orders to (800) **447-8438**. For other book services, including chapter reprints and large quantity sales, ask for the Special Sales department.

Canadian customers should call (800) **665-1148**, or fax (800) **665-0103**. For all other calls originating outside of the United States, please call (410) **528-4223** or fax us at (410) **528-8550**.

Visit Williams & Wilkins on the Internet: http://www.wwilkins.com or contact our customer service department at **custserv@wwilkins.com**. Williams & Wilkins customer service representatives are available from 8:30 am to 6:00 pm, EST, Monday through Friday, for telephone access.

98 99 00
1 2 3 4 5 6 7 8 9 10

I dedicate this book to my husband David and my daughters Denali and Logan for their love, support, patience, and most of all, their wonderful sense of humor throughout this project.

Preface

My ultrasound experience began with soft tissue imaging in 1979, when ultrasound was in its infancy within the field of veterinary medicine. That same year, echocardiography was introduced at Colorado State University's Veterinary Teaching Hospital. The dynamic presentation of heart disease on echocardiographic images and their varying morphologies fascinated me, and given the choice, I specialized in cardiac ultrasound. The field of ultrasound has evolved from the often challenging M-mode images to two-dimensional imaging and on to both spectral and color-flow Doppler. It is no longer a modality only used at universities and by specialists but is now widely available to the general practitioner. Three things motivated me to start this project: the struggle to obtain the proper images on my own in the early years, the current scarcity of available instruction, and having to obtain interpretive information from many different sources.

Chapter 1 provides a description of ultrasound and how it can best be used to generate images. The focus of this chapter is basic ultrasound physics and how it pertains to selecting transducers, understanding artifacts, and setting equipment controls.

Chapter 2 provides detailed instructions for obtaining the standard echocardiographic imaging planes. Obtaining quality images is vitally important for accurate interpretation. Poor technique not only provides inadequate information but often inaccurate information. The guidelines within this chapter are based on years of personal experience in working with veterinarians and veterinary students on scanning techniques. These techniques consistently result in good echocardiographic examinations and accurate interpretations; although, other methods do work as well and are just as accurate. Additionally, common mistakes made while trying to obtain the standard images are described, illustrated, photographed, and corrected.

Chapter 3 provides the basis for applying echocardiographic information. A foundation for interpreting echocardiograms is built on an understanding of what cardiac disease does structurally and hemodynamically to the heart. This text is not intended to be a cardiology book, but provides sufficient physiologic and hemodynamic information to understand the echocardiographic presentation of each disease. Chapter 3 discusses what constitutes abnormal appearance, how to make measurements, and comprehending the quantitative information.

Chapters 4 and 5 cover the echocardiographic features of acquired and congenital cardiac diseases. The classic appearance of each disease as well as the many variations of each disorder are presented.

I tend to be very thorough in my examinations to fully evaluate each animal's disease and status. I know, however, that often the diagnosis can be made with much less quantitative information and attention to detail, and that not every examination requires the same depth. I do feel that the attention to detail makes further medical or surgical management of the patient much easier. I hope that as examinations become easier and faster for you that more of this information will be applied.

It is my sincere wish that this book will be used as an instructional manual and comprehensive resource for the veterinary echocardiographer. To this end, I have provided an extensive review of the veterinary echocardiographic literature as well as pertinent human references within each chapter.

Acknowledgements

I would like to thank and acknowledge Dr. E. Christopher Orton. The knowledge I have gained from you, your confidence in me, and your support throughout this project are sincerely appreciated.

I would also like to thank Dr. Wayne E. Wingfield and Dr. Charles W. Miller for giving me the opportunity 18 years ago to learn about echocardiography and to help develop the cardiac ultrasound program at Colorado State University Veterinary Teaching Hospital.

The imaging planes and instructions are illustrated beautifully by Gale Mueller, and I am indebted to her for patiently drawing and redrawing the images until they were perfect.

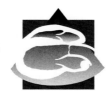

Contents

Chapter 1

PHYSICS OF ULTRASOUND   1

Basic Physics   2
Transducers and Resolution   8
Doppler Physics   13
Summary   32

Chapter 2

THE ECHOCARDIOGRAPHIC EXAMINATION   35

Introduction   35
Patient Preparation   36
Patient Positioning   37
Transducer Selection   40
Two-Dimensional Echocardiography   41
M-Mode Echocardiography   103
Spectral Doppler   112
Color-Flow Doppler   128

Chapter 3

EVALUATION OF SIZE, FUNCTION, AND HEMODYNAMICS   151

Evaluation of Size and Flow Profiles   151
Left Ventricular Function   186
Hemodynamic Information   210
Exercises   236

Chapter 4

ACQUIRED HEART DISEASE   261

Mitral Insufficiency   261
Aortic Insufficiency   286
Tricuspid and Pulmonic Insufficiencies   298

Endocarditis   301
Hypertrophic Cardiomyopathy   304
Dilated Cardiomyopathy   320
Restrictive Cardiomyopathy   332
Myocardial Infarction   337
Pulmonary Hypertension   342
Systemic Hypertension   352
Pericardial Effusions, Pericardial Disease, and Cardiac Masses   355
Miscellaneous Conditions Affecting the Heart   371

Chapter 5
CONGENITAL HEART DISEASE   383

Obstructions to Flow   383
Cardiac Shunts   409
Miscellaneous Congenital Defects   431

Appendix I: EFFECT OF ANGLE OF INCIDENCE (Θ) ON DOPPLER-DERIVED VELOCITY   447
Appendix II: EFFECT OF TRANSDUCER FREQUENCY ON THE NYQUIST LIMIT   449
Appendix III: EFFECT OF SAMPLE DEPTH ON THE NYQUIST LIMIT   451
Appendix IV: ECHOCARDIOGRAPHIC REFERENCE VALUES   453

Index   475

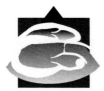

1

THE PHYSICS OF ULTRASOUND

Echocardiography (cardiac ultrasound) permits noninvasive and nonionizing visualization of the inside of the heart including the aorta, the ventricles and atria, the auricular appendages, and all the cardiac valves. Dynamic images of the contracting heart are created with two-dimensional and M-mode (motion-mode) images while blood flow through the heart can be seen and measured with Doppler ultrasound. Defects also can be seen, including valvular lesions, cardiac shunts, cardiac and thoracic masses, pleural and pericardial effusions, myocardial diseases, and stenotic lesions. More importantly, echocardiography allows assessment of cardiac chamber sizes, cardiac function, and blood flow, all of which provide information on hemodynamic status and extent of the disease process.

All this is possible because of sound. Sound is sent into the body and reflected from soft tissue structures. The reflected sound waves are analyzed, and an image is generated on a monitor. Sending out many sound waves side by side will produce an image with depth and width. The result is a two-dimensional image (Fig. 1.1). When the sound waves are continuously and rapidly sent out in sequence, many two-dimensional images can be generated per minute, and a moving image of the heart is made called real-time ultrasound. By sending out only one sound beam instead of many, only the structures associated with that one beam are seen, producing an M-mode image (Fig. 1.2). The structures associated with that one line through the heart continue to scroll on the screen as the heart continues to contract and relax. The M-mode image displays depth on the vertical axis and time on the horizontal axis.

Doppler is used in diagnostic ultrasound to provide information on blood flow through the heart and its vessels. Specific locations within the heart can be selected, and a spectral display of blood flow is created as it accelerates, reaches a maximum velocity, and then decelerates. As in M-mode, the horizontal axis represents time and the vertical axis represents velocity (Fig. 1.3).

This chapter focuses on the physical principles of sound waves that allow ultrasound to be used as a diagnostic tool. The physics of ultrasound involves an understanding of the basic properties of sound waves and how these properties affect transducer selection, image quality, and diagnostic interpretation. Only the principles needed to make knowledgeable technical decisions and diagnostic interpretations are presented in this chapter. More detailed information can be found in books dedicated to the physics of diagnostic ultrasound.

Uses of Echocardiography

- See internal cardiac structures
- Evaluate function
- Evaluate size
- See defects
  - Valvular lesions
  - Shunts
  - Myocardial abnormalities
  - Masses
  - Effusions
  - Stenotic lesions

FIGURE 1.1 Many sound waves sent into the body side by side will create an image with depth and width. The result is a two-dimensional echocardiographic image. This is a right parasternal long-axis four-chamber view of the heart. *RV*, right ventricle; *TV*, tricuspid valve; *RA*, right atrium; *IVS*, interventricular septum; *LV*, left ventricle; *LVW*, left ventricular wall; *LA*, left atrium; *MV*, mitral valve; *CT*, chordae tendinae.

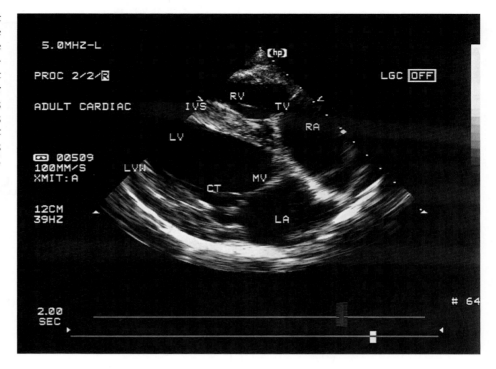

FIGURE 1.2 When one of the sound beams used to create the two-dimensional image is selected to generate an image, only the structures associated with that one beam are seen. The two-dimensional image at the top right of this figure shows a cursor representing the one beam. A one-dimensional M-mode image is created. The vertical axis represents depth and the horizontal axis represents time. Here, the structures of the left ventricle are seen as they change throughout three cardiac cycles. *RV*, right ventricle; *IVS*, interventricular septum; *LV*, left ventricle; *LVW*, left ventricular wall; *D*, diastole; *S*, systole.

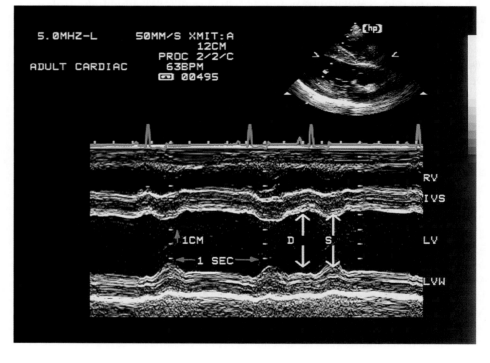

BASIC PHYSICS
Cycles and Wavelengths

Sound waves travel in longitudinal lines within a medium. The molecules along that longitudinal course of movement are alternately compressed (molecules move closer together) and rarefied (molecules are spread apart). The time required for one complete compression and rarefaction to occur is one cycle (Fig. 1.4). The distance in millimeters that the sound wave travels during one cycle is its wavelength.

Sound Waves

- Alternately compress and spread apart the molecules in their pathway
- 1 cycle = one complete compression and expansion
- Wavelength = the distance traveled during 1 cycle

The source of the sound wave determines the length of a cycle. Transducers, which will be discussed in detail later, generate the sound in diagnostic ultrasound. The wavelength is constant for each individual transducer, but there are many different transducers.

Frequency

The number of cycles per second is the frequency of the sound wave (Fig. 1.5). Frequency is measured in Hertz (Hz), where 1 Hz equals 1 cycle per second. Ultrasound has a frequency greater than 20,000 Hz and is beyond the range of human hearing. Because frequency is the number of complete cycles per second, the higher the frequency of the sound wave, the shorter the wavelength must be.

$$\uparrow \text{frequency} = \downarrow \text{wavelength}$$

A 5-megahertz (MHz) transducer transmits 5 million cycles/sec at 0.31 mm/cycle, whereas a 2-MHz transducer transmits only 2 million cycles/sec at 0.77 mm/cycle. Table 1.1 lists wavelengths for sound generated at various frequencies.

Frequency
- The number of cycles per second = frequency
- High frequency = shorter wavelengths
- Low frequency = longer wavelengths

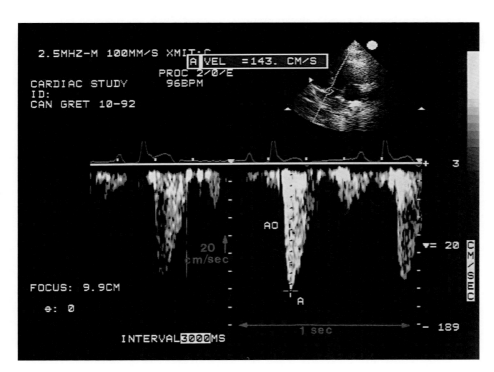

FIGURE 1.3   Doppler images display flow velocities on the vertical axis and time on the horizontal axis. Blood flow for specified areas in the heart is seen as it accelerates, reaches a maximum velocity, and then decelerates throughout the cardiac cycle. This CW Doppler tracing of aortic flow (*AO*) in a dog has a velocity of 143 cm/sec (*A*).

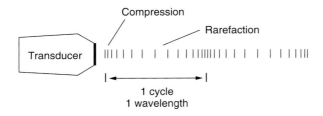

FIGURE 1.4   Sound waves cause compression and rarefaction of the molecules along the path of the sound waves. The time for one complete compression and rarefaction to occur is called a cycle. The distance sound travels during one cycle is measured in millimeters and is its wavelength.

TABLE 1.1
WAVELENGTHS OF SOUND AT COMMONLY USED FREQUENCIES

Frequency (MHz)	Wavelength (mm)
2.0	.77
3.5	.44
5.0	.31
7.5	.21

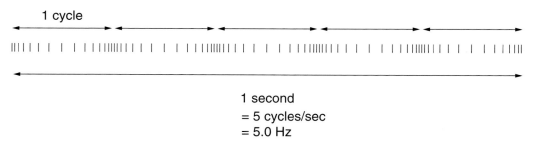

1 second
= 5 cycles/sec
= 5.0 Hz

FIGURE 1.5   The number of cycles per second is the frequency of the sound wave. Frequency is measured in Hertz (Hz) and 1 Hz equals 1 cycle per second.

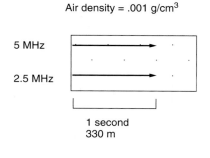

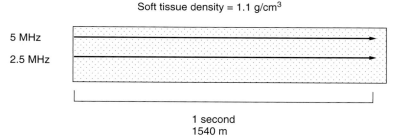

FIGURE 1.6   Increased tissue density allows sound to travel faster. Sound generated by a 2.5-MHz transducer and a 5-MHz transducer will have the same velocity within the same tissues because the speed of sound is not affected by frequency.

Speed of Sound

The speed of sound (V) depends on the density and stiffness of the medium through which it is traveling. Increased density allows sound to travel faster. The velocity of sound does not change within a homogeneous substance and is independent of frequency (Fig. 1.6). Table 1.2 lists the speed of sound in various tissues. The speed of sound through air is very slow because of the low density and stiffness of the air, whereas bone allows sound to travel at relatively high speeds.

The average velocity of a sound wave in soft tissue is 1540 m/sec regardless of transducer frequency (Fig. 1.7). Velocity is calibrated into the ultrasound machine, which then calculates the distance (D) to cardiac structures based on the time it takes to receive reflected echoes (T):

$$D = V \times T/2 \qquad \text{(Eq. 1.1)}$$

The time (T) required to travel 1 cm is 6.5 microseconds or 13 microseconds round trip. Although sound must travel through various tissues with slightly different velocities during an echocardiographic examination, the equipment is calibrated for the average speed of sound in soft tissues (1540 m/sec). Structures are displayed on a monitor at the calculated depth and an image of the heart is created. This always creates some degree of error in calculating true structure depth, but the error is nominal.

Acoustic Impedance

Acoustic impedance is the opposition or resistance to the flow of sound through a medium. Impedance depends on the density and stiffness of the medium and is independent of frequency. Stiff or hard materials are difficult to compress and rarefy. Although increased density increases the speed of sound, if the ability to compress and rarefy sound waves is limited, the impedance or resistance to sound transmission is high.

$$\text{acoustical impedance} = \text{density} \times \text{speed} \qquad \text{(Eq. 1.2)}$$

Contradictory as it sounds, the higher the density and greater the velocity of sound through a medium, the greater the resistance to sound transmission. Table 1.3 lists the acoustical impedance of sound in various tissues. Because of the stiffness and

TABLE 1.2
THE SPEED OF SOUND IN SOFT TISSUES

Tissue	Speed (m/sec)
Air	330
Fat	1440
Brain	1510
Liver	1560
Kidney	1560
Muscle	1570
Blood	1570
Bone	4080

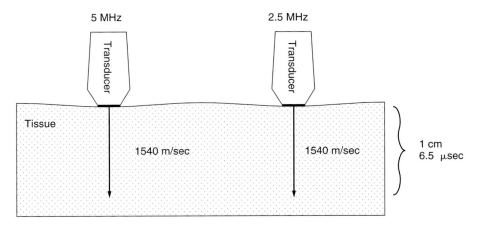

FIGURE 1.7   Sound travels through soft tissues at an average velocity of 1540 m/sec regardless of transducer frequency. The time required to travel 1 cm at 1540 m/sec is 6.5 μsec one way and 13 μsec round trip.

inability to compress and rarefy molecules easily, bone has a high impedance. Air, because the molecules are compressed and rarefied easily, has a low impedance. Acoustical impedence produces a high degree of sound reflection at bony interfaces, creating a shadow on the ultrasound image beyond the bone because of lack of further transmission.

Reflection, Refraction, and Scattering

Reflection is sound that is turned back at a boundary within a medium. These reflected echoes are called specular echoes. When two tissues with different acoustical impedances interface, a portion of the sound is reflected back to the transducer and the rest of the sound continues through the tissues. The greater the acoustical impedance, the greater the degree of reflection. By the same token, if two boundaries have little acoustical mismatch, they will not be identified as two different tissues. Therefore, interfaces between muscle and fluid, as in the heart, will reflect sound while the cells within the homogeneous muscle itself will not.

All interfaces between muscle and blood-filled chambers in the heart have slightly brighter boundaries on the ultrasound image because of this increased reflection. The interface between tissue and air has an even greater difference in acoustical impedance, and therefore, the pericardial sac around the heart is always one of the brightest structures in the ultrasound image. The gel placed between the transducer and skin surfaces prevents the large degree of reflection ordinarily seen between a tissue and air interface.

The angle at which sound strikes the reflective surface (the angle of incidence) determines the angle of reflection. The angle of reflection is equal to the angle of incidence (Fig. 1.8). When sound is directed perpendicular to a structure, the angle of incidence is zero, and the sound is reflected straight back to the transducer. If the angle of incidence is 50°, then the angle of reflection also will be 50°. When the angle of incidence is 90° or parallel to the interface, no sound will be reflected back to the source. This principle tells us that the best two-dimensional and M-mode cardiac images are obtained when sound is directed perpendicular to the tissues.

Not all sound is reflected however, and some continues on through the tissues. These sound waves are refracted if the two tissues are different (Fig. 1.8). Refraction is the change in direction of sound as it travels from one medium to another, which is similar to what happens when light waves in water create a distorted image. The greater the mismatch in acoustical impedance between the two tissues, the greater the degree of refraction. As the refracted sound beam travels in a new direction, the angle of reflection, with respect to the original source, is different. Thus, positional errors can result because the transducer thinks the received sound is coming from the same direction as the sound waves it generated earlier.

The errors produced by refraction during an examination create few problems, unless the refracted beam has to travel a great distance. A 1 or 2° angle at the top of the refracting tissue can result in a several millimeter error in position by the time the sound beam reaches the far side of a deep structure. When the two mediums differ enough to create a refractive angle of greater than 90° (as with soft tissue and bone), an image is not generated beyond the second structure.

Reflection of Sound

- Depends on acoustical mismatch
  - The greater the difference in acoustical properties, the greater the degree of reflection
- Depends on angle of incidence
  - Sound striking an organ perpendicularly will have almost all its sound reflected straight back to the transducer
- Depends on the size of the reflecting structure
  - Must be at least one-quarter the size of the wavelength
    - Higher-frequency transducers can reflect sound from smaller structures

TABLE 1.3
ACOUSTICAL IMPEDANCE OF VARIOUS TISSUES

Tissue	Impedance (g/cm^2/sec)
Bone	7.80×10^5
Muscle	1.70×10^5
Kidney	1.62×10^5
Blood	1.61×10^5
Brain	1.58×10^5
Fat	1.38×10^5
Air	$.0004 \times 10^5$

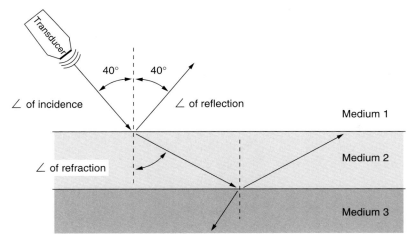

FIGURE 1.8 The angle of reflection is equal to the angle at which sound strikes the tissue. Sound that is directed perpendicular to the tissue is reflected straight back to the transducer, producing the best images. Sound is refracted when it crosses a boundary between two different tissues. The greater the difference in acoustical properties between the two tissues, the greater the degree of refraction.

Reflection of sound not only depends on the acoustical mismatch of two tissues but also the size of the structure. The structure must be at least one-quarter the size of the wavelength for reflection to occur. The short 0.21-mm wavelengths of a 7.5-MHz transducer can be reflected off structures that are as small as 0.05 mm in thickness, whereas structures must be at least 0.19 mm thick for the 0.77-mm wavelengths of a 2-MHz transducer to be reflected. High-frequency transducers, therefore, provide higher resolution images because smaller structures reflect their sound waves.

Structures that are small and irregular with respect to the sound wave do not reflect sound, but rather scatter it in all directions without regard for the angle of incidence (Fig. 1.9). Some of this scattered sound is directed back to the sound source and is what allows ultrasound to give us information about tissue character. Scattered sound is important for generating images from objects with large angles of incidence to the sound beam or from small structures like cells.

Attenuation

Sound traveling through a medium is weakened by reflection, refraction, scattering, and absorption of heat by the tissues. This loss of energy is called attenuation. High-frequency sound attenuates to a greater degree than low-frequency sound because its wavelength allows the sound to interact with more structures. This is the reason the deep bass sounds of an orchestra carry farther than the high-pitched sounds. The large degree of attenuation with high-frequency sound leaves less energy available for continued transmission through the medium.

↑ Frequency = ↓ Depth
↓ Frequency = ↑ Depth

The half-power distance of a tissue is the distance sound will travel through it before half of the available sound energy has been attenuated. Table 1.4 lists the half-power distances of various tissues at two different frequencies. The data in this table clearly show that low-frequency sound waves are able to penetrate tissues deeper than high-frequency sound waves.

Air attenuates half of the sound energy within 0.05 cm when a 2-MHz transducer is used. Therefore, although the density of air creates less impedance for sound, little sound energy is left to generate an image from soft tissues after 0.05 cm. Gel is used to eliminate the air between the transducer and skin, which otherwise would attenuate sound dramatically.

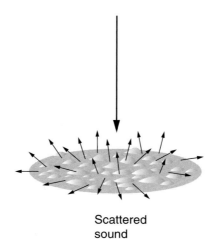

Scattered
sound

FIGURE 1.9   Structures that are small and irregular with respect to the wavelength cause sound to scatter in all directions. Some of this scattered sound will be directed back to the transducer for image generation. Scattered sound is important in tissue characterization.

TABLE 1.4
HALF-POWER DISTANCES OF VARIOUS TISSUES

Tissue	Distance (cm)	
	2.0 MHz	5.0 MHz
Water	380	.54
Blood	15	3
Soft tissue	1.5	.5
Muscle	.75	.3
Bone	.1	.04
Air	.05	.01

TRANSDUCERS AND RESOLUTION

Transducers are the source of sound in diagnostic ultrasound. Transducers contain piezoelectric crystals, which are deformed by electrical voltage and generate sound. These crystals, often called elements, also are able to receive sound and convert it back into electrical energy. The thickness of the crystals dictate the basic operating frequency of the transducer. Wavelength will be one-half of the element thickness, so decreased crystal thickness produces shorter wavelengths and higher frequencies.

Pulse Repetition Frequency

Transducers used in pulsed echo applications do not transmit sound continuously, but send sound waves out in short bursts and receive sound the remainder of the time. This is called pulsed ultrasound. The number of pulses per second is referred to as the pulse repetition frequency (PRF), which is also measured in Hertz. The PRF, for example, would be 10 Hz if there are 10 pulses per second (Fig. 1.10). Each pulse may have any number of cycles, but in diagnostic ultrasound there are 2 or 3 cycles per pulse. The number of cycles per pulse is controlled by damping materials within the transducer.

   The pulse duration (measured in microseconds) and pulse length (measured in millimeters) decrease if the sound wave frequency increases because the wavelengths are shorter (Fig. 1.10). Likewise, lower-frequency sound waves have longer wavelengths, thus pulse duration and length are increased. Accurate ultrasound images only can be generated if all reflected and scattered echoes are received at the transducer before the next pulse is generated. The transducer assumes that the echoes it receives are products of its last burst. If an echo has not been received before the next burst and it arrives at the transducer shortly after the second burst, then the instrument "thinks" that little time has elapsed since it was transmitted and received. Because time is used along with the speed of sound in tissues to determine structure depth, a structure that actually is deeper will be displayed closer to the body surface (Fig. 1.11). Pulse repetition frequency must decrease as deeper structures are imaged for accurate depth assessment.

Sound Beams

Sound beams generated by transducers are three dimensional. They not only have pulse length and duration, but also have beam widths and thicknesses. Beam diameter determines the width within the scan plane and the thickness perpendicular to the scan plane.

Sound beams do not remain the same width as they travel through a medium. In an unfocused transducer, the sound beam starts out with a width equal to the transducer diameter, and as the sound beam travels through the tissues, it diverges (Fig. 1.12). The distance from the transducer element to where the sound beam diverges is the near field of the beam. The area beyond the near field is the far field. Near field length is directly proportional to the beam diameter and inversely proportional to wavelength (Fig. 1.12). For two transducers of the same frequency, the near field will be longer for the transducer with the larger diameter. For two transducers with the same diameter, the near field will be longer for the higher-frequency transducer.

Far field divergence also depends on transducer size. Larger diameter transducers produce less divergence in the far field. High-frequency transducers with large diameters, therefore, produce the longest near field and the narrowest far field (Fig. 1.12).

If a curved element or lens is used, the beam can be focused, and beam width will decrease throughout the entire near field and create a focal zone; however, beam width will diverge rapidly beyond this focal point (Fig. 1.13). Many transducers have variable focal zones that the examiner can set. Focal zones, however, cannot be selected beyond the near field length of the transducer.

If multiple pulses are generated and each pulse is set to a different focal zone, then

Near field = radius² / wavelength
Larger beam width = longer near field
Shorter wavelength = longer near field

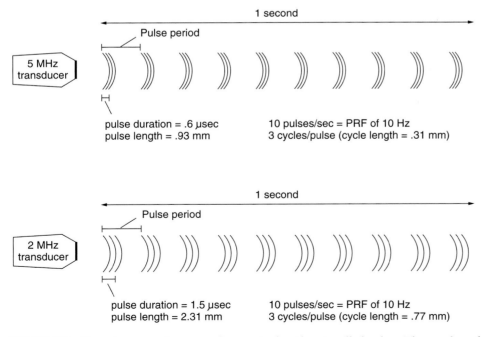

pulse duration = .6 µsec
pulse length = .93 mm

10 pulses/sec = PRF of 10 Hz
3 cycles/pulse (cycle length = .31 mm)

pulse duration = 1.5 µsec
pulse length = 2.31 mm

10 pulses/sec = PRF of 10 Hz
3 cycles/pulse (cycle length = .77 mm)

FIGURE 1.10 Transducers send out sound waves in short bursts called pulses. The number of pulses per second is called the pulse repetition frequency (*PRF*) measured in Hz. Each pulse has a duration based on the wavelength and number of cycles.

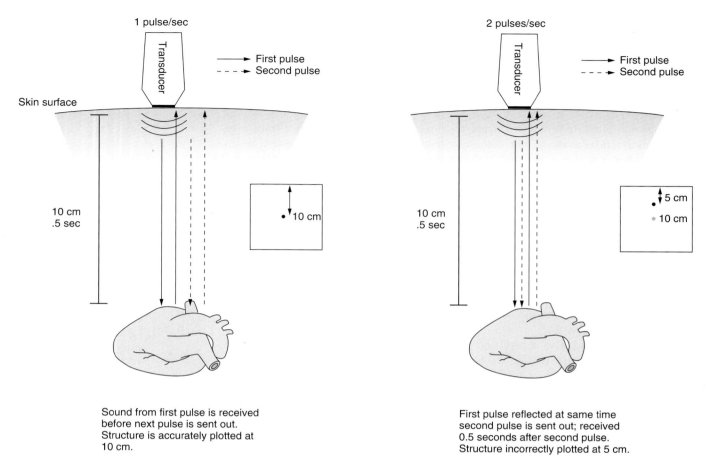

FIGURE 1.11   A sound wave must be transmitted, reflected, and received by the transducer before the next pulse is generated. The number of pulses per second is the pulse repetition frequency. Pulse repetition frequency must decrease for accurate structure localization when interrogating deeper structures.

an elongated focal zone can be created. The transducer simply ignores echoes returning from depths other than the focal depth for any given pulse.

Up to this point, only single sound beams have been considered. A single sound beam is used to generate an M-mode image of the heart. The beam travels through the cardiac structures and generates a one-dimensional image. Real-time or two-dimensional imaging uses an array (group) of crystals that are either mechanically or electronically triggered to generate sound waves. Each sound beam generated by a two-dimensional transducer is affected by pulse length, beam width, focal length, and PRF.

Mechanical transducers have one crystal that rapidly moves back and forth in an arc to create the two-dimensional sector image. Linear array transducers have multiple elements arranged in a row, whereas annular array transducers have multiple crystals arranged in a ring. Sequences of elements are electronically stimulated at one time (i.e., elements 1–4, then elements 2–5, etc.), with each group producing one scan line. This produces a high-quality image with increased line density within the generated image. Linear array transducers typically are not used in cardiac ultrasound.

Phased array transducers stimulate each crystal with a small time interval (less than a microsecond) between them and are directed through the tissues at slightly different angles (phased), producing a sector image (Fig. 1.14). These transducers

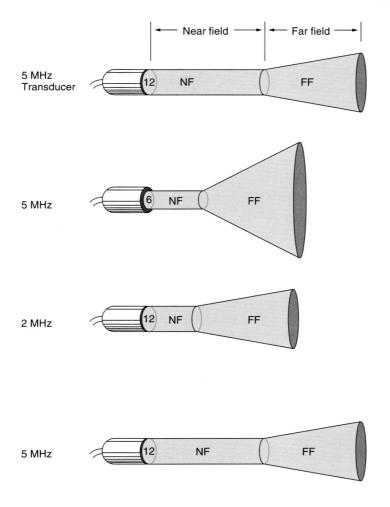

Near Field = r²/wavelength

∴ ↑ beam diameter = longer near field for transducers of the same frequency

∴ ↑ frequency = longer near field for transducers of the same diameter

∴ ↑ diameter = less far field divergence for same frequency

FIGURE 1.12   Sound beams have a diameter equal to transducer diameter and diverge as they travel out through a tissue. The distance from a transducer element to where the beam diverges is referred to as the near field. The area beyond that is the far field.

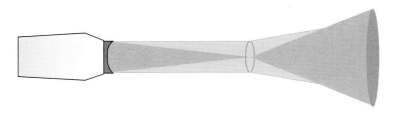

FIGURE 1.13   A sound beam can be focused by using a curved element or lens. This decreases beam width within the near field.

often are called electronic sector transducers. Rapidly stimulating these elements over and over again in sequence produces the moving cardiac images we call real-time ultrasound.

Annular phased array transducers have crystals arranged in rings. The rings are stimulated from the outside in. An entire ring can be focused both within the scan plane (longitudinally) and perpendicular (laterally) to the scan plane (Fig. 1.15), decreasing beam width in both dimensions. This tremendously enhances image resolution.

Axial Resolution

Resolution is the ability to identify two objects as different. Pulse length, beam width, beam diameter, focal length, and PRF are important physical aspects of transducers that affect the axial, lateral, and temporal resolution of ultrasound images.

Axial resolution is the ability to differentiate between two structures along the length of the sound beam. Axial resolution also is called depth or longitudinal resolution. The smaller the axial resolution, the better the detail of the image.

Transducer frequency plays an important role in axial resolution. Axial resolution is equal to half the pulse length, that is, two structures cannot be closer than half the pulse length to each other to be distinguished as two separate structures. Remember that pulse length depends on the wavelength of the sound and the number of cycles per pulse. When one or both of these is reduced, axial resolution improves (Fig. 1.16). Wavelength decreases as frequency of sound increases; therefore, axial resolution is better with 7.5-MHz frequency sound than with 3.5-MHz frequency sound. Pulse length and duration are shortened by adding damping materials within the transducer or electrical damping within the equipment.

Lateral Resolution

Lateral resolution is the ability to resolve two structures as distinct and different in a plane perpendicular to the sound wave. Lateral resolution is equal to beam width and improves with smaller beam widths. Beam width is affected by the following:

1. Focus of transducer-generated sound waves

2. Transducer diameter

3. Transducer frequency

The narrower the beam width, the better the ability to differentiate between two structures in a plane perpendicular to the sound beam (Fig. 1.17). Beam width varies along the length of the sound wave, but is narrowest at the focal zone in focused transducers. Lateral resolution is best (smallest) at the focal zone. Two structures that are side by side within the boundaries of the beam width will not be resolved as two different structures (Fig. 1.17). However, if they are offset a little in depth, they may be resolved as two different structures based on axial resolving powers of the transducer (Fig. 1.17).

Lateral resolution of an image is also best within the near field where beam width

---

Resolution

Axial: The ability to differentiate between two structures along the length of the sound beam.

Lateral: The ability to resolve two structures as different in the plane perpendicular to the sound beam.

Temporal: The ability to resolve structures with respect to time, keeping up with the actual events.

Pulse Length

- A pulse may have any number of cycles (generally 2–3 in echocardiography).
- Pulse length decreases with higher-frequency sound because of shorter wavelengths and increases with lower-frequency sound.

Axial Resolution

- Better axial resolution = better image detail
- Equal to one-half the pulse length
  - Higher-frequency transducers have better axial resolution

Lateral Resolution

- Improves with narrower beam widths
- Usually narrowest at focal zones of focused transducers
- Best within near field where beam width is narrowest

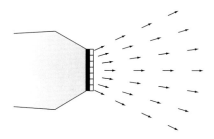

FIGURE 1.14   Phased array transducers have elements that are stimulated in sequence creating a slightly different angle of transmission through the tissues. This produces a rapidly moving real-time sector image.

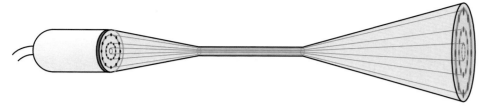

FIGURE 1.15   Annular phased array transducers have crystals arranged in a ring. Each ring is focused longitudinally within the image plane and perpendicularly (laterally) to the scan plane, enhancing resolution.

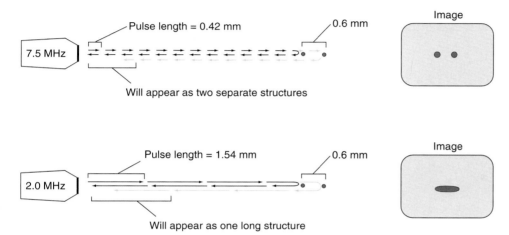

FIGURE 1.16   Axial resolution improves with increased frequency and decreased pulse length. Two objects must be further apart than one-half the pulse length to be identified as two different structures.

is narrowest. A high-frequency transducer will have better lateral resolution than a low-frequency transducer of the same size because of its longer near field. Long, narrow near fields allow more specific areas of the heart to be imaged, creating less ambiguity about the source of returning echoes (lateral position errors).

Longer near field length, focused transducer beams, and less far field divergence also improve image quality by increasing beam strength. Stronger beams increase the degree of reflection and can travel farther before all the sound is attenuated.

Temporal Resolution

The frame rate is the number of real-time images produced per minute depending on the PRF. The faster the frame rate, the faster the PRF. Faster frame rates produce better temporal resolution (resolution with respect to time). Logically, rapidly moving structures require fast frame rates to prevent blurred images and freeze-frame images of cardiac motion.

Sector transducers that emit multiple pulses with varying focal zones per scan line must wait until all sound has returned before generating the next set of pulses; otherwise, range or depth ambiguity results. In doing so, the frame rate and temporal resolution of the generated real-time image is reduced. Interrogation of deep structures also requires a slower frame rate, possibly resulting in less temporal resolution. PRF in both of these settings can be increased by reducing sector width, because less time is required before the next frame can be produced.

DOPPLER PHYSICS

Doppler dramatically has increased the diagnostic capabilities of cardiac ultrasound. This modality allows detection and analysis of moving blood cells and tells us about

Temporal Resolution

• Depends on frame rate
  • Reduce sector width to improve the frame rate

↑ Frequency = ↑ Resolution
↓ Frequency = ↓ Resolution

Doppler Ultrasound

Allows detection and analysis of moving blood cells and provides hemodynamic information
  • Direction
  • Velocity
  • Character
  • Timing

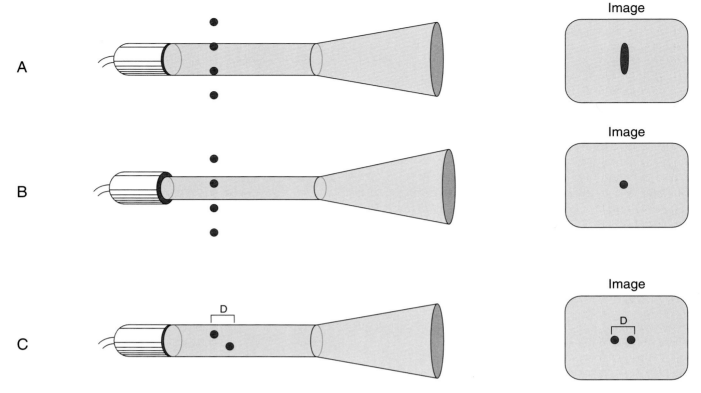

FIGURE 1.17   The ability to resolve two structures as different in a plane perpendicular (lateral resolution) to the sound beam depends on beam width. **A.** Two structures that fall within beam width will not be differentiated. **B.** Two structures that are farther apart than the beam width will be identified as separate. **C.** The axial resolving powers of the system may differentiate two structures that fall within beam width when they are offset in depth. *D*, depth.

the direction, velocity, character, and timing of blood flow. The hemodynamic information provided by Doppler echocardiography allows definitive diagnosis in most cardiac examinations.

Three types of Doppler may be used during an echocardiographic examination:

1. Pulsed-wave (PW)
2. Continuous-wave (CW)
3. Color-flow (CF)

Pulsed-wave (PW) Doppler is site specific, in which it can be directed and set to sample flow at specific places within the heart. However, PW Doppler is limited in its capacity to detect higher frequency (velocity) shifts. Continuous-wave (CW) Doppler can detect high-frequency shifts and, therefore, high-flow velocities with virtually no limits. Because sound is transmitted and received continuously, it is not possible to select and interrogate at specific depths within the heart. Although this may sound disadvantageous, the information provided is valuable. Color-flow (CF) Doppler is a form of pulsed-wave Doppler. Frequency shifts are encoded with varying hues and intensities of color. Flow information is graphic, and detection of abnormal flow is easier with CF Doppler; however, quantitative information is limited. These various forms of Doppler ultrasound and the factors that influence them are discussed in the following sections.

The Doppler Shift

Christian Johann Doppler (1803–1853), an Austrian physicist and mathematician, was the first to describe the Doppler effect. He found that all types of waves (light, sound, etc.) change in wavelength when the position between the source of the wave

---

Pulsed-Wave (PW) Doppler

- Allows flow to be examined at very specific sites
- Is limited in the maximum velocity that it can record accurately

Continuous-Wave (CW) Doppler

- There is no limit to the maximum velocity it can record
- Is not site specific; blood cells are examined all along the sound beam

Color-Flow (CF) Doppler

- Is a form of pulsed-wave Doppler
- Color codes the various velocities and directions of flow

The Doppler Shift

Wavelength (pitch and frequency) changes when the position between the sound source and the reflecting structure (blood cells in this case) changes.

and the receiver of the wave changes. For example, if you move toward a sound source, the pitch or frequency of that sound increases, and if you move away from that sound source, the frequency decreases. The change in frequency between sound that is transmitted and sound that is received is the Doppler shift.

When the source and the reflecting surface are both stationary, the transmitted (incident) and reflected wavelengths are equal (Fig. 1.18). When the reflecting structure is moving toward the source, sound waves are encountered more often, increasing the number of waves (↑ frequency) reflected back toward the source. When the reflecting structure is moving away from the source, sound waves travel

Cells moving toward the transducer reflect an increased number of sound waves and thus the received frequency is greater than the transmitted frequency.

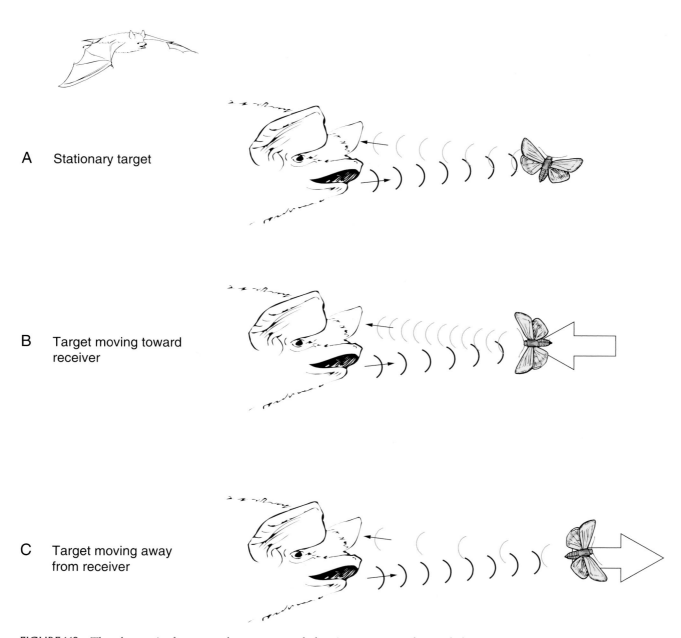

A   Stationary target

B   Target moving toward receiver

C   Target moving away from receiver

FIGURE 1.18   The change in frequency between sound that is sent out and sound that is reflected is called the Doppler shift. Bats use this principle when searching for food. **A.** Sound reflected from a stationary target will have the same frequency as the transmitted sound. **B.** Sound reflected from an object moving toward the bat will have a higher frequency than that sent out because the object encounters the incident waves more often. **C.** The object encounters the transmitted wavefront less often and a decrease in frequency is perceived when an object moves away from the bat.

Cells moving away from the transducer reflect less sound waves and thus the received frequency is less than the transmitted frequency.

ahead of the transmitted wavefront and are encountered less frequently, decreasing the number of sound waves (↓ frequency) reflected back to the source.

Everyday examples of Doppler shifts include any loud sound moving toward or away from you, such as sirens, trains, marching bands, etc. The sound of a siren as it approaches you will increase in pitch (frequency increases) and as it passes you will decrease in pitch (frequency decreases). Doppler radar uses this principle when police officers determine the speed of a car, because the frequency shift is used to determine velocity. Doppler radar also is used in forecasting weather. The Doppler shift that we use in diagnostic ultrasound is the difference in frequency transmitted by the transducer and received frequency reflected from blood cells.

Doppler Tracing

The Doppler-derived frequency shift (f_d) is equal to reflected frequency minus transmitted frequency; therefore, objects moving toward the source result in positive frequency shifts, whereas objects moving away from the source result in negative frequency shifts. The site (gate) for Doppler flow interrogation is selected by the examiner and is represented on the Doppler display as a line (baseline). Positive frequency shifts (flow moving toward the transducer) produce waveforms up from the baseline, whereas negative frequency shifts (flow moving away from the transducer) produce downward deflections on the Doppler tracing (Fig. 1.19). These images are called spectral tracings.

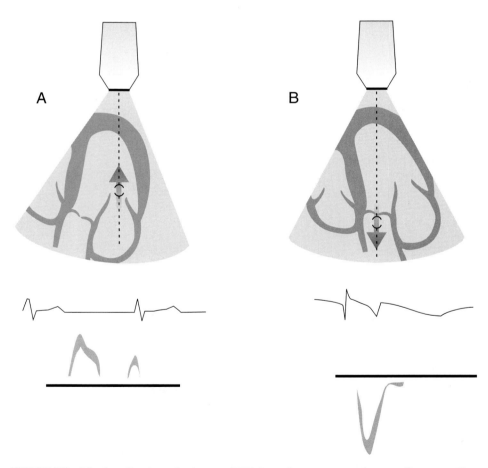

FIGURE 1.19   The baseline in pulsed-wave (PW) Doppler represents the sampling gate. Flow moving toward the transducer creates a positive frequency shift, and velocity will be plotted above the baseline. **A.** Mitral valve flow in this apical five-chamber view is toward the transducer and its flow profile is seen above the baseline. **B.** Aortic flow, moving away from the transducer in this apical five-chamber view, creates a negative frequency shift and its flow profile is shown below the baseline.

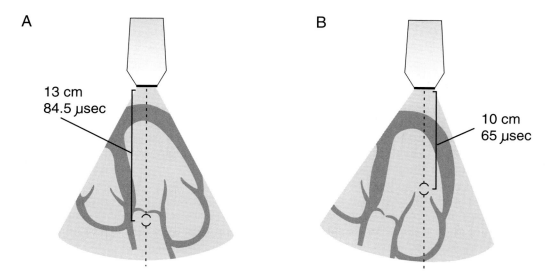

FIGURE 1.20   Frequency shifts are recorded only during the time interval indicated by the depth of the sample gate. Deeper gates require more time. **A.** A gate depth of 13 cm requires 169 μsec, whereas a gate of 10 cm (**B**) requires only 130 μsec to receive reflected sound at the transducer. Lower pulse repetition frequency is required for deeper structures.

Pulsed-Wave (PW) Doppler

Pulsing the sound waves allows a transducer to act as a receiver for the signal only during the time interval specified by a sample depth. With PW Doppler, the transducer will record frequency shifts only during the time interval dictated by the depth of the sample site, ignoring all other returning echoes (Fig. 1.20). New sound waves will not be transmitted until the transducer has received the echoes from the previous burst. Range resolution is the ability to measure velocity within a small cell at a specified depth along the ultrasound beam. The gate is the site at which sampling is set to occur. The examiner manually sets the gate while watching a two-dimensional image.

Continuous-Wave (CW) Doppler

CW Doppler continuously sends out sound and continuously receives sound. It is not possible to range gate CW Doppler because the transducer has no way of detecting the depth of the reflected signal. CW Doppler detects frequency shifts all along the ultrasound beam with no range resolution and is steered in one of two ways. Imaging CW systems use a cursor representing the Doppler sound beam. The cursor is placed over the two-dimensional image, and frequency shifts are calculated all along the beam in imaging CW systems. Nonimaging CW systems use a dedicated CW probe without a two-dimensional image. These systems require recognition of characteristic flow profiles.

Velocities along the beam vary, and a full spectrum of frequency shifts are detected with CW Doppler. When CW Doppler is used properly, the highest velocities along the line of interrogation are recorded. (Fig. 1.21). The highest flow velocities are what is of interest and diagnostically important. Lower velocity flows are hidden within the higher flow profiles. Flow patterns for the various valves and vessels in the heart are characteristic and usually are identified easily with both PW and CW Doppler.

The Doppler Equation

Doppler ultrasound can determine blood cell velocity within the heart or in peripheral vessels based on the Doppler shift. Blood cell velocity (V) is determined using the following formula:

$$V = \frac{C \times f_d}{2\,(f_o) \times \cos\theta} \tag{Eq.1.3}$$

Equation 1.3 shows that V is equal to the speed of sound in tissues (C) times the frequency shift (f_d) in kHz, divided by the transmitting frequency of the transducer (f_o [2.5, 3.5, 5.0, etc.]), times the cosine of θ, where θ is equal to the intercept angle of the ultrasound beam with blood flow.

The speed of sound in tissues is a constant (1540 m/sec), leaving the interrogation angle, θ, and transducer frequency as variables that can be controlled. Let's consider these two variables and how they affect the way a Doppler examination should be conducted and interpreted.

Angle of Interrogation

An important part of the Doppler equation is the cosine of the intercept angle. The closer to parallel the transmitted wave is with the direction of the interrogated blood flow, the more accurate the velocity measurement (Fig. 1.22).

When the Doppler equation is changed to calculate for the frequency shift, you can see that the cosine of the intercept angle directly affects the frequency shift (f_d).

$$f_d = \frac{V \times (2\,f_o) \times \cos\theta}{C} \tag{Eq. 1.4}$$

Because the speed of sound in tissues (C) and the transmitting frequency (f_o) are known, the calculated frequency shift and, therefore, the calculated flow velocity directly depend on the cosine of the intercept angle. The cosine of 0° is 1. The value of the cosine decreases as the angle of interrogation increases, and by the time an angle of 90° is reached, the cosine is zero. Table 1.5 lists the cosines for several angles. Larger intercept angles and cosines of less than 1 falsely decrease the recorded frequency shift of blood flow. Interrogation angles greater than 15° are considered unacceptable. The graph in Figure 1.23 shows the relationship between the cosine of the angle of incidence with respect to blood flow and the calculated velocity for a 5-MHz transducer.

Appendix 1 shows the mathematics involved in deriving flow velocities as the intercept angles with respect to blood flow increase.

Velocity Measurement

- Accurate measurements are affected by:
  - Transducer frequency
  - Intercept angle

Intercept Angle and Velocity Measurements

Velocity cannot be overestimated, just underestimated when interrogation angles with respect to flow become larger than zero.

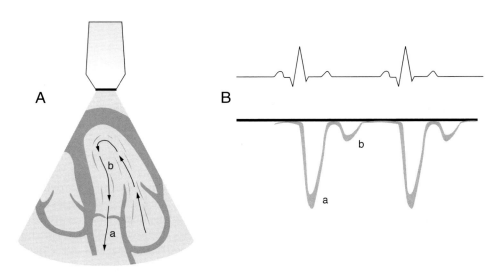

FIGURE 1.21   Continuous-wave Doppler detects frequency shifts all along the transmitted sound beam. All velocities are recorded. **A.** The highest velocity during systole is flow out of the aorta, and lower velocities during this time period are recorded but hidden within the aortic flow profile. **B.** The CW sound beam also records flow during diastole near the apex of the heart.

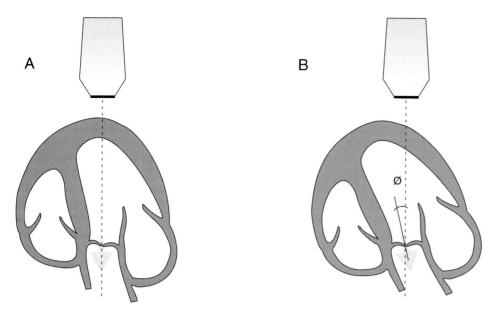

FIGURE 1.22 Frequency shifts directly depend on the cosine of the interrogation angle. **A.** The closer to parallel the transmitted Doppler signal is to blood flow, the more accurate the velocity will be because the cosine of 0° is 1. **B.** As the intercept angle, θ, deviates from 0, velocity will be underestimated.

TABLE 1.5
COSINES OF SELECTED ANGLES

Angle (Θ)	Cosine Θ
0	1.000
5	.996
10	.985
15	.966
20	.940
25	.906
30	.866
50	.643
75	.259
90	.000

Effect of Transducer Frequency

PW Doppler measures the frequency shift at specific locations within the heart. Just like two-dimensional and M-mode imaging, the reflected signal must be received before the next pulse is transmitted or the recorded signals will be ambiguous. The time interval between pulses, also referred to as the pulse repetition frequency (PRF), must be two times the sample depth. The time between pulses must increase as sample depth increases, resulting in decreased PRF. Decreased PRF decreases the Doppler frequency shift that can be measured accurately. Figure 1.24 shows how sampling frequency affects the perception of events. As the sampling frequency decreases, information is lost. Time on the clock in Figure 1.24 is perceived correctly until the sampling frequency decreases to two times per minute. At that rate, it is not possible to determine whether the hand on the clock is moving clockwise or counterclockwise. At a lower PRF of three times every 2 minutes, the hand seems to be moving counterclockwise. This is similar to what happens in movies when wheels on vehicles seem to rotate backward. The sampling rate (PRF) must be at least two times the frequency shift for the transducer to receive unambiguous flow information. Equation 1.5 states that the maximum Doppler shift that can be recorded accurately is equal to one-half the PRF.

Transducer Frequency and Velocity Measurement

The best Doppler recordings at any given depth are obtained with lower-frequency transducers.

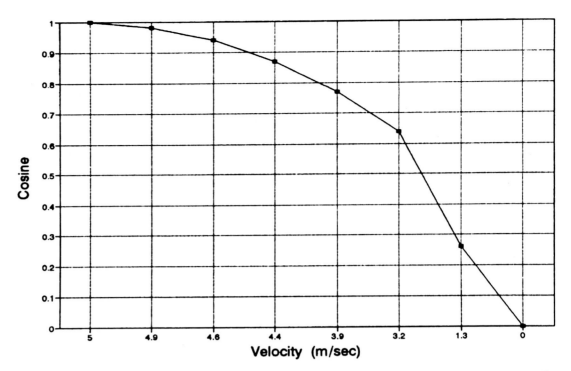

FIGURE 1.23   The effect of interrogation angle on maximum velocity. Cosine becomes smaller than 1 as intercept angles increase and falsely decrease recorded blood velocities. Angles greater than 15° are considered unacceptable because they greatly underestimate the true velocity.

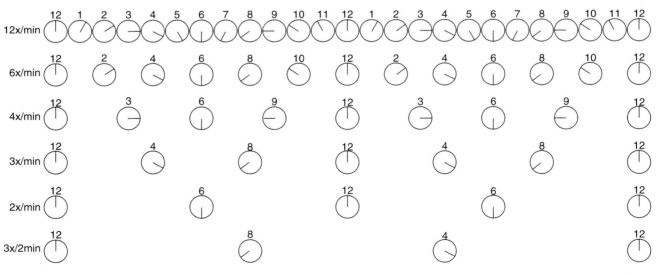

FIGURE 1.24   When sampling frequency (PRF) is not enough, the information obtained may not represent accurately what is occurring. In this diagram, the top line has a sampling frequency of 12 times per minute, and the time is displayed accurately. As sampling frequency decreases to 2 times per minute, it is not possible to decide if time is moving clockwise or counterclockwise. With an even lower sampling frequency of 3 times every 2 minutes, the events are erroneously perceived as moving counterclockwise. This is similar to what happens in PW Doppler when a signal aliases, creating ambiguity in the perceived direction of flow.

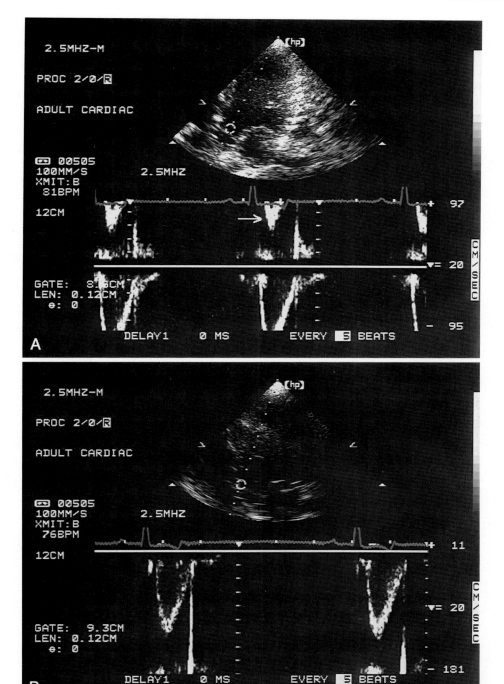

FIGURE 1.25   When the Nyquist limit is exceeded, aliasing occurs. **A.** When the Nyquist limit is not exceeded by a great degree, we can still see the typical flow profile; however, it wraps around the image. **B.** This type of aliasing can be eliminated by moving the baseline up or down to see the entire flow profile.

$$\text{Doppler shift} = \tfrac{1}{2}\,\text{PRF} \qquad\qquad \text{(Eq. 1.5)}$$

One-half the PRF is referred to as the Nyquist limit. When the Nyquist limit is exceeded, signal ambiguity results called aliasing. Figure 1.25 shows an aliased Doppler display. When the Nyquist limit is barely exceeded, the flow profile wraps around the image. This can be corrected by moving the baseline up or down on the monitor, allowing the entire profile to be recorded accurately. When the Nyquist limit is exceeded by larger degrees, the aliased signal no longer displays the characteristic flow profile, and direction can no longer be determined (Fig. 1.26). Switching to CW Doppler allows flow velocities that exceed the Nyquist limit to be recorded accurately. Equation 1.6 is used to determine the maximum velocity that a pulsed wave system can record accurately without aliasing for a given transducer frequency (f_o) and sampling depth (D).

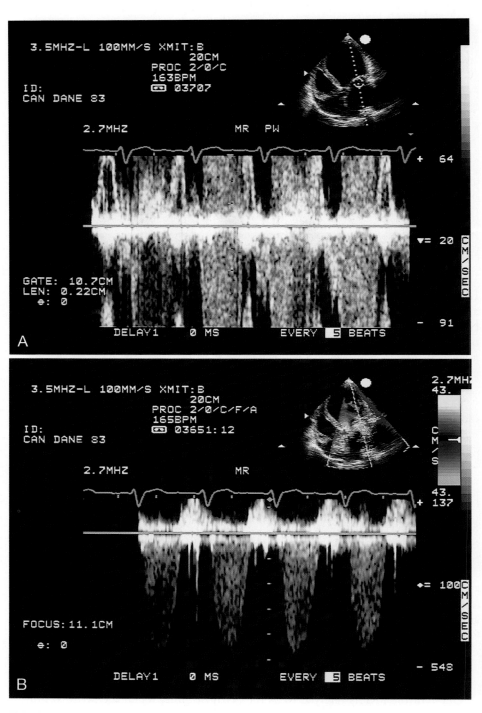

FIGURE 1.26   **A.** When velocities dramatically exceed the Nyquist limit, normal flow profiles are lost and it is impossible to determine flow direction or velocity. **B.** Switching to CW Doppler allows the high-velocity flow of mitral regurgitation to be recorded accurately. *PW,* pulsed-wave Doppler; *MR,* mitral regurgitation.

TABLE 1.6
**MAXIMUM VELOCITIES DETECTABLE AT SPECIFIC GATE DEPTHS FOR
SEVERAL TRANSDUCER FREQUENCIES**

Frequency	V at 7 cm	V at 12 cm	V at 20 cm
7.5	.56	.33	.20
5.0	.85	.49	.30
3.5	1.21	.71	.42
2.5	1.70	.99	.59

V, velocity in m/sec.

$$Vmax = \frac{(1540 \text{ m/sec})^2}{8(f_o) \times D}$$

(Eq. 1.6)

The equation shows that the maximum velocity that can be recorded at any given depth with no ambiguity is inversely proportional to transducer frequency.

The best recordings of higher-velocity jets at any given depth are obtained from lower-frequency transducers. This is opposite to what produces the best M-mode and two-dimensional examinations in which higher-frequency transducers produce the best images.

Table 1.6 lists the maximum velocities that can be recorded accurately at a variety of depths and transducer frequencies. Application of Equation 1.6 in determining the maximum velocity and Nyquist limit at set depths for several transducer frequencies is shown in Appendix 2.

Effect of Sampling (Gate) Depth

Equation 1.6 also shows that the maximum velocity that can be recorded without aliasing is inversely proportional to depth for any given transducer frequency. The Nyquist limit is exceeded far sooner at deeper gates for a given interrogation frequency. Table 1.6 lists the maximum velocity that can be accurately recorded for a given transducer frequency at varying depths. Appendix 3 shows mathematically the effect of gate depth on the Nyquist limit when transducer frequency is kept constant.

Blood Flow

Normal blood flow is typically laminar. All blood cells within a vessel, outflow tract, or chamber move in the same direction with similar flow velocities. Vessel and chamber walls create friction for the blood cells moving adjacent to wall surfaces, and velocities are somewhat slower along the periphery of the flow stream than in the center of the flow stream. Nevertheless, velocities are similar enough that a velocity profile is produced that has little variance.

PW Doppler appears hollow with little spectral broadening when flow is laminar, intercept angles are close to zero, and the Nyquist limit is not exceeded (Fig. 1.27). Spectral broadening is the filling in of the typically hollow waveform (Fig. 1.28). Spectral broadening in a pulsed-wave signal may be a result of improper gain settings, large intercept angle, or nonlaminar (turbulent) flow.

When flow becomes abnormal, it is turbulent. Turbulent flow has blood cells moving in many directions at various velocities. This kind of flow is seen with stenotic lesions, shunts, and valvular regurgitation. Doppler signals produced from turbulent flow have a lot of spectral broadening because of the many velocities and flow directions present in the jet. CW Doppler shows spectral broadening even when flow is laminar because flow velocities detected all along the transmitted sound beam vary tremendously (Fig. 1.28).

Color-Flow (CF) Doppler

CF Doppler is a form of pulsed-wave Doppler. Real-time images and color-flow mapping are done at the same time with alternating scan lines dedicated toward real-time image generation and Doppler signals.

Gate Depth and Velocity Measurement

For any given transducer frequency, the lesser the gate depth, the higher the velocity that can be measured.

What to Do about Aliasing

- Move the baseline up or down.
- Find a plane where less depth is necessary.
- Use a lower transducer frequency.
- Switch to CW Doppler.

Spectral Broadening in a PW Signal Results from

- Improper gain settings
- Large intercept angle
- Nonlaminar (turbulent) flow

CF Doppler

Aliasing occurs at lower velocities because of sampling time requirements.
- Therefore, aliasing may be seen even when flow is normal.

FIGURE 1.27 Pulsed-wave Doppler signals are hollow when flow is laminar because there is little variance in velocity.

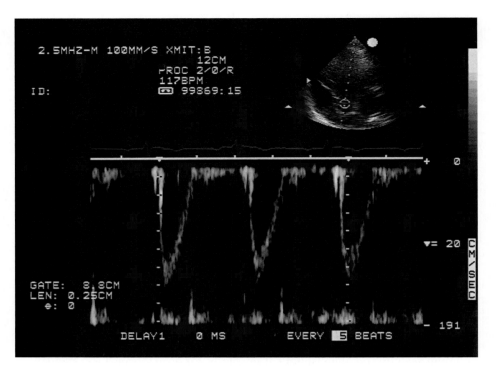

FIGURE 1.28 Spectral broadening is the filling in of a Doppler flow profile. CW Doppler displays always show spectral broadening because of the many velocities detected along the CW sound beam. PW Doppler may show spectral broadening when gain is too high, intercept angles are large, or flow becomes turbulent.

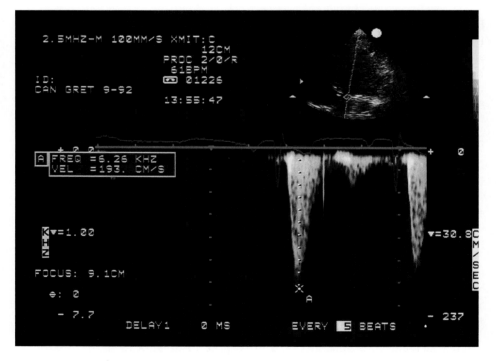

Remember that pulsed-wave ultrasound is range gated in that a specific sampling site is chosen and the ultrasound machine ignores signals that come back from any other point along the line of interrogation. This can be done by knowing the speed of sound in tissues and the depth of the gate. Color-flow mapping involves the analysis of information all along multiple interrogation lines, each with hundreds of gates, until a wedge is filled with color. Each gate sends frequency shift information back to the transducer (Fig. 1.29). This frequency shift information is sent to a processor that calculates the mean velocity, direction, and location of blood cells at each gate. Information from each gate is assigned a color and position on the image.

Blood flow in color mapping is perceived by the machine as either moving toward the transducer or away from it via a negative or positive frequency shift. Flow moving toward the sound source is plotted in hues of red, and flow moving away from the transducer is mapped in shades of blue (Fig. 1.30). No flow generates no frequency shift, thus no color is assigned. Enhanced color maps, available in most equipment, display flow velocity information as well as direction. Colors range from deep red for slow blood flow to bright yellow for rapid blood flow toward the transducer. Slow blood flow away from the transducer is mapped in deep blue colors, whereas more rapid flow away from the transducer is mapped in shades of light blue and white.

CF Doppler depends on two important factors: pulse repetition frequency and frequency of the transducer. As with spectral Doppler, the sound source frequency dictates the maximal velocity that can be accurately mapped at any given depth before aliasing occurs. Aliasing in CF Doppler involves a reversal of color, resulting in a mosaic or mixing of the blue and red hues (Fig. 1.31). Aliasing can occur while using high-frequency transducers when, in actuality, there is normal flow and the aliasing is only a function of transducer frequency. The aliasing would be eliminated if a lower-frequency transducer was used.

Many ultrasound machines have variance maps (Fig. 1.32). These machines map turbulent flow in hues other than blue or red. All color-flow images reproduced in this book use enhanced color maps.

Frame rate refers to the number of times a real-time or color-flow image is generated per minute. A frame rate of at least 15 times per minute is required for smooth transitions and the appearance of a continuously moving image. Color-flow information is superimposed on a two-dimensional image as a sector. Frame rate in CF Doppler is equal to PRF divided by scan lines per color sector. The operator can alter the width of this sector. Decreasing the color wedge decreases the amount of time necessary for sampling and increases the frame rate (Fig. 1.33). The operator also can eliminate the real-time image that extends beyond the width of the color sector. This also decreases the time necessary for image generation and enhances color-flow mapping.

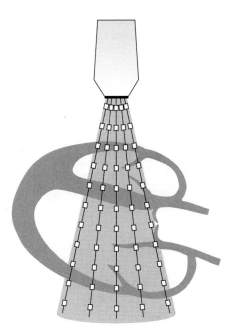

FIGURE 1.29   CF Doppler involves a sector filled with many lines of interrogation. Each line of sound contains a multitude of gates, each of which send frequency information back to the transducer. Color is then assigned to each gate based on direction and velocity of flow.

Optimize CF Imaging

- Decrease transducer frequency
- Decrease color sector width
- Eliminate real-time image
- Increase packet size
  - Decreases frame rate, however
- Decrease packet size
  - Decreases sampling time and is good for high heart rates, but may lose information

Many machines allow the operator to decrease the depth of the color wedge. This has no effect on frame rate because total image depth is unchanged; it merely decreases the information the mind has to process.

The number of times a line of sound is sampled is referred to as its packet size (Fig. 1.34). Increasing packet size improves image quality and fills in the color display but at the expense of frame rate. Packet sizes usually can be selected by the operator. Decreasing packet size will increase the frame rate but decrease sampling time. Information may be lost with short sampling times; however, this may be necessary with rapid heart rates. Increasing packet size will increase the time required for sampling and will decrease the frame rate, but it results in greater accuracy in measuring velocities and map color.

FIGURE 1.30 By convention, blood flow moving toward the transducer will be mapped in hues of red and yellow, in which deep red represents slower flow and bright yellow represents faster flow. Blood moving away from the transducer is mapped in hues of blue to white, in which deep blue represents slower flow and bright white represents faster flow. No flow or flow that is perpendicular to the interrogation line has no color assigned and will appear black.

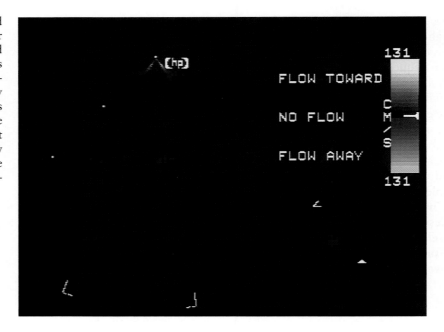

FIGURE 1.31 Aliasing secondary to high velocities or turbulent flow is displayed as a mosaic of color in CW Doppler. The turbulent flow of mitral regurgitation is shown as a multicolored jet (*arrow*) within the left atrium (*LA*) on this parasternal, long-axis, left ventricular outflow view through the heart. *RV*, right ventricle; *LV*, left ventricle; *AO*, aorta.

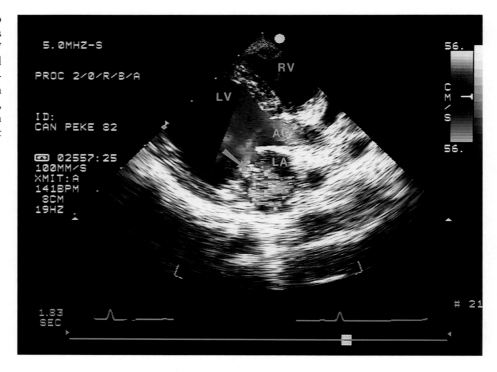

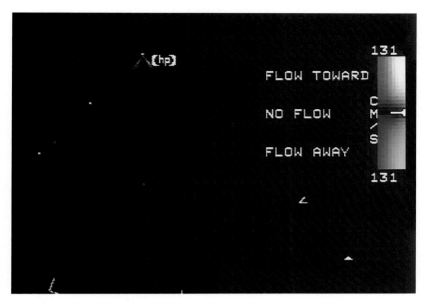

FIGURE 1.32   Variance maps are available on many machines. Turbulent flow is displayed in colors other than a mixture of blue and red.

ARTIFACTS

An artifact is anything seen on the echocardiographic image that is in the wrong place, is the wrong size, is the wrong shape, or is missing. Several artifacts already have been discussed, including two structures not resolving as separate entities both in the lateral and longitudinal planes; timing artifacts related to temporal resolution; and aliasing. Selecting the most appropriate transducer for the application will minimize these artifacts.

Other artifacts are created as a result of patient movement and respiration, improper gain settings, peripheral sound beams, or strong reflectors.

Patient Movement and Breathing Artifacts

Patient movement is a common problem when imaging animals because cooperation is sometimes difficult to obtain. Spending a few minutes calming the small animal before the examination while it is in lateral recumbency is often all that is necessary to quiet the patient. Even puppies and kittens often fall asleep during the examination.

The luxury of telling a patient to hold its breath or exhale deeply and hold it for a few seconds is nonexistent in veterinary medicine, thus respiratory artifact is a common problem. Holding a panting animal's mouth shut or blowing in its face for a moment or two while obtaining an M-mode image or a Doppler recording is imperative to obtaining good information. Allow the animal to pant between image acquisitions for continued cooperation. An extremely dyspneic animal often needs to be examined while in sternal position or standing.

Respiratory motion moves the transducer farther from and closer to the cardiac structures. The resulting M-mode image will have excessive cardiac motion simply because of this perceived cardiac motion by the equipment when it is actually only movement of the transducer with respect to the heart (Fig. 1.35).

Temporal artifact is the inaccurate timing of color-flow Doppler information. Temporal inaccuracy often is created secondary to respiratory movement. Color is encoded for a chamber or vessel at a location on the screen that has moved before the information is processed (Fig. 1.36). This usually appears as a sheet of color.

Side-Lobe Artifact

All transducers produce a central beam, which has been the basis of our discussion. They also all produce peripheral beams, which are directed laterally with respect to

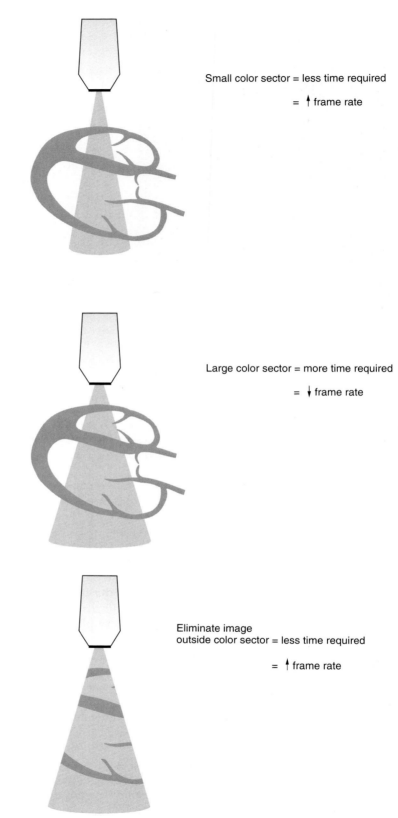

FIGURE 1.33 Decreasing the size of the color wedge sector reduces the time necessary for color sampling and increases the frame rate. Better temporal resolution is then possible. Eliminating the real-time image outside the color sector also decreases the amount of time necessary to generate an image and enhances color flow mapping.

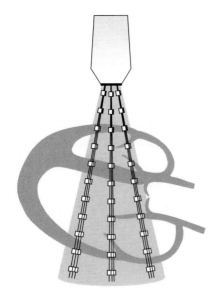

Large packet size = more time required

= ↓ frame rate

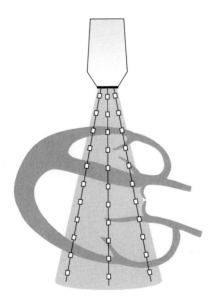

Small packet size = less time required

= ↑ frame rate

FIGURE 1.34   Packet size is the number of times each line within a color sector is sampled. Large packet sizes produce better color images because more samples can be taken. This is at the expense of frame rate, however, because more time is necessary. Smaller packet sizes decrease the number of times each scan line is sampled, so color information is not as complete, but frame rate is higher.

the central beam. When peripheral beams intercept structures and are reflected back to the transducer, the equipment cannot recognize that the information presented did not come from the central beam. Lateral structures are then superimposed on centrally located structures (Fig. 1.37). Side lobes are much weaker than central beams and thus returning echoes also are weaker. Often the potential artifact is not seen because main beam structures have stronger reflections. When other structures are not present to overshadow the artifact, however, the artifacts are easily visible. The most common place to see a side-lobe artifact is within dilated left atriums. This

FIGURE 1.35   Transducer movement secondary to breathing causes structures on this left ventricular M-mode to show excessive motion (*arrows*). Movement of the transducer closer to and farther from the heart is interpreted by the equipment as cardiac motion. *IVS*, interventricular septum; *LV*, left ventricle; *LVW*, left ventricular wall.

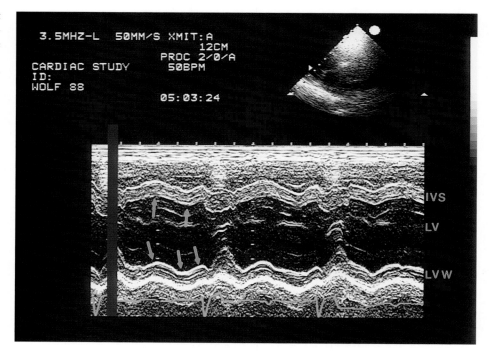

FIGURE 1.36   CF Doppler will be ambiguous when there is too much respiratory movement. An ambiguous sheeting effect is created as structures move before flow information is processed accurately.

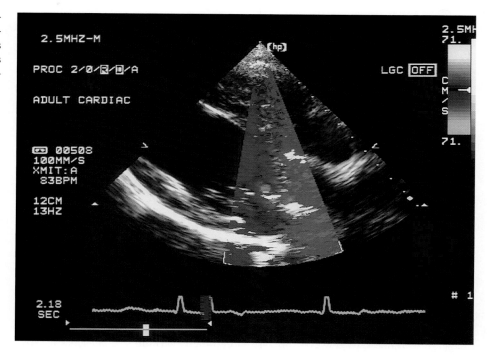

empty space allows weaker side lobe echoes to be displayed (Fig. 1.38). Side lobe reflections typically appear as a curved line extending from the side of the sector to the center. Make sure you see a structure in several imaging planes to eliminate possible misinterpretation of these reflections.

Reverberation Artifact

Reverberation artifact occurs when strong reflectors are encountered within the thorax. These structures send such strong echoes back to the transducer that the sound is both received by the transducer and reflected from it. The same sound beams travel through the heart again and when they are sent back to the transducer for a

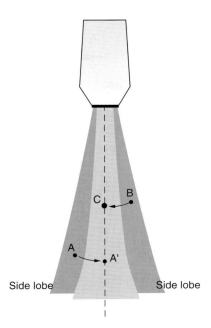

FIGURE 1.37 All transducers generate sound beams lateral to the central beam. Reflections from structures along these side lobes reach the transducer but are erroneously thought to have been generated by the central beam. Weak reflectors (**B**) in the periphery do not interfere with the true image (**C**). Reflectors (**A**) that are stronger than a true structure or that would be placed within an echo-free space (like a chamber) will create an artifactual structure on the real-time image (**A¹**).

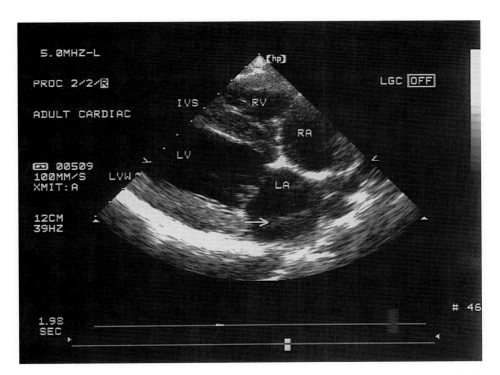

FIGURE 1.38 A side-lobe artifact (*arrow*) is seen within the left atrium (*LA*) of this right-parasternal four-chamber view of the heart. This artifact actually is produced from lateral structures. *RV*, right ventricle; *IVS*, interventricular septum; *RA*, right atrium; *LA*, left atrium; *LV*, left ventricle; *LVW*, left ventricular wall.

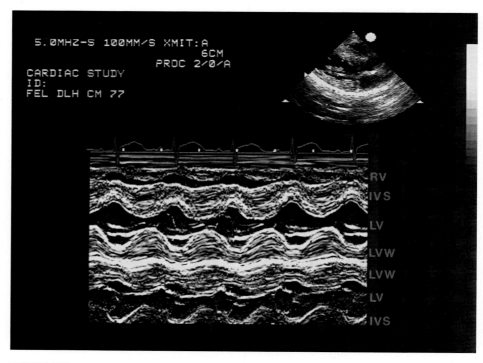

FIGURE 1.39   Strong reflections may bounce off the transducer and travel through the heart again. A duplicate image of the heart is created below the first one from the sound waves that return from the second reflections, because twice as much time has elapsed since the sound beam was generated originally. *RV*, right ventricle; *IVS*, interventricular septum; *LV*, left ventricle; *LVW*, left ventricular wall.

second time, they are perceived as having taken twice as long. This produces a mirror image below the first image (Fig. 1.39) and occurs often in cardiac imaging when strong reflectors like the pericardium and lung interface cause echoes to bounce back and forth. Reverberation artifact can be minimized by making sure depth settings are adequate for the heart size and not so deep as to produce a double image.

Reverberation artifact also can be produced between two strong reflectors within the thorax or heart. The sound may bounce back and forth between these two highly dense structures one to several times before traveling back to the transducer. Multiple images of the same structures are created, each equally spaced and deeper in the image.

Mirror-Image Artifact on Doppler Display

When spectral Doppler flow shows up on both sides of the baseline, it is referred to as a mirror-image artifact (Fig. 1.40). Depending on where blood flow is being sampled, it is still possible to determine which flow direction is the correct one. This artifact is created by high gain settings creating a situation similar to reverberation artifact. Mirror-image artifact also may be caused by large angles of incidence with respect to blood flow.

SUMMARY

Transducers send out sound waves that travel in cycles. The number of cycles per second determines transducer frequency. High-frequency transducers generate more cycles per second and thus have shorter wavelengths.

The average speed of sound in soft tissue is 1540 m/sec and is independent of transducer frequency. Acoustic impedance increases with increased tissue density and stiffness. This also is independent of transducer frequency. An acoustical difference between two tissues causes sound to be reflected back to the transducer.

Because bone is stiff and dense, it impedes the flow of sound tremendously and reflects almost all sound. Scattered sound generates the images from within homogeneous tissues where acoustical properties are similar and structures are small and irregular with respect to wavelength.

A structure must be at least one-quarter the size of the wavelength to be reflected. High-frequency sound with shorter wavelengths can reflect sound from smaller structures and produce better images. Sound attenuates rapidly with these short wavelengths, however, because the wavelengths interact with more structures. High-frequency transducers, therefore, create high-resolution images but lose strength rapidly and cannot penetrate as far into tissues as sound from low-frequency transducers.

Transducers contain piezoelectric crystals that generate sound and receive sound. The sound is sent out in pulses, and the number of pulses per second is the pulse repetition frequency of the transducer. One of the factors affecting axial resolution is the pulse length of a transducer. Higher-frequency transducers will have better axial resolution since their short waves and pulse lengths can differentiate smaller structures. Lateral resolution depends on several factors, one of which is beam width. The wider the beam width, the poorer the lateral resolving power because structures must be farther apart than the beam width to be differentiated. Therefore, lateral resolution is best with smaller diameter transducers. High-frequency transducers have longer near fields before the beam diverges; this enhances the lateral resolution of deeper structures.

Current technology allows multiple focal points along each sound beam in a phased array or annular array transducer. Correct timing of cardiac motion and flow depends on temporal resolution. As multiple focal zones are used or as deeper structures are imaged, the pulse repetition frequency is decreased, which may not allow information to process fast enough and temporal resolution will suffer. Decreasing the width of the real-time sector or decreasing the depth of interrogation will increase the PRF.

The change in frequency between sound transmitted by the transducer and sound received by the transducer is the Doppler shift. Blood cells moving toward the

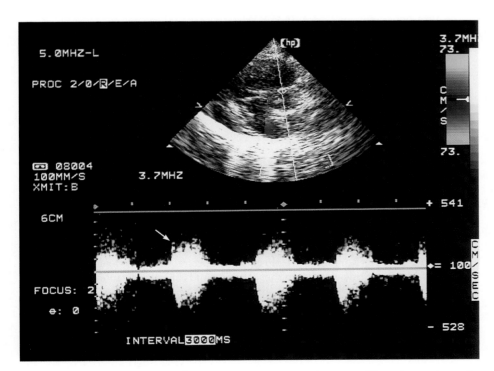

FIGURE 1.40   Mirror-image artifacts (*arrow*) are common in spectral Doppler tracings when gain settings are too high or intercept angles are large.

transducer will create a positive frequency shift and flow will be displayed above the baseline, whereas blood moving away from the transducer produces a negative frequency shift and flow profiles below the baseline.

Pulsed-wave Doppler is range gated in that it samples blood at indicated sites within the heart; however, it is limited in the highest velocity it is capable of measuring accurately. Continuous-wave Doppler samples blood flow all along the sound beam and, although not site specific, it has no Nyquist limit.

The Nyquist limit depends on PRF and thus transducer frequency. The Nyquist limit decreases as blood flow is sampled at increasing depths for any given transducer frequency. Lower-frequency transducers can record accurately higher flow velocities at any given depth before aliasing occurs. Accurate velocity measurements also depend on having an angle of interrogation that is parallel with flow. Deviations of the Doppler beam away from parallel result in underestimation of flow velocities.

Laminar flow creates a Doppler signal with little variance in velocity and little spectral broadening. Spectral broadening is seen when flow becomes turbulent or when CW Doppler is used because the transducer receives many frequency shifts.

Color-flow Doppler is a form of pulsed-wave Doppler. Frequency shift information is encoded with color. The most commonly used color map uses a blue (away) and red (toward) format. Aliasing typically occurs at lower velocities in CF Doppler because of the increased time needed for flow analysis at multiple gates. Aliasing in CF Doppler results in a mosaic of color. As in spectral Doppler, lower-frequency transducers will increase the Nyquist limit.

Artifacts are common in diagnostic ultrasound and may be created by the physical properties of transducers, patient-related factors, tissue characteristics, or operator-related errors. Selecting the most appropriate transducer for the examination, calming the patient, and realizing the limitations of diagnostic ultrasound will help eliminate many of these problems or allow intelligent decision making.

SUGGESTED READING

Burns PN. Principles of Doppler and color flow. Radiol Med (Torino) 1993;85(Suppl 1):3–16.

Darke PGG. Doppler echocardiography. J Small Anim Pract 1992;33:104.

Evans RG. Medical diagnostic ultrasound instrumentation and clinical interpretation: report of the ultrasonography task force. JAMA 1991;265:1155.

Goldstein A. Overview of the physics of ultrasound. Radiographics 1993;13:701.

Herring DS, Bjornton G. Physics, facts, and artifacts of diagnostic ultrasound. Semin Vet Med Surg (Small Anim) 1989;4:2.

Kirberger RM. Doppler echocardiography: facts and physics for practitioners. Compendium 1991;13:1679.

Kremkau FW. Doppler ultrasound: principles and instruments. 2nd ed. Philadelphia: WB Saunders, 1995.

Kremkau, FW. Diagnostic ultrasound: principle, instruments, and exercises. 4th ed. Philadelphia: WB Saunders, 1993.

Kremkau FW: Artifacts in ultrasound imaging. J Ultra Med 1986;5:227.

Miller MW, Knauer KW, Herring DS. Echocardiography: principles of interpretation. Semin Vet Med Surg (Small Anim) 1989;4:58.

Park RD. B-mode gray-scale ultrasound: imaging artifacts and interpretation principles. Vet Radiol 1981;22:204.

Powis RL. Ultrasound science for the veterinarian. Diagn Ultra 1986;2:3.

Rantanen NW. Principles of ultrasound application in animals. Vet Radiol 1981;22:196.

Voiculescu M, Pop A, Romosan I. Conventional spectral Doppler and color Doppler ultrasound imaging. Principles, limitations, artifacts and clinical indications in hepatology. Rom J Intern Med 1992;30:139.

Ziskin MC. Fundamental physics of ultrasound and its propagation in tissue. Radiographics 1993;13:705.

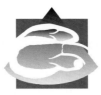

2

THE ECHOCARDIOGRAPHIC EXAMINATION

▼

INTRODUCTION

M-mode echocardiography was first described as a clinically useful tool in veterinary medicine in 1977 when Pipers reported its use in the horse (1). M-mode echocardiograms in animals were difficult to obtain and up to that time were used primarily in medical research with the aid of invasive methods such as implanted catheters and catheter-tipped transducers, removal or displacement of lung lobes, and transducer placement directly on the cardiac surface (2–6). As noninvasive methods of imaging dogs improved (7–10), early descriptive articles appeared documenting the echocardiographic appearance of cardiac disorders in animals (11–18). The need for quantitative information became apparent as the practicality and applicability of echocardiography in veterinary medicine became evident. Normal M-mode reference values were determined rapidly for the dog (19–24), cat (25–33), horse (1,34–38), cow (39), and pig (40). More reference values have been published since that time, with many articles directing specific attention to the effects of various physiologic and chemical influences on the echocardiogram.

The popularity of ultrasound increased with the advent of real-time imaging and its easy to understand two-dimensional images of the heart. Normal two-dimensional cardiac anatomy and some quantitative two-dimensional information in the dog (41–46), the cat (46,47), the horse (48–54), and the cow (55) have been described. A wide variety of cardiovascular disorders detectable by echocardiography has been presented in the literature. Recently, standards for imaging planes and terminology have been recommended for the dog and cat (41).

Doppler information regarding flow direction and velocity has increased the diagnostic accuracy of echocardiography. The normal appearance of cardiac flow profiles and the technique required for Doppler ultrasound in horses (49,56–58), dogs (59–66), and sheep (67) have been described.

Examination technique is less frequently described, and even then, often lacks the detail necessary for the novice ultrasonographer to obtain appropriate cardiac images. This chapter describes normal two-dimensional, M-mode, and Doppler images and the scanning techniques necessary to obtain those images correctly. The importance of correct technique, measurement, and assessment cannot be overemphasized. A methodical approach to scanning and interpretation should be used to increase technical proficiency and diagnostic accuracy. Try to perform the ultrasound

FIGURE 2.1 Shave between the right 4th to 6th intercostal spaces, from the costochondral junction to the sternum in small animals.

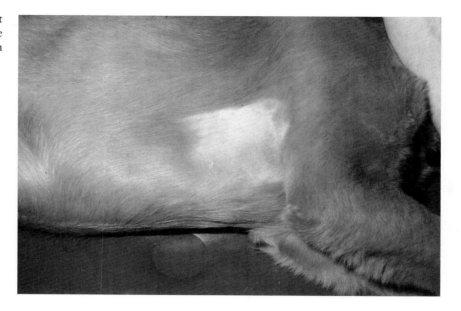

FIGURE 2.2 Large animals should be shaved if coats are thick. Clip from several inches above the olecranon to several inches below it in the right 3rd to 5th intercostal spaces.

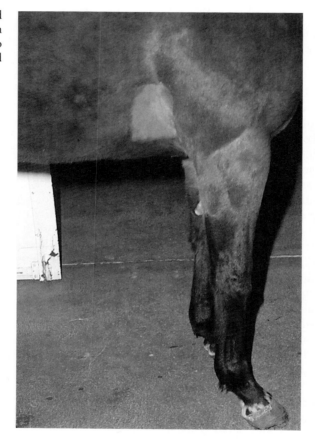

examination the same way each time. Consistency in patient placement, transducer orientation, table height, and equipment location with respect to the patient, allows the examination technique to become almost automatic.

PATIENT PREPARATION

Most animals require shaving on both the right and left sides of the thorax to minimize the effects of air on sound transmission. Shave the right 4th to 6th intercostal spaces in dogs and the 3rd to 5th intercostal spaces in horses, cows, and cats (Fig. 2.1). The left side should be shaved from approximately the 4th to 7th intercostal spaces in all animals. The clipped area should extend from the costo-chondral junction to the sternum in small animals and from several inches above the olecranon to several inches below it in the horse and cow (Fig. 2.2). Some animals with thin hair coats may be examined by simply moving aside the hair and applying generous amounts of ultrasonic transmission gel. Applying alcohol before the transmission gel helps eliminate air and improve skin contact when the animal is not shaved.

PATIENT POSITIONING
Small Animal Positioning

Most echocardiographers use a scanning table similar to that seen in Figure 2.3. The animal is placed in right lateral recumbency with the right 3rd to 6th intercostal spaces positioned over a cut-away section in the table. Gently restrain the animal by standing behind its back and placing your arms over the animal's hips and neck while holding the legs (Fig. 2.4).

Images are obtained by scanning from beneath the table because this method of examining the heart routinely produces better images. The heart drops down toward the thoracic wall, decreasing the problem of lung interference on echocardiographic images. It also allows a higher-frequency transducer to be used during many examinations because less depth penetration is necessary. Although good images can be obtained from the right side with the animal placed in left lateral recumbency, it

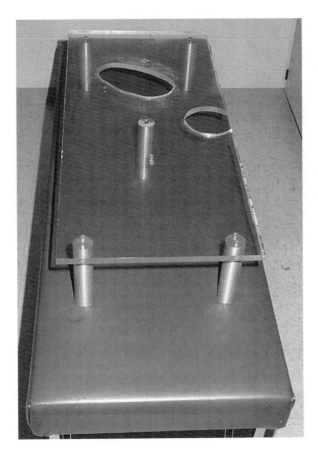

FIGURE 2.3   A scanning table with a cutout allows imaging from below the small animal and improves image quality.

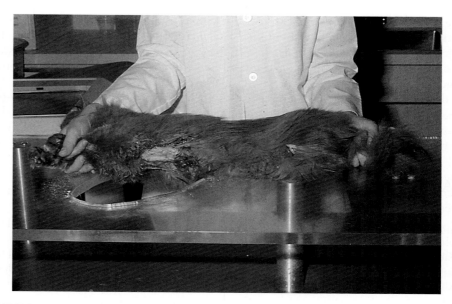

FIGURE 2.4   Hold the animal in a recumbent position with the shaved area over the cutout in the examination table. Place your arms over the animal's neck and hips while holding its legs extended.

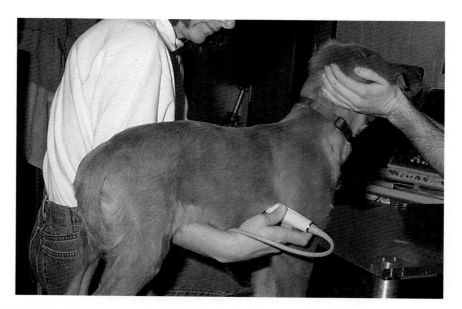

FIGURE 2.5   When an animal cannot tolerate a recumbent position, examinations can be preformed with the patient standing. Stand on the left side and place your arm under the animal to keep the animal up. The transducer is placed on the animal's right side for standard images.

takes more experience to become proficient at obtaining these images consistently. Air interference in the lungs is common in this position.

Construction of an examination table has been described (68). Important design considerations are length of the table, placement of the cutout, and table height. Enough length should be provided so the animal's head does not extend past the edge of the table when the thorax is positioned properly over the cutout. The cutout should also extend toward the edge of the table near the examiner so that deep-chested or large dogs do not feel as though they are falling off the back of the table. Cats and smaller animals can be held so the sternum extends just beyond the edge of the cutout and they will feel secure. Tables do not need to have an incline nor do they have to have adjustable cutouts. An oval cutout section oriented as in Figure 2.3 is necessary when using longer transducers to tilt the transducer into the more horizontal positions required for some images. The table should be high enough to hold the transducer vertically without restricted movement.

Occasionally, an animal will not tolerate a recumbent position because of discomfort or dyspnea. These animals are easier to examine when they are standing on a table or on the floor. To prevent an animal from lying down, position yourself on the animal's left side and place your arm under the animal to scan from the right side (Fig. 2.5). Transducer positions and manipulations are similar to those used when the animal is in lateral recumbency. Scanning with the animal in sternal recumbency is possible, but it is difficult to obtain some images. Sometimes it is necessary to hold a small animal in your lap to obtain an image.

Large Animal Positioning

Horses and food animals are examined while they are standing in a stall, chute, or stanchion. Imaging still takes place from the right side of the animal for all standard long- and short-axis views. The examination is then completed on the left side if the entire heart cannot be imaged from the right side. Many Doppler studies require examination from the left side of the thorax.

Most standard images require that the right front leg is pulled forward and slightly abducted (Fig. 2.2). Imaging becomes difficult when the horse, cow, or llama does not cooperate with leg placement because the transducer has to be pushed forward into the leg (Fig. 2.6). Imaging from the left side is also easier when the left fore limb is positioned forward.

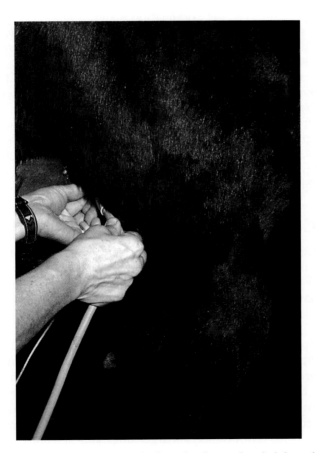

FIGURE 2.6   When a horse will not keep the front leg forward and abducted, the transducer has to be pushed forward into the leg and imaging becomes strenuous. Keep the transducer perpendicular to the chest wall when sliding the transducer forward.

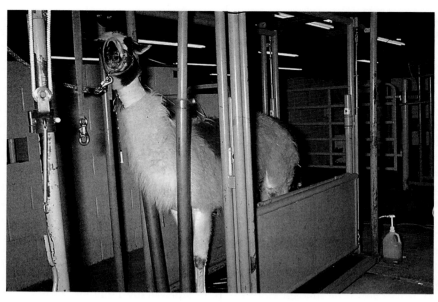

FIGURE 2.7   Llamas are placed in a chute that keeps the head up and prevents them from lying down.

Cows usually are placed in a head stanchion, but sometimes a squeeze chute is required. The front leg on the side where the examination will take place must be pulled forward and abducted, which usually requires tethering the leg in place. When this cannot be accomplished, the examination is almost impossible. A food animal surgery table has been used successfully by strapping the animal left side down, tilting the table slightly upward, and pulling the right front leg forward so that the ultrasonic window (transducer location) is exposed.

Llamas typically are placed in a chute that holds their head up and prevents them from lying down (Fig. 2.7). Imaging their hearts also requires their legs to be placed forward abducted.

All neonate food animals and foals are examined similarly to small animals in which they are placed on the scanning table in right lateral recumbency for standard imaging planes. Restraint is similar to that in small animals, which prevents unnecessary movement. A faster and more accurate examination usually can be performed in this manner.

TRANSDUCER SELECTION

High-Frequency Transducers Create High-Resolution Images

- Try higher-frequency transducers to see if it will work before selecting a lower one.
- Use a high-frequency transducer to obtain clearer images of near field structures.

Transducer frequency is an important consideration because it affects depth of penetration and resolution of the image. Higher-frequency transducers, because of their shorter wavelengths, allow better resolution of structures but less depth penetration. Low-frequency transducers, with longer wavelengths, allow sound waves to travel deeper into tissues before weakening, at the expense of resolution.

Although depth and resolution are inverse components of transducer frequency, when an appropriate transducer is used, the loss in resolution is not appreciated because structures are larger. High-frequency transducers should be used for cats and small dogs. A high-frequency transducer also can be used in larger animals to improve the resolution of near field structures like the tricuspid valve.

Switch to a lower-frequency transducer when starting the Doppler part of your examination to obtain better-quality Doppler information.

Medium-sized animals in the range of approximately 30 to 50 pounds often can be imaged with 5-MHz transducers. Larger dogs and newborn foals and calves usually require a 3.5 or lower frequency transducer. It is a good habit to try higher-frequency transducers before selecting a lower one just to see if it works. This allows you to create the best images for diagnostic purposes. Although an animal weighs 60 pounds, for example, a narrow thorax may allow the use of a 5-MHz transducer, which produces excellent images. Large animals, such as the adult horse or cow, almost always require a 2.5-MHz or lower transducer frequency for the sound beams to reach the far wall of the heart.

Apical four- and five-chamber examination planes sometimes require changing the probe to a lower frequency than used for imaging the patient's heart for standard right or left parasternal planes through the heart. Imaging from the apex of the heart to its base requires much more depth penetration than views that image the width of the heart. Even when all imaging planes can be obtained with one transducer, change to a lower transducer frequency when obtaining Doppler flow information. Lower-frequency transducers provide increased signal strength at greater depths and reduce aliasing during pulsed-wave interrogation. Lower transducer frequencies often are required to produce a strong enough spectral signal from small regurgitant volumes. Most equipment automatically switches to a lower frequency when Doppler is used, but often is not low enough.

TWO-DIMENSIONAL ECHOCARDIOGRAPHY
Controls

Basic two-dimensional echocardiographic controls are discussed in this section. Refer to your owner's manual for more detailed information and discussion of options specific to your equipment.

Depth
Depth controls adjust the field of view. Adjust the depth setting until the real-time image fills the field to reduce the amount of lung field and reverberation artifact seen at the bottom of the sector. A cursor or other calibration system is displayed alongside the sector image (Fig. 2.8). Each mark usually represents 1 cm of depth.

Gain
Gain, often called power or transmit on some machines, is used to control the output power or signal strength of the transducer. The entire sector image is affected by this control. A gain setting that is too high will produce a white distorted image, whereas a setting that is too low will produce a weak signal that will not generate a good image (Fig. 2.9). Set the gain so the image is clearly seen with no "blooming" of structures and the chambers contain no extraneous echoes.

Time-Gain Compensation
Equipment may have time-gain compensation (TGC) levers, which control the gain settings at specific depths on the real-time image (Fig. 2.10). Gain increases by sliding the lever to the right and decreases by sliding the lever to the left. This allows the stronger reflections from near field structures to be toned down (attenuated) and deeper structures that reflect weaker sound can be intensified on the monitor. Ultrasound machines without TGC sliding levers have TGC curves that are adjusted with three or four knobs. Each knob adjusts the slope and gain of the curve that represents various depths on the real-time image. Adjust each level until the image is pleasing without losing information in the near or far fields.

Compress
Compress adjusts the dynamic range of the displayed image. Increasing the compress level allows weaker echoes to be displayed and more shades of grey are visible; a softer-looking image is created. Decreasing compress reduces the dynamic range, eliminates weaker signals, resulting in a higher contrast image, and reduces background noise.

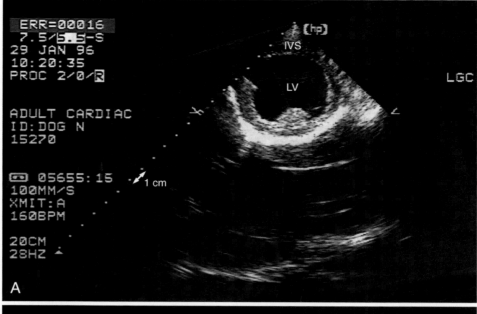

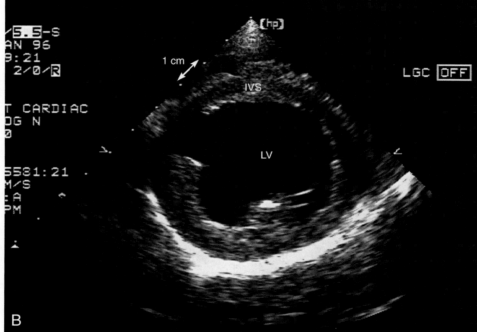

FIGURE 2.8   Depth can be adjusted to (**A**) enlarge or (**B**) decrease the field of view. A scale is displayed on the side of the sector image. Each mark represents a centimeter (*arrow*). *LV,* left ventricle; *IVS,* interventricular septum.

Persistence

The persistence control averages imaging frames by mixing information from old frames with new frames, resulting in a smoother image with less speckling. Cardiac imaging uses little, if any persistence, because the real-time effect becomes blurred with frame averaging.

Sector Width

Sector widths are adjustable from approximately a 120° angle to a narrow width of approximately 45° (Fig. 2.11). The smaller the sector angle, the faster the frame rate and the higher the resolution of the real-time image.

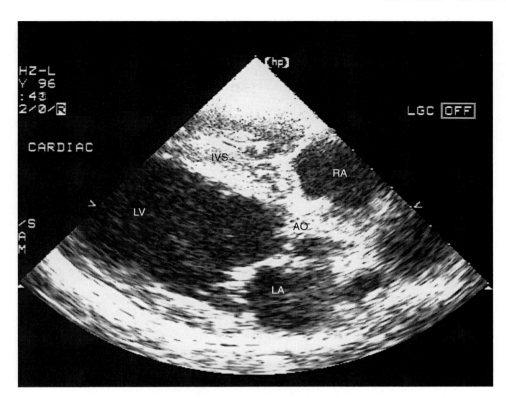

FIGURE 2.9   Gain controls the signal strength for the entire sector image. Here, the gain is set too high, producing a very white image with "blooming" of structures and too many echoes within the cardiac chambers. *RA*, right atrium; *IVS*, interventricular septum; *LV*, left ventricle; *LA*, left atrium; *AO*, aorta.

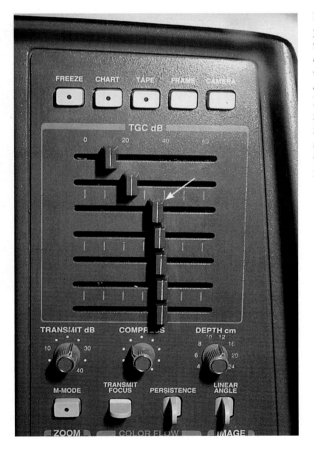

FIGURE 2.10   Each time-gain compensation (TGC) lever (*arrow*) controls the gain level at specific depths on the sector image. Moving the lever to the right will increase the intensity of the display, whereas moving the lever to the left will attenuate the magnitude of gain on the displayed image. The "knee" (*arrow*) corresponds to the level of the interventricular septum on the real-time image.

FIGURE 2.11 Small sector widths (**A**) increase the frame rate because less sampling time is required, producing a higher resolution image than when larger sector angles (**B**) are selected.

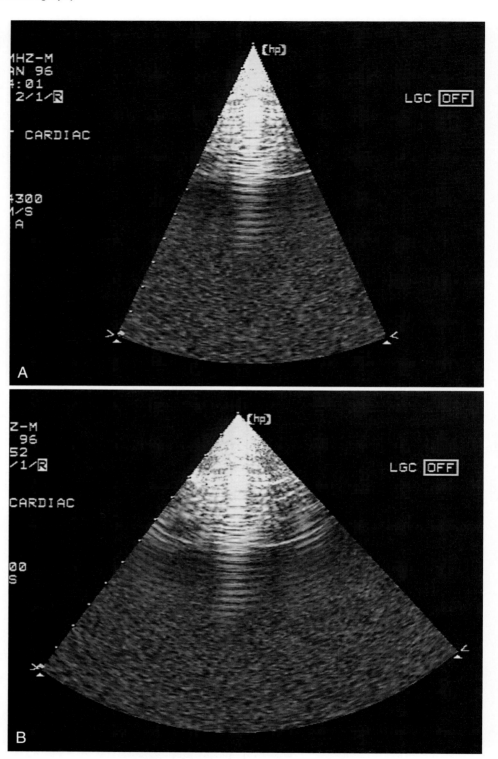

Two-Dimensional Images

Two-dimensional echocardiography uses transducers that transmit multiple beams of sound in the form of a sector or pie. The sector has width, depth, and thickness. Although section thickness is sometimes a factor in image quality, it is not considered when describing real-time anatomy. As the sector of sound is sent through the heart, solid tissue reflects sound back to the transducer and appears white on the monitor.

The fluid-filled spaces of the cardiac chambers lack the density to reflect sound. These areas appear black on the ultrasound monitor.

Terminology and image orientation are adapted from human echocardiography. The Committee on Standards for Veterinary Echocardiography have set recommendations to produce uniform views and they also have devised common terms for use when discussing an imaging plane (24).

Imagine cutting the heart into slices like a loaf of bread. The slice may follow the length of the loaf, the width of the loaf, or any angle between these planes. Each slice is representative of an echocardiographic plane. The imaging planes described in the following sections are recommended for standard examinations and represent identifiable and consistently recognizable landmarks within the heart. Many other imaging planes can be obtained, and structure identification is made as the image changes from a standard view to a nonstandard plane through the heart.

Standard cardiac images showing longitudinal and transverse sections of the heart are obtained from the right side of the thorax. Longitudinal images, referred to as long-axis views, are those in which the imaging plane follows the length of the heart from base to apex (Fig. 2.12). Transverse images, referred to as short-axis views, are those in which the imaging plane follows the width of the heart from right to left (Fig. 2.13). There are several angled or oblique views of the heart that show some structures in their length and others in a plane between the long and short axis.

Apical two-, four-, and five-chamber images, and several longitudinal and oblique planes require imaging from the left side of the animal. These planes can be obtained in dogs and cats by leaving the animal on the table in right lateral recumbency and scanning from above. Or the animal may be placed in left lateral recumbency on the

Long axis: Sagittal imaging planes that follow the length of the heart.
Short axis: Transverse imaging planes that follow the width of the heart.

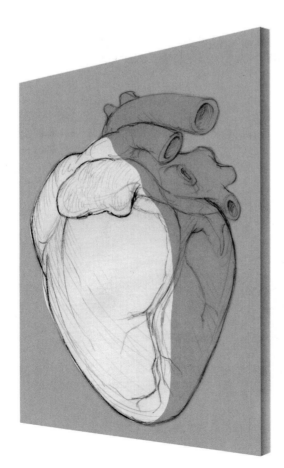

FIGURE 2.12   Longitudinal or long-axis views follow the length of the heart from base to apex.

Image Orientation

Long axis: Base of the heart to the right side of the sector image.
Short axis: Pulmonary artery to the right side of the sector image.
Apical: Left ventricle to the right side of the sector image.

examination table with transducer placement under the table. Obtaining the left parasternal views in thin, narrow, or deep-chested animals is easier when they are placed in left lateral recumbency on the table.

Standard left and right parasternal long-axis views of the heart are imaged with the base of the heart toward the right side of the monitor and the apex to the left. Transverse images are displayed so that the pulmonary artery is seen on the right side of the screen when a sweep from apex to base of the heart is made. Apical four- and five-chamber planes obtained from the left side of the thorax are oriented with the left side of the heart on the right side of the sector image.

Right Parasternal Long-Axis Images

The images obtained from the right side of the thorax in both large and small animals are similar. Terminology and image orientation are those recommended by the Echocardiography Committee of The Specialty of Cardiology, American College of Veterinary Internal Medicine (41). These recommendations were made for the dog and cat, but to remain consistent and avoid confusion the same terminology will be used for similar images in other animals including the horse, cow, and exotics. Long's article regarding standardized imaging technique in the horse will be referred to for cardiac images differing from those found in small animals (49).

Left Ventricular Outflow.   Right parasternal long-axis images always show the right ventricle (RV) at the top of the image (Fig. 2.14). The left ventricular outflow view shows a portion of the right atrium (RA) on the top right side of the image. Below the right ventricle and atrium are the interventricular septum (IVS) on the left, and the aorta (AO) on the right of the image. The left ventricular chamber (LV) and left ventricular wall (LVW) are seen at the bottom left of the image, and the left atrium (LA) is seen below the aorta on the right. The pericardium (P) is seen as an echodense bright line around the heart. This echogenicity is caused by the great difference in acoustical impedance between pericardial tissue and lungs.

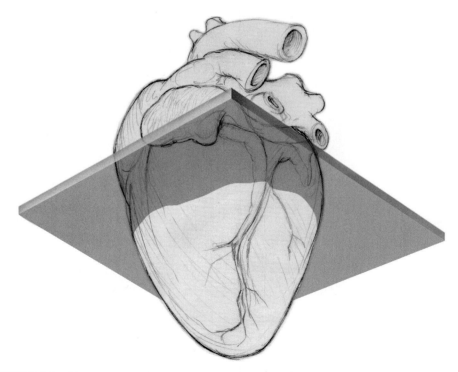

FIGURE 2.13   Transverse or short-axis images follow the width of the heart from right to left.

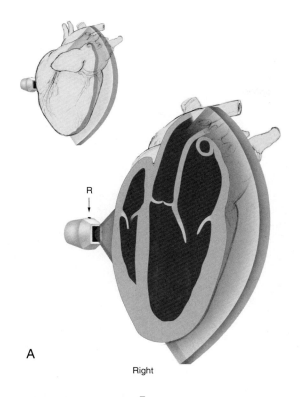

A

Right

FIGURE 2.14   **A.** This shows the spatial orientation of the sound plane for the right parasternal long-axis left ventricular outflow view of the heart. The heart is positioned as seen from above the animal while the animal is in right lateral recumbency. The transducer is placed under the animal on the right side of the thorax and the plane transects the heart along its length from right side to left side and base to apex. **B.** An illustration of the cardiac structures seen in this plane is shown. The image is displayed on the monitor so that the top of the sector corresponds to the skin surface and transducer location. **C.** The real-time two-dimensional image of this plane through the heart. *R,* reference mark; *T,* transducer; *RV,* right ventricle; *TV,* tricuspid valve; *RA,* right atrium; *AO,* aorta; *AOV,* aortic valve; *IVS,* interventricular septum; *LV,* left ventricle; *MV,* mitral valve; *LA,* left atrium; *RMPA,* right main pulmonary artery; *LVW,* left ventricular wall; *P,* pericardium.

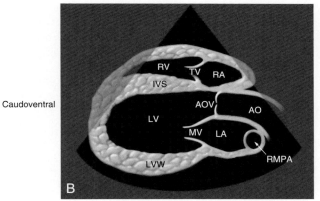

B

Caudoventral   Craniodorsal

Left

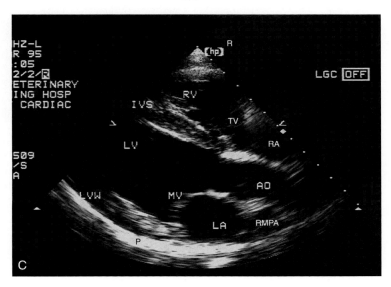

C

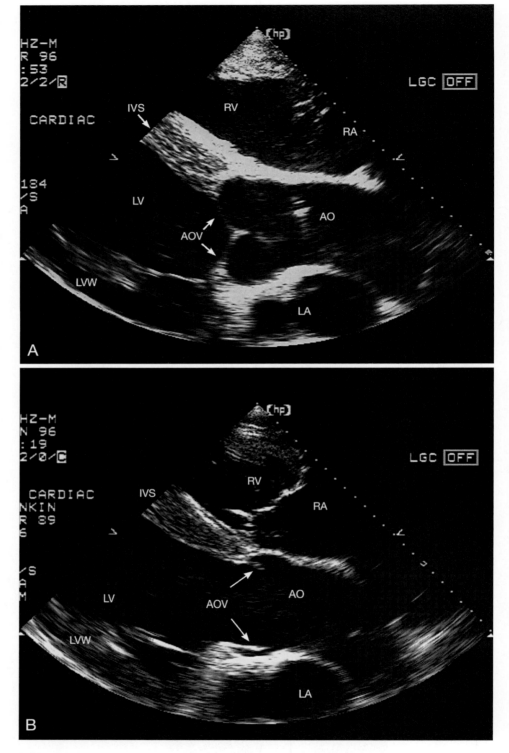

FIGURE 2.15   **A.** The aortic valves are clearly seen as semilunar cusps in this real-time long-axis image of the aorta in a horse during diastole. **B.** The semilunar valves (*arrows*) are pushed against the walls of the aorta during systole as blood flows past them. *RV*, right ventricle; *RA*, right atrium; *AO*, aorta; *AOV*, aortic valve; *IVS*, interventricular septum; *LV*, left ventricle; *LA*, left atrium; *LVW*, left ventricular wall.

The IVS and anterior aortic wall are continuous in this plane through the heart. The membranous portion of the IVS is seen where the muscular septum becomes a thin white line adjacent to the aorta. The aortic valves are seen just to the right of this junction as curved semilunar lines concave to the aorta (Fig. 2.15). The anterior mitral valve leaflet (MV) is a continuation of the posterior aortic wall as it extends into the left ventricular chamber. The shorter posterior MV cusp is seen at the junction of the muscular LVW and thin left atrial wall (Fig. 2.14).

The left ventricular wall and portions of the left atrium might not be seen in the horse depending on the size of the horse, the depth capabilities of the equipment, and the available transducers (Fig. 2.16). Also, the posterior leaflet of the mitral valve often is not in the image. Left parasternal imaging is necessary to see these structures.

Tipped long-axis views also are generated from this transducer location. The same structures are visible, but the apex of the heart is seen toward the top left of the sector image and the atria are seen at the bottom right (Figs. 2.17 and 2.18).

Four Chamber. A slight change in transducer orientation brings the right parasternal four-chamber plane of the heart into view (Fig. 2.19). The tricuspid valve and right atrium are more visible in this plane than in the left ventricular outflow plane. The RV and RA at the top of the sector are separated by the tricuspid valves. A clear interatrial septum (IAS) is seen on the right side of the image, separating the right atrium on top of the sector image from the left atrium at the bottom right of the

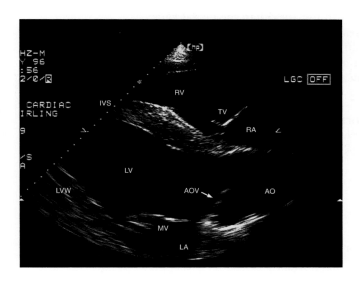

FIGURE 2.16   The right parasternal long-axis left ventricular outflow view in a horse. Portions of the left ventricular wall, left atrium, and mitral valves are not seen in large horses. *RV*, right ventricle; *TV*, tricuspid valve; *RA*, right atrium; *AO*, aorta; *AOV*, aortic valve; *IVS*, interventricular septum; *LV*, left ventricle; *MV*, mitral valve; *LA*, left atrium; *LVW*, left ventricular wall.

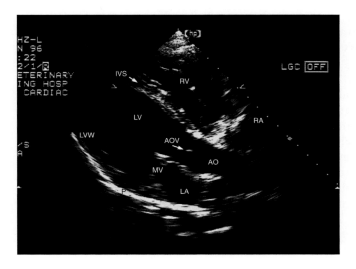

FIGURE 2.17   This is the right parasternal tipped long-axis left ventricular outflow view in a dog. *RV*, right ventricle; *AO*, aorta; *AOV*, aortic valve; *IVS*, interventricular septum; *LV*, left ventricle; *MV*, mitral valve; *LA*, left atrium; *LVW*, left ventricular wall; *P*, pericardium; *RA*, right atrium.

FIGURE 2.18   The right parasternal tipped long-axis left ventricular outflow view in a horse. *RV,* right ventricle; *AO,* aorta; *AOV,* aortic valve; *IVS,* interventricular septum; *LV,* left ventricle; *MV,* mitral valve; *LA,* left atrium; *LVW,* left ventricular wall.

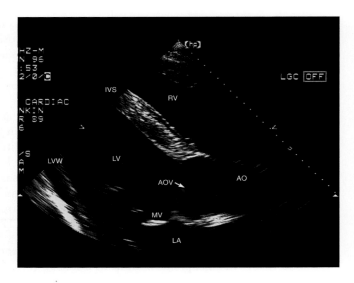

sector image. The left ventricle and interventricular septum are seen on the left side of the image.

The IAS and IVS are continuous with each other. The mitral and tricuspid valves are positioned at the junction of the IVS and IAS. The tricuspid valve annulus is located slightly more toward the apex than the mitral valve.

The entire left atrium and free wall of the left ventricle usually are not within the image in horses (Fig. 2.20). However, compared to the left ventricular outflow view, more of the mitral valve and left atrium are seen. Tipped four-chamber views show the same structures from a slightly different angle in both the small and large animal (Figs. 2.21 and 2.22).

Right Parasternal Short-Axis Images

Transverse images of the heart may be obtained at any level from the apex to the base. The five standard images (Fig. 2.23) that are taken in the transverse plane are as follows:

1. Left ventricle
2. Chordae tendinea
3. Mitral valves
4. Heart base with aorta
5. Heart base with pulmonary artery

An additional angled view through the long axis of the pulmonary artery with an oblique view of the left ventricle is also presented in Figure 2.23. This plane is between the longitudinal and short axis. As with the right parasternal long-axis views of the heart, these transverse or short-axis planes are similar in both large and small animals.

Left Ventricle with Papillary Muscles and Chordae Tendinea.

Images toward the apex of the heart at the level of the papillary muscles (Fig. 2.24) show a crescent-shaped right ventricular chamber at the top of the sector image. A circular left ventricle is seen below the interventricular septum. Symmetrically shaped papillary muscles are seen within the left ventricular cavity at approximately the 4- and 9-o'clock positions or the 3- and 8-o'clock positions. The shape of the left ventricular chamber in this plane often is described as a mushroom. Slight movement toward the base of the heart shows chordae tendinea at their attachment points to the papillary muscles (Fig. 2.25).

The free wall of the left ventricle may not be seen in the horse unless the images are obtained close to the apex of the heart (Fig. 2.26). Images from most normal

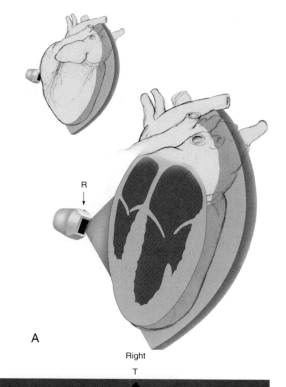

A

Right

FIGURE 2.19   **A.** The spatial orientation of the sound plane for the right parasternal long-axis four-chamber view of the heart is shown. The heart is positioned as seen from above the animal while the animal is in right lateral recumbency. The transducer is placed under the animal on the right side of the thorax and the plane spans the heart along its length from right side to left side and base to apex. **B.** This illustration of the resulting real-time image shows the relative positions of the cardiac structures. The top of the sector corresponds to the skin surface and transducer location. **C.** This is the real-time two-dimensional image of the four-chamber plane through the heart. *R,* reference mark; *T,* transducer; *RV,* right ventricle; *TV,* tricuspid valve; *RA,* right atrium; *IVS,* interventricular septum; *LV,* left ventricle; *MV,* mitral valve; *LA,* left atrium; *LVW,* left ventricular wall; *P,* pericardium.

T

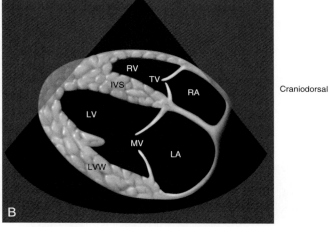

Caudoventral   Craniodorsal

B

Left

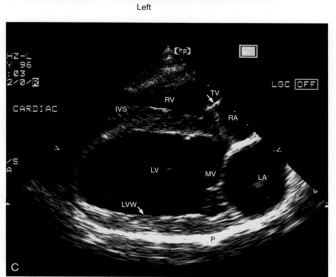

C

FIGURE 2.20   The right parasternal long-axis four-chamber view in a horse. Portions of the left ventricular wall and left atrium are not seen in large horses. *RV*, right ventricle; *TV*, tricuspid valve; *RA*, right atrium; *IVS*, interventricular septum; *LV*, left ventricle; *MV*, mitral valve; *LA*, left atrium; *LVW*, left ventricular wall.

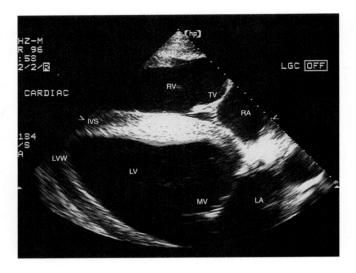

FIGURE 2.21   This is the right parasternal tipped long-axis four-chamber view in a dog. *RV*, right ventricle; *TV*, tricuspid valve; *RA*, right atrium; *IVS*, interventricular septum; *LV*, left ventricle; *MV*, mitral valve; *LA*, left atrium; *LVW*, left ventricular wall; *CT*, chordae tendinea; *P*, pericardium.

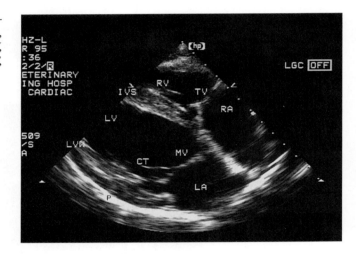

FIGURE 2.22   This is the right parasternal tipped long-axis, four-chamber view in a horse. *RV*, right ventricle; *TV*, tricuspid valve; *RA*, right atrium; *IVS*, interventricular septum; *LV*, left ventricle; *MV*, mitral valve; *LA*, left atrium; *LVW*, left ventricular wall.

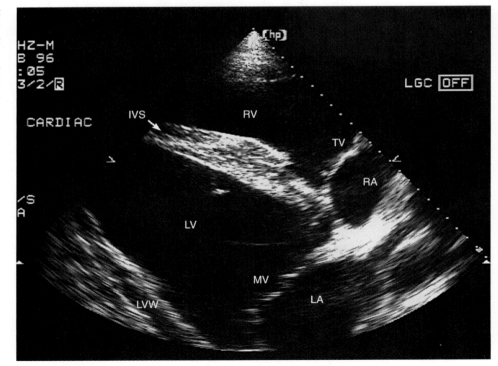

hearts will fit on a 24-cm depth sector image with the free wall completely visible during systole and only partially visible during diastole. The left ventricular chamber in the horse is somewhat more triangular in shape than the left ventricle in dogs and cats.

Mitral Valve. Tilting the transducer crystals toward the base of the heart brings the mitral valve into view. The leaflets when open will appear as an oval within the left ventricular chamber and as touching lines when they are closed during systole (Fig. 2.27). Movement of the mitral valves in this imaging plane is referred to as the "fish mouth." A larger portion of the right ventricle can now be seen above the left ventricle at the top of the sector image. Slower heart rates and longer diastolic filling periods in the horse make the mitral valve appear "floppier" than the valve motion seen in dogs and cats. Figure 2.28 shows this view in the horse.

Heart Base—Aorta. Toward the base of the heart, the aorta is seen as a circle or clover shape in the middle of the sector image (Figs. 2.29 and 2.30). All three valve cusps are present in this view of the heart. The image of closed valve leaflets in this plane is often called the "Mercedes sign" because of its resemblance to that manufacturer's logo. Above this circle, at the top of the sector, as always when transducer placement is on the right side of the thorax, is the right ventricle. The right ventricle extends from approximately the 11-o'clock position where the tricuspid valves are seen to the right side of the image where the pulmonary artery is seen. The pulmonic valve (PV) may be seen anywhere from the 3- to 5-o'clock position. The pulmonary artery (PA) extends downward from the valves, but only a portion of it is seen because the left auricle (LAU), a wedge-shaped extension of the LA, is seen just below the PV. The interatrial septum, seen at the left side of the image, separates the two atria.

Coronary arteries usually are seen leaving the sinus of Valsalva in the horse if the transducer is tilted just past the level of the aortic valves. Slight rotation of the transducer allows both cross-sectional and longitudinal images of the artery to be seen (Figs. 2.31 and 2.32).

Heart Base—Pulmonary Artery. Slightly further toward the base of the heart is the fourth plane that shows the length of the PA up to and including its bifurcation into the right and left main pulmonary arteries (Figs. 2.33 and 2.34). Only a small portion of the LA is now visible between approximately the 8- and 9-o'clock position on the image. The bifurcation usually is seen between the 5- and 6-o'clock position on the monitor. The right main pulmonary artery extends from right to left under the

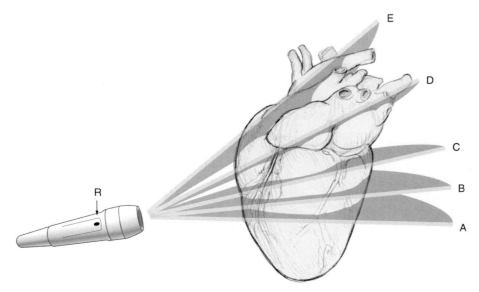

FIGURE 2.23 There are five standard transverse images of the heart. All are obtained from the same transducer location on the right side of the thorax. The transducer is pivoted from apex to base (caudal and ventral to cranial and dorsal) to obtain these views. **A.** Left ventricle with papillary muscles. **B.** Left ventricle at chordae tendinea. **C.** Left ventricle at mitral valves. **D.** Heart base—aorta. **E.** Heart base—pulmonary artery. *R*, reference mark.

FIGURE 2.24 **A.** The spatial orientation of the sound plane within the
heart is shown for the right parasternal short-axis left ventricle with papillary muscles view. The heart is positioned as seen from above the animal
while the animal is in right lateral
recumbency. The transducer is placed
under the animal on the right side of
the thorax and the plane traverses
the heart from right side to left side.
B. This illustration of the resulting
real-time image shows the relative
positions of the cardiac structures.
The top of the sector corresponds to
the skin surface and transducer location. **C.** This is the real-time two-
dimensional image of this plane
through the heart. *R*, reference
mark; *T*, transducer; *RV*, right ventricle; *IVS*, interventricular septum;
LV, left ventricle; *LVW*, left ventricular wall; *PM*, papillary muscle; *APM*
and *PPM*, anterior and posterior
papillary muscle; *P*, pericardium.

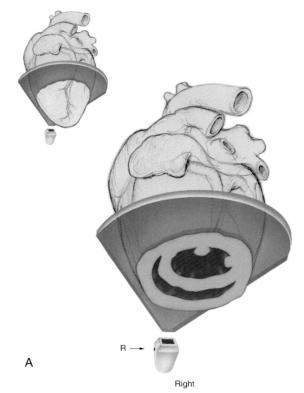

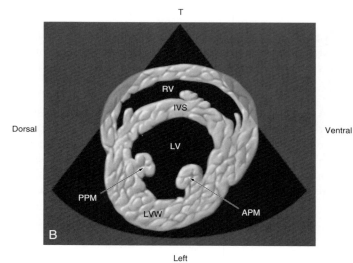

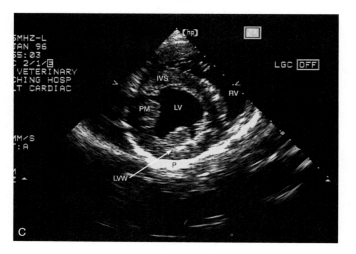

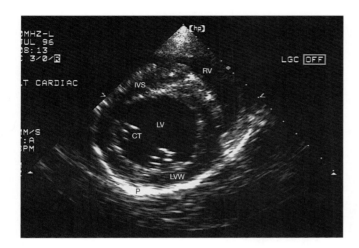

FIGURE 2.25   Slight movement of the transducer toward the base of the heart shows chordae tendinea at their attachment points on the papillary muscles. *RV*, right ventricle; *IVS*, interventricular septum; *LV*, left ventricle; *CT*, chordae tendinea; *LVW*, left ventricular wall; *P*, pericardium.

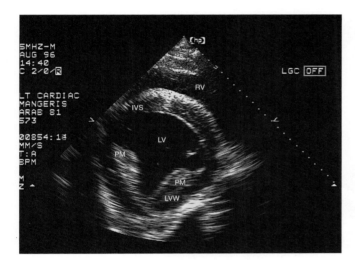

FIGURE 2.26   This is the right parasternal short-axis left ventricle with papillary muscles view in a horse. *RV*, right ventricle; *IVS*, interventricular septum; *LV*, left ventricle; *LVW*, left ventricular wall; *PM*, papillary muscle.

ascending aorta. Only a small portion of the left main pulmonary artery is seen as it extends into the lung field past the bifurcation.

Left Ventricle with Pulmonary Artery.   This oblique right parasternal image is generated at the level of the left ventricle. Slight twisting of the transducer allows us to see the pulmonary artery running along the right side of the image next to an egg-shaped left ventricle (Fig. 2.35). Long's right parasternal angled view in the horse is a modification of this plane (Fig. 2.36)(49). This image shows not only the pulmonic valve at approximately the 4- to 5-o'clock position, but also the right ventricular outflow above it and the main pulmonary artery below it. The pulmonary artery bifurcation is typically not seen in this plane.

Left Parasternal Apical Images

True apical images of the heart are difficult to obtain, and often what appears to be a true left ventricular apex is really part of the left ventricular lateral wall. Nevertheless, these images are used for many two-dimensional quantitative studies of function and are excellent planes for Doppler interrogation of the mitral and aortic valves. These views in the horse are severely foreshortened because depth and anatomical restrictions make apical images impossible to obtain.

Five Chamber.   The apical five-chamber long-axis image is generated with the transducer placed near the apex of the heart close to the sternum. The sound plane is directed dorsally and cranially along the length of the heart (Fig. 2.37). The apex of the LV is seen at the top right side of the image. The LA is seen at the bottom right

FIGURE 2.27 **A.** The spatial orientation of the sound plane within the heart is shown for the right parasternal short-axis left ventricle with mitral valves. The heart is positioned as seen from above the animal while the animal is in right lateral recumbency. The transducer is placed under the animal on the right side of the thorax and the plane crosses the heart from right side to left side. **B.** This illustration of the resulting real-time image shows the relative positions of the cardiac structures. The top of the sector corresponds to the skin surface and transducer location. **C.** This is the real-time two-dimensional image of this plane through the heart with open mitral valves. *R,* reference mark; *T,* transducer; *RV,* right ventricle; *PM,* papillary muscle; *IVS,* interventricular septum; *LV,* left ventricle; *LVW,* left ventricular wall; *AMV,* anterior mitral valve leaflet; *PVM,* posterior mitral valve leaflet.

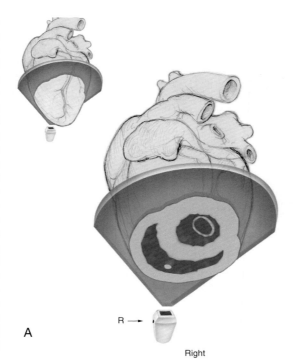

A

Right

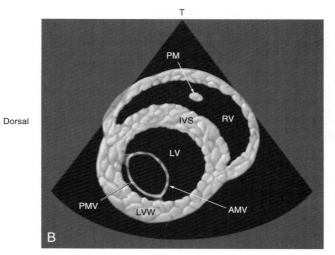

B

Left

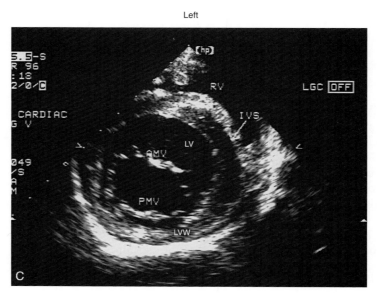

C

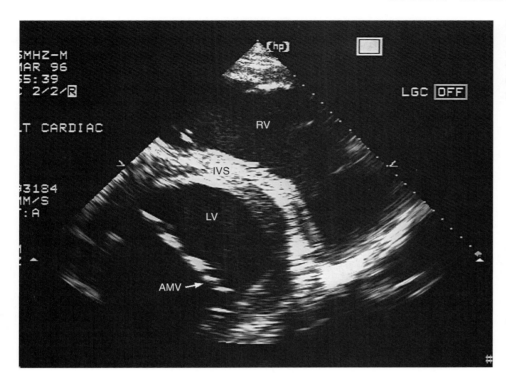

FIGURE 2.28 This is the right parasternal short-axis left ventricle with mitral valve image in a horse. *RV,* right ventricle; *IVS,* interventricular septum; *LV,* left ventricle; *AMV,* anterior mitral valve leaflet.

side of the image with mitral valves opening up into the left ventricular chamber. On the left side of the image the RV is seen at the top of the sector and the RA at the bottom of the image. Between the two atria, a longitudinal view of the aorta is seen as it leaves the left ventricle in a downward direction.

Despite a severely foreshortened left ventricle at the top of the sector image in the horse, the left atrium is seen at the bottom right side of the image with the mitral valves opening upward into the left ventricle as in the dog and cat (Fig. 2.38). The aorta is located centrally and extends downward on the image. Long described and labeled this imaging plane as the left parasternal angled view with left ventricular outflow and aorta (49).

Four Chamber. Remaining in the same intercostal space near the apex of the heart, sight movement of the transducer allows visualization of much more of the right side of the heart as the apical four-chamber plane is seen (Fig. 2.39). The aorta is no longer seen; instead, the IAS is now located between the left and right atria. The mitral and tricuspid valves are seen at the junction of the IAS and the IVS and open upward into the ventricles.

Left Parasternal Long-Axis Images

The first three left parasternal long-axis views described here are found in small animals from a cranial position on the left side of the thorax. Only slight manipulation of the transducer is required to move from one plane to the next. The last two left parasternal long-axis views described in this section are found in the large animal. These two planes are similar to the right parasternal left ventricular outflow and four-chamber, long-axis views except the left side is seen at the top of the sector image, and the right side is seen at the bottom of the sector image. Although not described by the Echocardiography Committee, these imaging planes can also be found in dogs and cats.

Left Ventricular Outflow (Small Animal). The left parasternal, left ventricular outflow view is the reference plane for this side of the thorax. This image is obtained from a cranial transducer position and looks similar to the right parasternal long-axis left ventricular outflow view except the tricuspid valves are not seen (Fig. 2.40).

FIGURE 2.29 **A.** The spatial orientation of the sound plane within the heart is shown for the right parasternal short-axis view of the heart base with aorta. The heart is positioned as seen from above the animal while the animal is in right lateral recumbency. The transducer is placed under the animal on the right side of the thorax and the plane spans the heart from right side to left side. **B.** This illustration of the resulting real-time image shows the relative positions of the cardiac structures. The top of the sector corresponds to the skin surface and transducer location. **C.** This is the real-time two-dimensional image of this plane through the heart. *R,* reference mark; *T,* transducer; *RV,* right ventricle; *RA,* right atrium; *TV,* tricuspid valve; *IAS,* interatrial septum; *NC,* noncoronary aortic valve cusp; *RC,* right coronary aortic valve cusp; *LC,* left coronary aortic valve cusp; *PV,* pulmonic valve; *LA,* left atrium; *LAU,* left auricle.

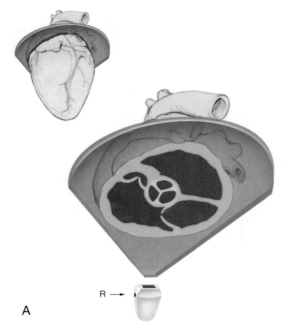

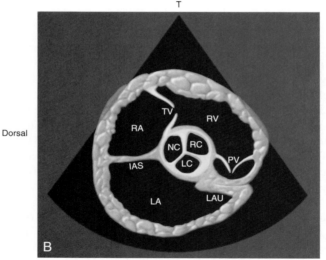

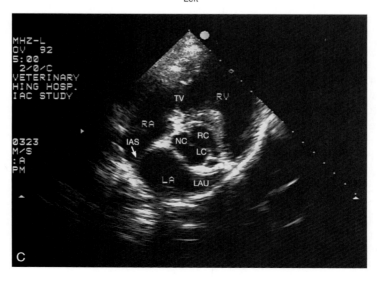

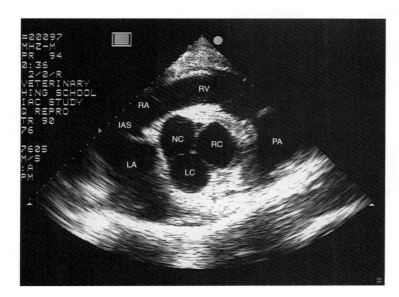

FIGURE 2.30   The right parasternal short-axis view of the heart base with aorta in a horse shows the aortic valve cusps clearly. *RV*, right ventricle; *RA*, right atrium; *IAS*, interatrial septum; *NC*, noncoronary aortic valve cusp; *RC*, right coronary aortic valve cusp; *LC*, left coronary aortic valve cusp; *LA*, left atrium; *PA*, pulmonary artery.

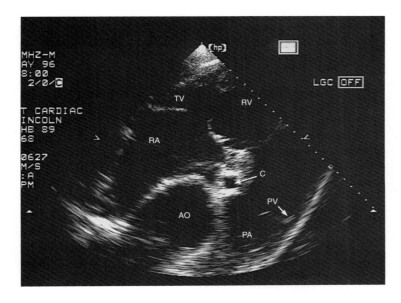

FIGURE 2.31   A transverse view of the coronary artery in the right parasternal short-axis view of the heart base with aorta in a horse. *RV*, right ventricle; *RA*, right atrium; *TV*, tricuspid valve; *PV*, pulmonic valve; *PA*, pulmonary artery; *AO*, aorta; *C*, coronary artery.

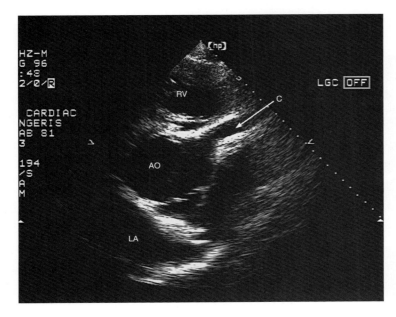

FIGURE 2.32   This transverse plane through the heart base in a horse shows a sagittal view of the coronary artery as it leaves the aorta. *RV*, right ventricle; *AO*, aorta; *LA*, left atrium; *C*, coronary artery.

FIGURE 2.33 **A.** The spatial orientation of the sound plane within the heart is shown for the right parasternal short-axis view of the heart base with pulmonary artery. The heart is positioned as seen from above while the animal is in right lateral recumbency. The transducer is placed under the animal on the right side of the thorax and the plane traverses the heart from right side to left side. **B.** This illustration of the resulting real-time image shows the relative positions of the cardiac structures. The top of the sector corresponds to the skin surface and transducer location. **C.** This is the real-time two-dimensional image of this plane through the heart. *R,* reference mark; *T,* transducer; *RV,* right ventricle; *RA,* right atrium; *TV,* tricuspid valve; *IAS,* interatrial septum; *PA,* pulmonary artery; *PV,* pulmonic valve; *RMPA,* right main pulmonary artery; *LMPA,* left main pulmonary artery; *AO,* aorta; *LA,* left atrium.

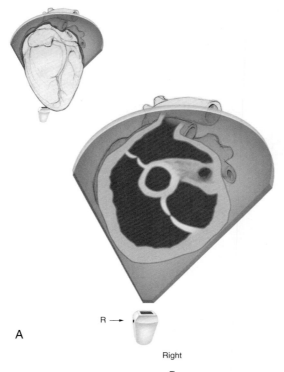

A

Right

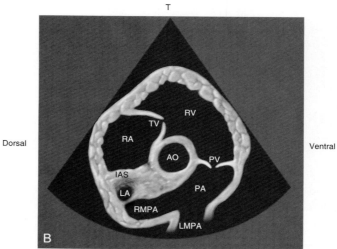

B

Left

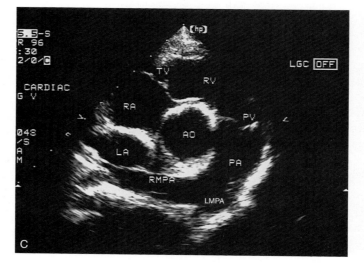

C

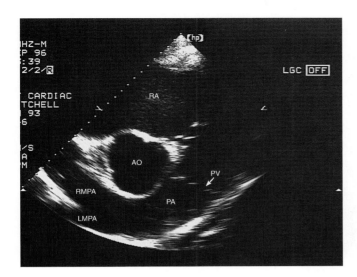

FIGURE 2.34 The right parasternal short-axis view of the heart base with pulmonary artery in a horse. *PV*, pulmonic valve; *PA*, pulmonary artery; *RMPA* and *LMPA*, right and left main pulmonary artery; *RA*, right atrium; *AO*, aorta.

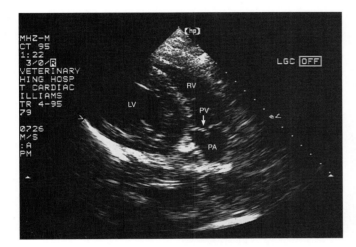

FIGURE 2.35 An oblique right parasternal view of the left ventricle shows the main pulmonary artery and pulmonic valve. *RV*, right ventricle; *PA*, pulmonary artery; *PV*, pulmonic valve; *LV*, left ventricle.

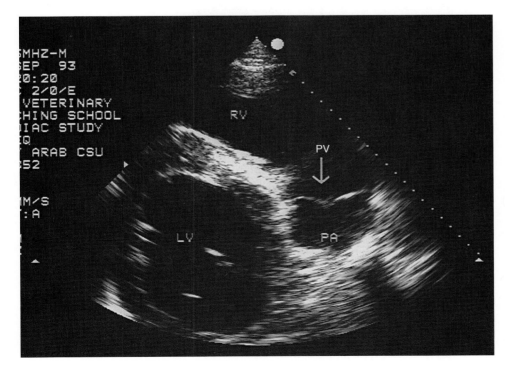

FIGURE 2.36 This is the left ventricle with pulmonary artery in the horse. *RV*, right ventricle; *PA*, pulmonary artery; *PV*, pulmonic valve; *LV*, left ventricle.

FIGURE 2.37 **A.** The spatial orientation of the sound plane within the heart is shown for the apical five-chamber view of the heart obtained from a left parasternal caudal transducer location. The heart is positioned as seen from above the animal while the animal is in left lateral recumbency. The transducer is placed on the left side of the thorax under the animal and the plane crosses the heart from apex to base. **B.** This illustration of the resulting real-time image shows the relative positions of the cardiac structures. The top of the sector corresponds to the skin surface and transducer location. **C.** This is the real-time two-dimensional image of this plane through the heart. *R*, reference mark; *T*, transducer; *RV*, right ventricle; *RA*, right atrium; *TV*, tricuspid valve; *LA*, left atrium; *LV*, left ventricle; *IVS*, interventricular septum; *AO*, aorta; *MV*, mitral valve; *AOV*, aortic valve.

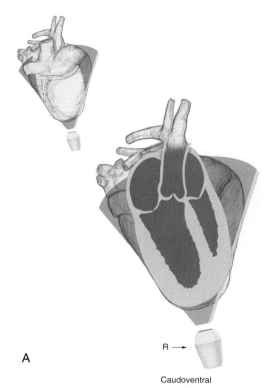

A

Caudoventral

T

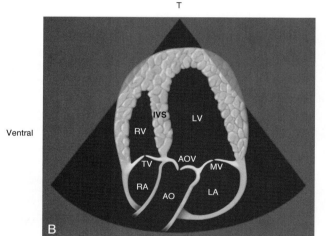

Ventral   Dorsal

B

Craniodorsal

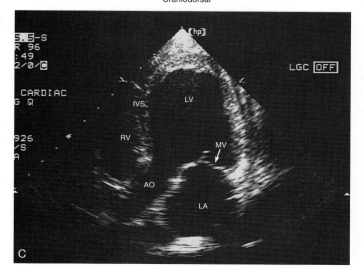

C

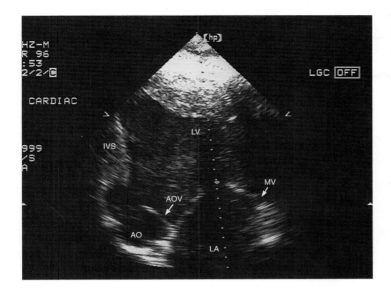

FIGURE 2.38 The left parasternal apical five-chamber view in a horse. The ventricle is severely foreshortened. *LA*, left atrium; *LV*, left ventricle; *IVS*, interventricular septum; *AO*, aorta; *MV*, mitral valve; *AOV*, aortic valve.

Instead, portions of the pulmonic valve are seen anterior to the ascending aorta. This view is excellent for observing the aortic valves and ascending aorta. Images still maintain the base of the heart to the right and apex to the left orientation.

Right Atrium and Auricle (Small Animal). Remaining in the cranial location and tilting the beam slightly results in a plane that transects the right atrium, tricuspid valve, and right auricle (Fig. 2.41). This image provides an oblique view of both ventricles, with an egg-shaped left ventricle on the left side of the image and the right ventricle on the top right of the sector image. The tricuspid valves open upward toward the right ventricle, and the right atrial appendage extends to the right and up from the atrium. The caudal vena cava (CVC) may be seen as it enters the right atrium from the left side of the image under the left atrium.

Right Ventricular Outflow (Small Animal). The third plane generated from the left cranial transducer position also requires slight tilting away from the left ventricular outflow plane. The right ventricular outflow tract and pulmonic valve are seen along the top of the image, with an oblique left ventricle and atrium along the bottom (Fig. 2.42). The pulmonary artery extends downward from the valve along the right side of the image. A small piece of the aortic valve is seen at the junction of the left ventricle and pulmonary artery. Manipulating this view slightly gives a more vertical plane through the pulmonary artery (Fig. 2.43). Other structures often are not clear in this more vertical image, but the pulmonic valves are imaged well, providing excellent alignment with flow for Doppler interrogation.

Four Chamber (Large Animal). This four-chamber view of the heart is obtained in the horse from a cranial location on the left side. It shows a tipped left ventricular chamber on the top left side of the image and the left atrium to the right and bottom of the image (Fig. 2.44). The left ventricular free wall is seen at the top of the sector image and the interventricular septum is seen below the left ventricular chamber. This plane through the heart offers a better look at the left ventricular free wall as well as the left atrium and mitral valves, which are often not completely seen on right parasternal images. A more horizontal image can also be obtained (Fig. 2.45).

Five Chamber (Large Animal). The aorta is seen in this left parasternal long-axis in the horse. This image is modified from the four-chambered parasternal long-axis view just described. Here, the aorta is included in the image (Fig. 2.46). Parts of the right ventricle and atrium are seen below the ventricular septum.

FIGURE 2.39 **A.** The spatial orientation of the sound plane within the heart is shown for the apical four-chamber view of the heart obtained from a left parasternal caudal transducer location. The heart is positioned as seen from above the animal while the animal is in left lateral recumbency. The transducer is placed on the left side of the thorax under the animal and the plane spans the heart from apex to base. **B.** This illustration of the resulting real-time image shows the relative positions of the cardiac structures. The top of the sector corresponds to the skin surface and transducer location. **C.** This is the real-time two-dimensional image of this plane through the heart. *R,* reference mark; *T,* transducer; *RV,* right ventricle; *RA,* right atrium; *TV,* tricuspid valve; *IVS,* interventricular septum; IAS interatrial septum; *LA,* left atrium; *LV,* left ventricle; *MV,* mitral valve.

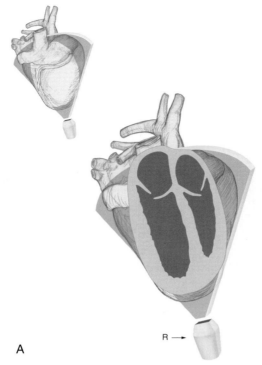

A

Caudoventral

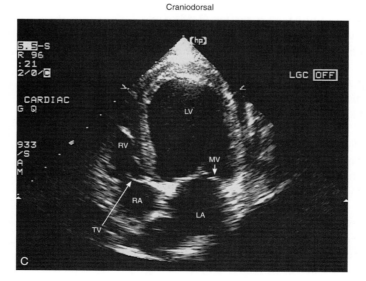

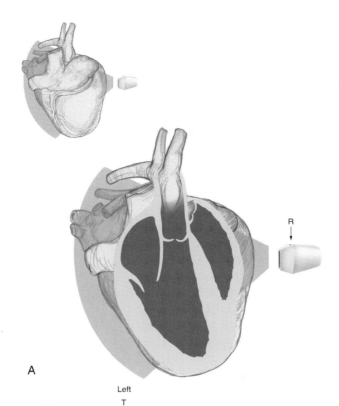

A

FIGURE 2.40   **A.** The spatial orientation of the sound plane within the heart is shown for the left parasternal long-axis left ventricular outflow view in a dog. The heart is positioned as seen from above the animal while the animal is in left lateral recumbency. The transducer is placed cranially on the left side of the thorax below the animal. The plane transects the heart from base to apex and left to right. **B.** This illustration of the resulting real-time image shows the relative positions of the cardiac structures. The top of the sector corresponds to the skin surface and transducer location. **C.** This is the real-time two-dimensional image of this plane through the heart. *R*, reference mark; *T*, transducer; *RV*, right ventricle; *PV*, pulmonic valve; *IVS*, interventricular septum; *LA*, left atrium; *LV*, left ventricle; *MV*, mitral valve; *AO*, aorta; *AOV*, aortic valve; *LVW*, left ventricular wall.

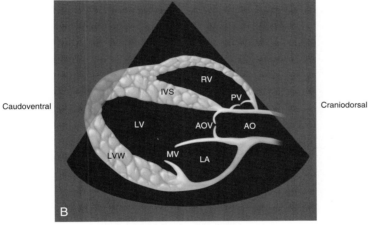

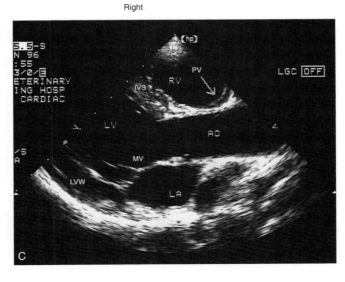

FIGURE 2.41 **A.** The spatial orientation of the sound plane within the heart is shown for the left parasternal long-axis right atrium and auricle view in a dog. The heart is positioned as seen from above the animal while the animal is in left lateral recumbency. The transducer is placed cranially on the left side of the thorax below the animal. **B.** This illustration of the resulting real-time image shows the relative positions of the cardiac structures. The top of the sector corresponds to the skin surface and transducer location. **C.** The real-time two-dimensional image of this plane through the heart looks like this. *R,* reference mark; *T,* transducer; *RV,* right ventricle; *RA,* right atrium; *RAU,* right auricle; *TV,* tricuspid valve; *IVS,* interventricular septum; *LV,* left ventricle.

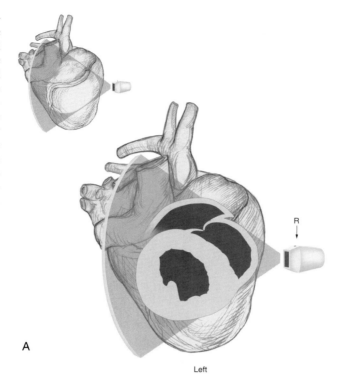

A

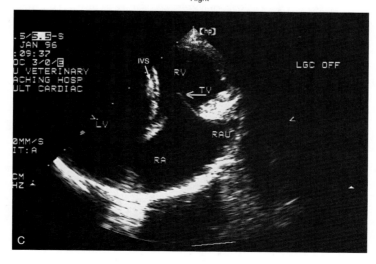

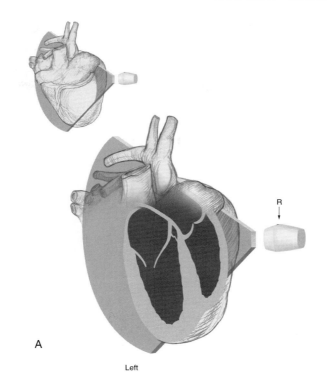

A

Left

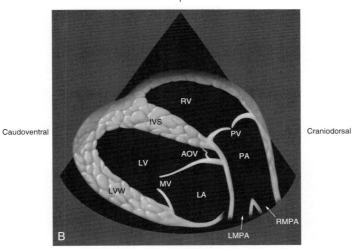

FIGURE 2.42   **A.** The spatial orientation of the sound plane within the heart is shown for the left parasternal long-axis right ventricular outflow view in a dog. The heart is positioned as seen from above the animal while the animal is in left lateral recumbency. The transducer is placed cranially on the left side of the thorax below the animal. **B.** This illustration of the resulting real-time image shows the relative positions of the cardiac structures. The top of the sector corresponds to the skin surface and transducer location. **C.** The real-time two-dimensional image of this plane through the heart. *R,* reference mark; *T,* transducer; *RV,* right ventricle; *PA,* pulmonary artery; *RMPA,* right main pulmonary artery; *LMPA,* left main pulmonary artery; *LV,* left ventricle; *LVW,* left ventricular wall; *PV,* pulmonic valve; *MV,* mitral valve; *AOV,* aortic valve; *LA,* left atrium.

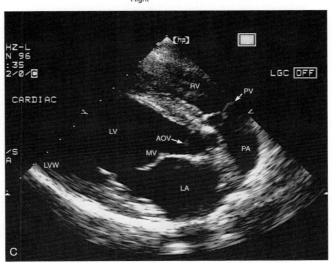

FIGURE 2.43   Slight modification of the left ventricular outflow view allows the pulmonary to be located centrally and more vertically in the image. *PA*, pulmonary artery; *PV*, pulmonic valve; *RV*, right ventricle.

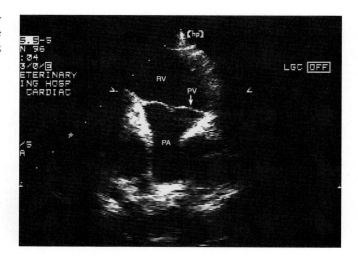

FIGURE 2.44   This is a tipped left parasternal four-chamber view of the heart in a horse. *LV*, left ventricle; *LVW*, left ventricular wall; *LA*, left atrium; *MV*, mitral valve; *IVS*, interventricular septum; *RA*, right atrium; *RV*, right ventricle.

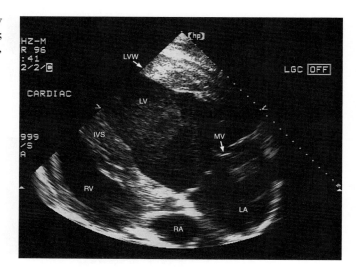

FIGURE 2.45   The transducer has been moved to a more dorsal and cranial location on the left side of the horse to obtain this more horizontally positioned four-chamber view of the heart. *LV*, left ventricle; *LVW*, left ventricular wall; *LA*, left atrium; *MV*, mitral valve; *IVS*, interventricular septum; *RA*, right atrium; *RV*, right ventricle.

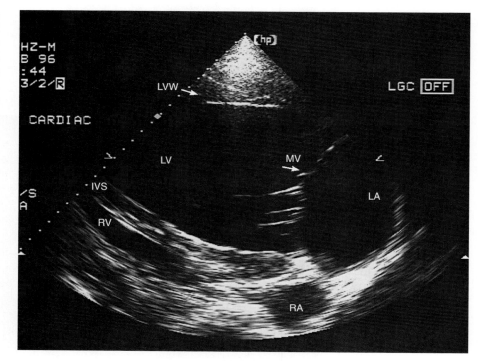

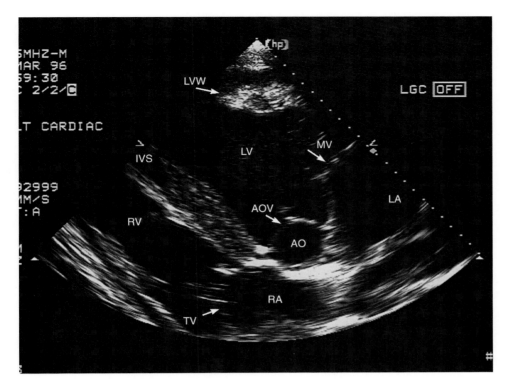

FIGURE 2.46   The tipped left parasternal five-chamber view of the heart in a horse includes the aorta. *LV*, left ventricle; *LVW*, left ventricular wall; *LA*, left atrium; *MV*, mitral valve; *IVS*, interventricular septum; *AO*, aorta; *AOV*, aortic valve; *RA*, right atrium; *RV*, right ventricle; *TV*, tricuspid valve.

Left Parasternal Short-Axis Images

These transverse images can be obtained in both the large and small animal. Structures are the same as those seen in the right parasternal images but have different locations.

Aorta, Right Atrium, Pulmonary Artery.   Remaining in the left 4th or 5th intercostal space and twisting the transducer toward a transverse plane through the heart creates the left parasternal short-axis view of the base of the heart (Fig. 2.47). The aorta is still seen as a circle or clover-shaped structure in the center of the image. The right atrium is seen at the bottom of the image with the right ventricle wrapping along the left side of the aorta. The tricuspid valves are found at approximately the 8- to 9-o'clock position. On the right side of the image, the pulmonary artery will wrap around the aorta as it does in right parasternal images, but the pulmonic valve is located at about 12 to 1 o'clock. The image can be manipulated to show a better view of the tricuspid valve at the expense of the pulmonary artery (Fig. 2.48). The image also may be adjusted to see a better view of the pulmonary artery and valve at the expense of the tricuspid valve (Fig. 2.49). This is often, but not always, a good plane for Doppler evaluation of the pulmonary artery and tricuspid valves.

In the horse, a plane similar to this is described and labeled by Long as the left parasternal angled view through the right ventricular inlet and outlet (Fig. 2.50)(49).

Left Ventricle.   The left ventricle is seen at the top right of the sector image. One papillary muscle may be lost within the near field at the top of the sector, whereas the other papillary muscle is located at approximately 4 to 5 o'clock on the sector image (Fig. 2.51). The interventricular septum separates the mushroom-shaped left ventricular chamber from the crescent-shaped right ventricular chamber. This imaging plane in the small animal provides great views of the right ventricular wall

FIGURE 2.47 **A.** The spatial orientation of the sound plane within the heart is shown for the left parasternal short-axis view of the heart base. The heart is positioned as seen from above the animal while the animal is in left lateral recumbency. The transducer is placed under the animal on the left side of the thorax and the plane spans the heart from left side to right side. **B.** This illustration of the resulting real-time image shows the relative positions of the cardiac structures. The top of the sector corresponds to the skin surface and transducer location. **C.** This shows the real-time two-dimensional image of this plane through the heart. *R*, reference mark; *T*, transducer; *RV*, right ventricle; *RA*, right atrium; *TV*, tricuspid valve; *PV*, pulmonic valve; *PA*, pulmonary artery; *RMPA* and *LMPA*, right and left main pulmonary artery; *AO*, aorta; *RC*, right coronary cusp; *NC*, noncoronary cusp; *LC*, left coronary cusp; *P*, pericardium.

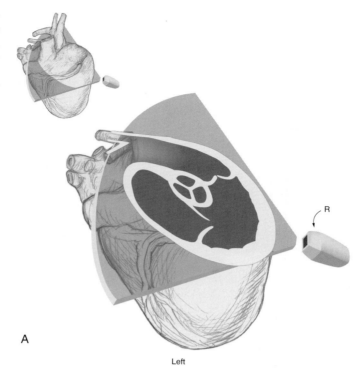

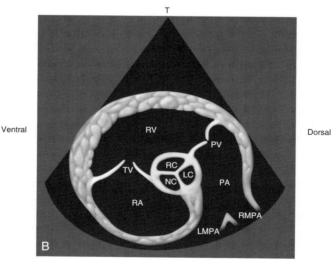

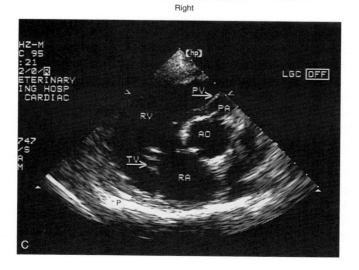

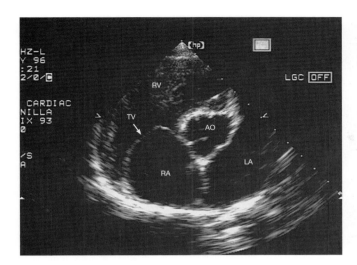

FIGURE 2.48   The left parasternal transverse image of the heart base can be manipulated to show clearer tricuspid valves. Distinct pulmonic valves are no longer seen. *AO*, aorta; *RV*, right ventricle; *RA*, right atrium; *TV*, tricuspid valve; *LA*, left atrium.

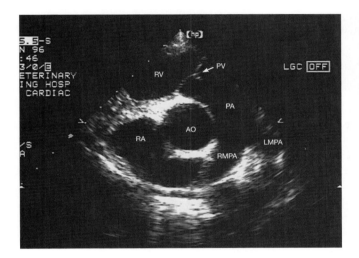

FIGURE 2.49   The left parasternal transverse image of the heart base also can focus on clear images of the pulmonary artery and its valve. The tricuspid valve loses its definition, however. *PV*, pulmonic valve; *PA*, pulmonary artery; *RV*, right ventricle; *RA*, right atrium; *AO*, aorta; *RMPA*, right main pulmonary artery; *LMPA*, left main pulmonary artery.

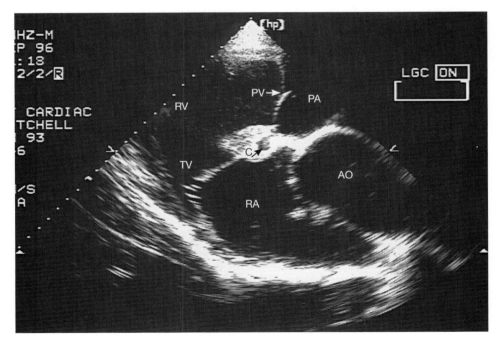

FIGURE 2.50   The real-time two-dimensional left parasternal oblique view of the heart in a horse shows well-defined pulmonic and tricuspid valves. *RV*, right ventricle; *RA*, right atrium; *TV*, tricuspid valve; *PV*, pulmonic valve; *PA*, pulmonary artery; *AO*, aorta; *C*, coronary artery.

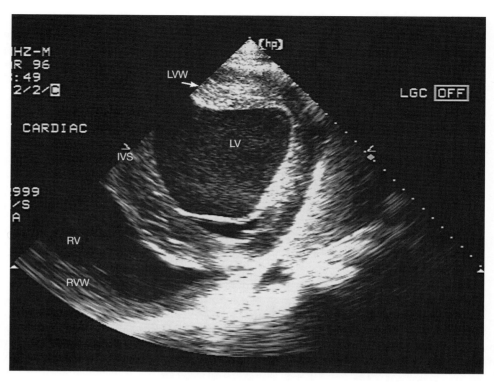

FIGURE 2.51   This real-time left parasternal transverse section of the left ventricle shows the left ventricular wall at the top of the sector image. *LV*, left ventricle; *LVW*, left ventricular wall; *IVS*, interventricular septum; *RV*, right ventricle; *RVW*, right ventricular wall.

that often is poorly seen in the near fields of right parasternal images. The right ventricular wall may not be seen in the horse because of depth limitations.

Subcostal Images

Small animals tolerate poorly the scanning to obtain these imaging planes. Sedation usually is required for good subcostal imaging planes. Subcostal images usually do not provide additional information because resolution often is inadequate for assessment of lesions, and Doppler interrogation with an imaging probe usually is not possible in medium to large dogs because of the increased depth needed for these views.

Two-Dimensional Imaging Technique

Several points and terms need to be clarified before describing the examination technique. All transducers have a reference mark, which may be a ridge or a colored or raised dot on the transducer (Fig. 2.52). The reference mark serves two purposes. First, it defines the plane in which sound waves leave the transducer. A two-dimensional sector of sound with width and depth is generated along the diameter of the transducer face indicated by the reference mark (Fig. 2.53). Second, all ultrasound machines display a symbol on the top right or left of the sector image (Fig. 2.54). Whatever the reference mark is directed toward during an examination will be seen on the side of the image with the symbol. For example, if the reference mark is directed toward the base of the heart while looking at a parasternal long-axis image, the atria and aorta will be seen on the side of the image with the symbol. The reference symbol is assumed to be on the right side of the sector for all imaging directions given in this book.

Terms used to describe transducer motion as imaging technique are discussed, including transducer face, rotate, lift or drop, and point. Transducer face refers to the crystal end of the probe. Directions will be given that orient the face in directions

---

Transducer Reference Mark

- Identifies how the sound beam leaves the transducer
- Provides orientation for structures on the sector image

Terms for Imaging Technique

Face: Crystal end of the transducer.

Rotate: Twisting the transducer clockwise or counterclockwise about its length.

Lift: Without changing the transducer location, lift it up toward the table, creating less of an angle between the animal and the transducer.

Drop: Without moving the transducer on the thorax, drop the transducer down away from the chest, creating a larger angle between the transducer and the animal.

Point: Aiming the transducer face toward the indicated anatomic structure (i.e., the lumbar spine).

relative to body parts. Rotating the transducer involves twisting it clockwise or counterclockwise along its long axis (Fig. 2.55). Pointing the transducer involves aiming the face toward the anatomical structure that is named (Fig. 2.56). The transducer should be held in the same plane with no rotation and no change in the angle between the dog and transducer. The cable will extend in the opposite direction. Lifting and dropping the transducer involves bringing it up toward the examination table or thorax or dropping it down away from the table without a change in transducer location or sound plane with reference to the animal (Fig. 2.57). When the probe is lifted up toward the table, the sound beams become more parallel to the animal, and a smaller angle is created between the transducer and the animal. Dropping the probe away from the table creates a larger angle between the animal and the transducer and orients the sound plane more perpendicularly to the animal.

When instructed to move the transducer in any of the indicated ways, it is important not to move it in any other manner. In other words, do not lift the probe inadvertently while rotating it, and don't lift the probe toward the table when instructed to point it in a different direction. Directions are given for scanning the right parasternal long-axis, left ventricular outflow plane first. Transducer movement to obtain all the other right parasternal planes are described as movements away from the transducer position necessary for this long-axis plane. Although every animal's heart is positioned a little differently within the thorax, once the long-axis left ventricular outflow plane is found, all other imaging planes through the heart are related to this plane in the same way, and transducer manipulation is similar. The directions given here, for small animals, are specifically directed toward obtaining images from below the animal while it is lying on a cardiac scanning table.

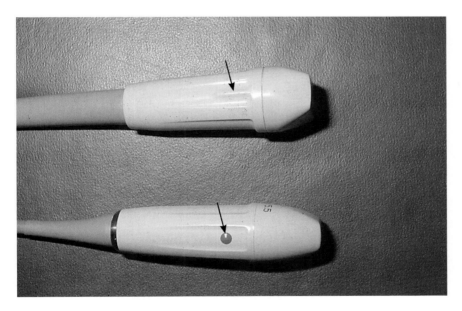

FIGURE 2.52 Every transducer has a reference mark (*arrows*) that helps orient the image on the monitor and defines the sound plane.

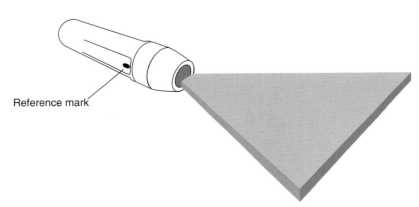

Reference mark

FIGURE 2.53 The sound plane is generated along the diameter of the transducer face indicated by the reference mark.

FIGURE 2.54 Every ultrasound machine displays a symbol (*arrow*) on the top right or left side of the sector image. Whatever the transducer reference mark is directed toward during the ultrasound examination will be seen toward the side of the real-time image with the symbol.

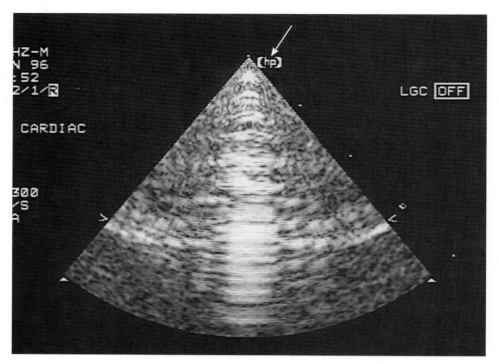

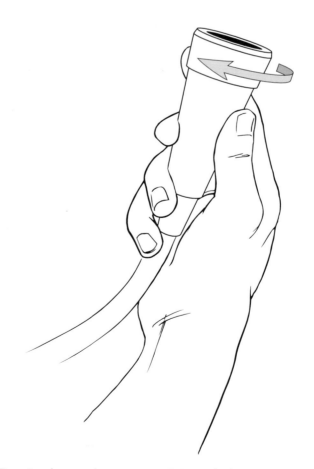

FIGURE 2.55   Rotating the transducer means twisting it clockwise or counterclockwise on its length.

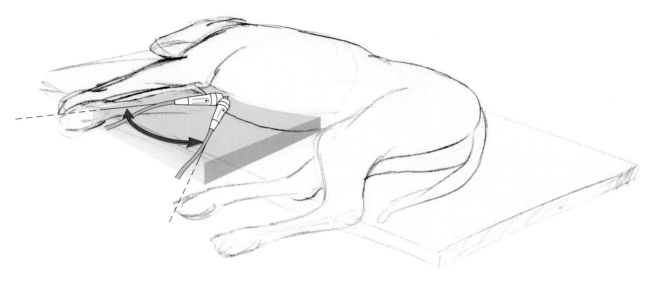

FIGURE 2.56 Pointing the transducer involves directing the transducer face toward the anatomic structure that is named. The cable will extend in the opposite direction. The transducer is not rotated during this movement; it remains in the same place on the thorax, and the same sound plane with reference to the animal is maintained.

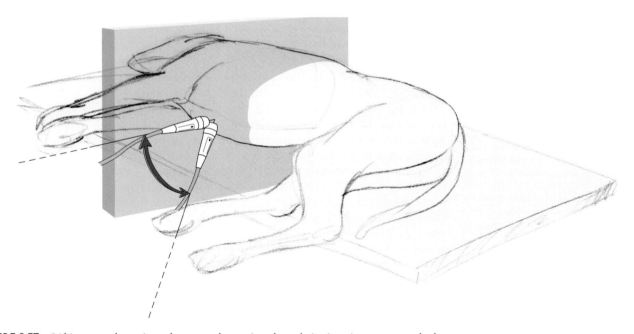

FIGURE 2.57 Lifting or dropping the transducer involves bringing it up toward the examination table or dropping it down away from the table. The transducer remains in the same location on the thorax; the face direction remains the same; the transducer is not rotated; and the sound plane with reference to the animal remains the same.

Small Animal

Right Parasternal Long-Axis Images

Left Ventricular Outflow.   This long-axis plane through the heart is obtained by placing the transducer within the 3rd to 6th intercostal space. The transducer usually is placed within the 5th or 6th intercostal space for larger dogs and in the 3rd to 5th intercostal spaces for smaller dogs and cats. The transducer is close to the sternum in cats and small dogs, but in larger dogs transducer placement usually is 1 to 3 inches away from the sternum toward the costochondral junction. Do not be afraid to move

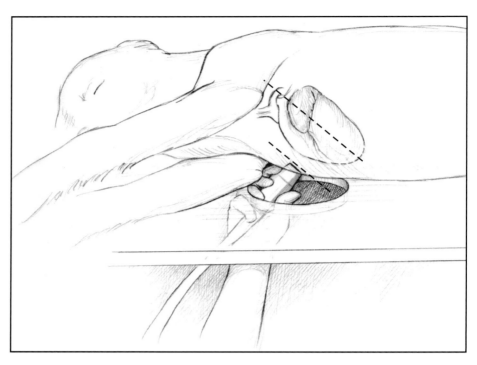

FIGURE 2.58   The long axis of the heart in the dog is aligned from approximately shoulder to xiphoid. The transducer face and sound plane should be aligned along an imaginary line connecting the base of the heart to the apex.

Small Animal
Right Parasternal Long Axis

Left Ventricular Outflow
View Imaging Technique
• 3rd to 6th intercostal space
• The transducer is close to the sternum in cats and small dogs, but 1 to 3 inches away from the sternum in larger dogs.
• Reference mark is toward the neck.
• Point the face toward the lumbar spine.
• Cable extends toward the elbow.
• Approximately a 45° angle is between the transducer and the animal.

the transducer once an image is found. Most animals have several echocardiographic "windows"; look for the one with the best resolution.

The transducer reference mark should be directed toward the scapular-humoral joint of the shoulder, and the transducer face (crystals) should be pointed dorsally and caudally toward the animal's lumbar spine. There should be an angle of approximately 45° between the transducer and the table. The sound plane should follow an imaginary line extending from the scapular-humoral joint to the xiphoid (Figs. 2.58 and 2.59). Hold the transducer in the following manner when searching for the heart (Fig. 2.60): Cradle the transducer in your hand with an index finger over the reference mark that is oriented along the plane of the scapula; extend the cable toward the elbows; direct the crystals toward the lumbar vertebrae; and then tilt transducer at approximately 45° to the table. Remember not to lift, drop, or rotate the transducer while searching for the best "window" so initial images will be close to a good long axis of the heart.

The feline heart is positioned so that its long axis is aligned more with the sternum. Because of this, the transducer is located very close to the sternum and horizontally, with an angle between the cat and the transducer that often approaches 10°. The reference mark is directed cranially and the face is pointing toward the thoracic spine instead of the lumbar spine (Fig. 2.61). The transducer in a cat also is located more toward the front leg than in dogs, and a front leg that is extended cranially aids in good image generation. The best images in cats are obtained when the cat is stretched out and the spine is kept straight. Once the long-axis left ventricular outflow view is obtained, all movements toward the other views are similar to those described in dogs.

The image should include the aortic root, left ventricular outflow tract, left ventricular chamber, mitral valves, and left atrium. If the image shows an interatrial septum and a short left ventricle instead of the aorta and a long ventricle (Fig. 2.62), rotate the transducer along its long axis in a counterclockwise direction so the reference mark moves toward the front legs. When the aorta is visualized, images that do not include a good left atrium and well-defined mitral valve (Fig. 2.63) should be adjusted by slowly lifting the probe into a plane more parallel to the examination

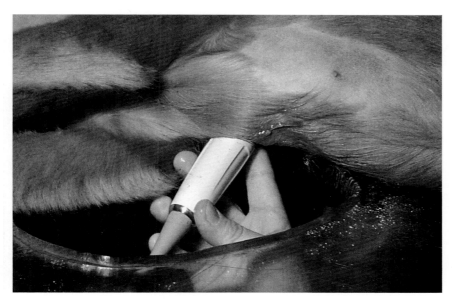

FIGURE 2.59   The right parasternal long-axis with left ventricular outflow view is obtained with the reference mark directed toward the animal's neck, the cable extended toward the animal's elbows, and the face directed toward the animal's lumbar spine. There should be an angle of approximately 45° between the transducer and the table.

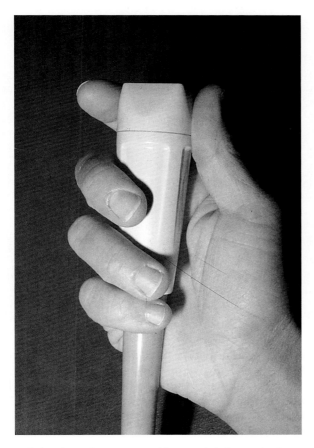

FIGURE 2.60   Search for the right parasternal long-axis left ventricular outflow view of the heart while the transducer is held in this manner and the image obtained will be close to the correct imaging plane. Cradle the transducer in your hand with the reference mark under the index finger. Hold it with the reference mark directed toward the animal's neck, the cable extended toward the animal's elbows, and the face directed toward the animal's lumbar spine. There should be an angle of approximately 45° between the transducer and the table.

FIGURE 2.61 The length of the heart in cats is aligned a little more along the sternum, and the transducer face is directed a little more toward the thoracic spine to obtain the long-axis left ventricular outflow view.

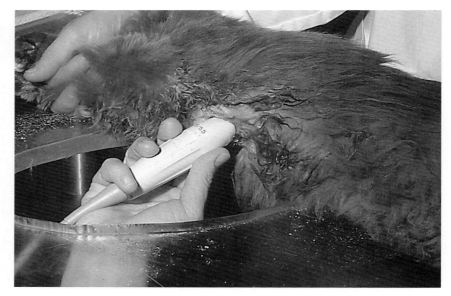

FIGURE 2.62 This image shows the interatrial septum and a short left ventricular chamber. Rotate the transducer counterclockwise so that the reference mark moves toward the sternum to lengthen the left ventricle and bring in the aorta. *RA*, right atrium; *RV*, right ventricle; *TV*, tricuspid valve; *LA*, left atrium; *LV*, left ventricle; *IVS*, interventricular septum; *IAS*, interatrial septum; *LVW*, left ventricular wall; *MV*, mitral valve.

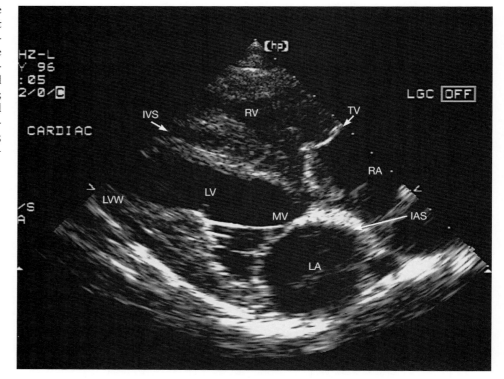

table. Stop the lifting motion when the mitral valves are clearly seen and they move well. Lifting too much will cause the aorta to disappear.

Often, a long-axis image shows all the correct structures but is severely foreshortened with no length to the left ventricular chamber (Fig. 2.64). There can be several reasons for this. Usually, it is because the sound plane does not cut through the ventricular long axis (Fig. 2.64). When this is the case, rotating the transducer on its axis in a clockwise or counterclockwise direction will lengthen the left ventricle. Sometimes, the plane of sound may not be pointed back toward the lumbar spine enough to line up with the length of the heart. Imagine a dog's heart on a lateral radiograph. The base of the heart is up toward the shoulder and the apex is down towards the xiphoid. The plane of sound should be directed along the imaginary line connecting these two reference points following the length of the heart (Fig. 2.58) and not cranial and caudal in line with the spine. Lastly, even if the sound plane is directed along the length of the heart correctly, it may not be traveling through the middle of the heart. Tilting the transducer up toward the table or down away from it will correct the image if this is the reason. Any or all three of these reasons may be a factor. Change one thing at a time, and after creating the best image with each movement, then change another thing. If the image becomes worse with any movement, reverse the movement and try another one. Each movement should be done slowly because the adjustments are usually very slight.

When none of the preceding transducer movements work, it usually is because the transducer is not positioned under the heart properly. Move the probe within the intercostal space toward the spine or toward the sternum until a larger ventricular chamber is seen and try again.

Once a long axis of the left ventricle is obtained, the image can be fine-tuned. Resolution improves by simply applying a little more pressure or by pressing the probe a little more against one rib or the other on each side of the transducer to "settle into the space" better.

The image can be manipulated to see more of the ventricles or more of the heart base. Without changing anything else, point the transducer face more dorsal toward the spine and away from the hip, while the cable moves away from the animal's front legs toward the sternum (Fig. 2.65). More of the atria and aorta will be seen as these structures move into the center of the sector image. Alternatively, directing the transducer face more caudally toward the hip, as the cable moves away from the sternum toward the head, allows the left and right ventricles to move into the center of the sector image (Fig. 2.66).

When the apex of the heart is seen toward the upper left side of the image and the base of the heart is seen at the lower right side of the image, the image is called a tipped long axis. These tipped images are the easiest to obtain and often have the best resolution.

To obtain a more horizontal left ventricular image move the transducer into the 3rd or 4th intercostal spaces and up toward the costochondral junction. Point the face caudal and move the cable toward the head away from the legs to generate a left ventricular image with good length (Fig. 2.67). After moving into this position, rotate the transducer on its long axis, clockwise or counterclockwise, to keep the aorta in view.

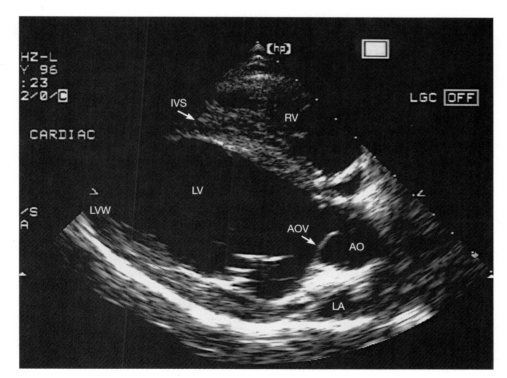

FIGURE 2.63 This image shows good length to the left ventricle and aorta, but the left atrium and mitral valves are not seen well. Lift the transducer up toward the dog into a plane more parallel with the examination table to bring the left atrium and mitral valve into view. *RV*, right ventricle; *LV*, left ventricle; *IVS*, interventricular septum; *AOV*, aortic valve; *AO*, aorta; *LVW*, left ventricular wall; *LA*, left atrium.

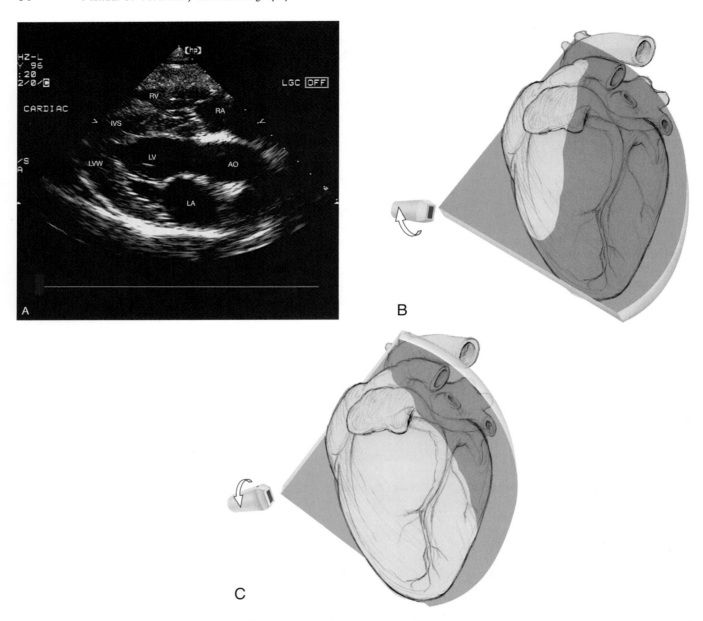

FIGURE 2.64   **A.** This image shows all the structures seen in a right parasternal long-axis left ventricular outflow view of the heart, but there is no length to the ventricular chamber. The sound plane may not be directed through the length of the ventricle. **B.** Here, the transducer is rotated too far clockwise, and in **C** the transducer is rotated too far counterclockwise. Either way, the sound plane slices through the top or bottom of the heart instead of through the middle. Rotate the transducer clockwise or counterclockwise to improve the plane. *RV,* right ventricle; *RA,* right atrium; *AO,* aorta; *LV,* left ventricle; *IVS,* interventricular septum; *LVW,* left ventricular wall; *LA,* left atrium.

Small Animal
Right Parasternal Long Axis

Four–Chamber View
Imaging Technique
- Start with left ventricular outflow view.
- Rotate the reference mark toward the spine until the aorta disappears.
- Lift and drop the transducer until left ventricular size is maximized.
- Point the face more caudally if the LV is still too short.

Four Chamber.   Parasternal four-chamber images of the heart are obtained by rotating the reference mark of the transducer toward the spine past the shoulder after the left ventricular outflow plane through the heart is seen (Fig. 2.68). Once the aorta has disappeared and the atrial septum is in view, tilt the transducer up toward the table or down away from it to maximize left ventricular size. If the ventricle still appears too short, point the transducer caudal to line the transducer face up along the length of the heart.

Right Parasternal Short-Axis Images.   Transverse or short-axis images of the heart are obtained by rotating the transducer toward the sternum with the reference mark turned 90° from its location for the long-axis plane. The mark is directed toward the animal's elbow. The same place on the thorax is used for transverse and long-axis images. The transducer is held more perpendicular (approximately 60 to 70°) with respect to the examination table for transverse images, however, and is pivoted from the base of the heart to the apex to obtain the various short-axis planes (Fig. 2.69). The cable still is directed ventrally because it is not held perpendicular to the thoracic wall, and the fanning motion is done with this 60 to 70° angle in mind. Depending on how the transducer is held, any of the transverse planes can be viewed first. As you point the transducer toward the apex of the heart, the face should be directed toward the xiphoid and the cable should extend cranially (Fig. 2.69). As you

Small Animal
Right Parasternal Short-Axis Views

Imaging Technique
- Remain in the same spot on the thorax as for the long-axis views.
- Rotate the reference mark toward the elbows.
- Drop the transducer down away from the animal slightly (approximately 60° between animal and transducer).
- The cable is still directed toward sternum.
- Pivot the transducer from xiphoid to shoulder to get all five transverse images.

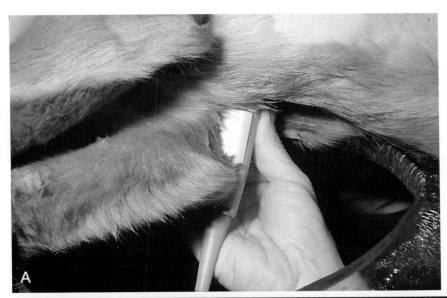

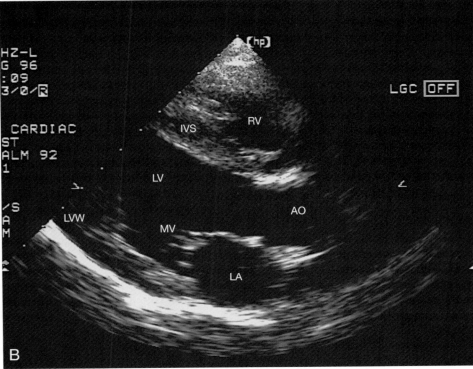

FIGURE 2.65   **A.** Pointing the transducer toward the spine and away from the hips will bring the base of the heart into the center of the sector image. **B.** The aorta and left atrium will be seen in the center of the image and only a portion of the left ventricle will be seen. *RV,* right ventricle; *IVS,* interventricular septum; *LV,* left ventricle; *AO,* aorta; *LVW,* left ventricular wall; *MV,* mitral valve; *LA,* left atrium.

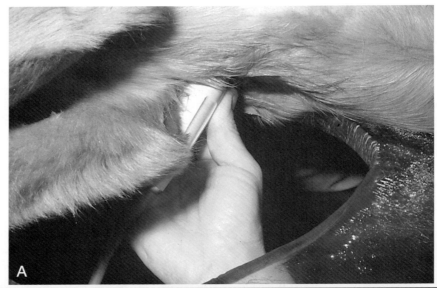

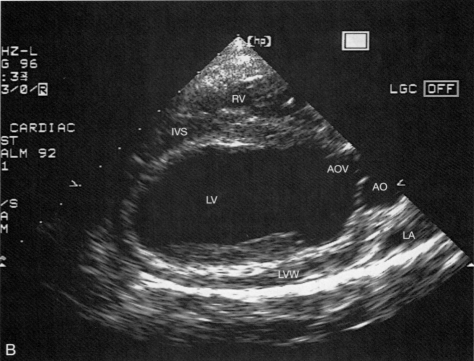

FIGURE 2.66   **A.** Pointing the transducer face toward the apex of the heart will bring the apex of the left ventricle toward the center of the image while the base of the heart moves out of the image to the right. **B.** More of the left ventricular chamber is seen when this is done, and very little of the base of the heart is seen in the image. *RV,* right ventricle; *IVS,* interventricular septum; *LV,* left ventricle; *AO,* aorta; *AOV,* aortic valve; *LA,* left atrium; *LVW,* left ventricular wall.

point the transducer face toward the base of the heart (the shoulder) the cable should move toward the xiphoid (Fig. 2.69). The fanning motion for scanning from base to apex should follow the length of the heart along an imaginary line extending from the shoulder to xiphoid (Fig. 2.58). Although these motions sound extreme, they are actually very slight. A small arc at the thoracic wall creates a large arc deep within the thorax.

When the sector image shows only part of the short-axis image and the rest is out of the sector to the left (Fig. 2.70), the transducer needs to be lifted up toward the

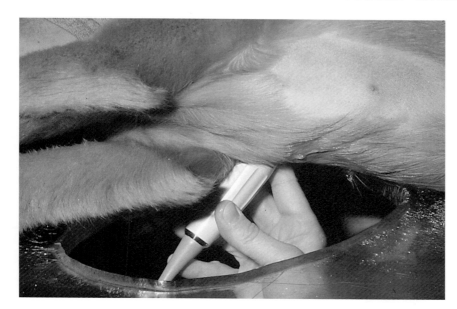

FIGURE 2.67 The transducer needs to move cranially one intercostal space and slide dorsally within that space. The face should be directed caudally to align the long-axis left parasternal images more horizontally across the sector image. If the aorta disappears or the left ventricle becomes smaller, rotate the transducer one way or the other. All these motions are needed to create a more horizontal image.

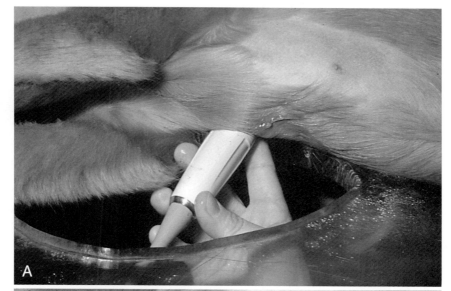

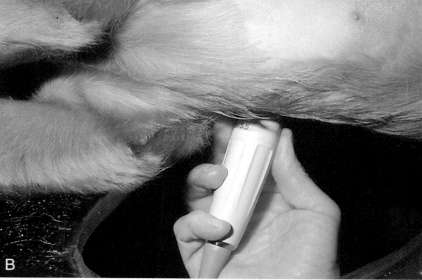

FIGURE 2.68 Parasternal long-axis four-chamber views of the heart are obtained by (**A**) leaving the transducer in the same location as for the left ventricular outflow view and (**B**) rotating the transducer clockwise until the reference mark is directed more toward the spine. The transducer may need to be pointed a little more caudally. Lift or drop the transducer slightly to maintain length to the ventricular chambers.

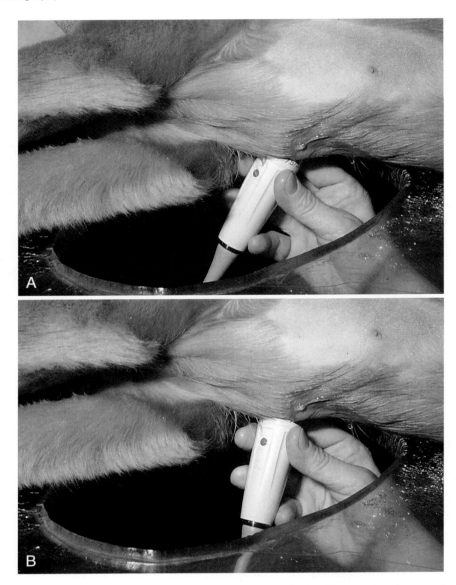

FIGURE 2.69   **A.** The left ventricular transverse view is obtained by rotating the transducer until the reference mark is directed toward the elbow or sternum and tilting the transducer slightly caudally and ventrally. Stop rotating when a symmetric circular left ventricle is seen. The cable should be directed slightly cranially. Because the transducer is not perpendicular to the thoracic wall for these images, the cable still should extend slightly ventrally toward the sternum or elbow. **B.** The transducer is pivoted and directed cranially and dorsally toward the shoulder to obtain the transverse mitral valve image. The cable should be directed down and ventrally toward the xiphoid.

table so the face points toward the spine or physically moved into the intercostal space toward the spine so that it is more directly under the heart. The opposite holds true for images that are partially out of the picture to the right (Fig. 2.71). In this case, the transducer face needs to be directed toward the sternum or physically moved toward the sternum.

Left Ventricle with Papillary Muscles.   Rotate the transducer until images of the left ventricle show a circular shape with symmetrical papillary muscles. The cable is directed slightly ventral and cranial (Fig. 2.69). An egg-shaped ventricle means the transducer has not been turned enough or it has been turned too much (Fig. 2.72). Rotate it back and forth until the most circular shape is seen.

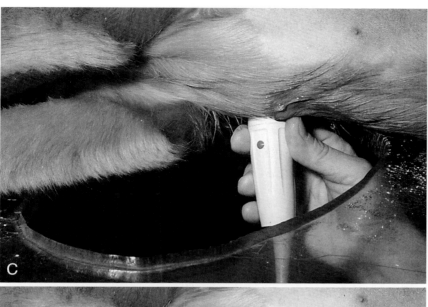

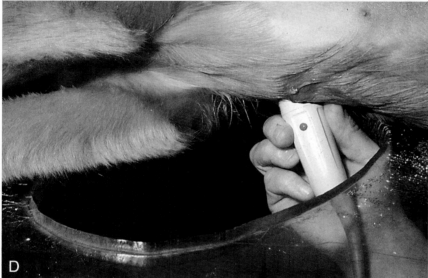

FIGURE 2.69 *(continued)*   **C.** Pivot the transducer even more toward the shoulder to obtain the transverse view of the aorta. The cable should be directed caudally and ventrally toward the xiphoid. The reference mark still is directed toward the elbows. Rotate the transducer slightly if necessary to view the aorta in the transverse circular plane. **D.** Once a transverse image of the aorta is obtained, pivot the transducer a little more cranially and dorsally to see the pulmonary artery and its bifurcation. Pivot the transducer in a circular motion until the clearest images of the pulmonary artery are seen.

When obtaining transverse sections, the further back the transducer is positioned toward the apex of the heart, the less you will see of the right ventricle, and the smaller the left ventricle will appear. This usually happens when the long-axis plane you started with was a very tipped view. Move forward an intercostal space and slightly dorsal to direct the sound plane through a larger section of the left and right ventricles.

Mitral Valves.   Pivot the transducer very slightly toward the neck. The cable should move toward the xiphoid if the LV was imaged first and away from the xiphoid if the heart base was imaged first (Fig. 2.69). At the level of the mitral valves, both sides of the valve should be attached to the lateral walls. Rotate the transducer back and forth until a symmetrical oval-shaped valve is seen within the left ventricular chamber.

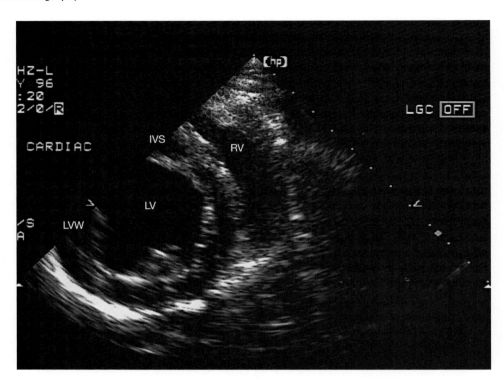

FIGURE 2.70   When the heart moves off the sector image to the left side of the monitor, the transducer is located too close to the sternum. Either physically move the transducer in the intercostal space toward the spine or point the transducer face toward the spine by lifting the transducer toward the table. *LV,* left ventricle; *RV,* right ventricle; *IVS,* interventricular septum; *LVW,* left ventricular wall.

Heart Base—Aorta.   Pivot the transducer crystals more toward the neck and the aorta will appear in the middle of the image. The cable now extends toward the xiphoid (Fig. 2.69). Tilt the transducer back and forth until the aortic valves are seen. At this point, there is often air interference in the image. Try to clean up the image by slowly pointing the transducer in various directions. Systematically pointing the crystals in a complete 360° arc around its axis may produce a clearer image. Sometimes the transducer needs to be moved forward an intercostal space to improve the image. When you move the transducer forward, be sure to move dorsally toward the spine at the same time. The pulmonic valve and pulmonary artery may not be seen well in this plane even when images of the aorta are excellent. The pulmonary artery is seen better with either of the two imaging planes described next.

Heart Base—Pulmonary Artery.   Once a good image of the heart base with aorta, left atrium, and left auricle is seen, the transducer is tilted slightly further toward the neck to bring the main pulmonary artery into view (Fig. 2.69). The image of the pulmonic valve and the bifurcation should be clear, although the rest of the image may not be. Clearer images of the pulmonary artery and valve may require pointing the transducer slightly toward the sternum. This move simply involves directing the crystals away from the spine to the sternum. In this move, the cable should move slightly away from the sternum and be directed caudally.

Left Ventricle with Pulmonary Artery.   Start with the right parasternal long-axis left ventricular outflow view. From this plane, drop the transducer down away from the table into a more vertical position until the mitral valves are no longer in view and the aorta and left ventricle still are clearly visible. No rotation of the transducer should have occurred and the ventricle should not have lost its length. From this plane, slowly rotate the transducer reference mark toward the elbow (Fig. 2.73). The pulmonary artery will be seen on the right side of the sector image and the left ventricle will become egg shaped. Once the artery is seen, point the transducer in

Small Animal
Right Parasternal Short Axis
_____

Left Ventricle with Pulmonary Artery
Imaging Technique
- Start with the tipped long-axis left ventricular outflow view.
- Drop the transducer away from the animal until the mitral valves do not move, but the aorta and its valves still are clearly seen.
- Rotate the reference mark toward the sternum.
- Stop when the pulmonary artery is seen on the right side of the image.
- Point the transducer face in different directions until the longest pulmonary artery is seen.

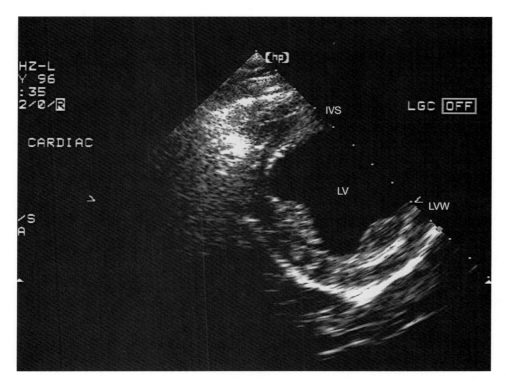

FIGURE 2.71   When the heart moves off the sector image to the right side of the monitor, the transducer is located too close to the spine. Either physically move the transducer in the intercostal space toward the sternum or point the transducer face toward the sternum. *LV*, left ventricle; *IVS*, interventricular septum; *LVW*, left ventricular wall.

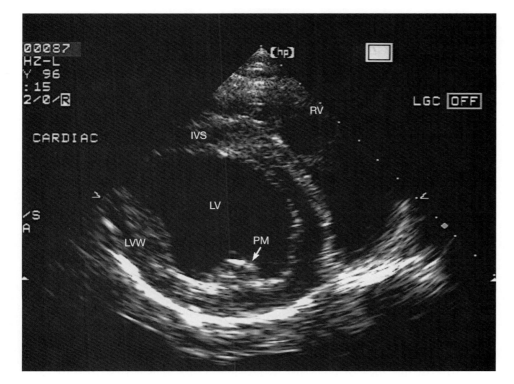

FIGURE 2.72   An egg-shaped left ventricular chamber means the transducer has either been rotated too much or not enough. Rotate it clockwise and counterclockwise until a symmetric circular chamber is obtained. *RV*, right ventricle; *LV*, left ventricle; *IVS*, interventricular septum; *LVW*, left ventricular wall; *PM*, papillary muscle.

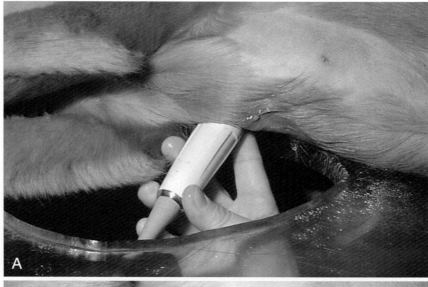

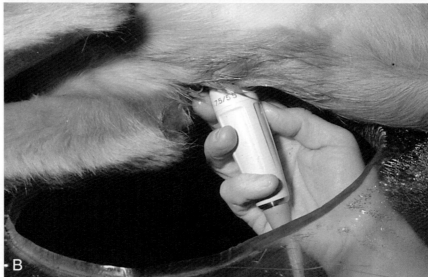

FIGURE 2.73   Starting with the left ventricular outflow view (**A**), tilt the transducer down away from the dog (**B**) until the mitral valves are not seen moving anymore. At that point, rotate the transducer counterclockwise toward the sternum until the pulmonary artery comes into view along the right side of the sector.

Small Animal
Left Parasternal Apical Views

Imaging Technique
- The reference mark is dorsal and caudal toward the lumbar spine.
- The sound plane is parallel with the table.
- The face is pointed toward the neck.
- The cable extends toward the knees.
- Start with the liver and move forward along the sternum until the heart is seen.
- Move away from sternum, dorsally, if the image is not clear.
- Lift the transducer up toward the animal for the five-chamber view; drop it down for the four-chamber view.

slightly different cranial directions and from side to side until the longest pulmonary artery is seen.

Left Parasternal Apical Images

Four- and Five-Chamber Views. Transducer positions for four- and five-chamber views are similar and will be discussed together. The reference mark should be directed dorsally and caudally with the transducer face directed cranially toward the shoulder and base of the heart (Fig. 2.74). The transducer should be placed as far back toward the apex of the heart as possible. Often it is easiest to start in an intercostal space near the xiphoid and find the liver. Move cranially and dorsally, space by space, until the heart is seen. Be sure to hold the transducer parallel to the body. If the image is not clear, first slide the probe dorsally in the space; if it is still not clear, move forward one more space. More pressure is applied to the transducer for these images than for any other because the probe is so parallel to the body wall and effort is needed to direct the sound beams under the ribs. An image may become clearer simply by pushing a little harder.

One of the two apical planes should be visible at this point. A four-chamber view is seen if the transducer is not parallel enough to the body wall (Fig. 2.74). Lift the transducer up toward the thorax and the aorta will come into view for the five-chamber plane (Fig. 2.74). Conversely, if the five-chamber view is visible, drop the transducer away from the body wall (cable goes down) and the four-chamber view will appear. Rotate the transducer slightly counterclockwise when imaging from five- to four-chamber planes to maintain ventricular length and obtain the best mitral valve motion. When the apex of the heart is not at the top of the sector, but off to the right side of the image (Fig. 2.75), that indicates that the transducer face is directed toward the spine too much and needs to be redirected toward the base of

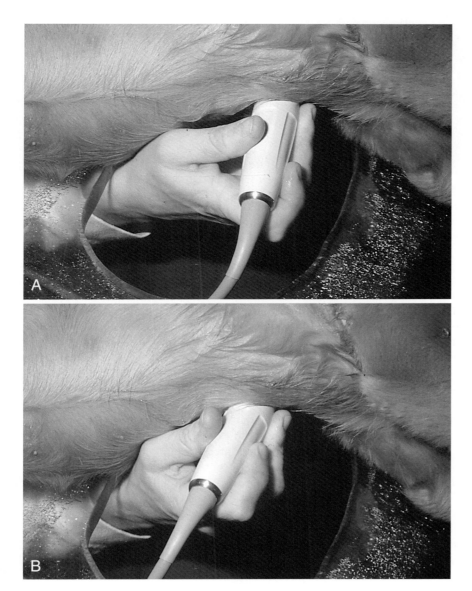

FIGURE 2.74   **A.** With the reference mark directed dorsally and caudally, and the face directed toward the shoulder and base of the heart, a four-chamber view of the heart is imaged. A transducer angle of less than 30° from the body wall is common. **B.** Tilt the transducer up toward the body wall to bring the aorta into view and obtain the apical five-chamber plane through the heart. Rotate the transducer back and forth slightly when moving from one plane to the next to maximize left atrial size and mitral valve motion.

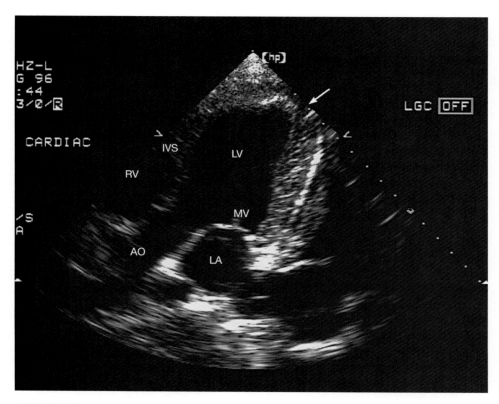

FIGURE 2.75   When the apex of the heart is located to the right side of the image (*arrow*) instead of at the top of the sector, the transducer face is directed too much toward the spine; it should be pointed more toward the head and legs. *LV,* left ventricle; *RV,* right ventricle; *IVS,* interventricular septum; *AO,* aorta; *LA,* left atrium; *MV,* mitral valve.

the heart. Point the crystals more toward the shoulder and front legs. The movement should involve sweeping the crystals in an arc, with respect to the body, from the spine, toward the head, and then the legs without changing the sound plane. The cable should be moving in an arc from the xiphoid to the knees. This movement will bring the length of the ventricle into view as well as move the apex of the heart to the top of the sector image.

Left Parasternal Long-Axis Images.   As with the right parasternal long-axis views, directions for the left-sided views are given as movements away from the left parasternal long-axis with left ventricular outflow view. Pay particular attention to obtaining good images for that view and the other views will come easily. Directions are given for small animals placed in left lateral recumbency that are imaged from below through a cutout.

Left Ventricular Outflow.   The left 3rd to 4th intercostal spaces are used for the left ventricular outflow image. With the reference mark directed cranially, the transducer face and sound beam should almost line up along the long axis of the body with the crystals pointing toward the spine and slightly caudal. The cable will extend out from the sternum and, because the face is pointed slightly caudal, the cable is extending slightly cranial toward the elbows (Fig. 2.76). The transducer itself is almost parallel to the body or the examination table with an angle of approximately 30°. Move the transducer dorsally and cranially until a clear image is obtained. Your hand will be touching the animal's front leg if you are forward enough. Then tilt the transducer up toward the table then down away from the table until the left ventricular outflow tract is seen. If the left atrium and ventricle are too small (foreshortened), rotate the transducer slightly clockwise or counterclockwise on its axis to lengthen them.

Small Animal
Left Parasternal Cranial Long Axis

Left Ventricular Outflow View
Imaging Technique
- Use the 3rd to 4th intercostal space; your hand should be touching the front leg.
- The reference mark is cranial.
- The sound plane is parallel with the examination table.
- The face is directed slightly caudally toward the thoracic spine.
- The cable extends toward the elbows.
- The transducer is 2 to 3 inches away from the sternum.

Right Atrium and Auricle.   Without changing the location, position, or sound beam direction drop the transducer down away from the examination table to bring the right atrium and auricle into view (Fig. 2.76). Lift and drop the transducer until the largest and clearest right auricle, atrium, and tricuspid valves are seen. The clearest and largest views of the right auricle may not show the best tricuspid valve motion. Rotate the transducer back and forth to obtain clear images of the tricuspid valve; this may be at the expense of clear auricular images.

Right Ventricular Outflow.   From the transducer position used for the left parasternal long-axis left ventricular outflow view, the transducer is lifted up toward the examination table. It will be almost horizontal and parallel with the table for this plane (Fig. 2.76). As the transducer is raised up, the left ventricular outflow tract will disappear from view, and the pulmonic valve and right ventricular outflow tract will be seen at the top of the sector image. More of the left atrium is seen and only a glimpse of the aortic valve is seen, if it is seen at all. Move the transducer up and down slightly until the clearest pulmonary valve is seen. Slightly rotating the transducer in a clockwise or counterclockwise direction and pointing the transducer a little more caudal will bring more of the pulmonary artery into view at the expense of other structures, which will lose their definition (Fig. 2.76).

Left Parasternal Short-Axis Images

Aorta, Right Atrium, Pulmonary Artery.   This view of the heart is seen with the transducer held almost perpendicular to the thoracic wall (approximately 70 to 80° with respect to the table). The cable should extend toward the sternum and slightly caudal. The reference mark is directed dorsally (approximately 90° from its location for imaging the cranial long-axis images) at approximately the 3-o'clock position (Fig. 2.77). Rotate the transducer until the aorta is seen as a circle in the center of the image. If rotation does not produce a circular aorta, move cranially and dorsally into another intercostal space. Lift the transducer up toward the dog or down away from the dog to improve the pulmonic valve image at the top right side of the sector image. The transducer also may be pointed dorsally or ventrally to see a better pulmonic valve image. The more cranial the transducer is placed on the thorax, the better the right atrium and tricuspid valve images will be. The valves will open almost straight up toward the top of the sector in these images.

Large Animal

The normal equine heart barely fits onto the sector image of equipment with a maximum depth of 24 cm. The entire left atrium rarely is visible in the adult horse in either the transverse or long-axis planes. Better images of the left atrium and left ventricular wall can be obtained by imaging from the left side of the horse.

Two-dimensional echocardiographic images may be obtained from both the left and right parasternal positions as in small animals. All M-mode images usually are derived from the right parasternal real-time images. When the heart size exceeds the depth capabilities of the equipment, left ventricular M-modes are obtained from the left parasternal position. There is no statistically significant difference in M-mode measurements obtained from the left versus the right parasternal planes. Most CW and PW Doppler spectral tracings are obtained from the left parasternal position, with the exception of the pulmonary artery and sometimes the tricuspid valve, whose spectral tracings are obtained from the right parasternal images.

When describing reference mark location in the horse, it is done with reference to time on a clock. The clock should be imagined on the right or left side of the thorax with 12 o'clock straight up toward the spine, 3 o'clock cranial toward the front leg, and 9 o'clock caudal toward the tail. The left ventricular, long-axis with outflow view will be used as a reference plane; all other views will be movements away from this plane. Technique is described in this manner for consistency. The most complete reference to date on imaging technique in the horse uses a right parasternal, four-chamber view of the heart as its reference plane (49). All terms for transducer movement are the same as those used when describing small animal technique. Figure

---

Small Animal
Left Parasternal Cranial Long Axis

Right Atrium and Auricle
Imaging Technique
- Remain in the same location as for the left ventricular outflow view.
- Drop the transducer down away from the animal.

Small Animal
Left Parasternal Cranial Long Axis

Right Ventricular Outflow View
Imaging Technique
- Remain in the same location as for the left ventricular outflow view.
- Lift the transducer up toward the animal.

Small Animal
Left Parasternal Short Axis

Heart Base
Imaging Technique
- Remain in the same location as for the cranial long axis images.
- Rotate the transducer until the reference mark is toward the thoracic spine.
- Drop the transducer down away from the animal until the transducer is almost perpendicular to the thorax.
- The face should point slightly cranially and the cable extends slightly caudally.
- If the aorta is not a circle, rotate the transducer clockwise and counterclockwise until it is a circle. If that does not work, move forward or back a space.

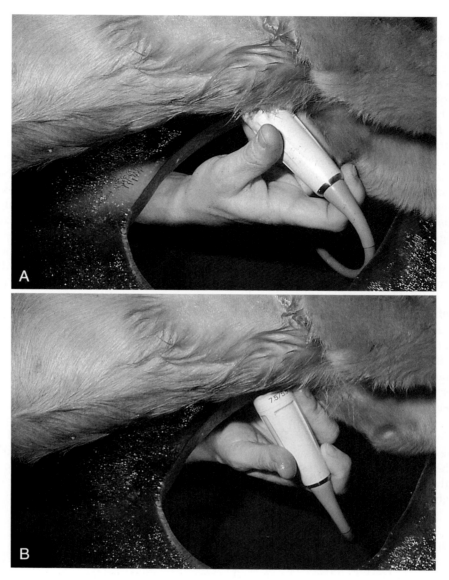

FIGURE 2.76   **A.** With the transducer precisely positioned cranially in the left 3rd or 4th intercostal space, the reference mark directed cranially, and the sound plane directed along the length of the body, the left parasternal long-axis left ventricular outflow view is obtained. The transducer is lifted up toward the table, then down away from the table, and is held at approximately a 30° angle away from the table until the aorta is seen. **B.** Without changing transducer location, drop the transducer down away from the thoracic wall and the right atrium and auricle will come into view.

2.78 shows the orientation of the heart in the equine thorax. The base of the heart is directed toward 1 o'clock and the apex toward 7 o'clock.

Right Parasternal Long-Axis Images

Left Ventricular Outflow.   Place the transducer within the 3rd to 5th intercostal space, approximately 2 to 3 inches dorsal to the olecranon. Start with the transducer at a right angle (perpendicular) to the thoracic wall. The transducer reference mark should be dorsal and slightly cranial, at approximately 1 o'clock when looking down the length of the transducer (Fig. 2.79). The transducer should be pushed forward into the horse's leg until a clear cardiac image in obtained. This requires some effort because often a clear image is not obtained because the transducer is not far enough forward. As you move the transducer forward, hold it perpendicular to the thoracic

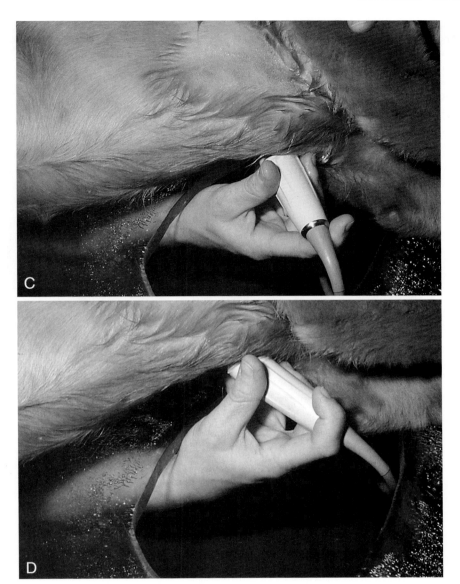

FIGURE 2.76 *(continued)*   **C.** Lifting the transducer toward the thoracic wall away from the left ventricular outflow view will bring the right ventricular outflow tract and pulmonary artery into the image. **D.** The pulmonary artery can be centered more within the image by lifting the transducer a little more and pointing the face more caudally.

wall; do not point it forward. If the leg is not positioned cranially and is not abducted slightly, it will require a lot of work to obtain a clear image (Fig. 2.6). If sliding forward does not result in a clear image of the left ventricle, the transducer should be moved (not pointed) up or down in a dorsal to ventral position until an image with good resolution is obtained. Remember to keep the transducer perpendicular to the chest wall. At this point, the image may lack a good aortic image and have a severely shortened left ventricular chamber image (Fig. 2.80). To bring the aorta or more of the aorta into view, rotate the transducer clockwise toward 1 or 2 o'clock until most of the ascending aorta comes into view. Don't worry about what is happening to the ventricle or mitral valves at this point and just rotate until the aorta is completely in view. Keep the transducer perpendicular to the thorax; don't point the transducer forward while rotating. Once a good aorta image is seen, but the mitral valve and left atrium are not seen well (Fig. 2.80), improve the image by holding the transducer in the same place (this can be done by using your other hand to hold the face of the probe

Large Animal
Right Parasternal Long Axis
___

Left Ventricular Outflow View
Imaging Technique
- 3rd to 5th intercostal space
- Approximately 2 to 3 inches above the olecranon
- Keep the transducer perpendicular to the chest wall.
- The reference mark is directed toward 1 o'clock.
- Push the cable end of the transducer into the leg so the crystal face points slightly caudally to lengthen the LV.
- Rotate the transducer so the reference mark moves more toward the leg to keep the aorta in the image if necessary.

FIGURE 2.77   The reference mark should be directed dorsally and the transducer should be held almost perpendicular to the dog at approximately 70 to 80° away from the chest to obtain the left parasternal short-axis view. The cable should extend slightly ventrally and caudally and the face should be directed slightly cranially.

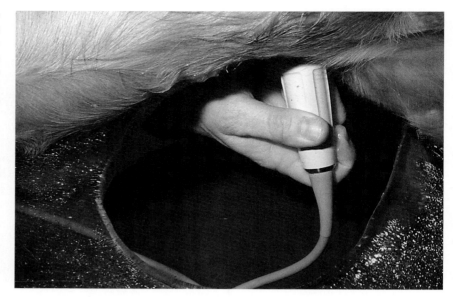

FIGURE 2.78   The base of the heart is located cranially and dorsally in the horse. If 12 o'clock is imagined as straight up in a line drawn perpendicular to the ground, the base of the heart is found at approximately 1 o'clock. The apex of the heart is located at approximately 7 o'clock. The sound beam should be aligned along an imaginary line from 1 to 7 o'clock for the long-axis left ventricular outflow view.

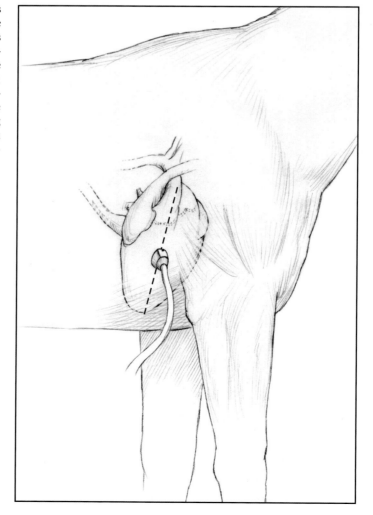

in position against the animal's skin surface) and pointing it in a slightly caudal direction (Fig. 2.80). This will move the cable of the transducer toward the horse's leg. Often, it feels as though the cable cannot be pushed into the leg any further when an adequate image is obtained. At this point, do not rotate, just point. The transducer will no longer be perpendicular to the thorax at this time.

Depending on how ventrally or dorsally the transducer is placed on the thoracic wall, the image may be a tipped long axis with aorta or it may be the standard long-axis image in which the septum and anterior aortic wall run horizontally across the sector image from right to left. A tipped long axis is obtained when the transducer is positioned ventrally on the thorax. The apex of the heart is up toward the top left side of the sector indicating that the probe is positioned closer to the apex of the heart. If the transducer is perpendicular to the thorax and pointed directly into the chest, move the transducer cranially and dorsally (into the leg and up) to see the horizontal standard long-axis with outflow view. You are moving the probe up toward the base of the heart. Try not to lose the image as you slide the transducer over the skin surface. For both of these movements, if the ventricle becomes shortened again, direct the probe in a slightly more caudal direction (cable moves into the leg) to lengthen the chamber. Make sure the reference mark is still at 1 to 2 o'clock.

When a standard long axis with outflow is seen, pointing the crystals toward the base of the heart (up toward 1 o'clock) will bring more of the heart base structures into view, and pointing the crystals toward the apex (down toward 7 o'clock) will bring more of the ventricle into view.

Four Chamber.   Starting at the right parasternal long-axis with left ventricular outflow view, rotate the transducer counterclockwise so that the reference mark moves toward 12 o'clock (Fig. 2.81). Continue to rotate the transducer until the aorta has disappeared and an interatrial septum is seen. Keep the transducer pointed slightly caudal with the cable pushed into the leg to keep length to the left ventricular chamber. This motion toward the four-chamber plane works from both the tipped long-axis and the standard long-axis views of the heart.

Right Parasternal Short-Axis Images.   Transverse views of the heart are obtained by rotating the transducer clockwise toward the olecranon with the

Large Animal
Right Parasternal Long Axis
_____

Four–Chamber
Imaging Technique
- Remain in the same location as for the left ventricular outflow view.
- Rotate the transducer counterclockwise until the reference mark is at about 12 o'clock.
- Keep the cable pushed into the leg for a long LV.

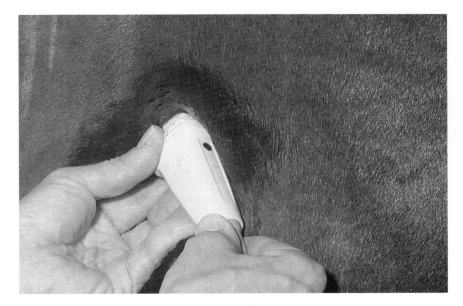

FIGURE 2.79   Right parasternal long-axis left ventricular outflow views of a horse's heart are obtained in the 3rd to 5th intercostal space. The reference mark should be directed toward 1 o'clock, the transducer should be pushed forward into the leg, and the face should be directed slightly caudally.

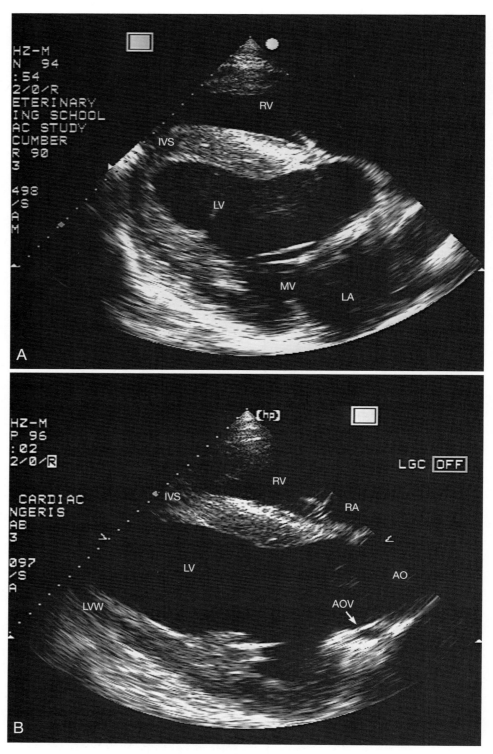

FIGURE 2.80   **A.** This long-axis image lacks an aorta and has a severely foreshortened left ventricular chamber. Rotate the transducer clockwise until a long aorta is seen. **B.** When the aorta is seen clearly but the mitral valves are not, lengthen the left ventricular chamber by holding the transducer face in the same location with the left hand and pushing the cable toward the leg to direct the face caudally and slightly dorsally without moving on the skin surface (**C**). *RV*, right ventricle; *RA*, right atrium; *IVS*, interventricular septum; *LV*, left ventricle; *LVW*, left ventricular wall; *AO*, aorta; *AOV*, aortic valve; *LA*, left atrium; *MV*, mitral valve.

FIGURE 2.80 *(continued)*

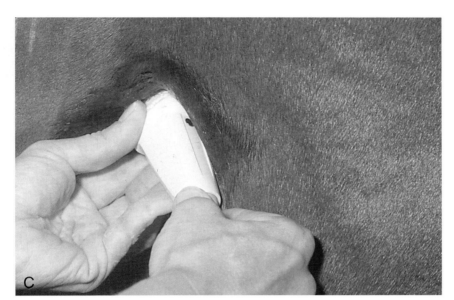

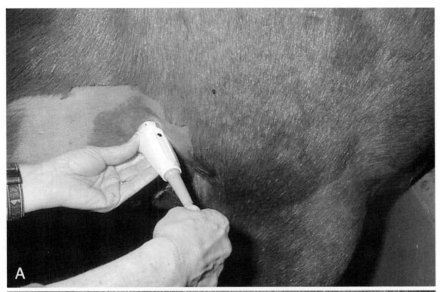

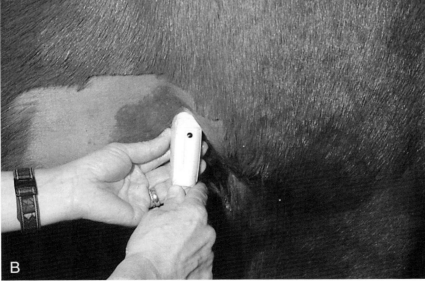

FIGURE 2.81 **A.** Rotate the transducer counterclockwise until the reference mark is directed toward 12 o'clock to see the right parasternal four-chamber view of the heart. The cable should still be pushed into the leg and the transducer face should be directed slightly caudally to keep length to the left ventricle. **B.** Pointing the face dorsally will produce a tipped four-chamber view of the heart.

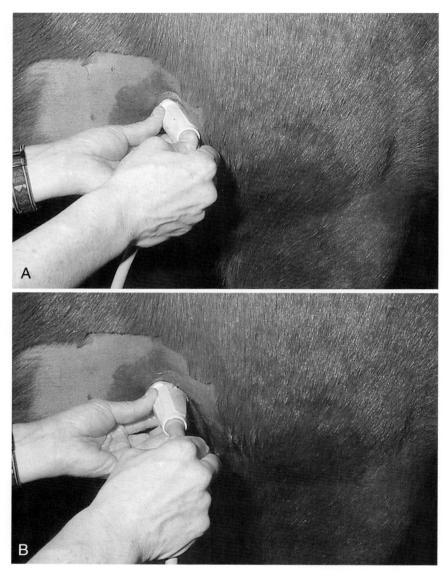

FIGURE 2.82 **A.** Transverse images of the left ventricle are obtained by rotating the transducer toward the olecranon 90° from its location for the long-axis planes at approximately 4 o'clock. Rotate until a symmetric circular left ventricular chamber is seen. The face is almost perpendicular to the thorax but may be pointing slightly ventrally and caudally. **B.** Pivot the transducer face upward so the sound plane is directed a little more dorsally and cranially to see the short-axis view of the mitral valves. The cable will move down toward the floor.

Large Animal
Right Parasternal Short-Axis Views

Imaging Technique
- Remain in the same location as for the long-axis views.
- Rotate the transducer until the reference mark is at approximately 4 o'clock and a circular LV or aorta is seen.
- Pivot the transducer face down to the sternum for the LV and up to the neck for the heart base.

reference mark at approximately 4 to 5 o'clock, 90° from its direction in the long-axis plane. The transducer is pivoted in dorsal to ventral directions, from base to apex, to obtain the various short-axis planes. The heart base is dorsal and cranial at approximately 1 o'clock and the apex is sternal and caudal at approximately 7 o'clock.

Left Ventricle.   Rotate the transducer clockwise away from the long-axis plane until the reference mark is located at about 4 o'clock (Fig. 2.82). The left ventricle is seen as a circle, and the papillary muscles should be similar in appearance and size. If one papillary muscle appears to be larger than the other, and the chamber is slightly egg shaped, the transducer has been rotated too much or too little. The transducer should be almost perpendicular to the thoracic wall with the face pointed in a slightly

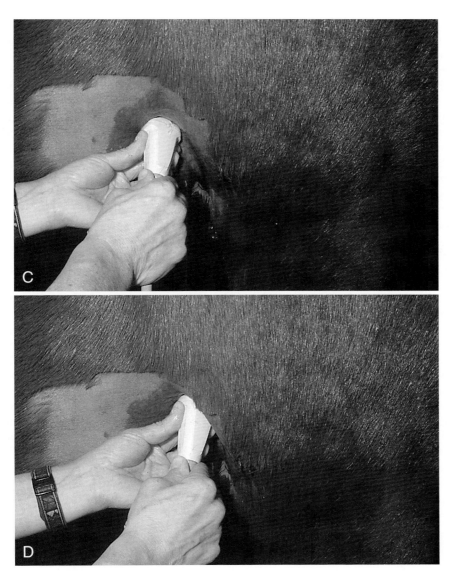

FIGURE 2.82 *(continued)*   C. Continue pointing the transducer face in a cranial and dorsal direction to see the base of the heart with aorta. Rotate the transducer clockwise and counterclockwise if necessary (if the image does not show a closed circular structure) to see the aorta in a true transverse section. D. The face is pointed even more cranially and dorsally to image the pulmonary artery. The angle between the transducer and the thoracic wall is small by the time this view is obtained. The transducer should be rotated back and forth until clear images of the artery are obtained.

caudal and ventral direction. Pivot the transducer in a line joining 7 to 1 o'clock to find the largest, most symmetric image for a true transverse plane through the left ventricle.

Mitral Valve.   The mitral valves are located just above the level of the papillary muscles and should be seen as a symmetric oval extending across the ventricular chamber. Movement up from the apex of the heart toward the base requires pivoting the transducer dorso-cranially (Fig. 2.82). Just before the mitral valves are visible, chordae tendinea will be seen at their attachment sites on the papillary muscles. The ventricular chamber should still be circular. If it becomes oval, rotate the transducer clockwise or counterclockwise until the ventricular chamber becomes circular again. At the mitral valve level, both sides of the valve should be attached to the lateral walls. Images that do not show this kind of symmetry require either less or more transducer rotation to improve the scan plane. Often, the transducer needs to be rotated slightly counterclockwise as it moves up from the level of the papillary muscles toward the mitral valves.

Heart Base—Aorta.   Continue pointing the transducer face up toward the base of the heart in a dorsal and cranial direction (Fig. 2.82). A clover-shaped aorta will appear in the center of the image. The transducer face should be pointed dorsally and cranially toward approximately 1 o'clock with the reference mark located anywhere from 4 to 5 o'clock. The transducer should be rotated clockwise and counterclockwise until a symmetric aorta is imaged.

Heart Base—Pulmonary Artery.   Clear images of the pulmonary artery and valve often require pointing the transducer slightly more dorsal and cranial toward 1 o'clock and fan the face right and left (cranial and caudal) once the heart base is seen to create the best image possible (Fig. 2.82). Rotate the transducer clockwise and counterclockwise as necessary to see the valves distinctly.

Left Parasternal Long-Axis Images.   Images from this side of the thorax, though not more difficult to obtain, are often not as clear as those obtained from the right side of the thorax. Nevertheless, images are usually good enough to assess the mitral valves and left ventricular wall, which will be positioned at the top of the sector image instead of at the bottom.

Four Chamber.   This is the reference view for imaging from the left side. Long refers to this view as the left ventricular inlet view (49). Transducer movement to all other planes are referenced from this view. The horse's leg should be abducted and pulled forward. Transducer placement is in the left 4th to 5th intercostal space approximately 2 inches above the olecranon (Fig. 2.83). The reference mark should be straight up toward the spine at the 12-o'clock position, and the transducer should be almost perpendicular to the chest wall, but pointed slightly cranially and dorsally until the longest and widest left ventricular chamber is seen. The mitral valves should open well and chordae tendinea should be seen. As with the long-axis planes on the right side, depending on the starting location, a tipped view or a more horizontal view may be seen. If the view is tipped, it is because the transducer has been placed in a more ventral and caudal location, so the apex is closer to the transducer than the

Large Animal
Left Parasternal Long Axis
_____

Four–Chamber
Imaging Technique
• Use the 4th to 5th intercostal space.
• The transducer is 2 to 3 inches above the level of the olecranon.
• The reference mark is at 12 o'clock.
• Keep the transducer almost perpendicular to the thoracic wall.
• Point the face dorsally and cranially until the largest LV is seen.

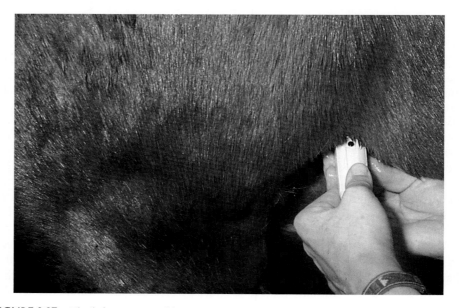

FIGURE 2.83   The left parasternal long-axis images of the heart in a horse are obtained from the 4th or 5th intercostal space just dorsal to the olecranon. The reference mark is directed straight up at 12 o'clock, and the face is titled slightly cranially and dorsally until the longest left ventricular chamber is seen. Pivot the transducer cranially and caudally to lengthen the left ventricle.

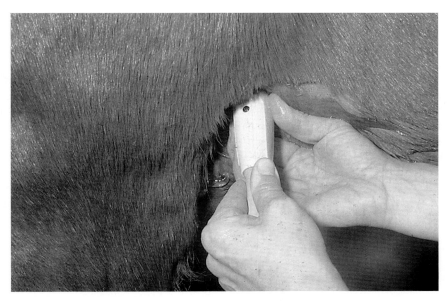

FIGURE 2.84   Once the tipped left parasternal long-axis four-chamber image of the heart is obtained, rotate the transducer counterclockwise until the aorta comes into view. The reference mark will be located at approximately 10 or 11 o'clock.

base. The transducer is directed cranially and dorsally for the tipped view to include the left atrium and mitral valves well. Rotate the transducer on its axis until the best view of the left atrium is obtained. Move the transducer up on the thorax, toward the spine, and forward a space to change a tipped view into a more horizontal image.

Five Chamber.   Move from a horizontal four-chamber view to a tipped view by positioning the transducer more ventrally and caudally. Point the transducer face cranially and dorsally to keep the left atrium and mitral valves in the image. Once the tipped view is obtained, rotate the transducer counterclockwise until the aorta is seen (Fig. 2.84). This will bring the reference mark to approximately 10 or 11 o'clock on the thorax.

Left Parasternal Short-Axis Images.   Although only two short-axis views are described in the horse for the left parasternal position, many views can be obtained. Pivot the transducer from base to apex in a ventral to dorsal direction, just like on the right side, to see the transverse images. Follow the structures along from one plane to the next to identify cardiac features.

Left Ventricle.   Starting with the left parasternal long-axis four-chamber horizontal view, rotate the transducer until the left ventricle is seen as a circular structure at the top of the sector image. The reference mark will be located at approximately 3 to 4 o'clock on the thorax (Fig. 2.85). The papillary muscles should be very equal in size, and the left ventricular chamber should not be oblong if the transducer has been rotated enough. Pivot the transducer face slightly in every direction until the size of the left ventricular chamber is maximized.

Heart Base—Right Ventricle, Pulmonary Artery.   This view is not a true transverse section and pivoting from the left ventricular transverse view up to the base of the heart will not be enough. Instead, the transducer must be located as far forward as possible and more ventral. (Fig. 2.86). When the left front leg is pulled as far forward as possible, this view is easier to obtain. Once the base of the heart is seen, point the transducer face caudally and dorsally to image the pulmonary artery, its valve, the tricuspid valve, and right atrium as they wrap around the left side of the image. The transducer reference mark should be located at approximately 1 or 2 o'clock. Point in caudo-dorsal and caudo-ventral directions until the best images are obtained.

Large Animal
Left Parasternal Long Axis

Five–Chamber
Imaging Technique
- Remain in the same location as for the four-chamber view.
- Rotate the transducer counterclockwise until the aorta is seen; the reference mark should be at approximately 10 or 11 o'clock.

Large Animal
Left Parasternal Short Axis

Left Ventricle
Imaging Technique
- Start with the four-chamber view.
- Rotate the transducer until the reference mark is at 3 to 4 o'clock and a circular left ventricle is seen.
- Pivot transducer about its location in multiple directions to find the largest symmetrical LV chamber.

Large Animal
Left Parasternal Short Axis

Heart Base
Imaging Technique
- Move the transducer down on the thorax to the level of the olecranon.
- Move as far cranially as possible.
- The reference mark is at 12 to 1 o'clock.
- Point caudally and slightly dorsally until both pulmonic and tricuspid valves are seen.

Large Animal
Left Parasternal Apical View

Five–Chamber
Imaging Technique
- Slide the transducer down to just above the level of the olecranon and caudally a couple of intercostal spaces from where the parasternal four- and five-chamber views were obtained.
- The reference mark is at 2 to 3 o'clock.
- The face is directed cranially and dorsally toward 10 or 11 o'clock.
- There is a small angle between the transducer and thorax (less than 30°).
- Pivot the transducer toward thorax and away from it until clear images are seen.

Left Parasternal Apical Images.   This is not a true apical image in the horse because the left ventricular chamber is severely foreshortened. However, this view allows the aorta to be seen in somewhat of a long axis as it leaves the ventricle and also may be used for Doppler studies.

Five Chamber.   The transducer needs to move into a more ventral position on the thoracic wall than is required for the horizontal four-chamber view. The reference mark needs to be directed to approximately 11 or 10 o'clock (Fig. 2.87). The transducer is angled dramatically for this image as the face is directed in a cranial and dorsal direction. Pivot the transducer toward the body and away from the body until clear images of the mitral valves and aortic root are seen. The aorta will be located centrally in the image and the left atrium and mitral valves will be to the right.

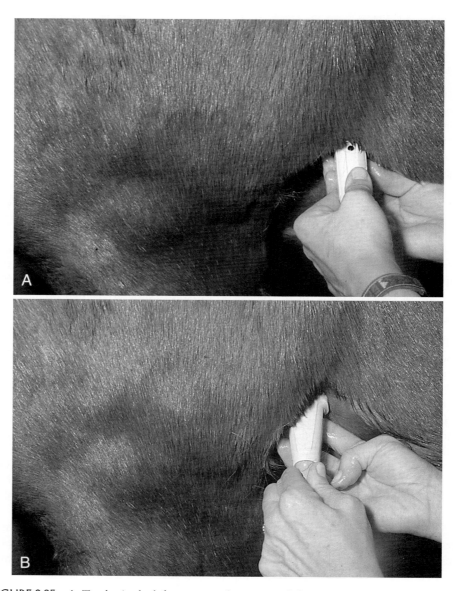

FIGURE 2.85   **A.** To obtain the left parasternal transverse left ventricular view, start with the long axis. **B.** Rotate the transducer clockwise until the reference mark is located at approximately 3 or 4 o'clock. Rotate the transducer back and forth until the left ventricle is circular with papillary muscles. The transducer face should be pivoted cranially and caudally until the left ventricular chamber size is maximized.

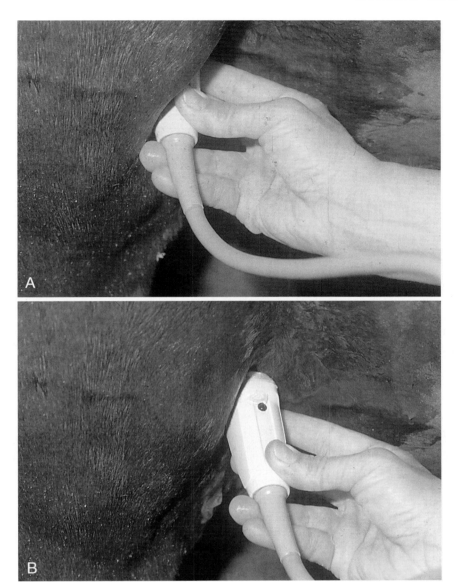

FIGURE 2.86   **A.** Place the transducer as far forward as possible at the level of the olecranon to obtain the left parasternal short-axis view of the heart base. The reference mark is at 12 to 1 o'clock, and the face is directed slightly caudally and dorsally. **B.** Here, the transducer is pulled away from the leg to better show how the sound plane is oriented.

M-MODE ECHOCARDIOGRAPHY

M-mode refers to motion mode. This type of image displays cardiac structures in a one-dimensional plane. M-mode images are obtained from the real-time, long-axis left ventricular outflow plane or from the left ventricular transverse plane by placing a cursor over the structures you want to see. The cursor represents one beam of sound. This imaging method is referred to as an "ice pick" view of the heart. Only the structures associated with the cursor are seen in the M-mode image (Figs. 2.88, 2.89, and 2.90). The features associated with that one line of sound through the heart scroll across the monitor and change in thickness or position as the heart fills and contracts. The resulting M-mode image has depth through the heart on the Y axis and time on the X axis.

M-mode Images

- One-dimensional image of structures
- Only structures associated with the cursor are seen
- Depth on the Y axis
- Time on the X axis
- Record subtle changes in wall and valve motion
- Used for accurate measurements of size

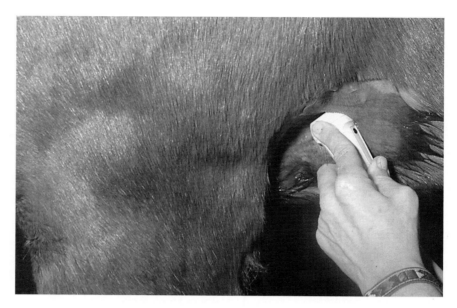

FIGURE 2.87   To obtain the left parasternal apical five-chamber view of the heart in a horse, the reference mark needs to be located at approximately 1 to 2 o'clock. The transducer is sharply angled with the face directed cranially and dorsally from a ventral location on the thoracic wall. Placement should be near the level of the elbow. Pivot the transducer toward and away from the body until the clearest images are obtained.

Controls

Once a good quality real-time image is obtained, only two main controls are needed to obtain an M-mode image—cursor positioning and sweep speed.

Cursor

The M-mode image depends on where the cursor is positioned on the real-time image. A track ball or joy stick moves the cursor over the two-dimensional image. Whatever structures the cursor transects will display on the M-mode image.

Sweep Speed

The M-mode image can be compressed or expanded along the X axis. The sweep speed controls how fast an image moves across the screen. Typical sweep speeds are 25, 50, and 100 mm/sec. At 25 mm/sec, many cardiac cycles are included on one frozen frame. At a sweep speed of 100 mm/sec, fewer cardiac cycles are seen per frame. With the high heart rates of cats, a sweep speed of 100 mm/sec is often necessary to separate better the events of diastole and systole. The slow heart rates of horses require a slower sweep speed of 50 or 25 mm/sec to obtain a few cardiac cycles per frozen image.

M-mode Images

M-mode echocardiography has a high sampling rate when compared with two-dimensional imaging and is superior to real-time images in recording subtle changes in wall and valve motion. M-mode images used for accurate assessment of size and function are obtained at the left ventricle, mitral valve, and aortic root levels.

Left Ventricle

Left ventricular images are obtained by placing the cursor perpendicular to the interventricular septum and left ventricular free wall at the chordae tendinea level, between the tips of the mitral valve leaflets and the left ventricular papillary muscles (Figs. 2.88 and 2.91). Imaging planes include the right parasternal long-axis left

M-mode
Left Ventricle

Imaging Planes
- Right parasternal transverse LV
- Right parasternal long-axis LV outflow view
- The left parasternal transverse left ventricle and right parasternal four-chamber views may be used in the horse.

Imaging Technique
- Place the cursor perpendicular to the septum and wall on all views.
- The cursor should be between tips of the mitral valve and the papillary muscles at the level of the chordae and the largest LV dimension.
- On transverse views the ventricle should be divided into equal and identical halves.

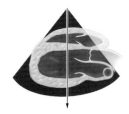

Diastolic

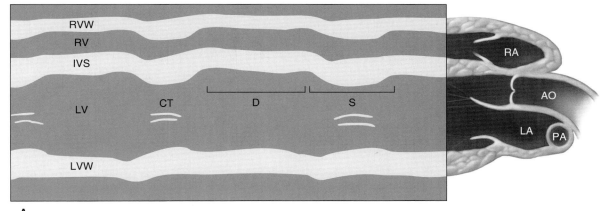

A

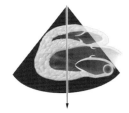

Systolic

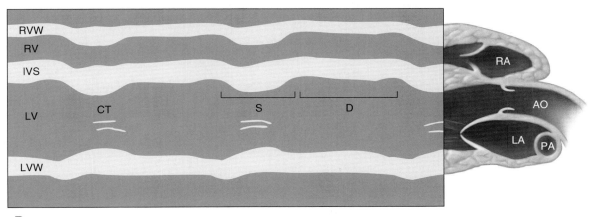

B

FIGURE 2.88   With the cursor placed over the left ventricle, the right ventricle is seen at the top of the image. The septum, left ventricular chamber, and left ventricular wall are below the right ventricle. **A.** During diastole, the wall and septum become thinner and the chamber enlarges. **B.** During systole, the wall and septum become thicker and the left ventricular chamber becomes smaller. The right ventricle and wall also exhibit these changes, but they may not be seen as clearly. The same part of the left ventricle is seen as it fills and empties. Here, three cardiac cycles are seen. *RVW,* right ventricular wall; *RV,* right ventricle; *IVS,* interventricular septum; *LV,* left ventricle; *LVW,* left ventricular wall; *CT,* chordae tendinea; *D,* diastole; *S,* systole; *RA,* right atrium; *AO,* aorta; *LA,* left atrium; *PA,* pulmonary artery.

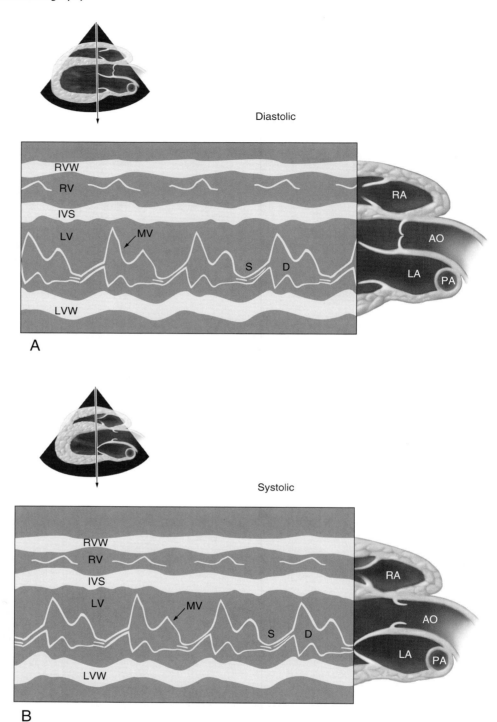

FIGURE 2.89   The mitral valves are seen as an M shape when the cursor is placed over the tips of the mitral valves. **A.** Rapid ventricular filling during early diastole forces the valves open and up toward the septum. As pressures equalize between the left atrium and ventricle, flow decreases and the valves move toward an almost closed position. As the atrium contracts and flow into the left ventricle increases again, the mitral valve moves up toward the septum again. **B.** Closure of the mitral valve occurs after atrial systole, and the leaflets appear as several lines within the ventricular cavity. Four diastolic filling periods are seen on this diagram. *RVW,* right ventricular wall; *RV,* right ventricle; *IVS,* interventricular septum; *LV,* left ventricle; *LVW,* left ventricular wall; *MV,* mitral valve; *S,* systole; *D,* diastole; *RA,* right atrium; *AO,* aorta; *LA,* left atrium; *PA,* pulmonary artery.

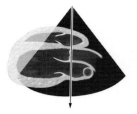

Diastolic

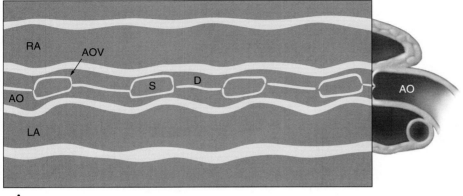

A

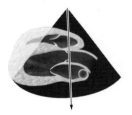

Systolic

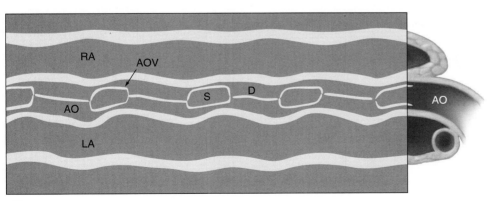

B

FIGURE 2.90   A cursor placed over the aorta displays the aorta as two parallel lines. **A.** The aorta moves downward with diastole and the left atrium becomes smaller as it empties during diastole. A line in the middle of the aorta represents the closed cusps during diastole. **B.** The aorta moves upward during systole and the left atrium enlarges as it fills during this time period. The aortic valve opens toward the walls of the aorta with the onset of systole, remains there for the duration of systole, and then moves rapidly to a closed position at the end of systole. *RA*, right atrium; *AO*, aorta; *LA*, left atrium; *AOV*, aortic valve; *S*, systole; *D*, diastole.

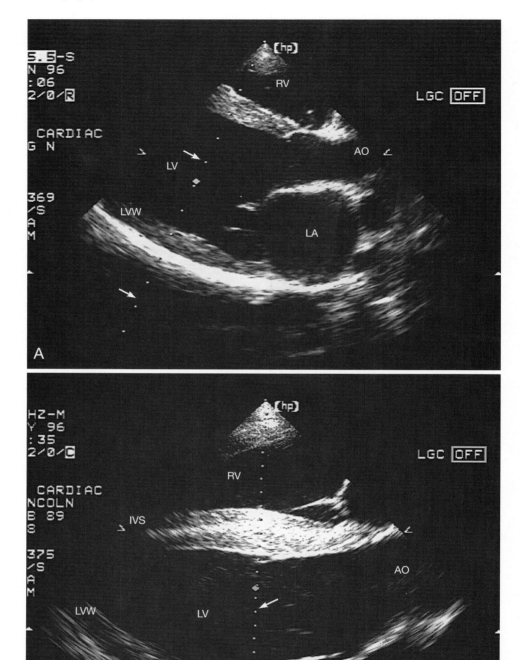

FIGURE 2.91 Left ventricular M-modes may be obtained from several real-time views. The right parasternal long-axis left ventricular outflow view in the dog (**A**) and in the horse (**B**).

ventricular outflow plane and transverse plane at the chordae level (46,69–71). In the horse, the left parasternal transverse plane at the chordae level and right parasternal four-chamber planes also are used (49,50).

An M-mode cursor placed through a tipped left ventricular outflow plane is often diagonal through the ventricle. The image should be corrected so that the interventricular septum and anterior aortic wall line up almost horizontally across the sector image. The M-mode cursor then can be placed perpendicular to the

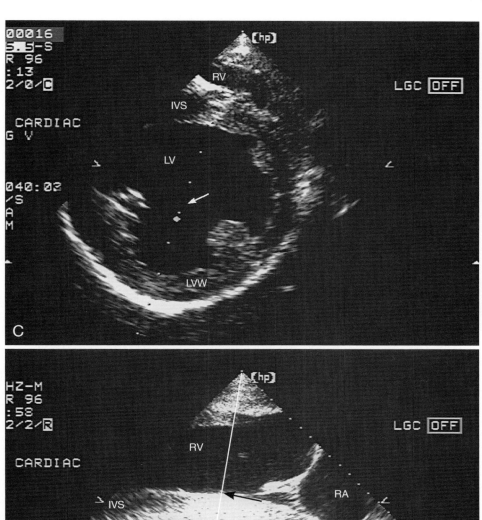

FIGURE 2.91 *(continued)*   C. Right parasternal transverse images of the left ventricle at the level of the chordae tendinea in large and small animals also may be used. **D.** Right parasternal four-chamber views also are used in the horse. The M-mode cursor *(arrow)* is placed perpendicular to the septum and left ventricular wall and should be located between the tips of the mitral valve leaflets and the papillary muscles over the chordae tendinea in both long-axis and transverse planes. *RV,* right ventricle; *LV,* left ventricle; *IVS,* interventricular septum; *AO,* aorta; *LA,* left atrium; *LVW,* left ventricular wall; *RA,* right atrium.

interventricular septum and left ventricular wall, below the tips of the mitral valves at the largest ventricular chamber size. Perpendicular placement of the cursor and use of the right parasternal long-axis left ventricular outflow view will produce the best M-mode image with the most reproducible and accurate size and

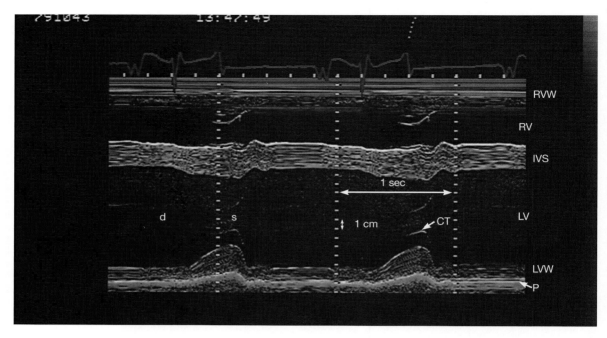

FIGURE 2.92 This is an M-mode of the left ventricle in a horse. The left ventricular M-mode displays the right ventricular wall and right ventricle at the top of the image. The interventricular septum, left ventricular chamber, and left ventricular wall are below. *RVW,* right ventricular wall; *RV,* right ventricle; *IVS,* interventricular septum; *LV,* left ventricle; *LVW,* left ventricular wall; *CT,* chordae tendinea; *P,* pericardium; *d,* diastole; *s,* systole.

function measurements. Care should be taken to generate the M-mode from the best longitudinal image possible. The ventricle should not be foreshortened, and mitral valve motion should show good excursion toward the septum. If transverse images are used to generate the M-mode image, the cursor should still be placed perpendicular to the septum and free wall as if dissecting the image into perfect right and left halves (Fig. 2.91). Imaging should move from mitral valve to papillary muscle, and the desired plane for generating an M-mode image of the left ventricle is the plane that is intercepting the chordae tendinea between both of these standard planes.

The M-mode will show a right ventricle at the top of the image, followed by the interventricular septum, the left ventricular chamber, and then the left ventricular free wall at the bottom of the image (Figs. 2.92 and 2.93). The pericardium on an M-mode image is always a bright line just below the left ventricular free wall. The right ventricular wall may not be clear on M-mode images. The normal septum and left ventricular wall move away from each other as the ventricle is filling during diastole and they move toward each other as the heart contracts during systole (Fig. 2.88). The wall and septum thicken during ventricular contraction and become thinner as they relax during ventricular filling. The free wall of the left ventricle should continue its slight downward or filling motion until just before ventricular systole. In many cases, there is a slight downward dip of the posterior wall and a small upward motion of the ventricular septum just before contraction.

Mitral Valve

Cursor position over the tips of the mitral valve leaflets produces an M-shaped structure on the M-mode image. The cursor should be positioned perpendicular to the septum and mitral valve leaflets. The right parasternal long-axis left ventricular outflow view or transverse view at the level of the mitral valve may be used (Fig. 2.94)(46,49,50,69–71). Initial motion of the valve reflects rapid ventricular filling,

M-mode
Mitral Valve

Imaging Planes
- Right parasternal long-axis left ventricular outflow view
- Right parasternal transverse mitral valve view

Imaging Technique
- Place the cursor perpendicular to the septum over the tips of the mitral valve.
- On transverse views, place the cursor perpendicular to the valves as it divides the image into equal and similar halves.

and this "E" point (first peak of the "M") should almost touch the septum as it does on real-time images (Figs. 2.89 and 2.95). The rapid ventricular filling phase of diastole is driven by a pressure gradient. The left ventricle has just finished emptying while the left atrium has just completed its filling phase. As the left ventricle fills and the pressure differential decreases, flow through the valve decreases. This creates the downward motion seen after the E point. The valve remains partially open during middiastole as blood flows slowly through them into the ventricle. Toward the end of diastole as the atria contract, the valve is again forced up toward the septum by the rush of blood into the left ventricle associated with atrial systole. Because volume is less during this phase, the amplitude of the second peak of the M, referred to as the A point, should always be lower than the E point. Following atrial contraction, the valves move toward a closed position. Rapid heart rates will result in a mitral valve that does not have M-shaped motion because the rapid ventricular filling and atrial contraction phases of diastole coincide (Fig. 2.96). Slow heart rates spread out the two phases of filling (Fig. 2.97).

Aortic Root

Positioning the cursor perpendicular to both aortic walls and directing it through the largest portion of the left atrium produces an M-mode of the base of the heart. This is obtained from the right parasternal long-axis left ventricular outflow or transverse view (Fig. 2.98)(46,49,50,69–71). Aortic valve motion, though not necessarily left atrial size, is easier to record from short-axis images. The right atrium is seen at the top of the image, followed by the anterior and posterior aortic walls, which move parallel to each other (Figs. 2.90 and 2.99). Below the aorta is the left atrium. The left atrium fills during ventricular systole, which is one reason the aorta moves anteriorly at that time. There should be little posterior left atrial wall motion.

During diastole, the aortic valves are displayed as a line in the center of the aorta. With systole, the valve cusps move rapidly toward each wall and remain there until the end of outflow. This creates a boxlike image on the M-mode.

M-mode
Aorta and Left Atrium

Imaging Planes
• Right parasternal long-axis LV outflow view
• Right parasternal transverse aorta

Imaging Technique
• Place the cursor perpendicular to the aortic walls over the aortic valves.
• Make sure the cursor is over the atrium and not the auricle on transverse planes.

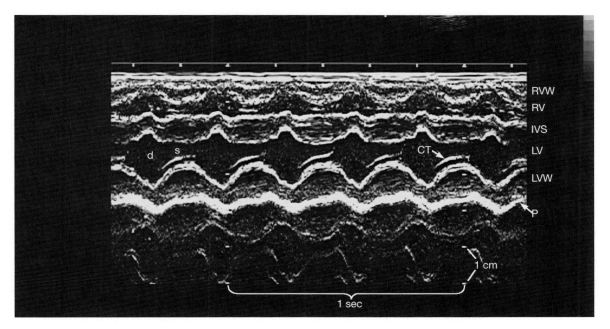

FIGURE 2.93 M-modes in cats require increased sweep speeds to spread out the events of diastole and systole. *RVW,* right ventricular wall; *RV,* right ventricle; *IVS,* interventricular septum; *LV,* left ventricle; *LVW,* left ventricular wall; *CT,* chordae tendinea; *P,* pericardium; *d,* diastole; *s,* systole.

FIGURE 2.94 Two views may be used to obtain good M-modes of the mitral valves. **A.** A cursor (*arrow*) may be placed over the tips of the mitral leaflets on the left ventricular outflow view. **B.** Alternately, the cursor may be placed over the mitral valves on the transverse right parasternal image. The cursor should bisect the ventricle into perfect right and left halves and be aligned perpendicular to the septum and free wall in both of these views. *RV*, right ventricle; *IVS*, interventricular septum; *LV*, left ventricle; *MV*, mitral valve; *LVW*, left ventricular wall; *LA*, left atrium; *AO*, aorta.

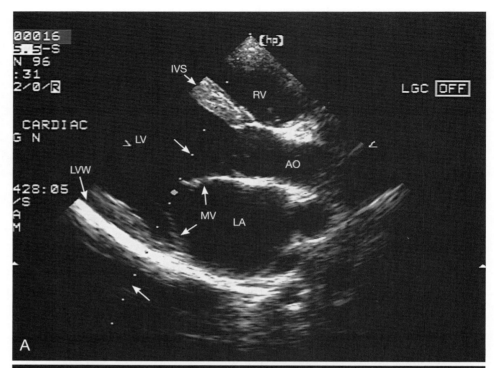

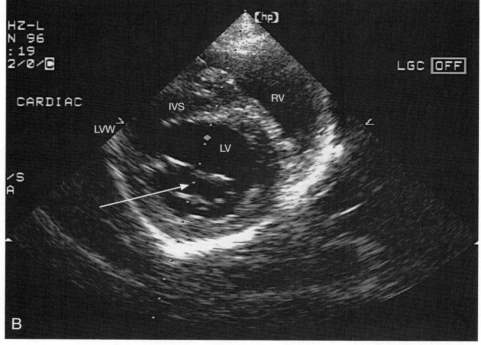

SPECTRAL DOPPLER

Doppler Interrogation

- For quantitative information
  - use images that align the Doppler beam parallel with flow
- For nonquantitative information
  - parallel alignment with flow is not necessary

Doppler examination of the heart uses imaging planes that align the sound beam as parallel as possible with the direction of flow. This is the opposite of sound beam alignment, which will produce the best two-dimensional images. Remember that sound is reflected directly back to the transducer if it strikes the structure with a 0° angle of incidence. Doppler, however, depends on the angle of incidence in a different manner. The farther away from parallel the sound beam is to flow, the greater the error introduced into the maximum velocity. Apical views are therefore the

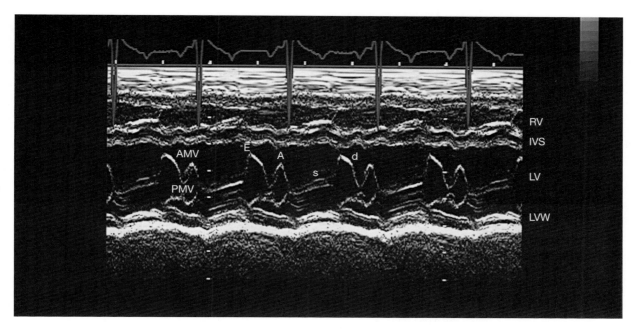

FIGURE 2.95   The mitral valve is seen as an "M" on M-mode images. The "E" point represents maximum opening with rapid ventricular filling. The "A" point represents maximum excursion following atrial contraction. The valve is displayed as multiple lines during systole. *RV*, right ventricle; *IVS*, interventricular septum; *LV*, left ventricle; *AMV*, anterior mitral valve; *PMV*, posterior mitral valve; *LVW*, left ventricular wall; *d*, diastole; *s*, systole.

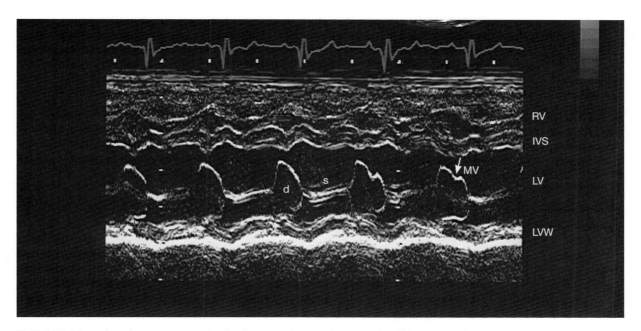

FIGURE 2.96   When heart rates are high, the two phases of ventricular filling coincide as in the first three beats on this M-mode, and the mitral valve is no longer displayed as an "M." The latter two beats have a slightly slower heart rate, and flow secondary to atrial contraction is just beginning to be visible on the back side of the E peak. *RV*, right ventricle; *IVS*, interventricular septum; *LV*, left ventricle; *MV*, mitral valve; *LVW*, left ventricular wall.

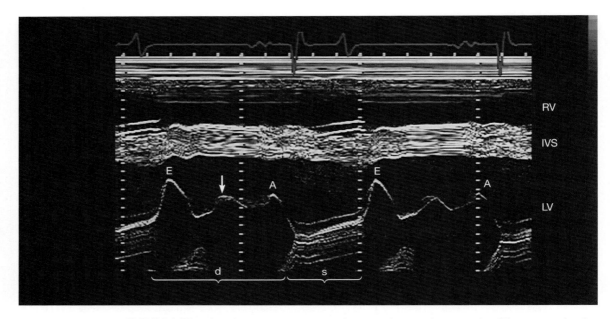

FIGURE 2.97   Slow heart rates separate the two phases of ventricular filling. Mitral valve motion in this horse with a heart rate of 35 shows extra undulations during middiastole (*arrow*). *RV,* right ventricle; *IVS,* interventricular septum; *LV,* left ventricle; *d,* diastole; *s,* systole.

appropriate views for obtaining flow information for mitral and aortic valves. Parasternal long-axis planes are useful when interrogating the pulmonary artery or sometimes the tricuspid valve.

When simply determining the presence or absence of a regurgitant jet or stenotic lesion is important, then parasternal images may provide that information. It is possible to interrogate the left atrium (for instance, from parasternal long-axis images) and determine the extent of a regurgitant jet into the atrium. Measurement of regurgitant fractions, cardiac outputs, or pressure gradients, however, requires parallel alignment with flow. These are the planes described in the following section (49,56,57,59–67).

Controls

Cursor

A cursor is placed along the predicted line of flow to record velocities (Fig. 2.100). The direction of flow usually can be determined with color-flow Doppler. Without color guidance, however, the flow direction must be determined by interrogating the area carefully.

The crystals in mechanical scanners stop in the direction that the cursor is directed before switching to Doppler imaging. Phased array transducers will record Doppler information from where the cursor is placed on the sector.

Gate

The gate is represented by a marker on the cursor line and corresponds to the sampling site (Fig. 2.100). Its depth can be adjusted along the cursor with a track ball, toggle switch, or joy stick.

Gate Size

The sample volume size can be adjusted to include more or less area. Increasing the gate size too much will lead to some ambiguity as to exact location of flow information, but may allow small regurgitant jets to be found with greater ease.

Angle Correction

Most machines have a separate cursor originating from the Doppler cursor that is used to correct for angle when the Doppler cursor cannot be placed parallel to flow (Fig. 2.100). The equipment will take the angle into account when calculating flow velocity and plot the flow profile accordingly. It is always better to try to align the cursor as parallel as possible to flow instead of using the angle correction because flow velocity alignment errors in the third dimension can be magnified with angle correction.

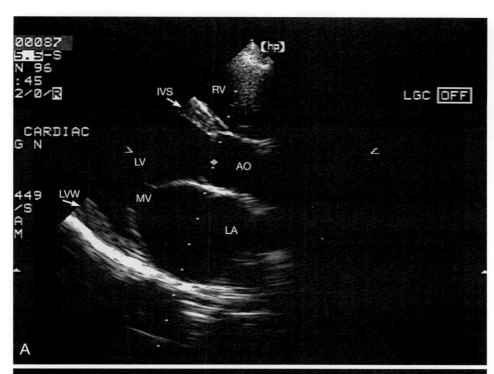

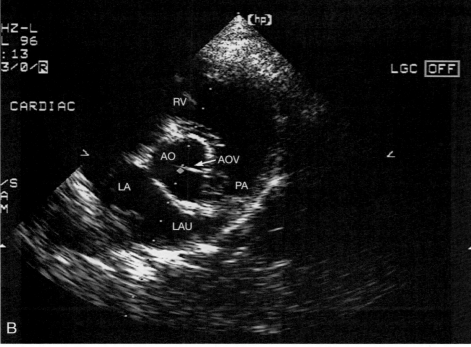

FIGURE 2.98 The aortic root M-mode may be obtained by placing the cursor perpendicular to the aortic walls and through the largest part of the left atrium on either the long-axis left ventricular outflow view (**A**) or the transverse view at the level of the aorta (**B**). *RV*, right ventricle; *IVS*, interventricular septum; *LV*, left ventricle; *AO*, aorta; *AOV*, aortic valve; *MV*, mitral valve; *LVW*, left ventricular wall; *LA*, left atrium; *LAU*, left auricle; *PA*, pulmonary artery.

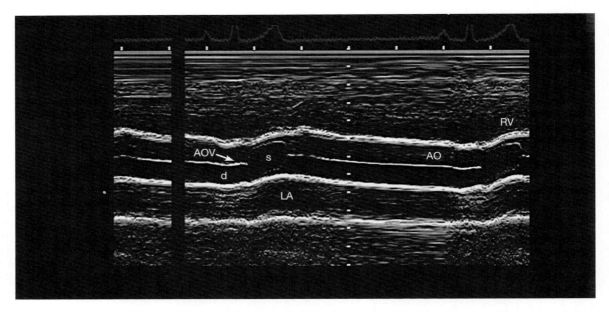

FIGURE 2.99   The M-mode at the base of the heart shows the right ventricle at the top of the image followed by the aorta and left atrium. The aortic valves are seen between the two parallel walls of the aorta. *RV*, right ventricle; *AO*, aorta; *AOV*, aortic valves; *LA*, left atrium; *d*, diastole; *s*, systole.

FIGURE 2.100 Doppler interrogation involves placing a cursor representing the Doppler sound beam over the area of interest (*thin arrow*). A gate placed anywhere along the interrogating Doppler sound beam indicates where blood flow is to be sampled (*thick arrow*). Angle correction may be used to align flow with the Doppler beam (*curved arrow*).

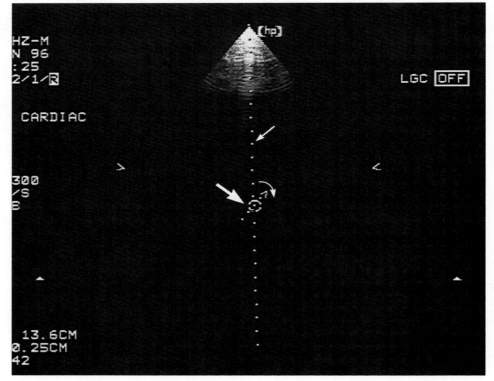

Baseline

The baseline corresponds to zero velocity. The gate in pulsed-wave Doppler is represented by the baseline and flow moves up or down away from zero velocity. The baseline can be shifted up or down to unwrap mildly aliased signals (Fig. 2.101). A baseline positioned at the top of the Doppler spectrum will only display flow away from the gate or transducer, but at twice the velocity before aliasing occurs. The baseline also may be moved down on the spectrum.

Scale

The range of velocities may be changed in both pulsed-wave and continuous-wave displays. Increasing the scale setting will increase the velocity limits on each side of the baseline, and decreasing the scale will decrease the velocity limits. The flow profile will decrease as the velocity limits are increased and will increase as the scale is decreased. The maximum velocity limit in PW Doppler increases with lower-frequency transducers or less sampling depth.

Doppler Gain

Similar to other gain controls, this intensifies or decreases image intensity. Increasing Doppler gain will increase the strength of the returning signal. Turn the gain on high enough to be sure that all the signal is recorded. Then turn it down until associated noise and mirror-image artifacts are removed.

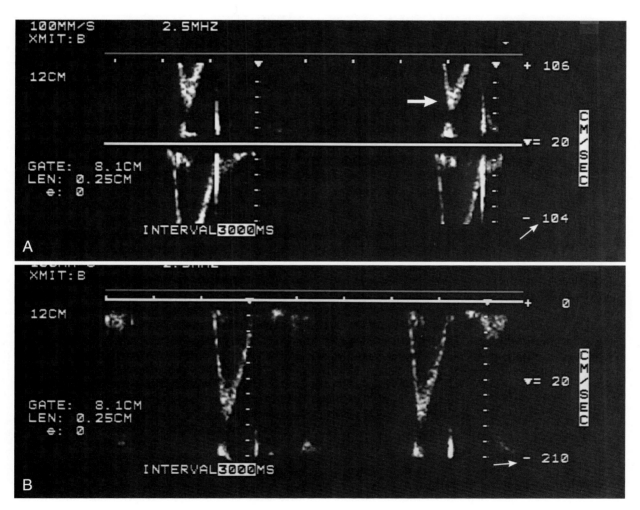

FIGURE 2.101   The baseline may be adjusted up or down to reduce the amount of aliasing. **A.** Flow exceeding the velocity limit of −104 cm/sec (*thin arrow*) aliases or "wraps around" the image (*thick arrow*). **B.** When the baseline is moved up, higher flow velocities of −210 cm/sec away from the gate may be recorded (*arrow*) before aliasing or "wrap around" occurs. The baseline also may be moved down to increase maximum positive flow velocities.

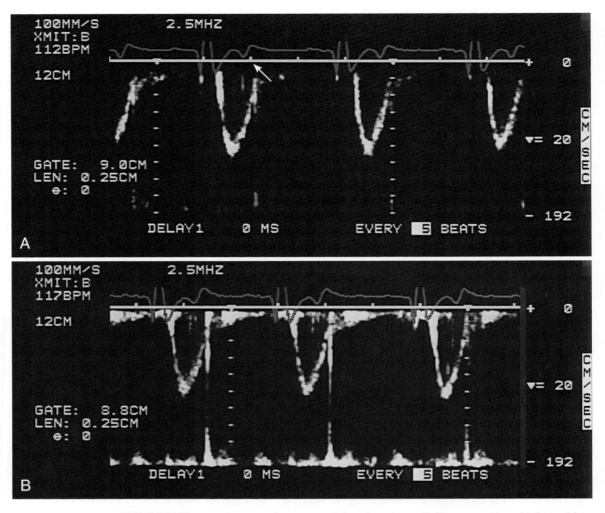

FIGURE 2.102   **A.** This Doppler image of flow has the wall filters turned up high, and low velocities near the baseline are not recorded (*arrow*). **B.** Decreasing the filter allows low-velocity flow signals at the beginning and end of systole to be displayed.

Wall Filters

Doppler wall filters decrease the amount of low-frequency noise that is recorded from slow-moving structures such as cardiac walls. Turning the wall filter up too high, however, eliminates the start and end of flow information because these are the slowest flow velocities (Fig. 2.102).

Sweep Speed

This control is the same as the one used for M-mode displays of the heart. Doppler signals can sweep across the display monitor at a rate of 25, 50, or 100 mm/sec.

Normal Doppler Flow Profiles

Quantitative information regarding the severity of regurgitation or measurement of left ventricular or systemic pressures is not possible without specifically aligning the Doppler beam as parallel as possible with flow. The imaging planes described for recording the following Doppler flow images, if obtained correctly, will align the Doppler beam as parallel as possible with flow.

Several planes are available for recording flow and each should be interrogated to assure the most accurate Doppler recordings. Some imaging planes are difficult to obtain and keep while recording flow. More force is needed to obtain these images.

At first, image quality may be poor because of hand fatigue, but practice will improve technique and your hand will develop the strength to maintain the image while Doppler flows are recorded.

As already discussed, the presence or absence of abnormal flow can be recorded from many real-time images. This information is useful and Doppler interrogation should be attempted in as many planes as possible.

These instructions assume the use of an imaging pulsed-wave or continuous-wave (CW) probe. If a nonimaging CW probe is used, the transducer should be placed in the same position as the imaging probe. It is helpful to record the two-dimensional images first to localize and orient in your mind the direction necessary to record aortic flow. Tracing should be evaluated for the crispest sound and the highest velocity.

Aortic Flow

Imaging Plane Used

Small Animal.   The optimal plane for recording accurate aortic flow is the apical five-chamber view. The Doppler gate is positioned just distal to the aortic valve and sinus of Valsalva (Fig. 2.103). Move the transducer in and out of the imaging plane to make sure that the highest velocity is being recorded. Remember, the image seen on the monitor is two dimensions, and the Doppler sound beam must interrogate the third dimension by moving side to side and up and down as you scan the aorta.

Large Animal.   Published aortic flow velocities are available for Doppler obtained from the right parasternal long-axis left ventricular outflow view. Aortic flow may be aligned more parallel to flow using the left parasternal apical five-chamber view of the heart (Fig. 2.104).

Appearance.   Flow in the aorta is away from the transducer, so flow profiles are negative. The beginning of flow starts toward the end of the QRS complex and ends

---

Spectral Doppler
Aortic Flow

Imaging Plane
- Left parasternal apical five-chamber view
- Place the gate distal to the aortic valves and sinus of Valsalva.

Appearance
- Rapid acceleration
- Slower deceleration
- Asymmetric appearance
- Flow starts toward the end of the QRS complex

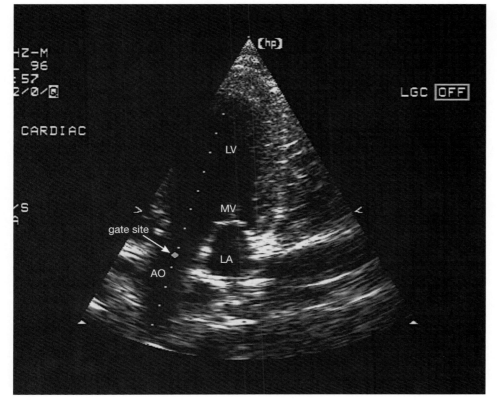

FIGURE 2.103   The optimal recording plane for aortic flow in the small animal is the left parasternal apical five-chamber view. The gate is placed just distal to the aortic valves and sinus of Valsalva (*arrow*). *AO*, aorta; *LV*, left ventricle; *LA*, left atrium; *MV*, mitral valve.

FIGURE 2.104 Aortic flow in the horse is interrogated from the left parasternal apical five-chamber view. The gate is placed just distal to the aortic valves and sinus of Valsalva (*arrow*). *LV,* left ventricle; *IVS,* interventricular septum; *AOV,* aortic valve; *AO,* aorta; *LA,* left atrium; *RV,* right ventricle.

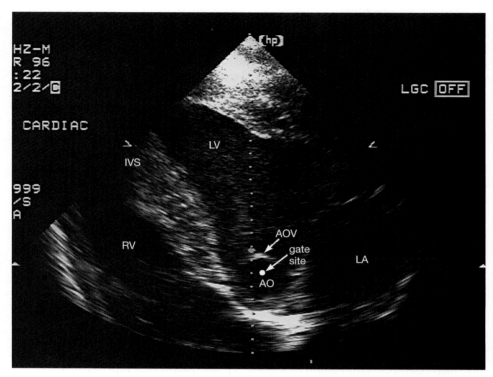

just after the T wave (Fig. 2.105). There is rapid acceleration so that peak velocity is reached within the first third of systole. Little spectral broadening occurs with PW Doppler until just after peak velocity is reached. Flow decelerates slower than it accelerates, giving the aortic flow profile an asymmetric appearance. Upward flow can be recorded, which is probably mitral flow as the annulus moves toward the gate during contraction.

Left Ventricular Outflow Tract

Imaging Plane Used
Small Animal.   Flow within the left ventricular outflow tract also uses the apical five-chamber plane. The gate is positioned just proximal to the aortic valves between the ventricular septum and the open anterior mitral valve leaflet. If a discrete or dynamic subvalvular obstruction is suspected, move the gate up and down the outflow tract to record and localize any aliased signals.

Large Animal.   The right parasternal long-axis left ventricular outflow view was used for published reference values (57). The left parasternal apical five-chamber view aligns the Doppler beam more parallel with left ventricular outflow. The gate is positioned just proximal to the aortic valves between the ventricular septum and the open anterior mitral valve leaflet.

Appearance.   Outflow tract flow profiles are negative and similar in appearance to aortic flow except that velocities are lower. Negative and positive flow can be seen during diastole depending on the gate position with respect to mitral inflow. The further the gate moves away from the aortic valve, the more upward mitral flow is seen.

Pulmonary Flow

Imaging Plane Used
Small Animal.   Pulmonary flow may be accurately recorded from the right parasternal left ventricle with pulmonary artery view, the left parasternal short-axis

Spectral Doppler
Pulmonary Flow

Imaging Planes
• Right parasternal left ventricle with PA
• Left parasternal cranial long axis with right ventricular outflow
• Left parasternal short axis
• Place the gate distal to the valves.

Appearance
• Symmetric profile
• Peak velocity approximately midway during ejection

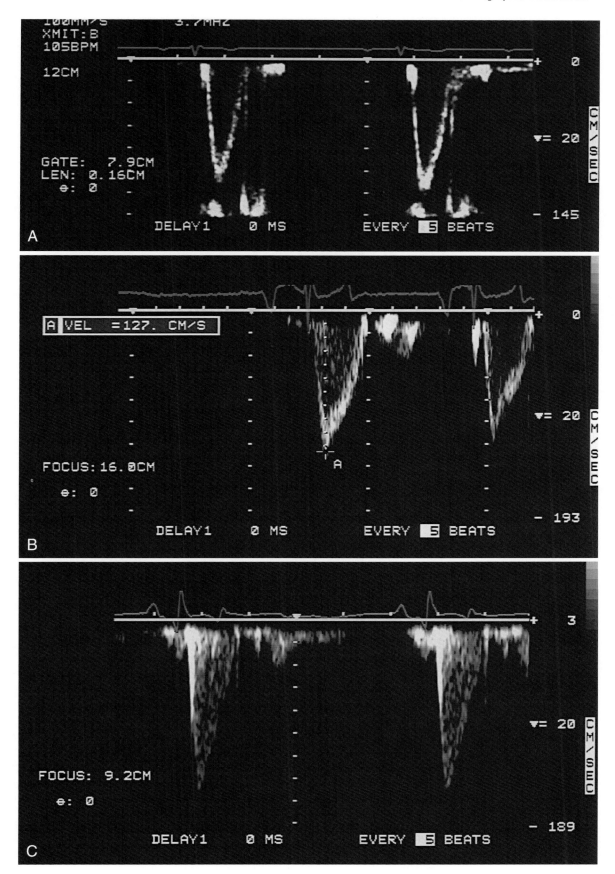

FIGURE 2.105 Aortic flow is negative, starts just after the QRS complex, and continues until after the T wave. Its acceleration phase is rapid and an asymmetric appearance is created because deceleration is slower. Shown here are PW aortic flow profiles in a dog (**A**), CW aortic flow profiles in a horse (**B**), and CW flow profiles in a dog (**C**). CW Doppler was used in the horse to obtain a stronger spectral signal and in the dog to eliminate an aliased signal.

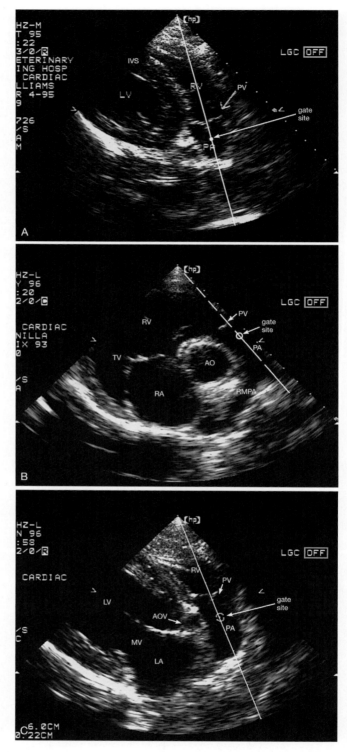

FIGURE 2.106   Pulmonary artery flow in the small animal is recorded from one of three possible views: (**A**) the right parasternal transverse view of the left ventricle with pulmonary artery, (**B**) the left parasternal short-axis view with aorta and pulmonary artery, or (**C**) the left parasternal long-axis right ventricular outflow view. The gate is placed distally to the pulmonic valve (*arrows*). *RV*, right ventricle; *PA*, pulmonary artery; *PV*, pulmonic valve; *LV*, left ventricle; *IVS*, interventricular septum; *RMPA*, right main pulmonary artery; *AO*, aorta; *AOV*, aortic valve; *LA*, left atrium; *MV*, mitral valve; *TV*, tricuspid valve.

plane with aorta and pulmonary artery, or the left parasternal long-axis right ventricular outflow view (Fig. 2.106). The gate is placed distal to the valve within the pulmonary artery.

Large Animal.   There is excellent alignment with the Doppler beam on the right parasternal transverse view with the left ventricle and pulmonary artery (Fig. 2.107). Although the angle for interrogation is good, depth is often a factor in preventing adequate flow recordings. Try CW Doppler if PW signals are not strong enough.

Appearance.   Flow moves away from the transducer in these planes and is negative. Flow starts toward the end of the QRS complex and continues through the T wave (Fig. 2.108). Acceleration time is slower than in the aorta and peak velocity is reached approximately midway through ejection. This gives the flow profile a symmetric and rounded appearance and is a good way to distinguish normal aortic from normal pulmonary flow on still images. Reduced vascular resistance may be the reason for decreased acceleration time in the pulmonary artery. As with aortic flow, spectral broadening does not occur until after peak velocity has been reached and flow begins to decelerate.

Peak velocities are lower than in the aorta probably because of the lower pressure gradient from right ventricle to pulmonary artery. Flow velocities vary with respiration secondary to increased venous return with inspiration. Therefore, inspiration increases velocity and expiration decreases flow velocities in the pulmonary artery.

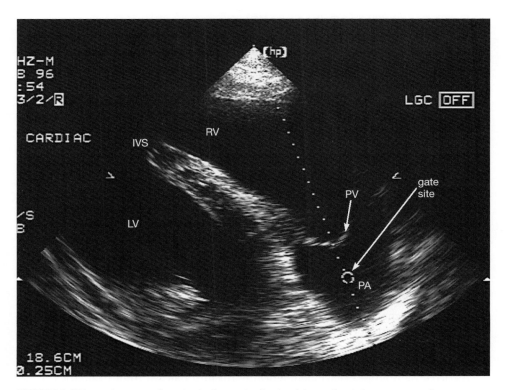

FIGURE 2.107   Pulmonary flow in the horse is obtained from the right parasternal transverse view of the left ventricle with pulmonary artery. *RV*, right ventricle; *PA*, pulmonary artery; *PV*, pulmonic valve; *LV*, left ventricle; *IVS*, interventricular septum.

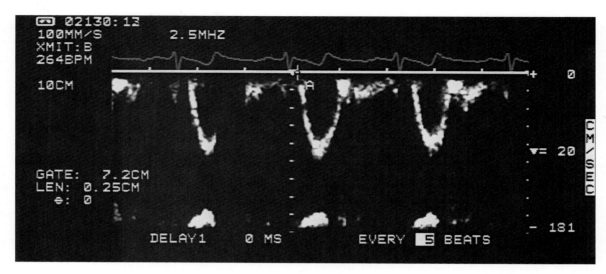

FIGURE 2.108   Pulmonary flow is negative on the Doppler tracing. It starts toward the end of the QRS complex and continues through the T wave. The flow profile is fairly symmetric because acceleration and deceleration times are similar, and peak velocity is reached approximately halfway through ejection.

Right Ventricular Outflow Tract

Imaging Plane Used

Small Animal.   Right ventricular outflow velocities are recorded from any of the three views used to interrogate pulmonary artery flow. The gate is positioned proximal to the pulmonic valve with the outflow tract between the right ventricular wall and septum.

Large Animal.   The right ventricular outflow tract view from the right side of the thorax is used in horses. The transducer is placed in the right 3rd intercostal space and tilted cranially to align the pulmonary artery and outflow tract well enough for Doppler (57).

Appearance.   Right ventricular outflow Doppler recordings are similar to pulmonary artery flow except velocities are lower. Depending on gate location with reference to the pulmonic valve and tricuspid valve, positive and negative diastolic flow may be recorded.

Mitral Inflow

Imaging Plane Used

Small Animal.   Left parasternal apical four- and five-chamber planes are used to record mitral inflow (Fig. 2.109). When deciding which imaging plane to use, look for the best flow profiles with highest velocities, least spectral broadening, and good definition to E and A peaks. The highest velocities are usually found when the sample gate is placed at the tips of the leaflets when they are wide open (Fig. 2.110). A mitral valve opening click should be heard clearly, and a closing click should be heard barely. Lack of an opening sound suggests that the gate is too far into the left ventricle, whereas too loud of a closing sound usually is heard when the gate is placed too close to the mitral annulus.

Incorrect sample gate placement will alter the mitral flow profile dramatically and create the appearance of diastolic functional problems. Samples placed too close to the mitral annulus will decrease E velocities and deceleration times.

When at all possible, PW Doppler should be used to assess mitral inflow profiles.

Spectral Doppler
Mitral Inflow
_____

Imaging Planes
- Left parasternal apical four chamber
- Left parasternal apical five chamber
- Place the gate at the tips of the mitral valve when open.

Appearance
- E higher than A
- Separation of E and A depends on heart rate
- Positive flow after A is secondary to annular movement

CW Doppler summates the velocities along the beam, and flow profiles do not differentiate between velocities found at the mitral leaflet tips or at the annulus.

Large Animal.   The left parasternal apical five-chambered plane through the heart is used to record mitral flow into the left ventricle of the horse (Fig. 2.111). Tilt the transducer until alignment is as good as possible. The gate should be placed at the tips of the mitral valve leaflets when they are wide open.

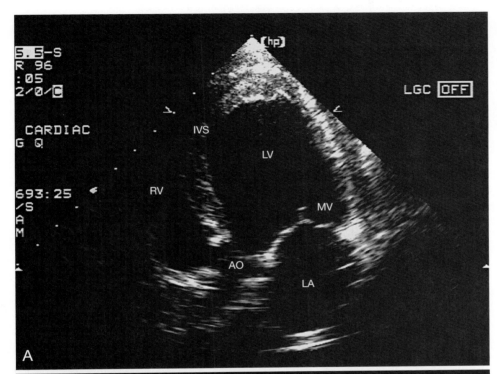

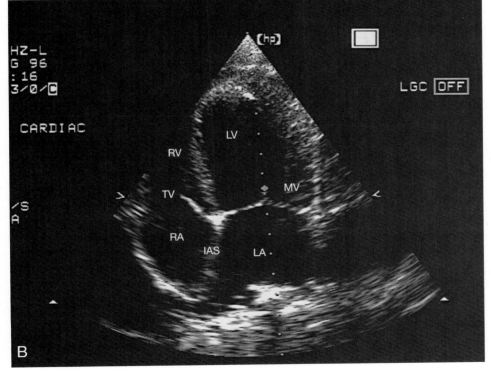

FIGURE 2.109   Mitral inflow in the small animal is recorded from either the left parasternal apical five-chamber view (**A**) or apical four-chamber view (**B**). *LV*, left ventricle; *MV*, mitral valve; *LA*, left atrium; *IVS*, interventricular septum; *RV*, right ventricle; *RA*, right atrium; *AO*, aorta; *IAS*, interatrial septum; *TV*, tricuspid valve.

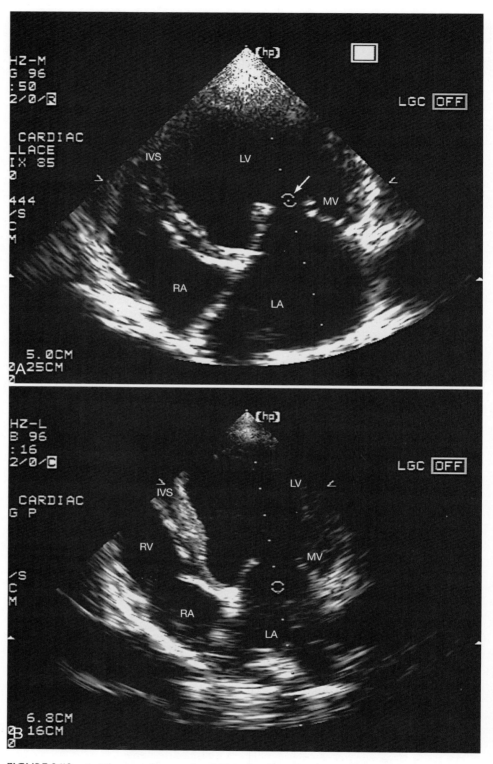

FIGURE 2.110   **A.** The sample gate should be placed at the tips of the leaflets when they are wide open (*arrow*). **B.** Gates placed too closely to the mitral annulus will decrease E velocities and deceleration times. *LV*, left ventricle; *IVS*, interventricular septum; *MV*, mitral valve; *RV*, right ventricle; *LA*, left atrium; *RA*, right atrium.

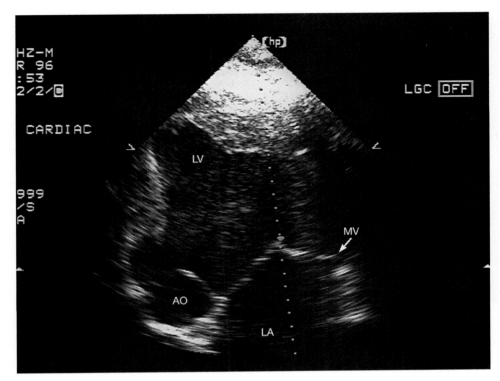

FIGURE 2.111   The left parasternal apical five-chamber view of the heart is used to record mitral inflow in the horse. The gate is placed at the tips of the mitral leaflets when they are wide open. *LV,* left ventricle; *AO,* aorta; *MV,* mitral valve; *LA,* left atrium.

Appearance.   Mitral valve flow profiles are positive and resemble the letter M, similar to M-mode images of mitral valve motion. The two phases of inflow are recorded (Fig. 2.112). Rapid ventricular filling is the E peak and corresponds to peak velocity. The second peak of the "M" occurs secondary to atrial contraction, and upward motion occurs just after the P wave on the electrocardiogram. Mitral inflow stops with the onset of systole after the beginning of the QRS complex.

The closeness of the E and A peaks depends on heart rate. Rapid heart rates will create more compact "Ms" and may even cause the two filling phases to overlap resulting in superimposed waveforms. (Fig. 2.113). This overlap will start to appear at heart rates approaching 125 beats per minute. Complete loss of separation always will be present when heart rates exceed 200 beats per minute. It is unusual for mitral inflow profiles in a cat to show two well-defined peaks. Slow heart rates may separate the two peaks dramatically (Fig. 2.114).

The E peak is always higher than the A peak in normal hearts, which creates an E:A ratio greater than 1. Positive flow may be seen after the A wave and is secondary to the mitral annulus movement toward the sternum after the valve closes. This motion pushes blood toward the transducer and is recorded after diastole is concluded.

Tricuspid Flow

Imaging Plane Used

Small Animal.   Standard right parasternal apical four- and five-chamber views of the heart usually do not align flow parallel to the Doppler sound beam. This is rectified by moving the transducer cranially and dorsally on the thorax until the tricuspid valve is seen opening in an upward direction. Correct alignment can

Spectral Doppler
Tricuspid Inflow

Imaging Plane
- Left parasternal cranial right atrium and auricle
- Left parasternal transverse
- View between the apical four-chamber and the transverse view
- Place the gate at the tips of the valve leaflets when they are open.

Appearance
- E usually higher than A, but may be reversed
- Beat to beat changes in velocity as a result of respiration

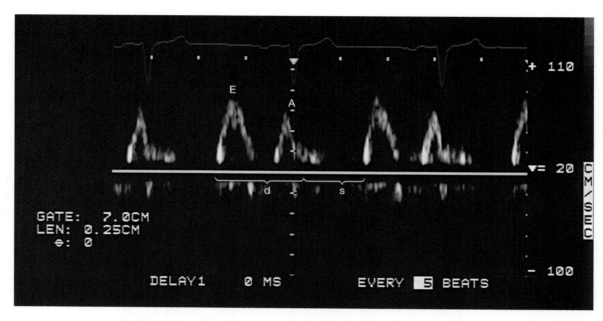

FIGURE 2.112   Mitral flow is positive and resembles the letter "M." The E point corresponds to rapid ventricular filling. The A peak represents flow associated with atrial contraction. Normally, the E:A ratio is greater than 1. *d*, diastole; *s*, systole.

therefore be seen in the left parasternal plane between the apical four-chamber and the transverse view, on heart base right atrium and auricle view, or the left parasternal transverse plane through the heart base view (Fig. 2.115). The gate should be placed at the tips of the tricuspid valve leaflets when they are wide open. Try to obtain flow profiles in all planes and search for the flow profile showing the highest velocities for both inflow phases with the least spectral broadening.

Large Animal.   Right parasternal four-chamber long-axis and left ventricular outflow long-axis views are used to record tricuspid flow profiles in the horse (Fig. 2.116). Sometimes the more oblique view through the right atrium is used. To obtain this view, rotate the transducer partially toward the transverse view and tilt the transducer dorsally and cranially until the longest right atrium is seen. Search for the best alignment with flow and the clearest spectral tracings with the least spectral broadening.

Appearance.   Tricuspid inflow appears similar to mitral inflow profiles. There is both a rapid ventricular filling phase resulting in an E peak and an A peak associated with atrial contraction as in mitral flow recordings (Fig. 2.117) Inspiration increases peak flow velocities, especially the E wave; therefore, the E:A ratio increases with inspiration and decreases with expiration. E:A ratios can be less than 1 for tricuspid inflow, and positive systolic flow may be greater than those seen in mitral flow tracings.

COLOR-FLOW DOPPLER

Color-flow Doppler has added an entirely new dimension to echocardiography. It has eliminated much of the time-consuming search for small insufficient jets, allows proper alignment with all valvular flows, and when properly used, echocardiographic interpretations can be made with the added confidence that nothing has been missed.

Controls

The most common color-flow controls are discussed here. Each manufacturer has its own specific set of color-flow features. Refer to the owner's manual for more detailed information regarding individual equipment.

Gain

Color-flow gain adjusts the system's sensitivity to received color information. Unlike gain or power controls for two-dimensional imaging, gain controls for color-flow

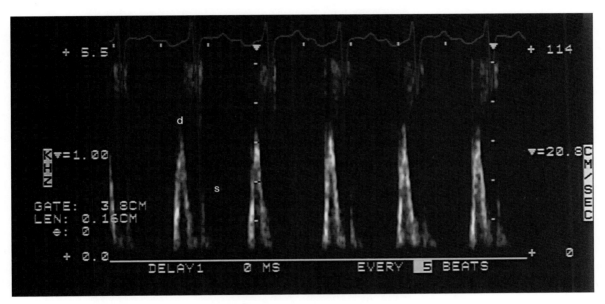

FIGURE 2.113   Rapid heart rates will result in a loss of separation between the two diastolic filling phases. Mitral flow in this cat with a heart rate of 193 shows only one peak during diastole. *d*, diastole; *s*, systole.

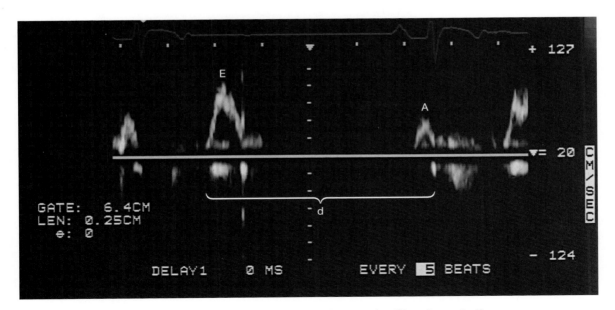

FIGURE 2.114   Slow heart rates separate the E and A peaks of ventricular filling dramatically. *d*, diastole.

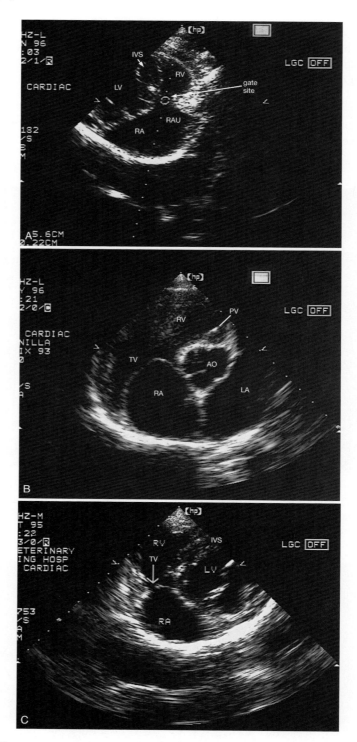

FIGURE 2.115   Tricuspid flow in the small animal may be recorded from several views including: (**A**) the left parasternal long-axis view with right atrium and auricle; (**B**) the left parasternal transverse view of the heart base; or (**C**) a plane somewhere between the apical four-chamber and the transverse plane. The sample site is located at the tips of the leaflets when they are wide open (*arrow*). *TV*, tricuspid valve; *IVS*, interventricular septum; *RV*, right ventricle; *LV*, left ventricle; *RA*, right atrium; *RAU*, right auricle; *AO*, aorta; *LA*, left atrium; *PV*, pulmonic valve.

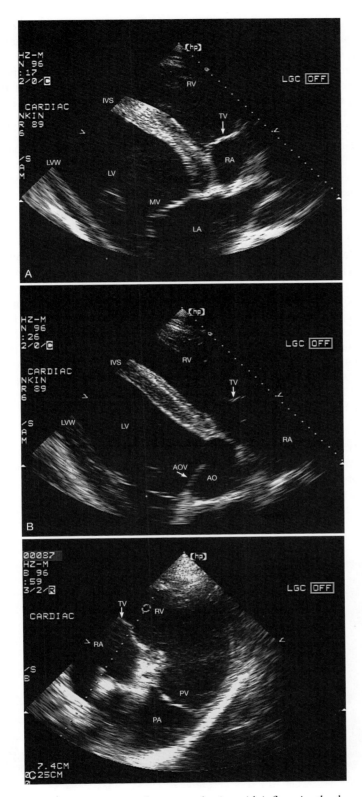

FIGURE 2.116   Several views are used to record tricuspid inflow in the horse: the right parasternal tipped four-chamber view (**A**), the right parasternal tipped left ventricular outflow view (**B**), or an oblique view of the right atrium obtained from the right parasternum (**C**). *IVS*, interventricular septum; *RV*, right ventricle; *RA*, right atrium; *TV*, tricuspid valve; *LV*, left ventricle; *LVW*, left ventricular wall; *MV*, mitral valve; *AO*, aorta; *AOV*, aortic valve; *LA*, left atrium; *PV*, pulmonic valve; *PA*, pulmonary artery.

Doppler do not affect output power, it just affects receiver gain. Increasing the color gain will increase the amount of color shown on the image. When the gain is turned up too high, speckling or noise will appear throughout the color wedge (Fig. 2.118) This speckling is different from the mosaic pattern seen with turbulent flow because the speckling is not a discrete jet and is not confined to the blood-filled areas of the heart and vessels. Adjust the gain until just before noise begins to appear.

Depth

The depth setting sets the depth of the color wedge over the two-dimensional image (Fig. 2.119). Reducing the depth to which color-flow information is superimposed on the real-time image allows the mind to focus on the area of interest. Reducing thedepth does not affect the pulse repetition frequency or the transmit power on most ultrasound machines.

Color Map

The color map allows selection of preconfigured color-flow presentations. As noted in Chapter 1, all information in this book will use the BART color map, which uses the blue/away and red/toward configuration.

Other maps include RABT (red/away and blue/toward) and pastel maps. Turbulent flow may be displayed with either an enhanced or a variance display. The underlying laminar flow is still encoded with a BART display, but the disturbed flow is displayed with different characteristics. An enhanced map encodes different velocities with different colors, producing a mosaic of reds, blues, yellows, and cyans. A variance map mixes green into the areas of disturbed flow (see Chapter 1). The result is yellow when green mixes with red and cyan when green mixes with blue.

Color-Flow Processing

The operator controls the way color information is acquired and processed. Each line of color-flow information may be sampled for variable lengths of time (see Chapter 1). A large packet size corresponds to a longer period, decreased frame rate, many color samples, and high-quality color. The reduced frame rate, how-

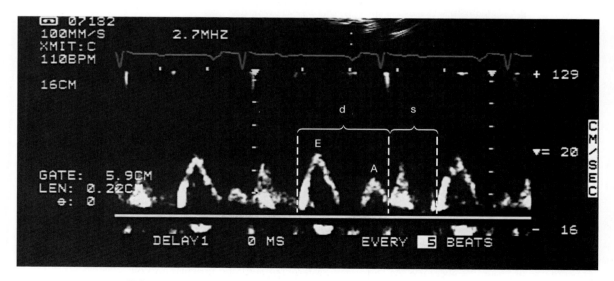

FIGURE 2.117   Tricuspid flow is positive and similar to mitral inflow. Rapid right ventricular filling is represented by the E peak, and flow associated with atrial contraction is represented by the A peak. The E:A ratio, though typically greater than 1, may also be less than 1. *d*, diastole; *s*, systole.

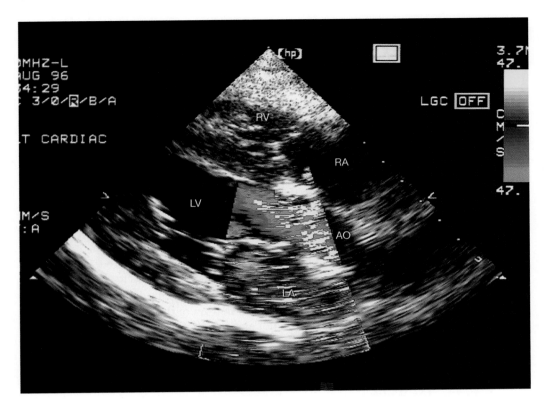

FIGURE 2.118 Color gain is too high when speckling is superimposed on the myocardium. *RV,* right ventricle; *RA,* right atrium; *LV,* left ventricle; *LA,* left atrium; *AO,* aorta.

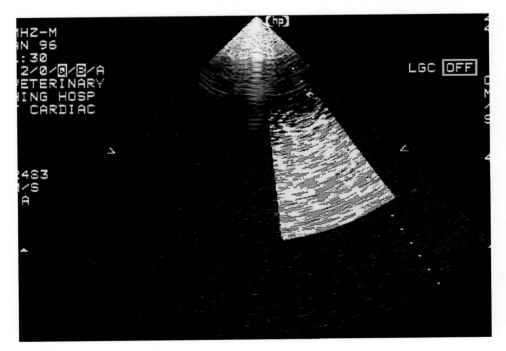

FIGURE 2.119 The depth of color superimposed on the two-dimensional image may be adjusted. Reducing the depth does not affect frame rate but does eliminate extraneous information beyond the area of interest.

ever, may create temporal artifacts with the high heart rates of cardiac imaging. Medium packet sizes produce faster imaging rates but shorter sampling times and a lower-quality color image; these are appropriate for cardiac imaging with average heart rates. Small packet sizes result in the fastest frame rates, but little time is spent gathering flow information. Select large packet sizes for high-quality color images and medium packet sizes for higher frame rates and excellent resolution.

Filters are also an operator-controlled feature of color-flow processing. Filters remove high-intensity, low-velocity information from the image. High filter settings remove most of the low-velocity signals and are often used to eliminate the strong signals received from wall and valve motion. Low filters only remove some of the high-intensity signals so that low flow velocities are seen well. Cardiac imaging requires medium to large packet sizes and medium to low filter settings.

Baseline

Adjusting the baseline on the color bar allows higher velocities to be displayed in one direction before aliasing occurs. This control is primarily used to "unwrap" aliased signals (Fig. 2.120). A number at the top and bottom of the color bar represents the maximum detectable velocity before color aliasing occurs. Moving the baseline up or down will double the maximum detectable velocity for blood flow away or toward the transducer.

Color Sector Width

The color sector width control adjusts the size of the color wedge (Fig. 2.121). The color wedge can be increased to fill the entire real-time sector. Reducing the color

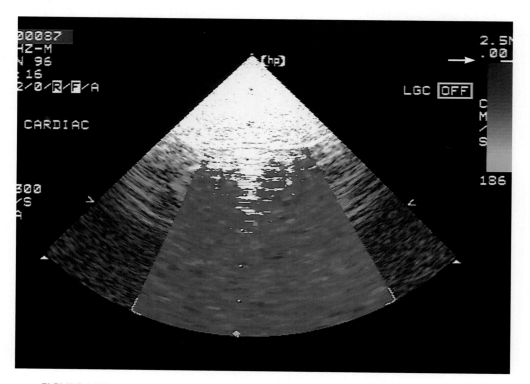

FIGURE 2.120   The zero line on the color bar can be adjusted so that higher velocities may be recorded in one direction or another before aliasing occurs. Here, the baseline has been moved up from its central position (*arrow*), and negative flow may reach velocities of 186 cm/sec before aliasing occurs.

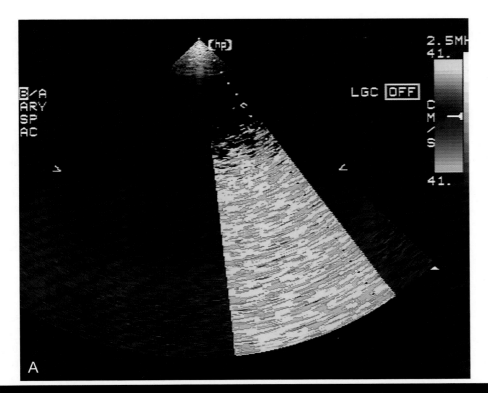

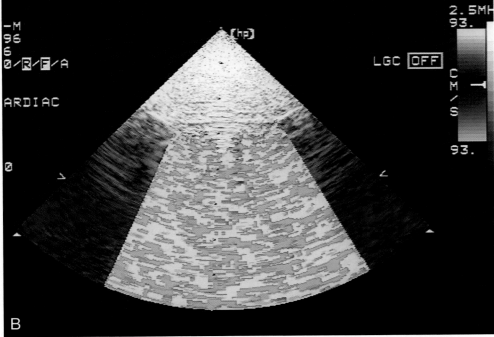

FIGURE 2.121   The width of the color sector can be adjusted. **A.** A small color sector increases the frame rate and improves color flow information. **B.** Larger color sectors decrease frame rate and diminish the accuracy of color information at high heart rates.

width increases frame rate because less time is required to process flow information. Alternately, increasing color width decreases frame rate and reduces the accuracy of color-flow information, especially in patients with high heart rates. The black-and-white image can be suppressed as well, leaving just the color wedge and the background real-time information.

Color Position

The color position control allows the color wedge to be moved across the sector image from right to left. The wedge can be kept small to improve the quality of the color information while placing it anywhere over the real-time image (Fig. 2.121).

Persistence

Persistence frame averages old information with new information to display smooth images, which reduces image noise. Too much persistence creates a blurred effect. This control is often used during real-time imaging of soft tissues.

Normal Color-Flow Imaging

Color-Flow Doppler

- Aliasing occurs at lower velocities than with spectral Doppler.
- Color aliasing may occur when flow is laminal.
- Use lower-frequency transducers for best color-flow imaging with less aliasing.
- Use a small color sector to reduce temporal artifacts.

Color-flow imaging is done best with low-frequency transducers. Try a lower-frequency transducer if color does not fill the chambers that are interrogated. In horses, color-flow imaging of the deeper structures may not be possible. Imaging from the left side to interrogate the mitral valve at a lesser depth is often necessary.

Aliasing occurs at lower velocities with color-flow Doppler because of the low PRF required. Normal flow may have aliased signals as a result, which causes a wrapping-around effect where the blues moving away from the transducer are layered with reds after the Nyquist limit is exceeded, and the reds moving toward the transducer are layered with blue. The layering is seen in the middle of the flow jet while the periphery of the color-flow profile remains true to its flow direction (Fig. 2.122). Figure 2.123 shows a series of images of flow in the pulmonary artery. Early flow velocities exceed the Nyquist limit and have almost completely "wrapped" to a red color even though flow is down away from the transducer. As flow velocity decreases toward the middle of systole and velocities start to equal the Nyquist limit, blues are shown in the image. The latter part of systole shows only blues when flow velocity has decreased and no longer exceeds the Nyquist limit.

Turbulent flow results in disorganized and greatly variant velocities. When turbulent flow is detected, green is added to the areas of disorganized flow and a mosaic pattern is seen (Fig. 2.124). This mosaic pattern is easy to detect and helps identify areas of abnormal flow. Low-velocity flows are not detected and no color is assigned. These areas will remain black.

Tipped long-axis views and apical four- and five-chamber views are the best for imaging color-flow Doppler. Images that are not tipped but align the interventricular septum horizontally across the sector also may produce good color images. The color-encoded, two-dimensional images will be different depending on the generated image. For example, a tipped view with the apex up will show color flowing through the heart with exactly the opposite colors of what would be seen if the image was generated with the apex down and base up toward the top right of the sector. Try several transducer positions to find the optimal plane for color-flow imaging of specific structures.

Mitral and Tricuspid Flow

Typical parasternal long-axis, four-chamber or left-ventricular outflow images, and apical four- and five-chamber views will show mitral inflow as red with a brighter central area. When the Nyquist limit is exceeded, the central area of flow may have a layer of blues superimposed on it (Figs. 2.125, 2.126, 2.127, and 2.128). The same is true for tricuspid flows (Figs. 2.129, 2.130, and 2.131). Because in the parasternal images tricuspid flow is not as deep, aliasing will not occur as readily, and the layering effect is seen less commonly. Trivial to mild amounts of tricuspid regurgitation are seen commonly in all animals (Fig. 2.132).

Aortic Flow

Aortic flow is seen as hues of blue and red as blood leaves the left ventricle in a downward direction in the apical five-chamber views (Fig. 2.133). The depth of the aorta in this view results in a low Nyquist limit and "wrap around" or aliasing is seen. Parasternal views of the aorta may have flow mapped as either red or blue, depending on the angle at which the aorta is aligned with the transducer (Figs. 2.134 and 2.135). The color changes as the aorta curves away from the heart.

Pulmonary Flow

Pulmonary artery flow encoded on the transverse image at the heart base in either the left or right parasternal views is usually blue as blood leaves the right ventricle in a direction away from the transducer. Because the artery curves, this plane typically has a layering of colors within the pulmonary artery flow profile (Figs. 2.136 and 2.137). Total reversal of color is often seen (Fig. 2.123) as flow progresses from high velocities during early systole to slower velocities at the end of systole. Trivial to mild amounts of pulmonic insufficiency are seen in both large and small animals (Fig. 2.138).

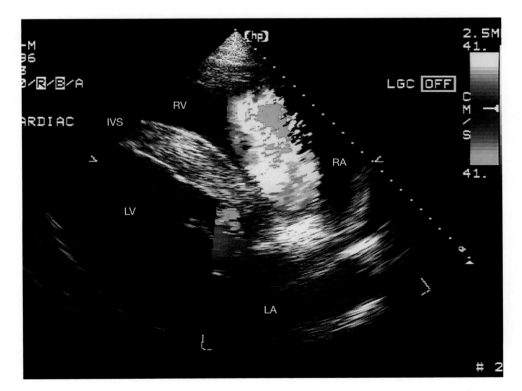

FIGURE 2.122   Color wraps around the color bar when velocities exceed the Nyquist limit. When flow is laminar but exceeds the limit, a layering effect is seen. Here, tricuspid inflow displays red at the periphery but has a middle yellow layer. As flow velocity increases in the center, color aliases to blue. *RV*, right ventricle; *IVS*, interventricular septum; *LV*, left ventricle; *RA*, right atrium; *LA*, left atrium.

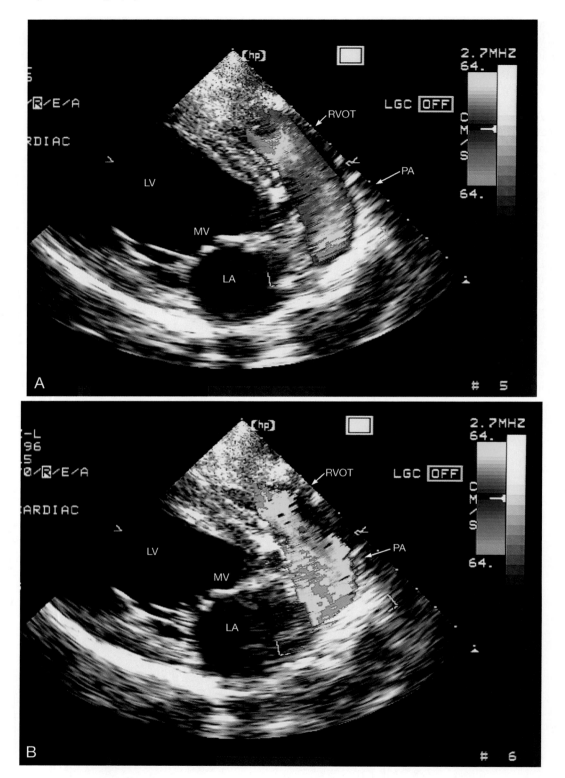

FIGURE 2.123   This series of images shows flow within the right ventricular outflow tract and pulmonary artery. **A.** Initial velocities exceed the Nyquist limit of 64 cm/sec (see color bar), and although flow is down and away from the transducer, it is primarily red. **B.** As flow starts to decelerate, blues start to be superimposed on the red.

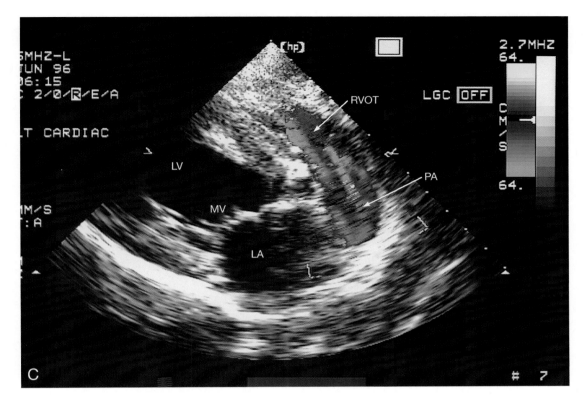

FIGURE 2.123 *(continued)*   C. Finally, toward the end of systole, when flow has decreased to less than 64 cm/sec, the aliasing is seen barely in the center of the artery. *RVOT*, right ventricular outflow tract, *PA*, pulmonary artery; *LV*, left ventricle; *MV*, mitral valve; *LA*, left atrium.

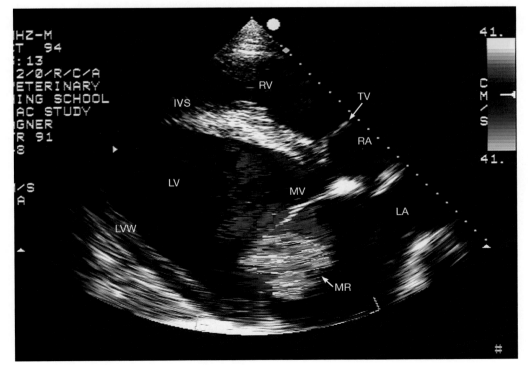

FIGURE 2.124 When turbulent flow is detected and it exceeds the Nyquist limit, the disorganized cellular movement creates a mosaic pattern on the color-flow image. Here, a mosaic jet of mitral insufficiency is displayed. *RV*, right ventricle; *RA*, right atrium; *TV*, tricuspid valve; *IVS*, interventricular septum; *LV*, left ventricle; *MV*, mitral valve; *LA*, left atrium; *MR*, mitral regurgitation; *LVW*, left ventricular wall.

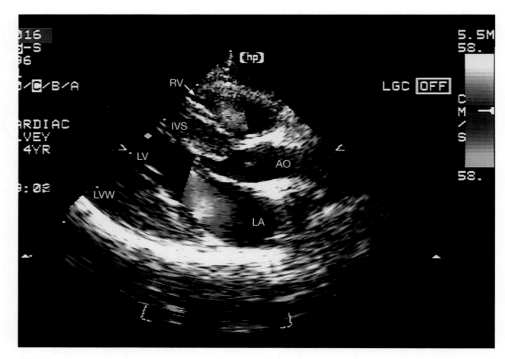

FIGURE 2.125   Flow from the left atrium into the left ventricle on this right parasternal long-axis left ventricular outflow view in a cat is red because flow is directed upward in this tipped view. *RV*, right ventricle; *IVS*, interventricular septum; *AO*, aorta; *LV*, left ventricle; *LVW*, left ventricular wall; *LA*, left atrium.

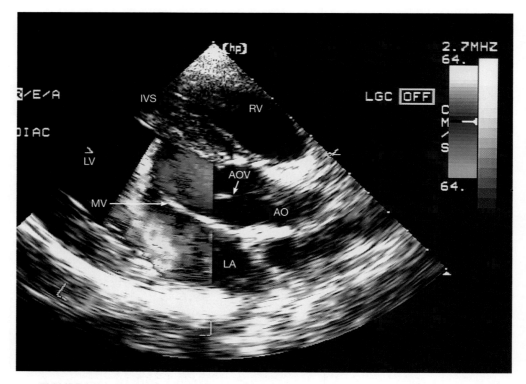

FIGURE 2.126   Flow from the left atrium into the left ventricle on the right parasternal left ventricular outflow view in this dog has a layered central flow area at the threshold of aliasing. *RV*, right ventricle; *LV*, left ventricle; *AO*, aorta; *AOV*, aortic valve; *LA*, left atrium; *IVS*, interventricular septum; *MV*, mitral valve.

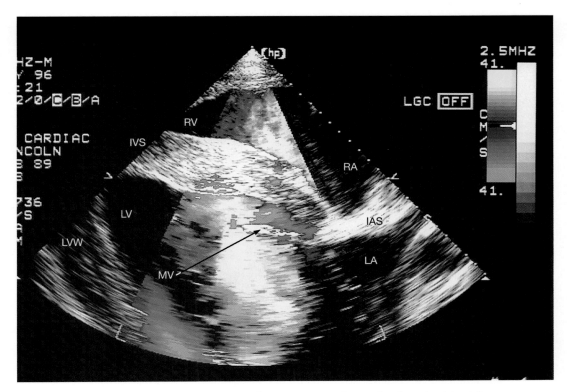

FIGURE 2.127   The depth required for color-flow mapping of mitral inflow in this right parasternal four-chamber view in the horse shows less color filling at the bottom of the sector. The Nyquist limit also is exceeded at lower velocities (41 cm/sec) because of the depth requirements. *RV*, right ventricle; *RA*, right atrium; *IAS*, interatrial septum; *IVS*, interventricular septum; *LV*, left ventricle; *LVW*, left ventricular wall; *MV*, mitral valve; *LA*, left atrium.

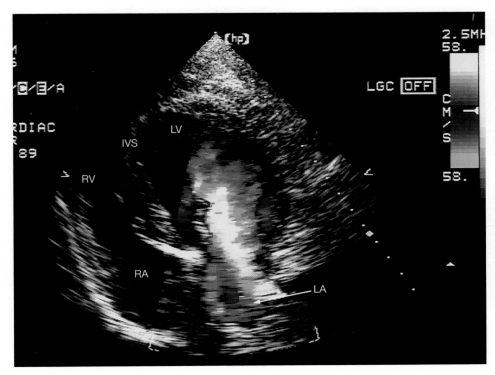

FIGURE 2.128   Mitral inflow is seen as a central bright yellow core superimposed on slower red flow at the periphery of the jet as it moves up from the left atrium into the left ventricle in this apical four-chamber view in a dog. *LV*, left ventricle; *IVS*, interventricular septum; *RV*, right ventricle; *RA*, right atrium; *LA*, left atrium.

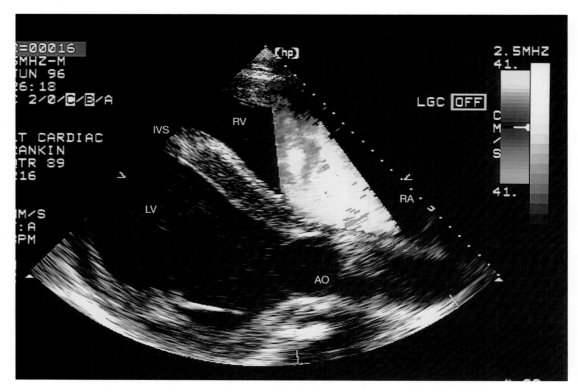

FIGURE 2.129   Tricuspid flow in this right parasternal tipped left ventricular outflow view in a horse shows central velocities that are starting to exceed the Nyquist limit of 41 cm/sec. *IVS*, interventricular septum; *RV*, right ventricle; *RA*, right atrium; *LV*, left ventricle; *AO*, aorta.

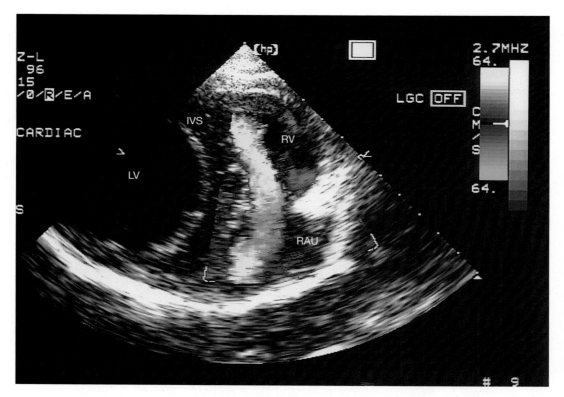

FIGURE 2.130   The left parasternal, cranial long-axis view of the right atrium and auricle do not show flow within the right auricle. *RV*, right ventricle; *RAU*, right auricle; *LV*, left ventricle; *IVS*, interventricular septum.

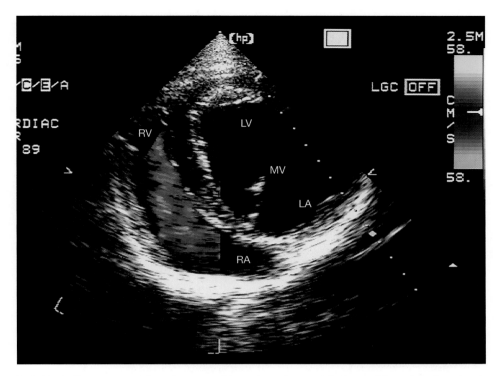

FIGURE 2.131   Tricuspid flow during middiastole in this modified apical four-chamber view is slow and well below the Nyquist limit of 58 cm/sec. *LV*, left ventricle; *RV*, right ventricle; *MV*, mitral valve; *LA*, left atrium; *RA*, right atrium.

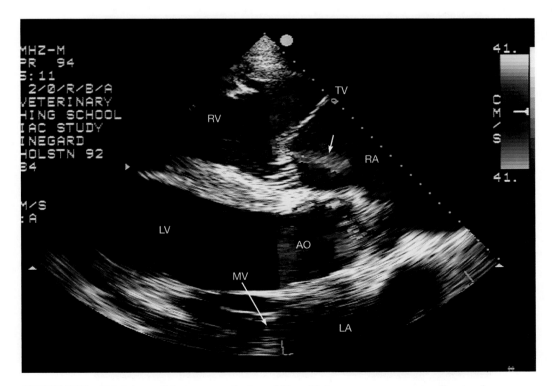

FIGURE 2.132   Trivial to mild amounts of tricuspid insufficiency are common in all animals. Here, a trivial amount of tricuspid regurgitation (*arrow*) is seen on this right parasternal long-axis left ventricular outflow view in a horse. *RV*, right ventricle; *RA*, right atrium; *TV*, tricuspid valve; *LV*, left ventricle; *AO*, aorta; *LA*, left atrium; *MV*, mitral valve.

FIGURE 2.133 Aortic flow is seen as an aliased signal because the Nyquist limit is almost always exceeded. **A.** Here, aortic flow in the horse on an apical five-chamber view shows bright yellow and red and aliased flows even though flow is away from the transducer. **B.** This apical five-chamber view in a dog during early systole when velocities are high shows an almost completely aliased signal. **C.** Later in systole during deceleration, much of the flow is accurately mapped as blue. *RV*, right ventricle; *LV*, left ventricle; *MV*, mitral valve; *LA*, left atrium; *TV*, tricuspid valve; *RA*, right atrium; *AO*, aorta.

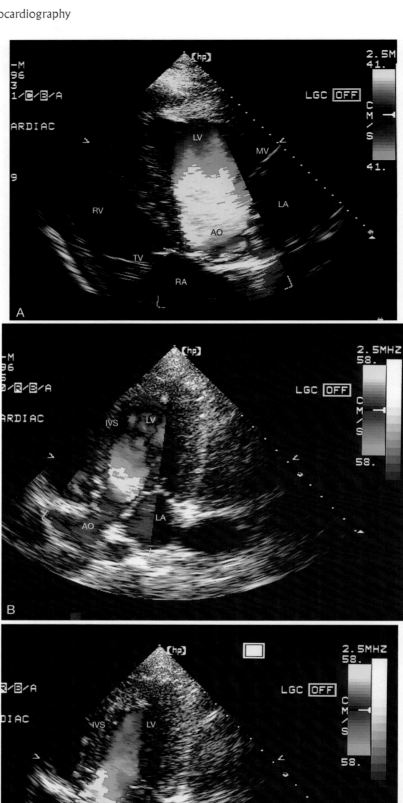

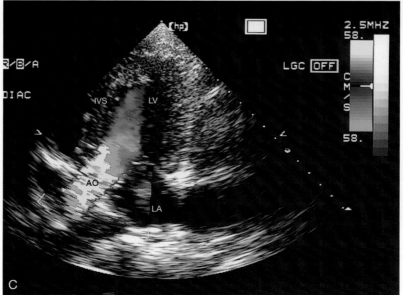

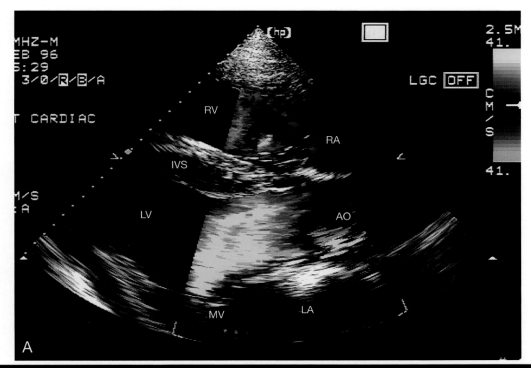

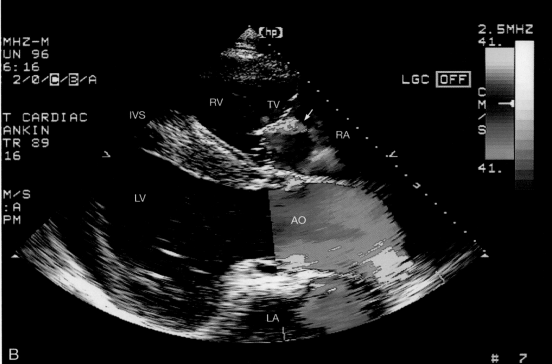

FIGURE 2.134   Aortic flow in this horizontal right parasternal long-axis left ventricular outflow view in a horse is red when flow enters the outflow tract (**A**) and blue when flow turns away from the transducer (**B**). A trivial amount of tricuspid regurgitation is seen (*arrow*). *RV*, right ventricle; *RA*, right atrium; *IVS*, interventricular septum; *LV*, left ventricle; *AO*, aorta; *LA*, left atrium; *MV*, mitral valve.

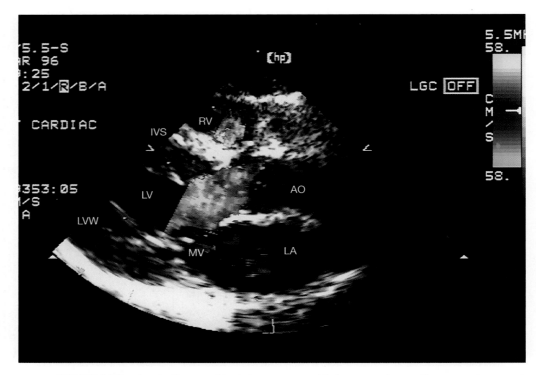

FIGURE 2.135   Aortic flow in this right parasternal left ventricular outflow view in a cat is shown accurately in reds and yellows. *RV*, right ventricle; *IVS*, interventricular septum; *LV*, left ventricle; *LVW*, left ventricular wall; *AO*, aorta; *LA*, left atrium; *MV*, mitral valve.

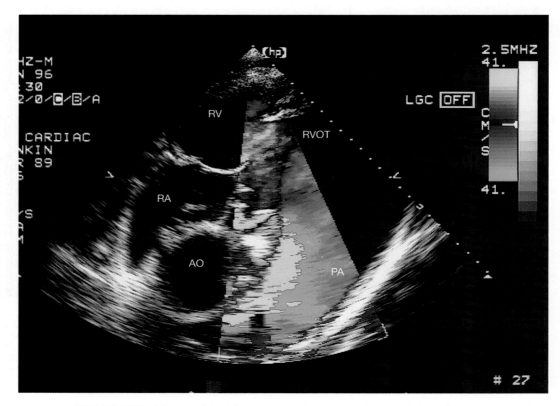

FIGURE 2.136   Flow in this right parasternal transverse image of the pulmonary artery in a horse shows mild aliasing (yellow) during late systole. *RV*, right ventricle; *RVOT*, right ventricular outflow tract; *RA*, right atrium; *AO*, aorta; *PA*, pulmonary artery.

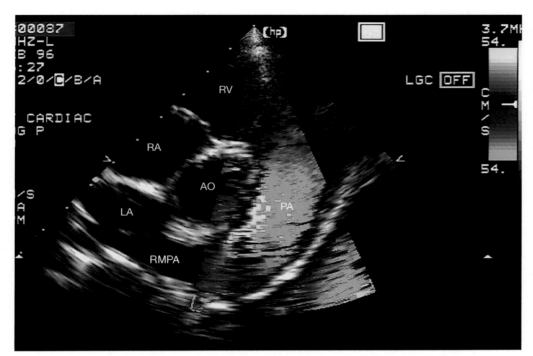

FIGURE 2.137 Early systolic flow mapping within the pulmonary artery shows an aliased signal as can be seen in this right parasternal transverse view of the artery in a dog. *PA*, pulmonary artery; *RV*, right ventricle; *RA*, right atrium; *LA*, left atrium; *AO*, aorta; *RMPA*, right main pulmonary artery.

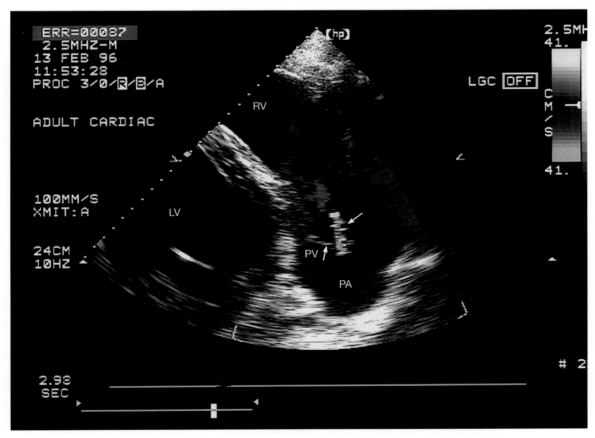

FIGURE 2.138 Trivial to mild pulmonic insufficiency is common in all animals. Here, a trivial amount of pulmonic insufficiency (*arrow*) is seen on the right parasternal transverse view of the pulmonary artery in a horse. *RV*, right ventricle; *LV*, left ventricle; *PV*, pulmonic valve; *PA*, pulmonary artery.

REFERENCES

1. Pipers FS, Hamlin RL. Echocardiography in the horse. JAVMA 1977;170:815–819.
2. Franklin TD, Weyman AE, Egenes KM. A closed-chest model for cross-sectional echocardiographic study. Am J Physiol 1977;233:H417–H419.
3. Kerber RE, Abboud FM. Echocardiographic detection of regional myocardial infarction: an experimental study. Circulation 1973;47:997–1005.
4. Kerber RE, Abboud FM, Marcus ML, Eckberg RL. Effect of inotropic agents on the localized dyskinesis of acutely ischemic myocardium: an experimental ultrasound study. Circulation 1974;49:1038–1046.
5. Landiano S, Yellen E, Kotler M, Levy J, et al. A study of the dynamic relations between the mitral valve echogram and phasic mitral flow. Circulation 1975;51:104–113.
6. Bishop VS, Horwitz HL, Stone HL, et al. Left ventricular internal diameter and cardiac function in conscious dogs. J Appl Physiol 1969;27:619–623.
7. Baylen BG, Garner DJ, Laks MM, et al. Improved echocardiographic evaluation of the closed-chest canine: methods and anatomic observations. J Clin Ultrasound 1980;8:335–340.
8. Mashiro I, Nelson RR, Cohn JN, et al. Ventricular dimensions measured noninvasively by echocardiography in the awake dog. J App Physiol 1976;41:953–959.
9. Stefan G, Bing RJ. Echocardiographic findings in experimental myocardial infarction of the posterior left ventricular wall. Am J Cardiol 1972;30:629–639.
10. Wyatt HL, Heng MK, Meerbaum S. Cross sectional echocardiography. I. Analysis of mathematical models for quantifying mass of the left ventricle in dogs. Circulation 1979;60:1104–1113.
11. Dennis MO, Nealeigh RC, Pyle RL, et al. Echocardiographic assessment of normal and abnormal valvular function in Beagle dogs. Am J Vet Res 1978;39:1591–1598.
12. Pipers FS, Bonagura JD, Hamlin RL, et al. Echocardiographic abnormalities of the mitral valve associated with left sided heart disease in the dog. JAVMA 1981;179:580–586.
13. Bonagura JD, Pipers FS. Echocardiographic features of pericardial effusion in dogs. JAVMA 1981;179:49–56.
14. Bonagura JD, Pipers FS. Echocardiographic features of aortic valve endocarditis in a dog, a cow, and a horse. JAVMA 1983;182:595–599.
15. Pipers FS, Rings DM, Hull BL, et al. Echocardiographic diagnosis of endocarditis in a bull. JAVMA 1978;172:1313–1316.
16. Lacuata AQ, Yamada H, Nakamura Y, et al. Electrocardiographic and echocardiographic findings in four cases of bovine endocarditis. JAVMA 1980;176:1355–1365.
17. Pipers FS, Hamlin RL, Reef V. Echocardiographic detection of cardiovascular lesions in the horse. J Equine Med Surg 1979;3:68–77.
18. Wingfield WE, Miller CW, Voss JL, et al. Echocardiography in assessing mitral valve motion in three horses with atrial fibrillation. Equine Vet J 1980;12:181–184.
19. Okamoto Y, Hasegawa A. Studies on canine echocardiography. Part I. Normal pattern of echocardiogram. J Jpn Vet Med Assoc 1977;30:588–594.
20. Yamada E. A basic study on echocardiography of the dog. Part I. Anatomical relationship between the heart and the direction of ultrasonic beams transmitted from the body surface. Bull Azabu Vet Coll 1978;3:225–234.
21. Boon J, Wingfield WE, Miller CW. Echocardiographic indices in the normal dog. Vet Radiol 1983;24: 214–221.
22. Pipers FS, Andrysco RM, Hamlin RL. A totally noninvasive method for obtaining systolic time intervals in the dog. Am J Vet Res 1978;39:1822–1826.
23. Jacobs G, Mahjoob K. Multiple regression analysis, using body size and cardiac cycle length, in predicting echocardiographic variables in dogs. Am J Vet Res 1988;49:1290–1294.
24. Lombard CW. Normal values of the canine M-mode echocardiogram. Am J Vet Res 1984;45:2015–2018.
25. Soderberg SF, Boon JA, Wingfield WE, et al. M-mode echocardiography as a diagnostic aid for feline cardiomyopathy. Vet Radiol 1983;24:66–73.
26. Allen DG. Echocardiographic study of the anesthetized cat. Can J Comp Med 1982;46: 115–122.
27. Allen DG, Downey RS. Echocardiographic assessment of cats anesthetized with xylazine-sodium pentobarbital. Can J Comp Med 1983;47:281–283.
28. Allen DG, Nymeyer D. A preliminary investigation on the use of thermodilution and echocardiography as an assessment of cardiac function in the cat. Can J Comp Med 1983;47:112–117.

29. Pipers FS, Hamlin RL. Clinical use of echocardiography in the domestic cat. JAVMA 1980;176:57–61.

30. Pipers FS, Reef V, Hamlin RL. Echocardiography in the domestic cat. Am J Vet Res 1979;40:882–886.

31. Fox PR, Bond BR, Peterson ME. Echocardiographic reference values in healthy cats sedated with ketamine hydrochloride. Am J Vet Res 1985;46:1479–1484.

32. Jacobs G, Knight DH. M-mode echocardiographic measurements in nonanesthetized healthy cats: effects of body weight, heart rate, and other variables. Am J Vet Res 1985;46:1705–1711.

33. Jacobs G, Knight D. Change in M-mode echocardiographic values in cats given ketamine. Am J Vet Res 1985;46:1712–1713.

34. O'Callaghan MW. Comparison of echocardiographic and autopsy measurements of cardiac dimensions in the horse. Equine Vet J 1985;17:361–368.

35. Lombard CW, Evans M, Martin L, Tehrani J. Blood pressure, electrocardiogram and echocardiogram measurements in the growing pony foal. Equine Vet J 1984;16:342–347.

36. Stewart JH, Rose RJ, Barko AM. Echocardiography in foals from birth to three months old. Equine Vet J 1984;16:332–341.

37. Lescure F, Tamazali Y. L'echocardiographie TM le cheval: la technique. Le Point Vet 1983;15:37–45.

38. Lescure F, Tamazali Y. Valeurs de reference en echocardiographie TM chez le cheval de sport. Rev Med Vet 1984;135:405–418.

39. Pipers FS, Reef V, Hamlin RL, et al. Echocardiography in the bovine animal. Bov Pract 1978;13:114–118.

40. Pipers FS, Muir WW, Hamlin RL. Echocardiography in swine. Am J Vet Res 1978;39:707–710.

41. Thomas WP, Gaber CE, Jacobs GJ, et al. Recommendations for standards in transthoracic two-dimensional echocardiography in the dog and cat. J Vet Int Med 1993;7:247–252.

42. O'Grady MR, Bonagura JD, Powers JD, et al. Quantitative cross-sectional echocardiography in the normal dog. Vet Radiol 1986;27:34–49.

43. Schiller NB, Skioldersbrand CG, Schiller EJ, et al. Canine left ventricular mass estimation by two-dimensional echocardiography. Circulation 1983;68:210–215.

44. Thomas WP. Two-dimensional, real-time echocardiography in the dog: technique and anatomic validation. Vet Radiol 1984;25:50–64.

45. Bonagura JD, O'Grady MR, Herring DS. Echocardiography: principles of interpretation. Vet Clin North Am Small Anim Pract 1985;15:1177–1194.

46. Lusk RH, Ettinger SJ. Echocardiographic techniques in the dog and cat. J Am Anim Hosp Assoc 1990;26:473–488.

47. DeMadron E, Bonagura JD, Herring DS. Two-dimensional echocardiography in the normal cat. Vet Radiol 1985;26:149–158.

48. Voros K, Holmes JR, Gibbs C. Measurement of cardiac dimensions with two-dimensional echocardiography in the living horse. Equine Vet J 1991;23:461–465.

49. Long KJ, Bonagura JD, Darke PGG. Standardized imaging technique for guided M-mode and Doppler echocardiography in the horse. Equine Vet J 1992;24:226–235.

50. Reef VB. Echocardiographic examination in the horse: the basics. Compendium 1990;12:1312–1320.

51. Carlsten J. Two-dimensional, real-time echocardiography in the horse. Vet Radiol 1987;28:76–87.

52. Voros K, Holmes JR, Gibbs C. Anatomical validation of two-dimensional echocardiography in the horse. Equine Vet J 1990;22:392–397.

53. Reimer J. Cardiac evaluation of the horse: using ultrasonography. Vet Med 1993;88:748–755.

54. Stadler P, Rewel A, Deegen E. M-mode echocardiography in dressage and show jumping horses of class "S" and in untrained horses. J Vet Med A 1993;40:292–306.

55. Yamaga Y, Too K. Diagnostic ultrasound imaging in domestic animals: two-dimensional and M-mode echocardiography. Jpn J Vet Sci 1984;46:493–503.

56. Stadler P, Weinberger T, Deegen E. Pulsed Doppler echocardiography in healthy warm blooded horses. J Vet Med A 1993;40:757–778.

57. Reef VB, Lalezari K, De Boo J, et al. Pulsed-wave Doppler evaluation of intracardiac blood flow in 30 clinically normal standardbred horses. Am J Vet Res 1989;50:75–83.

58. Long KJ. Doppler echocardiography in the horse. Equine Vet Ed 1990;2:15–17.

59. Brown DJ, Knight DH, King RR. Use of pulsed-wave Doppler echocardiography to

determine aortic and pulmonary velocity and flow variables in clinically normal dogs. Am J Vet Res 1991;52:543–550.

60. Yuill C, O'Grady MR. Doppler-derived velocity of blood flow across the cardiac valves in the normal dog. Can J Vet Res 1991;55:185–192.

61. Darke PGG, Bonagura JD, Miller M. Transducer orientation for Doppler echocardiography in dogs. J Small Anim Pract 1993;34:2–8.

62. Gaber CE. Normal pulsed wave Doppler flow velocities in adult dogs. Proc 5th ACVIM 1987:923.

63. Kirberger RM, Bland-van den Berg P, Darazs B. Doppler echocardiography in the normal dog: Part I. Velocity findings and flow patterns. Vet Radiol Ultrasound 1992;33:370–379.

64. Kirberger RM, Bland-van den Berg P, Grimbeek RJ. Doppler echocardiography in the normal dog: Part II. Factors influencing blood flow velocities and a comparison between left and right heart blood flow. Vet Radiol Ultrasound 1992;33:380–386.

65. Darke PG. An evaluation of transducer sites for measurement of aortic and pulmonary flows by Doppler echocardiography. Proc 9th ACVIM 1991:703–705.

66. Darke PGG. Two-dimensional imaging for Doppler echocardiography in dogs. Proc 8th ACVIM 1990:261–268.

67. Kirberger RM. Pulsed wave Doppler echocardiographic evaluation of intracardiac blood flow in normal sheep. Res Vet Sci 1993;55:189–194.

68. Huml RA. Radiography corner: tables for echocardiography and abdominal ultrasonography. Vet Tech 1994;15:170–171.

69. Bonagura JD. Echocardiography. JAVMA 1994;204:516–522.

70. Miller MW, Knauer KW, Herring DS. Echocardiography: principles of interpretation. Semin Vet Med Surg (Small Anim) 1989;4:58–76.

71. Sisson D, Schaeffer D. Changes in linear dimensions of the heart, relative to body weight, as measured by M-mode echocardiography in growing dogs. Am J Vet Res 1991;52:1591–1596.

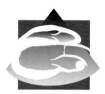

3

EVALUATION OF SIZE, FUNCTION, AND HEMODYNAMICS

The ability to identify cardiac chambers and valves via M-mode ultrasound was a major breakthrough in the cardiology field. Structure and function could be assessed noninvasively. The advent of two-dimensional echocardiography permitted easier diagnosis of disease because the relationships between structures were seen. Two-dimensional and M-mode ultrasound provide data regarding size and structure as well as hemodynamic information. However, Doppler ultrasound provides so much information about intracardiac pressures, stroke volumes, regurgitant fractions, shunt ratios, and systolic and diastolic function that most invasive cardiac tests are no longer necessary. Several general reference articles are published discussing the principles of echocardiography and its interpretation (1–13). This chapter discusses the assessment of cardiac structure, size, and function, as well as hemodynamics from M-mode, two-dimensional, and Doppler studies.

EVALUATION OF SIZE AND FLOW PROFILES
Assessment of Two-Dimensional Images

Subjective Determination of Size
Before accurate measurements are made from M-mode or two-dimensional images, impressions of size and function can be obtained from two-dimensional images. In most cases, it is possible to finish a two-dimensional examination without making any quantitative measurements and have a good assessment of size and function. What follows are guidelines for subjectively interpreting real-time images.

Right Parasternal Long-Axis Left Ventricular Outflow View.
When a clear right ventricular wall is seen, its thickness is approximately 1/3 to 1/2 the thickness of the left ventricular free wall. An increase in right ventricular wall thickness suggests the presence of right ventricular hypertrophy (Fig. 3.1). The interventricular septum is slightly thicker than the left ventricular free wall in dogs and cats, but can be much thicker than the free wall in horses, especially foals (Fig. 3.2)(14–19). If right ventricular hypertrophy is present, the interventricular septum also may be hypertrophied. These assessments are subjective; thus, if after careful quantitative

---

Left Ventricular Outflow View Assessment (Dogs)

- No bowing of the IVS
- IVS and LVW similar in size
- IVS does not protrude into LVOT
- RV wall approximately 1/2 thickness of LVW
- RV chamber size approximately 1/3 of LV chamber size
- LA and AO similar in size
- MV excursion almost to IVS
- No valvular lesions

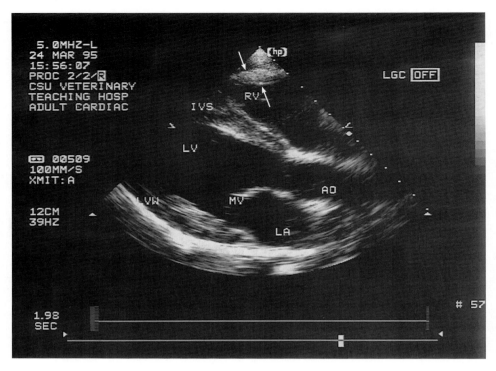

FIGURE 3.1 Right ventricular wall thickness (*arrows*) should be approximately 1/3 the thickness of left ventricular wall thickness in normal animals. The interventricular septum is typically about the same thickness as the left ventricular wall in dogs and cats. This ultrasound is of a canine patient. *RV*, right ventricle; *IVS*, interventricular septum; *LV*, left ventricle; *AO*, aorta; *MV*, mitral valve; *LA*, left atrium; *LVW*, left ventricular wall.

Left Ventricular Outflow View Assessment (Cats)

- No bowing of the IVS
- IVS and LVW similar in size
- IVS protrudes slightly into LVOT
- RV wall approximately 1/2 thickness of LVW
- RV chamber size approximately 1/3 of LV chamber size
- LA up to 1.7 times the size of the AO
- MV excursion almost to IVS
- No valvular lesions

measurements the left ventricular wall is thin, then the relationship of right ventricular wall thickness to left ventricular wall thickness should be reevaluated.

The interventricular septum should not bow toward the right or left ventricles during diastole. Displacement toward the right indicates left ventricular volume overload (Fig. 3.3). Displacement toward the left tends to indicate right ventricular volume or pressure overload, or in some cases, it may indicate a manifestation of left ventricular hypertrophy (Fig. 3.4). Biventricular dilation often keeps the pressure relationship between both ventricles the same and bowing of the septum will not be present. The relationship of right ventricular size to left ventricular size in a normal heart should be approximately 1 to 3 (Fig. 3.5).

The interventricular septum in all animals except cats also should not protrude into the left ventricular outflow tract. The width of the outflow tract should be the same as the width of the aortic root (Fig. 3.1). The interventricular septum in most healthy cats tends to deviate slightly into the outflow tract (Fig. 3.6).

The relationship of wall thicknesses and chamber sizes are different in neonates. Right ventricular wall thickness is as great or greater than left ventricular wall thickness in all neonates (14,15). Right ventricular chamber size is also larger in neonates and the volume may remain large for several weeks (14,15). Assessment of cardiac size in neonates is often a challenge, and if pathology is not clear, it may be necessary to re-evaluate the heart after the animal is 3 to 4 months old.

Although left atrial size may be slightly larger than aortic root size, visually, the left atrial to aortic root ratio should appear to be approximately 1:1 in the dog. Cats have larger atria with respect to the aorta than dogs in which the visual ratio of left atrium to aorta may be 1.6:1.0 in healthy cats (Fig. 3.7) (18,19). In horses, the entire left atrium often is not seen; therefore, the left atrium and aorta comparison cannot be made. The ratio of left atrium to aorta can be deceiving if the aortic root is small and is only a rough assessment of atrial size.

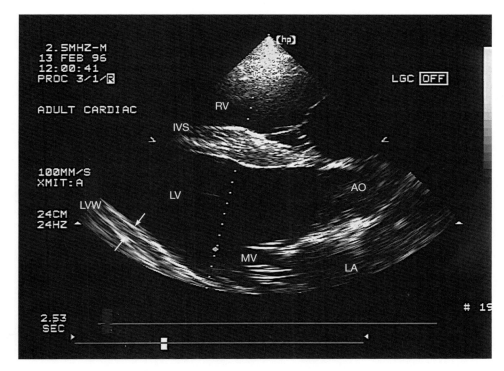

FIGURE 3.2   The normal interventricular septum in horses is usually much thicker than the left ventricular wall (*arrows*). *RV,* right ventricle; *IVS,* interventricular septum; *LV,* left ventricle; *AO,* aorta; *MV,* mitral valve; *LA,* left atrium; *LVW,* left ventricular wall.

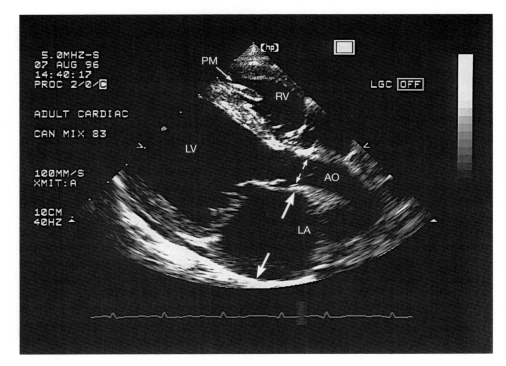

FIGURE 3.3   Bowing of the interventricular septum towards the right ventricle indicates left ventricular volume overload. This image also shows a dilated left atrium (*large arrows*) which should be approximately the same size as the aorta (*small arrows*). *RV,* right ventricle; *PM,* papillary muscle; *LV,* left ventricle; *AO,* aorta; *LA,* left atrium.

Enlargement of the left atrium may be seen in planes other than the long axis, as is discussed in the following sections. For this reason, measurements of left atrial size may be more accurate when taken from two-dimensional images. Any one echocardiographic modality should not be used solely to assess cardiac size (20,21).

Left atrial size decreases within hours after birth as the ductus and foramen close, resulting in decreased atrial volume. Therefore, echocardiographic examinations even at several weeks of age should show the same left atrial to aortic root ratio as that seen in mature animals (15). The newborn foal has a smaller LA/AO ratio than

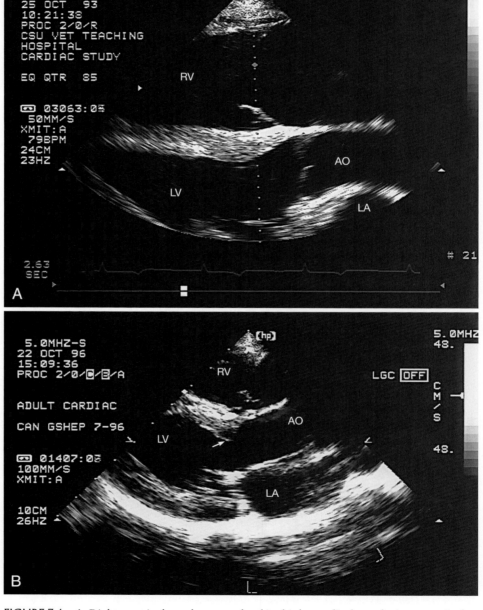

FIGURE 3.4   **A.** Right ventricular volume overload in this horse displaces the interventricular septum downward toward the left ventricle. **B.** Hypertrophy of the septum will cause it to extend further into the left ventricular chamber and outflow tract than normal (*arrow*) as seen in this dog with subaortic stenosis. *RV*, right ventricle; *LV*, left ventricle; *AO*, aorta; *LA*, left atrium.

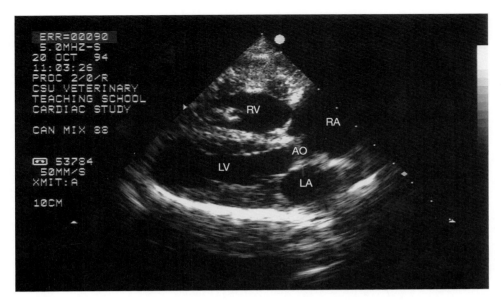

FIGURE 3.5   An approximate ratio of right ventricular chamber to left ventricular chamber that exceeds 1:3 indicates right ventricular volume overload as seen in this dog with pulmonic stenosis and insufficiency. The right ventricular wall also is hypertrophied. *RV*, right ventricle; *RA*, right atrium; *LV*, left ventricle; *AO*, aorta; *LA*, left atrium.

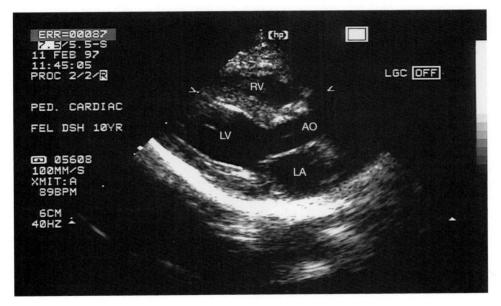

FIGURE 3.6   The base of the interventricular septum in normal cats tends to protrude into the left ventricular outflow tract slightly. *RV*, right ventricle; *LV*, left ventricle; *LA*, left atrium; *AO*, aorta.

humans, cats, or dogs (14,15).This suggests smaller left atrial size at birth and decreased atrial enlargement secondary to the ductus arteriosus.

The anterior mitral valve leaflet tips should almost touch the ventricular septum during diastole. The leaflet should extend straight out from the annulus. The leaflet should not have a convex or concave shape during diastole (Fig. 3.8). An abnormal shape during diastole could indicate decreased left ventricular ejection fraction, severe aortic insufficiency, or mitral stenosis. The valve itself should appear the same thickness throughout its length from the base of the leaflet, where it attaches near the aortic root, to its tip. This is assessed best during diastole when the valve is wide open,

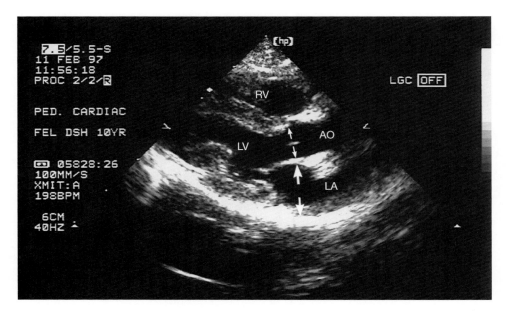

FIGURE 3.7 The left atrium (*large arrows*)in normal cats can be up to 1.6 times larger than the aorta (*small arrows*). *RV,* right ventricle; *LV,* left ventricle; *AO,* aorta; *LA,* left atrium.

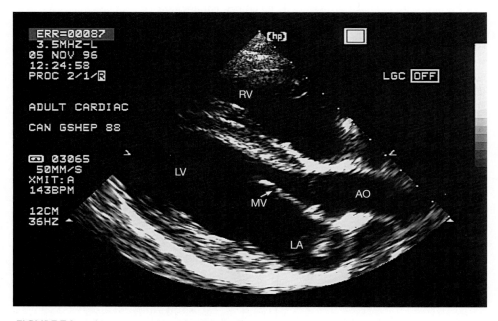

FIGURE 3.8 The anterior mitral valve leaflet should extend straight out to the ventricular septum during diastole with no bowing. *RV,* right ventricle ; *LV,* left ventricle; *AO,* aorta; *LA,* left atrium; *MV,* mitral valve.

Left Ventricular Outflow View Assessment (Horses)

- No bowing of the IVS
- IVS thicker than LVW
- RV wall approximately 1/2 thickness of LVW
- RV chamber size approximately 1/2 of LV chamber size
- LA smaller or the same size as AO
- MV excursion almost to IVS
- No valvular lesions
- Spontaneous contrast may be seen

and not during systole when the leaflet edges are touching each other and appearing thickened at their tips. Do not mistake chordae tendineae for lesions as they extend from the leaflets (Fig. 3.9).

Spontaneous contrast is seen within the right ventricular chamber and sometimes within the left ventricle of horses in all planes. This cloudlike swirling of visible intracardiac blood is reported in approximately 50% of horses examined echocardiographically and is considered a normal finding; however, it also is seen in horses with exercise-induced pulmonary hemorrhage (22). This contrast is especially prevalent in race horses, with a reported 93% occurrence. Increasing age, male gender, and pregnancy increase the occurrence of contrast. High heart rates increase the amount of contrast seen within these hearts (22).

The cloudlike echoes of circulating blood also have been reported in experimental healthy sedated dogs (23). Cloudlike echos are seen more readily with high-frequency transducers than low-frequency transducers in the same animal secondary to increases in both lateral and longitudinal resolution (23). The cloudlike echos have not been reported in clinically healthy dogs out of the research setting.

Right Parasternal Long-Axis Four-Chamber View.   Right ventricular chamber size appears slightly larger in right parasternal long-axis four-chamber views than in the right parasternal long-axis with outflow plane; however, the 1-to-3 relationship with the left ventricle should still predominate. The interventricular septum should extend straight to the apex of the heart from the mitral and tricuspid annuluses with only a slight deviation to the right at the septal base near the valvular annuluses (Figure 3.10).

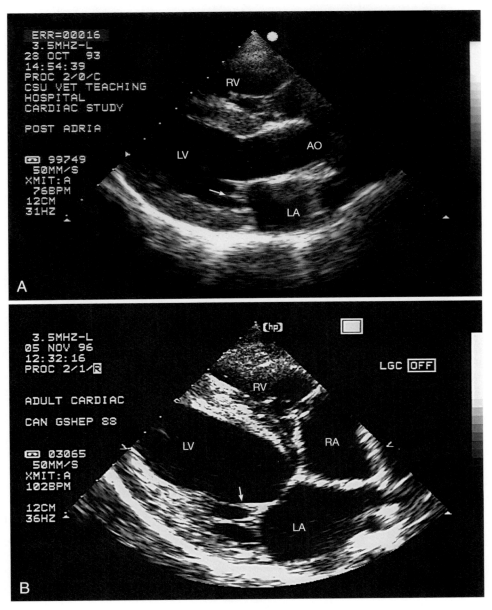

FIGURE 3.9   Chordae tendineae should not be mistaken for lesions when the mitral valves are closed (*arrow*) on both left ventricular outflow views (**A**) and four-chamber views (**B**). *RV,* right ventricle; *LV,* left ventricle; *AO,* aorta; *LA,* left atrium.

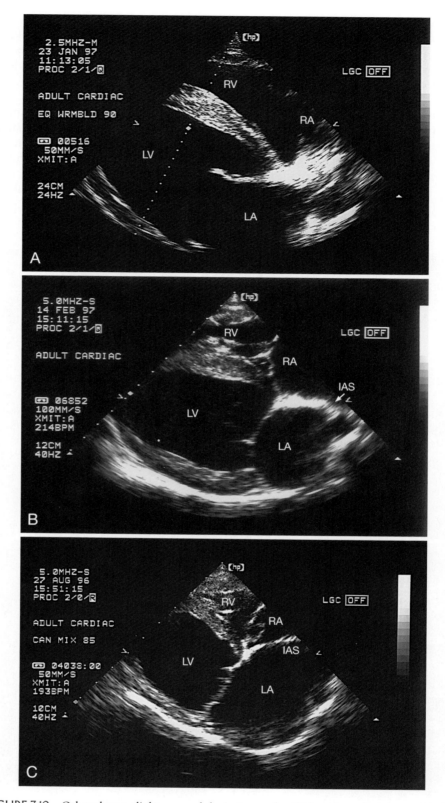

FIGURE 3.10   Other than a slight upward deviation at the AV junction, the interventricular septum should be straight with no bowing to the right or left on four-chamber views as seen in this horse (**A**) and this dog (**B**). The interatrial septum should also be straight with no deviation to the right or left. **C.** Bowing of the interventricular and interatrial septums to the right side of the heart is indicative of left ventricular and left atrial volume overload. *RV*, right ventricle; *RA*, right atrium; *LV*, left ventricle; *LA*, left atrium; *IAS*, interatrial septum.

The atrial septum also should be straight with no curvature to the right or left side of the heart. Often a thinner area of echoes exists midway along the atrial septum that at times appears as a defect (Fig. 3.11). This thin area of tissue is the membrane that closed the foramen ovale. The right atrium always appears smaller than the left atrium in this view. The tricuspid annulus is slightly closer to the apex of the heart than the mitral annulus by 1 to 2 mm. Right ventricular to left ventricular free-wall thickness ratios are often easier to visualize in this plane.

This four-chamber view of the heart is excellent for examining the atrioventricular valves. Valve thickness should remain the same from the base of the leaflet to the tip. The closed atrioventricular valve should have a slight convex shape with respect to the ventricle.

Right Parasternal Transverse Left Ventricle.

A good transverse view of the left ventricular chamber at the level of the papillary muscles should be round and symmetric. The papillary muscles should be similar in size and the septum should not be flattened. The left ventricular lumen should have a mushroom shape. Right-sided pressure or volume overload often flattens the septum, creating a triangular-shaped left ventricular chamber (Fig. 3.12). In small animals, the septum and free wall, excluding the papillary muscles, should be similar in size, whereas in horses, the septum is usually much thicker than the free wall. The right ventricular chamber should be crescent shaped in all animals. Cross sections of papillary muscles and irregularities on the right ventricular side of the septum are common and normal in this view (Figs 3.13, 3.14).

Right Parasternal Transverse Heart Base.

The aorta and pulmonary artery diameters at the level of their valves should be similar on right parasternal transverse images of the heart base (Fig. 3.15). Pulmonary artery enlargement may be seen with poststenotic dilations or volume overloads. The aorta and left atrium diameters in the dog also should be visually fairly close in size in this plane (Fig. 3.16). Pulmonic valves are not as bright as aortic valves and often have a slight upward curvature. The pulmonary artery diameter should not change from the level of the pulmonic valve to the bifurcation.

Four-Chamber View Assessment (All Animals)

- No bowing of the IAS or IVS
- No valvular lesions

Transverse Left Ventricle Assessment (Cats and Dogs)

- Uniform shortening
- Circular outer shape
- Mushroom LV internal shape
- Symmetric papillary muscles

Transverse Left Ventricle Assessment (Horses)

- Uniform shortening
- Triangular outer shape
- Triangular LV internal shape
- Symmetric papillary muscles

Transverse Heart Base Assessment (Dogs)

- Aorta and pulmonary artery similar in size
- Left atrium and aorta similar in size

Transverse Heart Base Assessment (Cats)

- Aorta and pulmonary artery similar in size
- Left atrium larger than aorta

Transverse Heart Base Assessment (Horses)

- Aorta and pulmonary artery similar in size
- Aorta clover shaped
- Left atrium smaller or the same size as aorta

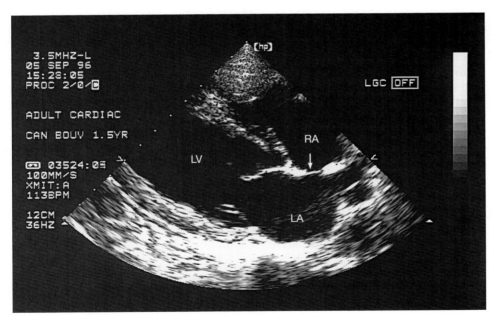

FIGURE 3.11   A thinner area of echogenicity midway along the atrial septum represents the membrane, which closed the foramen ovale (*arrow*). *RA*, right atrium; *LV*, left ventricle; *LA*, left atrium.

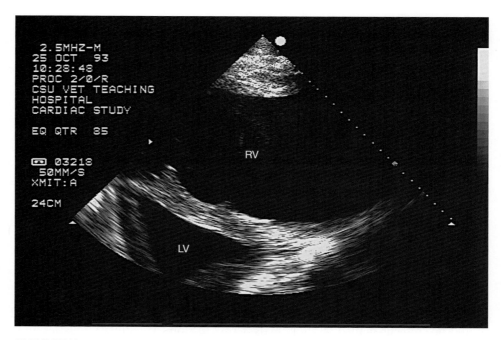

FIGURE 3.12   This horse's interventricular septum on the transverse plane is flattened and pushed toward the left ventricle, indicating elevated right ventricular diastolic pressure and volume overload. *RV,* right ventricle; *LV,* left ventricle.

Quantitative Assessment of Size

Two-dimensional measurements of size have been reported for the cat and dog (20,21). Instructions for measuring the various cardiac dimensions from two-dimensional images are described here and the reference values can be found in Appendix 4. Measurements from real-time images are a viable option when M-mode images are not of good diagnostic quality or the M-mode cursor cannot be aligned properly.

Measurements of cardiac size obtained from real-time images require freezing the image at end diastole and at end systole. End diastole is identified as the largest left ventricular dimension just before complete mitral valve closure. End systolic frames are identified as the smallest ventricular chamber size just before mitral valve opening. Measurements of chamber size are obtained from the endocardial surface of the ventricular septum to the endocardial surface of the left ventricular wall. This is called the trailing edge to leading edge method, which is slightly different from the leading edge method the American Society of Echocardiography (ASE) recommends. Left ventricular wall measurements are taken from the top of the wall, including the endocardial surface, to the top of the pericardial sac. Septal measurements, however, are taken from the trailing edge of the right side of the septum to the trailing edge of the left ventricular side of the septum. Measuring planes are similar for dogs and cats. The only exception involves measurement of the left ventricular wall, septal, and chamber sizes from the right parasternal long-axis view in the dog. The measurements in dogs were derived from images that do not have a well-defined aorta, whereas the measurements in cats were obtained from standard left ventricular outflow imaging planes (19,20).

Measurement

Left Ventricular Chamber, Wall, and Septum. Measurements of the minor dimension through the left ventricular chamber can be made from a right parasternal long-axis view, which includes part of the left ventricular outflow tract and aortic valve and the left atrium and mitral valve (Fig. 3.17). A line extending perpendicularly from the septum to the wall, just beyond the tips of the mitral valves when they

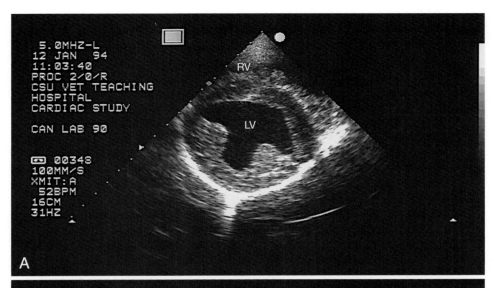

FIGURE 3.13   Both of these images show normal irregularities on the right ventricular side of the septum. *RV*, right ventricle; *LV*, left ventricle.

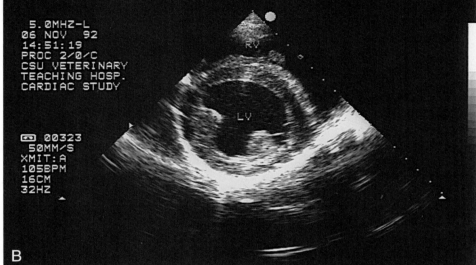

FIGURE 3.14   Right ventricular papillary muscles often are seen in cross section on transverse images of the left ventricle (*arrow*). *RV*, right ventricle; *LV*, left ventricle.

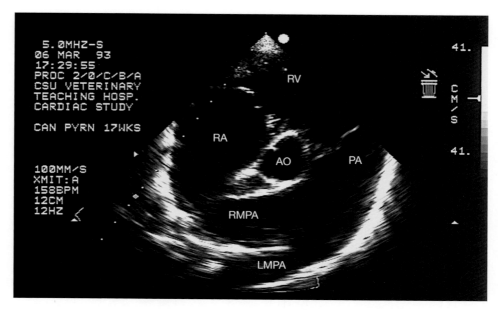

FIGURE 3.15 The pulmonary artery and aorta should have very similar dimensions on transverse images of the heart base. Here, the pulmonary artery is extremely dilated, and even the left main pulmonary artery is visualized easily. *RV,* right ventricle; *RA,* right atrium; *AO,* aorta; *PA,* pulmonary artery; *RMPA,* right main pulmonary artery; *LMPA,* left main pulmonary artery.

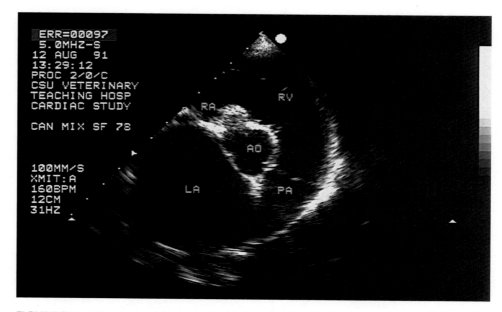

FIGURE 3.16 Diameters of the aorta and left atrium should be similar in size on transverse views. This dog with mitral insufficiency has a severely dilated left atrium. *RV,* right ventricle; *RA,* right atrium; *AO,* aorta; *PA,* pulmonary artery; *LA,* left atrium.

were wide open was used to identify the location for measuring the left ventricular minor diameter. The image is advanced until the largest and smallest chamber sizes corresponding to diastolic and systolic dimensions respectively are identified.

The minor chamber size also may be measured from the right parasternal short-axis view of the heart at the level of the chordae tendineae (Fig. 3.18). A line connecting the septum and wall, dividing the ventricle into equal and symmetric halves, is used to identify measuring points. The line should be perpendicular to a line connecting the chordae on each side of the image.

Wall and septal thicknesses are made from either imaging plane along the same lines that identified ventricular chamber dimensions. The trailing edge method is used for the septum and the leading edge method is used for the wall.

Left ventricular length is a measurement that does not have a corresponding M-mode parameter. This measurement may be obtained from the right parasternal long-axis four-chamber view or a modified right parasternal long-axis left ventricular outflow view where the left atrium is no longer visible and only a portion of the ascending aorta is seen. Both of these planes should clearly define the left ventricular apex. On the four-chamber plane, a line defining the mitral annulus is drawn (Fig. 3.19). The measurement of left ventricular length is made along a line connecting the apex to a point that bisects the annulus. On the modified view, two slightly different locations may be used to measure left ventricular length. A reference line defining the aortic annulus is drawn (Fig. 3.20). One measurement extends from the left ventricle apex to a point midway across the aortic valve. Another measurement can be taken along a line that extends from the apex to the point where the aortic valve and mitral valve meet.

Left parasternal apical four-chamber views also are used to measure left ventricular length (Fig. 3.21). A reference line is drawn along the ventricular side of the mitral annulus. The length is measured along a line extending from the apex to a point that bisects the reference line.

Aorta and Left Atrium.   Left atrial size is measured from the right parasternal long-axis four-chamber view (Fig. 3.19). A reference line connecting the mitral annulus is drawn on the atrial side of the valve. The anterior–posterior dimension of the left atrium is measured by drawing a line that bisects as closely as possible the

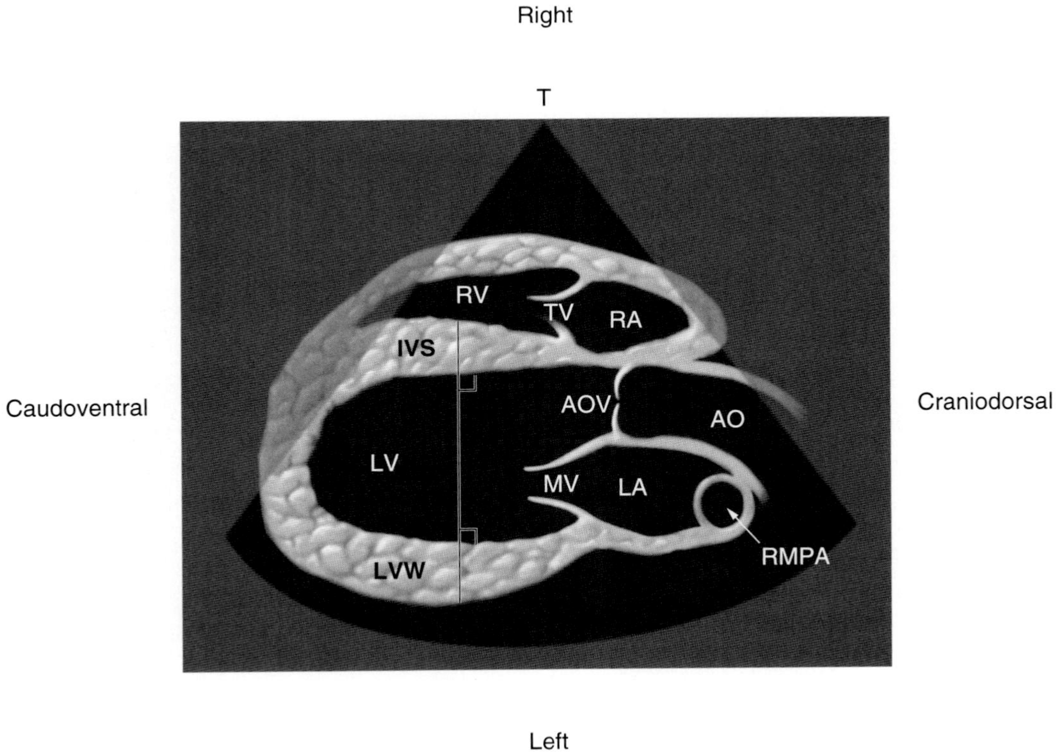

FIGURE 3.17   Measure the left ventricular chamber, septum, and wall from right parasternal long-axis left ventricular outflow views. At the tip of the mitral valves at their maximum extension into the ventricular chamber during diastole, a line is drawn perpendicular to the wall and septum. This line is used as the reference points for measurement both during diastole and systole. *RV*, right ventricle; *TV*, tricuspid valve; *RA*, right atrium; *IVS*, interventricular septum; *AOV*, aortic valve; *AO*, aorta; *MV*, mitral valve; *LA*, left atrium; *LVW*, left ventricular wall; *RMPA*, right main pulmonary artery.

atrium into equal halves and is parallel to the line defining the annulus. An apical–basilar dimension also may be measured on two-dimensional images. This is done by drawing a line perpendicular to the line defining the annulus and again dividing the atrium as closely as possible into equal halves (Fig. 3.19). The apical–basilar measurement extends from the base of the atrium to the reference line and not to the valve leaflets themselves.

The left atrium also may be measured on left parasternal apical four-chamber views, which maximize left atrial size (Fig. 3.21). This plane may be slightly different than the one used to measure left ventricular length because each chamber should be maximized for the parameter to be measured. A line connecting the mitral annulus on the atrial side is used as a reference for the other measuring points. The basal–apical measurement is made from a line that divides the atrium as closely as possible into equal halves and is perpendicular to the reference line. The basal–apical measurement starts at the base of the atrial septum and stops at the reference line. A lateral–medial measurement can also be made. This is done from a line that divides the atrium into equal halves and is parallel to the reference line at the annulus.

The area of the left atrium may be obtained from either of these planes (Fig. 3.22). Trace the endocardial surface of the left atrium along the inside of the mitral valves and exclude the pulmonary veins.

Aortic root measurements are made from a right parasternal long-axis view, which maximizes the aorta at the expense of the left atrium (Fig. 3.23). A well-defined aorta and valves should be seen. A line connecting the annulus is made and measured. In addition, the distance across the sinus of Valsalva is measured. The largest dimension is selected and is measured at a line parallel to the one defining the aortic annulus.

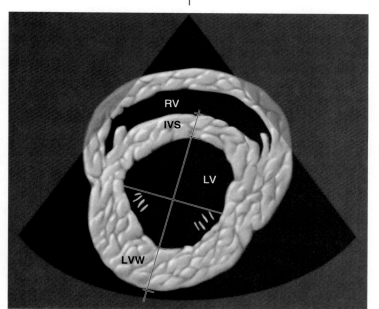

FIGURE 3.18 Left ventricular, septal, and wall dimensions also may be measured from transverse images at the level of the chordae tendineae. Using a reference line connecting the chordae on each side of the chamber, draw a line perpendicular to the reference line that bisects the ventricular cavity into symmetric and equal halves. Use this line as the reference points for measurement. *RV*, right ventricle; *IVS*, interventricular septum; *LV*, left ventricle; *LVW*, left ventricular wall.

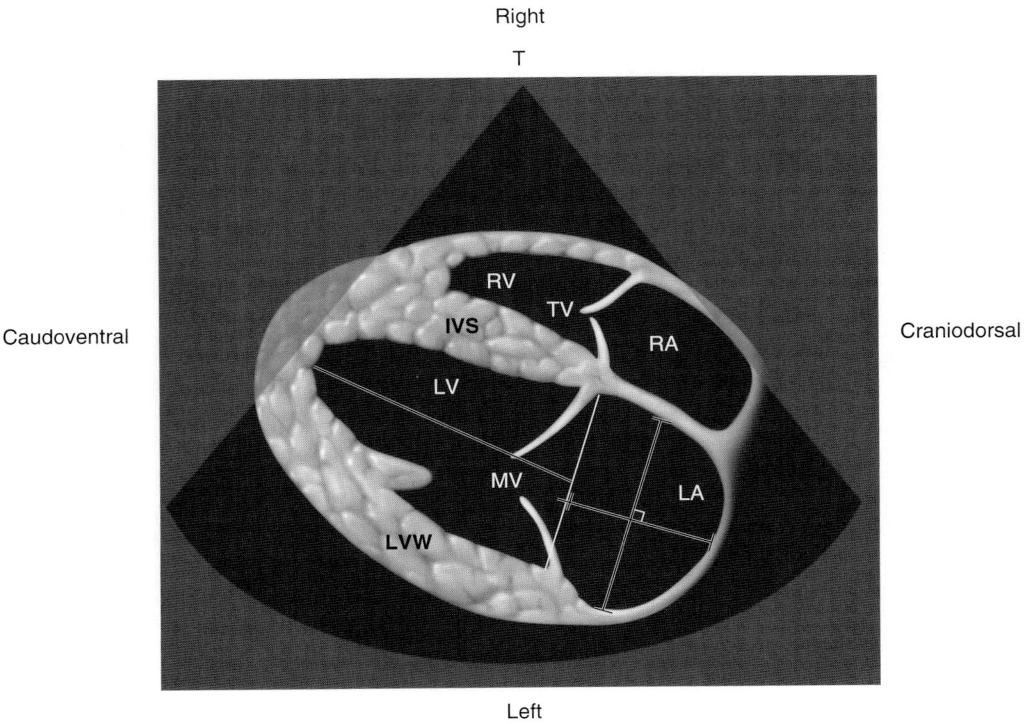

FIGURE 3.19   Right parasternal four-chamber views are used to measure ventricular length and atrial size. A line spanning the left atrial side of the mitral annulus is drawn for reference. Ventricular length is measured from the apex of the left ventricle to the midpoint of the reference line. Left atrial size is measured from anterior to posterior along a line parallel to the reference line that bisects the atrium as closely as possible into equal halves. An apical basilar measurement of the left atrium may be made along a line that is perpendicular to the reference line and also divides the atrium as closely as possible in half. *RV*, right atrium; *TV*, tricuspid valve; *RA*, right atrium; *LV*, left atrium; *MV*, mitral valve; *LA*, left atrium; *LVW*, left ventricular wall.

The left parasternal long-axis left ventricular outflow view also is used to measure aortic root size. The annulus is measured on the aortic side of the valve and this is also used as a reference line (Fig. 3.24). The sinus of Valsalva is measured at its largest dimension in a line parallel to the annulus, and the ascending aorta distal to the sinus also is measured. Divide the measurement of the sinus of Valsalva in half and measure the ascending aorta that is far away from the line that defined the measurement for the sinus.

Planimetry of the aorta is done on either the right or left parasternal transverse views of the aorta (Fig. 3.25). Trace along the internal surface of the aorta at the level of the aortic valve cusps.

Evaluation

Dogs.   All parameters of ventricular size correlate to body surface area (BSA). Left atrium to aorta ratios and wall thickness to chamber size ratios did not correlate with body size, nor did any parameter of function (21). The parameters of function are included in Appendix 4 and will be discussed in a later section specifically dedicated to function.

Systolic and diastolic dimensions derived from short-axis views are slightly greater than those obtained from long-axis views. However, the difference is not significant and the correlation between chamber sizes and wall thicknesses are high with correlation coefficients of .93 for diastolic dimensions, .88 for systolic dimensions, .95 for diastolic wall thickness, and .86 for systolic wall thickness. Septal

FIGURE 3.20 A right parasternal long-axis left ventricular outflow view, which is slightly modified so as not to visualize good mitral valves, is used to measure ventricular length. A line extending across the aortic valve is used for reference. Ventricular length may be measured along a line connecting the apex of the chamber to the midpoint of the aortic valves or to the aortic mitral valve junction. *RV*, right ventricle ; *TV*, tricuspid valve; *RA*, right atrium; *IVS*, interventricular septum; *AO*, aorta; *LA*, left atrium; *LV*, left ventricle; *LVW*, left ventricular wall.

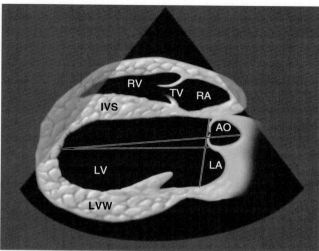

FIGURE 3.21 The left parasternal apical four-chamber view also may be used to measure ventricular length. A line extending from the apex to the midpoint of a reference line drawn on the ventricular side of the mitral annulus is used for measurement. *LV*, left ventricle; *RV*, right ventricle; *IVS*, interventricular septum; *MV*, mitral valve; *TV*, tricuspid valve; *LA*, left atrium; *RA*, right atrium; *IAS*, interatrial septum.

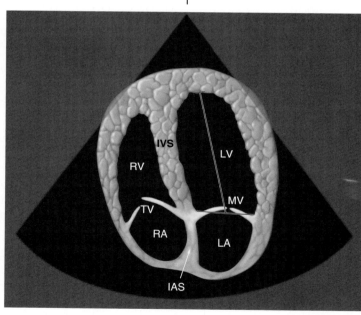

thicknesses also showed no significant differences between imaging planes but the correlation coefficients were slightly lower. There are also no significant differences between measurements taken from right or left parasternal imaging planes for the left atrium and aorta.

Ventricular lengths during diastole and systole showed no significant differences between any of the three measuring techniques on right parasternal images. The right parasternal images were much better than left parasternal images for measuring

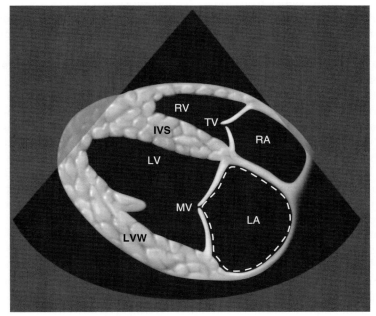

FIGURE 3.22 Left atrial area is measured by tracing the endocardial surface of the chamber from right parasternal four-chamber views or left parasternal apical four-chamber views. *RV,* right ventricle; *TV,* tricuspid valve; *RA,* right atrium; *IVS,* interventricular septum; *MV,* mitral valve; *LA,* left atrium; *LV,* left ventricle; *LVW,* left ventricular wall.

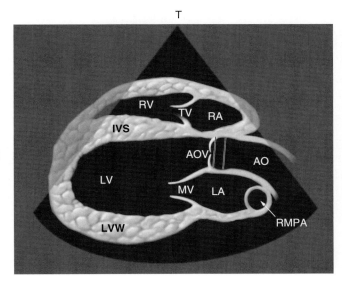

FIGURE 3.23 Aortic root size from right parasternal long-axis views are made at both the level of the valve and at the maximum distance across the sinus of Valsalva. *RV,* right ventricle; *TV,* tricuspid valve; *RA,* right atrium; *IVS,* interventricular septum; *AOV,* aortic valve; *AO,* aorta; *MV,* mitral valve; *LA,* left atrium; *LV,* left ventricle; *LVW,* left ventricular wall; *RMPA,* right main pulmonary artery.

length because the left parasternal images tended to foreshorten the ventricular chamber.

Cats.   Mean values from long-axis and short-axis planes are not significantly different. No significant correlation exists between body surface area or weight and parameters of cardiac size in the cat (20). This is because of the small range of weights within the adult cat population.

Two-dimensional measurements and M-mode measurements in cats have a close correlation, but the closest relationship appears between measurements taken from two-dimensional short-axis measurements and M-mode values (20). M-modes in the reported study, however, were not obtained with two-dimensional guidance.

Horses.   Two-dimensional measurements are available for the horse (24,25). One study validated the measurements for accuracy by postmortem echocardiographic measurement comparison (24). All values of echocardiographic size showed correlations greater than .87 with autopsy measurements. The second study found a significant correlation to body weight for the interventricular septum systolic thickness, aortic root dimension at end systole, and chordal lumen of the left ventricle at end systole (25).

Parameters were measured by the same methods as in the dog (21) in the following planes: right and left transverse planes of the left ventricle at the level of the papillary muscles and the chordae tendineae; left transverse images of the left ventricle at the level of the mitral valve and heart base with aorta; right-sided long-axis four-chamber; right-sided long-axis with left ventricular outflow; left-sided long-axis with left atrium and left ventricle; and left-sided long-axis with left ventricular outflow tract. This is sometimes the only way to measure some of the equine parameters, especially the left atrium.

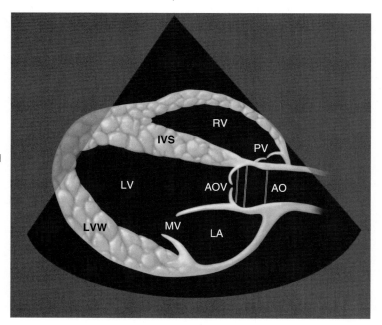

FIGURE 3.24   Left parasternal images of the left ventricular outflow tract also are used to measure the aorta. In addition to measuring the distance at the level of the valves and the sinus of Valsalva, the ascending aorta is measured at a point distant to the sinus and equal to half the measured size of the sinus. *RV,* right ventricle; *PV,* pulmonic valve; *IVS,* interventricular septum; *AOV,* aortic valve; *AO,* aorta; *MV,* mitral valve; *LA,* left atrium; *LV,* left ventricle; *LVW,* left ventricular wall.

Right

T

Dorsal

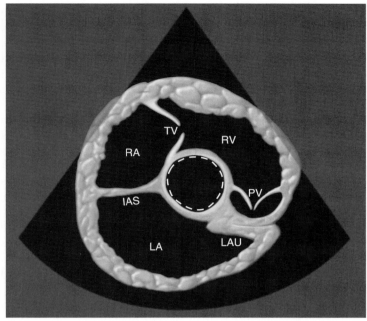

Ventral

TV

RV

RA

IAS

PV

LA

LAU

Left

FIGURE 3.25 Area calculation of the aortic root is made at the level of the valves on transverse images. *TV*, tricuspid valve; *RV*, right ventricle; *RA*, right atrium; *PV*, pulmonic valve; *IAS*, interatrial septum; *LA*, left atrium; *LAU*, left auricle.

Measurement and Application of M-mode Images

Basic Guidelines

The ASE sets recommendations for measurement of M-mode images in humans (26,27). The same guidelines are followed for veterinary species. The recommendations are not made because one location for measurement is necessarily better than another as far as predicting true cardiac size. The recommendations were made because they generated the least variability among human echocardiographs. The ASE recommends that all diastolic measurements be made at the onset of the QRS complex. Using the ECG for timing and measurement purposes assures consistency in measuring methods among examiners as well as provides greater accuracy in comparing measurements from serial examinations in the same patient. When an ECG is not recorded on the M-mode image, use the largest ventricular dimension for diastolic measurements. In humans, little difference is found between measurements made at the beginning of the QRS complex and those made at the largest ventricular dimension, except in children in which a greater increase in dimension exists at the very end of diastole.

The ASE also adheres to a measuring method referred to as the leading edge theory, which means that measurements are made from the leading or top edge of one structure to the leading edge of the next structure. This helps eliminate any variability in boundary thickness created by different ultrasound equipment as well as differences in gain settings, both of which may increase the perceived thickness of structures.

The ASE recommends that measurements be made at end respiration. Because no single measurement of wall or chamber size should be used, the effects of respiration have not been studied in veterinary medicine. At least three to five cardiac cycles should be used and averaged for each measurement. This should negate any effects of respiration and changes in filling secondary to sinus arrhythmias.

M-modes may be obtained and measured from long or short-axis views (6,20). Studies comparing M-mode values to real-time images found better correlation between measurements made from M-mode and measurements made from transverse left ventricular images; however, the M-modes were not obtained with real-time guidance (20). Carefully obtaining very specific sites and planes when placing the M-mode cursor over cardiac structures on either the long or short axis should yield similar values. Normal values have been generated using both methods. The goals when obtaining two-dimensional images for generating M-mode images is to maximize left ventricular size on long-axis left ventricular outflow views and to minimize it on transverse left ventricular views.

Some normal M-mode reference values are made within this section of text but complete reference tables for dogs (28–40), cats (18,19,28,41–49), horses (14–17,50–54), sheep (55), swine (56,57), llamas (58), and cows (59–62) are found in Appendix 4. All parameters of chamber size and wall thickness in the dog have a linear correlation with weight and body surface area. The correlation coefficients for these cardiac dimensions with weight or body surface area are similar. The difference in actual measurements is minimal with most predictions for normal ranges falling within 2 mm of each other when applying each method. To make data application easier in the adult dog, the Appendix includes charts with normal ranges for each parameter at each BSA. Weights corresponding to each BSA are included in the charts. Several breeds have been studied extensively enough to have their own normal reference values. Tables with values specific to the beagle (38), golden retriever (40), Afghan hound (40), Pembroke Welsh corgi (40), miniature poodle (40), greyhound (34,35), and English cocker spaniel (39) are available in Appendix 4.

Although a correlation exists between feline heart dimensions and body size, the correlation is weak because of the small degree of variation in weight. Values correlating the cardiac parameter to BSA or weight are not used. Instead, a single reference range for each variable is used for all cats (18,19,28,41–49).

Studies have attempted to correlate cardiac dimensions with weight, body surface area, and height in the horse, but the correlation is weak. Therefore, as in cats, a normal range for each parameter is used in all horses regardless of size or breed (14–17,50–54).

Cardiac dimensions obviously must increase as an animal grows. Several studies have been performed in foals, puppies, and calves that establish growth-related changes in cardiac dimensions and function as the animal grows (14,15,33,37,59–61). Only the left ventricular wall thickness increases with advancing age after the animal reaches maturity. All other parameters remain static during the aging process.

Several studies have been performed to determine the effects of heart rate and other variables on echocardiographic parameters of size. Inverse relationships exist for heart rate and weight, left ventricular systolic and diastolic dimensions, and left atrial size (18,30,31,44). The effect of heart rate on ventricular dimension is nominal.

The following discussions will emphasize technique for measuring M-mode echocardiograms. Important differences between breeds and species will be addressed and factors affecting the measurement will be discussed. Each individual M-mode measurement of size and function is just one piece of the puzzle and should not be used individually when making an echocardiographic interpretation. All the information should be put together and analyzed as a whole. The entire set of data should fit together logically. If some information does not fit logically, then technical error may be a factor; however, another cardiac problem may be present that has not been identified. Exercises included in this chapter show how to analyze the entire echocardiographic examination.

Left Ventricle

Measurement

Location.   Left ventricular measurements are obtained from real-time images with the cursor placed between the papillary muscles and the tips of the mitral valves (Fig. 2.91). This location is easier to locate on long-axis left ventricular outflow images. Maximize the length and width of the left ventricular chamber when using

---

Breeds with Their Own Reference Values

- Beagle
- Pembroke Welsh Corgi
- Afghan hound
- Greyhound
- Miniature poodle
- English cocker spaniel
- Golden retriever

Puppies with Their Own Reference Values

- Bullmastiff
- English pointer

M-Mode Measurement of the LV

- From Long Axis
  - left ventricular outflow view
  - maximize length and width of LV
- From Short Axis
  - level of chordae tendineae
  - smallest symmetric chamber

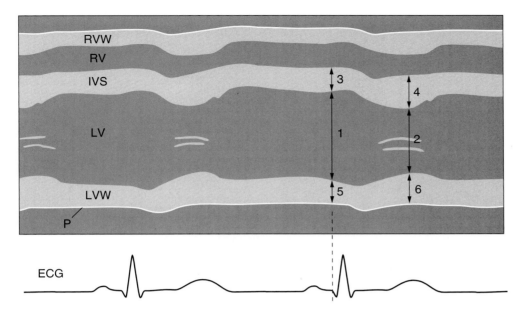

FIGURE 3.26 Measurement from left ventricular M-modes include the following: 1) left ventricular chamber during diastole; 2) left ventricular chamber during systole; 3) interventricular septum during diastole; 4) interventricular septum during systole; 5) left ventricular wall during diastole; and 6) left ventricular wall during systole. See the text and Appendix 4 for details. *RVW*, right ventricular wall; *RV*, right ventricle; *IVS*, interventricular septum; *LV*, left ventricle; *LVW*, left ventricular wall; *P*, pericardium.

the long-axis view. When using a transverse image, fan the transducer between the level of the papillary muscles and the mitral valves until good images of the chordae are obtained within a symmetric circular ventricular chamber. Obtain the smallest symmetric left ventricular chamber at the level of the chordae.

The M-mode image should show some chordae tendinea within the left ventricular chamber. In small animals like kittens and very young puppies, the relationship of mitral valve to papillary muscles is often much closer, and more mitral valve is recorded in M-modes of the left ventricle. The ASE recommends recording and measuring the left ventricle at the level of the mitral valve tips in young children and infants.

When left ventricular images do not allow perpendicular placement of the M-mode cursor to the septum and left ventricular free wall, more accurate measurements of size and function will be obtained from the two-dimensional image itself. This is best accomplished when a cine-loop is available, in which the image can be advanced frame by frame until the largest and smallest left ventricular dimensions can be frozen for measurements.

Although the ASE recommends measuring diastolic chamber dimensions at the beginning of the QRS complex, it recommends measuring systolic chamber size at the peak downward point of septal motion (Fig. 3.26). The free wall should be used when septal motion is abnormal. Measurements should be made straight up or down from whatever point is selected—do not move diagonally across the ventricular chamber from septum to wall. Diastolic and systolic left ventricular chamber sizes are taken from the left ventricular side of the septum to the top of the left ventricular free wall. The thickness of either the septum or wall is not included in chamber dimension measurements. Free wall and septal thicknesses are measured along the same lines that chamber dimensions are calculated. The interventricular septum is measured from the top of the septum to the bottom of the septum during both systole and diastole. Both the right and left ventricular boundaries are included in septal measurements. Left ventricular free wall measurements start at the top of the left ventricular wall and go down to the top of the bright line defining the pericardial sac.

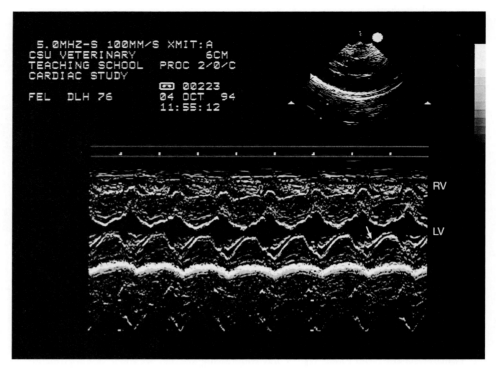

FIGURE 3.27   This represents an acceptable left ventricular M-mode image for measuring chamber dimensions. Some chordae are visible within the chamber (*arrow*). *RV,* right ventricle; *LV,* left ventricle.

Wall and septal excursion measurements are sometimes made from M-mode images. These measure the greatest distance the wall makes upward during systole and the septum makes downward during systole.

Figure 3.27 shows an appropriate M-mode image for measurement. Clear boundaries as well as chordae are present within the left ventricular chamber.

Measuring Pitfalls.   M-modes are easy to measure when the images are good; but during the learning phase when images are not optimum, there are several pitfalls to avoid. When images are not clear or you are not comfortable with the M-mode cursor angle through the heart, it is better not to make the measurement than to base a diagnosis on potentially erroneous information.

RESPIRATORY MOTION.   Breathing can create many artifactual motion abnormalities on the M-mode image. Figure 3.28 shows how wall and septal motions are altered secondary to respiration. This kind of motion is seen even if the animal is not panting. Placing a hand over the animal's nostrils momentarily while 3 or 4 cardiac cycles are recorded on the M-mode will usually eliminate this artifact.

DEFINING WALL AND SEPTAL BOUNDARIES.   The most common problem during measurement of left ventricular M-modes is defining septal and wall boundaries. The right ventricular side of the septum is the most difficult to define. Right ventricular hypertrophy, left ventricular dilation, or poor technique all contribute to ambiguity in identifying the right side of the septum. Hypertrophied right ventricles also result in hypertrophied papillary muscles and trabeculae within the right chamber (Fig. 3.3, 3.29). Care must be taken when obtaining the M-mode to identify and separate the right ventricular papillary muscle from the septum. This usually involves generating a long-axis real-time image that is positioned horizontally across the monitor. Sometimes looking carefully at the real-time image will allow identification of the true right side of the septum on M-mode images. When an M-mode has an ill-defined IVS, move the image into a more horizontal position across the monitor to define the septal boundaries better.

The left ventricular wall is usually easier to obtain on M-modes, but at times chordae tendineae or papillary muscles may create ambiguous measuring points. Chordae tendineae generally follow wall motion but have a slower upward rate of motion during systole. Figure 3.30 shows how chordae mistakenly may be included in wall thickness measurements if one doesn't look carefully at both the real-time image used to generate the M-mode and the details of the M-mode image itself. Papillary muscles appear as thickening above the free wall usually during systole, but sometimes throughout both phases of the cardiac cycle (Fig. 3.31). If wall thicknesses appear to be greater than septal thickness, and real-time images do not support this finding, papillary muscle is probably included in left ventricular wall thickness measurements. To eliminate the papillary muscles from the real-time image, elongate the left ventricular chamber by rotating the transducer or lifting the probe toward the table.

Assessment. The presence or absence of left ventricular volume overload is determined from diastolic dimensions. This measurement reflects maximum ventricular filling when the heart is relaxed. Systolic dimensions are a reflection of systolic function in the heart and should not be used to assess the presence or absence of dilation. The same principle applies to wall and septal thickness measurements. The presence or absence of hypertrophy should be determined from diastolic measurements of thickness. Systolic measurements are a reflection of systolic function, so increased thickness during systole may simply reflect increased function as opposed to hypertrophy. Hypertrophy does increase systolic thicknesses, but the effect of increased systolic function cannot be separated from the effects of hypertrophy. Specific application of these measurements will be made throughout the following chapters when the various cardiac disorders are discussed.

Right ventricular wall thickness and chamber size may be measured from left ventricular M-modes, but the measurements vary greatly because of varying right ventricular conformations between animals. Values are available, however, and may

---

Evaluation of Chamber Size
- Use diastolic LV dimension.

Assessment of Wall Thickness
- Use diastolic VS and LVW thicknesses.
- Use LVW to LVd ratio.

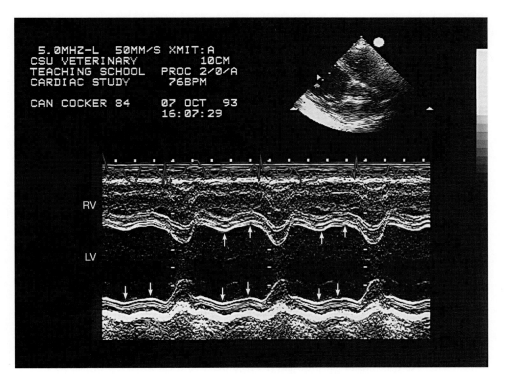

FIGURE 3.28 Respiratory motion causes artifactual wall and septal motion (*arrows*). *RV*, right ventricle; *LV*, left ventricle.

FIGURE 3.29 **A.** Papillary muscles within the right ventricle may create ambiguous definition of the right side of the septum. **B.** Hypertrophy of the septum or right ventricular wall also may make definition of the right side of the septum difficult.

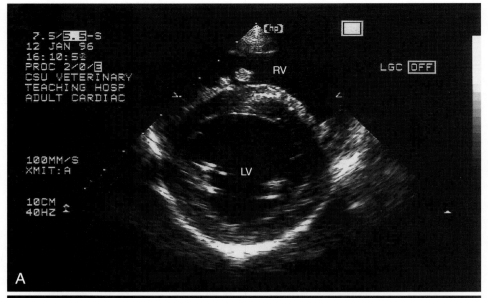

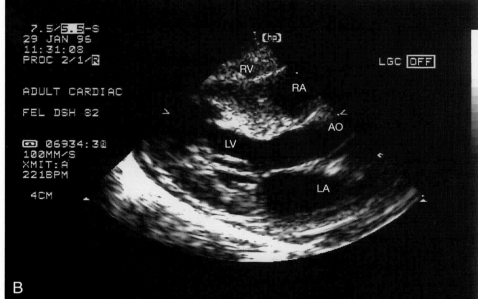

be found in Appendix 4. Measure the right ventricular wall and chamber sizes at the same point in the cardiac cycle in which left ventricular measurements are made. The leading edge theory of measurements is used.

The left ventricular diastolic chamber size to wall thickness ratio is used in humans to assess the extent of compensatory hypertrophy during disease processes (63). This assessment of wall thickness also has been done using the reverse ratio of wall thickness to chamber size (64). The normal heart will have a wall thickness that maintains normal systolic stress on the heart. As the ventricle dilates, wall thickness should increase to maintain normal systolic wall stress. Increases in chamber size to wall thickness relationships suggest inadequate hypertrophy, whereas decreases suggest excessive hypertrophy. In the presence of left ventricular volume overload, a normal ratio suggests appropriate compensatory hypertrophy. Dilated cardiomyopathies would show an abnormal ratio. Hearts with aortic stenosis or hypertension should have increased wall thickness to chamber size ratios; however, the hypertrophy is appropriate as a compensatory mechanism to deal with the high

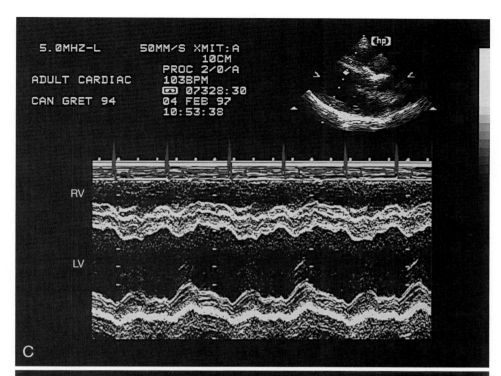

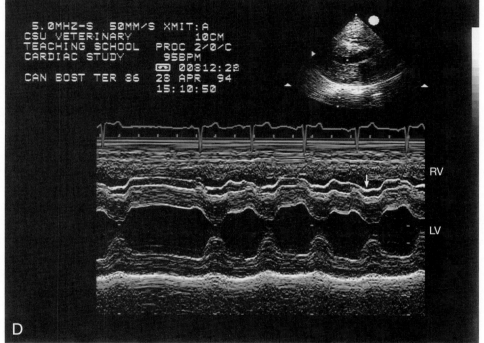

FIGURE 3.29 *(continued)* **C.** The right ventricular side of the septum is irregular and suggests that part of the tricuspid apparatus is included in the septal structures. **D.** The line on the right ventricular side of the septum (*arrow*) may be part of the septum or may be chordae. Look to the real-time image for help in defining the septal boundary. *RV*, right ventricle; *RA*, right atrium; *LV*, left ventricle; *AO*, aorta; *LA*, left atrium.

afterload. If no other pathology is present, the degree of hypertrophy often can be used to assess the severity of aortic stenosis when Doppler is not available to determine pressure gradients.

Several differences exist between species. In the dog and cat, the interventricular septum is slightly thicker than the free wall. The horse, however, has a much thicker septum than free wall. This difference is even more pronounced in dressage horses when compared to jumpers and untrained horses (17). The excessive septal thickness is no longer visible in endurance horses however (51,53). When these horses' hearts endure the stresses of exercise, the free wall has to deal with more stress because it is thinner than the septum and will hypertrophy accordingly until its thickness is comparable to the septum. These extremely fit horses also have increased ventricular chamber sizes caused by increased volume within the cardiac chamber and as a result of greater reserve for exercising periods.

Greyhounds have increased left ventricular dimensions and wall thicknesses compared to other dogs of the same weight (34). This difference exists whether the greyhound is a racing or nonracing animal. In humans, the effects of exercise on the heart regress after several weeks of not exercising. In greyhounds, however, the increased dimensions and hypertrophy persist despite a sedentary lifestyle. Generic values cannot be applied to the greyhound.

Measurements of wall and septal excursions are a reflection of volume changes within the ventricular chamber. Greater volume changes create greater wall and septal motion excursions than smaller volume changes. This measurement is not made routinely and its application is of limited use in diagnostics; however, they are supporting numbers when assessing the entire examination.

When the left ventricle is volume contracted for any reason, wall motion abnormalities become evident, which mimic cardiac disease. If ventricular size measurements are smaller than normal, and the animal is possibly dehydrated or has any reason to be in a volume-contracted state, repeat the echo examination after rehydration.

Left ventricular function is calculated from the measurements of left ventricular size during systole and diastole. This is discussed later in this chapter.

Mitral Valve

Measurement.   Before the advent of Doppler echocardiography, mitral valve M-modes were analyzed for rate of opening and closing as well as excursion distances. Normal ranges for these parameters were wide because the effects of heart rate and pressure differentials are very pronounced on how fast or slow the valve opens and closes. Two-dimensional and Doppler echocardiography provide greater accuracy in assessing valve movement as well as flow through the valve. Mitral valve M-modes are still valuable for detecting subtle movement alterations created by

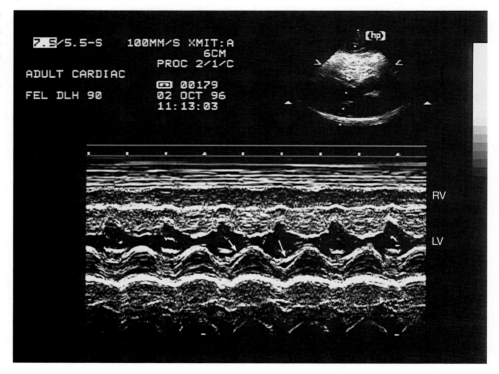

FIGURE 3.30 Chordae tendineae (*arrow*) mistakenly can be included in left ventricular wall measurements. Chordae generally have a slower rate of rise during systole and can be differentiated from the wall based on this slower motion. *RV,* right ventricle; *LV,* left ventricle.

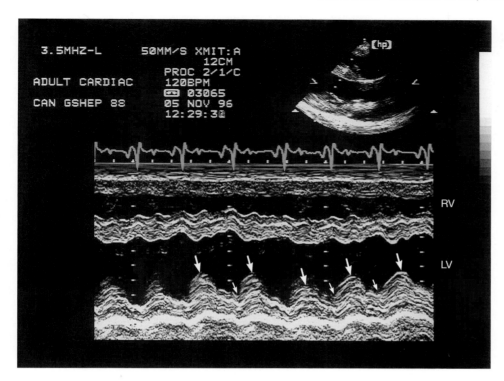

FIGURE 3.31 Papillary muscles appear as thickened areas along the top of the left ventricular wall. This is seen during systole and is discontinuous with the wall during diastole (*large arrows*). It also may be seen during diastole (*small arrow*) and mistakenly can be assessed as hypertrophy. *RV,* right ventricle; *LV,* left ventricle.

altered flow through and around the valve. Systolic anterior motion and diastolic flutter are two findings that are easily seen on M-mode images. In the absence of Doppler, M-mode images provide important hemodynamic information. They will be discussed in the following sections and chapters.

One consistent and popular mitral valve measurement is the E point to septal separation (EPSS) (Fig. 3.32). The EPSS is the shortest distance from the E point of the mitral valve to the ventricular septum.

Assessment.   The measurement is easy to make and is an indicator of left ventricular inflow and function. Cardiac pathology may increase, decrease, or not affect EPSS; but EPSS has strong negative correlation to ejection fraction in the absence of aortic and mitral insufficiencies (Fig. 3.33)(65). This correlation to ejection fraction is based on the fact that flow into the ventricle is equal to flow leaving the ventricle. In the presence of high end diastolic left ventricular pressures, such as in dilated cardiomyopathy, flow from the left atrium to the left ventricle is reduced secondary to reduced ventricular compliance. Consequently, flow out of the left ventricle also is reduced.

Studies in humans and dogs have shown that EPSS accurately separates normal from abnormal left ventricular function, regardless of left ventricular size when dilation is present (66). Hypertrophy, however, restricts valve motion and may decrease EPSS. EPSS is also valid for assessing left ventricular function in the presence of abnormal septal motion (67).

EPSS shows a very weak correlation to BSA and weight in some studies and no correlation in others; therefore, body size is generally not considered when assessing normal EPSS values. Although an inverse correlation of EPSS to heart rate has been shown in one study, another shows no effects of breed, age, sex, mass, or heart rate on EPSS (65). Any correlation is weak and is not significant enough to warrant adjustment of normal values for the animal's weight or heart rate.

Left Atrium and Aorta

Measurement.   The most common method of measuring the left atrium is on M-mode images at the largest left atrial dimension at end systole from the top of the

FIGURE 3.32   The only routinely measured parameter from mitral valve M-modes is the E point to septal separation (EPSS) (1). *RVW*, right ventricular wall; *RV*, right ventricle; *IVS*, interventricular septum; *LV*, left ventricle; *MV*, mitral valve; *LVW*, left ventricular wall; *A*, peak MV motion secondary to atrial contraction; *C*, point of MV closure; *D*, point of MV opening; *E*, maximum MV.

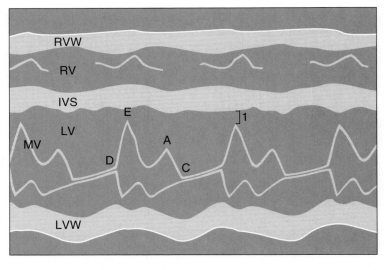

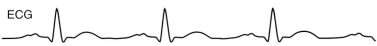

FIGURE 3.33   The large E point to septal separation (EPSS) (*arrows*) on this M-mode is indicative of poor cardiac output.

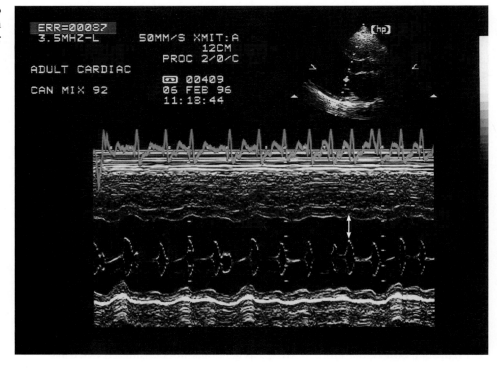

posterior aortic wall to the top of the pericardium (Fig. 3.34). Left atrial wall thickness is not recorded well, and the pericardium provides a consistent, easily visualized atrial boundary. Although the left atrium may enlarge in planes other than that recorded for M-mode images, it is a clinically useful indicator of left atrial size in dogs. The atria in cats tend to dilate in planes other than those used for this

M-mode measurement; therefore, the absence of dilation should not be based on this number alone. Two-dimensional measurements of left atrial size are more accurate in assessing atrial size.

The aorta is measured from the top of the anterior aortic wall to the top of the posterior wall at end diastole. Ideally, two aortic valve cusps should be seen to minimize angle problems; but if using two-dimensional echocardiography as an aid in deriving M-mode, two visible cusps are not as critical. Many normal values in animals have been generated with only one cusp visible on the M-mode echocardiogram.

Assessment.   A positive correlation exists between aorta and left atrial dimensions and weight and BSA in dogs and cats. Although specific values can be assessed, a ratio of left atrium to aortic root size may be used to indicate the severity of the atrial dilation. This is a reliable value because cardiac chambers usually maintain a fixed relationship with one another (68). It is important to assess aortic root size before using the ratio. A small aorta may be seen in animals with low output failure, and the left atrium to aortic root ratio will reflect greater left atrial enlargement than actually is present.

Left atrial size is similar to aortic root size in dogs (range LA/AO = 0.83–1.13). In cats, the left atrium may be much larger than the aorta (range LA/AO = 0.88–1.79). In horses, the left atrium is generally smaller than the aortic root (range LA/AO = 0.67–0.75). In neonate foals, left atrial size is larger than it is just hours later, after the ductus and foramen have closed. This trend is also seen in humans and presumably in other species as the volume load on the heart decreases (14). The aortic root size has been shown to be higher in endurance horses; whether this is secondary to increase ejection fraction is not known (53).

Measurement and Assessment of Spectral Doppler Flow

Doppler has dramatically increased the diagnostic capabilities of cardiac ultrasound. Its ability to provide information about direction, velocity, character, and timing of blood flow allows definitive diagnostics in most cardiac examinations.

Doppler information is scarce in animals, but most of what has been reported is similar to that seen in humans (69). Before values were available in dogs, human values were used as a reference, which were generally applicable. Several good

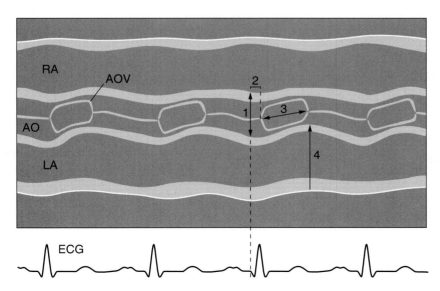

FIGURE 3.34   Measurements obtained from aortic root and left atrial M-modes include 1) the aorta, 2) the pre-ejection period, 3) the left ventricular ejection time, and 4) the left atrium. See the text or Appendix 4 for details. *RA,* right atrium; *AO,* aorta; *AOV,* aortic valve; *LA,* left atrium.

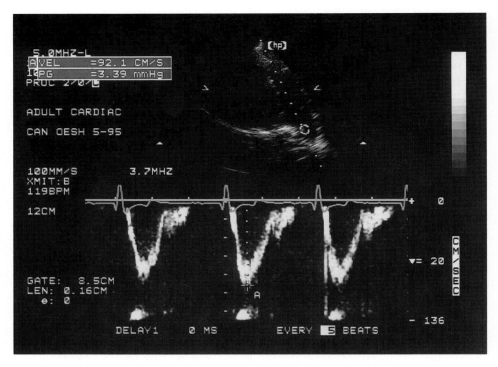

FIGURE 3.35   Peak velocity for aortic or pulmonary flow is made by identifying the maximum downward point. The peak velocity of pulmonary flow in this image is marked by point A and is calculated as 92.1 cm/sec.

reference articles have been published that review the principles of Doppler echocardiography and its uses in veterinary medicine (9,70–79). Although the measurements may appear intimidating, today's equipment performs all the calculations. Remember to interrogate multiple views when possible for all valvular flows because the imaging planes for best Doppler alignment varies from animal to animal. Following are directions for measurement and how to apply them.

Measurement

Peak and Mean Velocity.   Peak velocity is simply measured by placing a cursor at the apex of maximal upward or downward motion (Fig. 3.35). The velocity is measured automatically from the baseline to the cursor and may be displayed in cm/sec or m/sec. Tracing the flow profile provides a measure of mean velocity throughout the flow period (Fig. 3.36).

Flow Velocity Integral.   Flow velocity integrals (FVIs) are another component of flow that is directly proportional to stroke volume (79,80). The flow integral is calculated by tracing the flow profile with a trackball or joystick (Fig. 3.36). When the entire flow profile is traced, the FVI displays on the monitor in centimeters. The area under the flow velocity curve represents the distance a volume of blood travels; it will be used with the area of the vessel or valve the blood is flowing through to calculate stroke volume. Flow velocity integrals also are referred to as time velocity integrals (TVIs) or velocity time integrals (VTIs).

Systolic Time Intervals.   Acceleration and deceleration rates may be measured from flow profiles. The start of ejection needs to be marked, and peak velocity needs to be identified for the machine to determine the acceleration rate. The end of ejection and peak velocity needs to be identified to measure deceleration (Fig. 3.37).

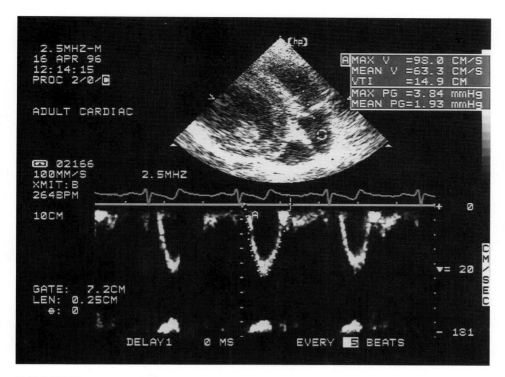

FIGURE 3.36   Tracing the aortic or pulmonary flow profile provides a measure of mean velocity (V) throughout systole. Here, mean velocity is calculated as 63.3 cm/sec. Peak velocity (MAX V) is measured automatically from flow traces as is the velocity time integral (VTI) of 14.9 cm.

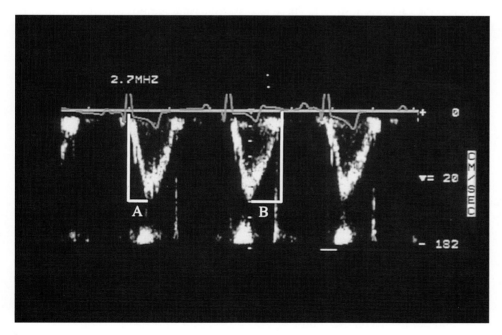

FIGURE 3.37   Acceleration rate is measured from the start of flow to the point of peak velocity (**A**), whereas deceleration rate is measured from the point of peak velocity to the end of flow (**B**). The equipment automatically will determine the rates. Time to peak flow (TTP) corresponds to the time interval represented by A.

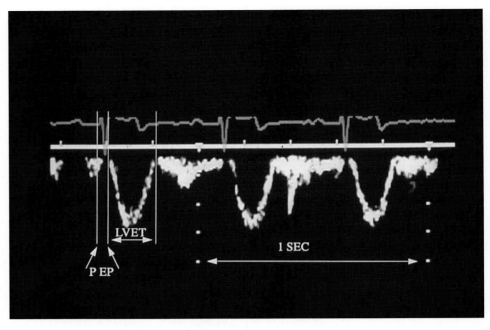

FIGURE 3.38 Systolic time intervals may be measured from pulmonary and aortic flow profiles. Pre-ejection period (PEP) is measured from the beginning of the QRS complex to the beginning of downward flow. Left ventricular ejection time (LVET) is measured from the start of downward flow to the end of flow.

Systolic time intervals also are measured from aortic and pulmonic flow profiles (Fig. 3.38) (75,80,81). Left ventricular ejection time (LVET) is measured from the onset of flow to the end of flow at the baseline. This is also called flow time (FT)(75). Time to peak flow (TTP) is measured from the onset of flow to the point of maximal velocity (Fig. 3.37) (75,80,81). These two systolic time periods are then divided to yield a variable that indicates the fraction of time spent in reaching maximal velocity (TTP/FT). Pre-ejection periods are measured from the onset of the QRS complex to the onset of systolic flow (75,80,81).

Evaluation

Little or no correlation exists between peak velocities for flow across the four valves and age, sex, or breed in the dog (75,80,82). Several studies have found that heart rate and weight affect flow velocities, whereas other studies have not (75,82–84). The studies that showed an effect of mass and heart rate on flow velocities revealed that decreases in mass and increases in heart rate increased flow velocities. This is discussed further in the following sections. The systolic time intervals will be discussed later in this chapter.

Aortic Flow. Aortic flow profiles are negative and have a rapid acceleration compared to the slower deceleration (71,74–83,85,86). This gives the normal aortic flow profile an asymmetric appearance. Peak velocity should be reached during the first third of systole. Dogs have a mean time interval of 55 msec from start of flow to peak, whereas in sheep, mean time to peak velocity is 50 msec. The ratio comparing the time it takes to reach peak velocity to the total time of flow is .30 in dogs and .23 in sheep (74,75,86).

Peak velocities obtained from PW and CW examinations are only slightly different. The discrepancy may be secondary to the Doppler angle (75). Most normal healthy dogs will not have aortic flow velocities exceeding 200 cm/sec. Flows above 250 cm/sec are considered normal, but flows that fall within the 200 to 250 cm/sec range are questionable. Other aspects of the echocardiographic examination will

---

Doppler Flow Profiles

- High velocity
  - = Increased volume
  - = Stenosis
- Low velocity
  - = Decreased stroke volume

Factors That Increase Doppler Flow Velocities

- Increasing HR
- Inspiration
- Decreasing weight
- Age, sex, and breed have no effect

have to be used to determine whether disease is present. Flow velocities are affected by heart rate. Increased heart rates will increase peak and mean velocities (75,82,86).

Doppler flow profiles are difficult to obtain in the horse primarily because of the large angles of incidence that are encountered. A study of 30 normal standard-bred horses had a range of 60 to 280 cm/sec with a mean of 101 ± 29 (80). The value of 280 was much higher than the rest of the population; the value closest to it was 170 cm/sec. In this study, it was postulated that the angle correction used during flow evaluation overestimated the velocity. Normally, Doppler cannot overestimate a velocity unless inaccurate angle correction is applied (80,86).

Pulmonary Flow.   Pulmonary flow profiles also are negative in all the views that can be obtained in the animal. The flow has a very symmetric profile with similar acceleration and deceleration rates (71,74,76–83,85,86). Often, it displays a rounded peak as opposed to the pointed peak velocity profile of aortic flow (75). Peak velocity is reached approximately halfway through ejection. The mean ratio of time to peak velocity to total ejection time is .43 in dogs and .42 in sheep (75,86).

Peak pulmonary flow velocity in the dog is typically less than 130 cm/sec, which is lower than peak aortic flow velocity because of lower resistance within the pulmonary system (74,75,81,82,86). It is interesting to note that this difference is not seen in horses (83). This was postulated to be secondary to erroneous flow velocity readings secondary to inaccurate angle correction. Pulmonary flow has a slightly longer ejection time and reduced pre-ejection period compared with aortic flow because of the reduced afterload (75,86).

Peak pulmonary flow velocity in the horse is reported as less than 700 cm/sec (80). Most of the population studied, however, had maximal flow velocities less than 160 cm/sec. This difference may again be an angle correction problem.

Respiration affects flow within the right side of the heart (74,75,80,81–83,86). Increased venous return during inspiration increases pulmonary flow velocities. Heart rate like aortic flow also affects maximal velocities. Faster heart rates in the dog increase velocities as faster heart rates do on the left side of the heart (75). There is also a mass effect on the right side of the heart. Increased mass decreases the mean velocity and is speculated to be secondary to decreased heart rate in larger dogs (75).

Mitral Valve Flow.   Mitral flow profiles in all planes are positive. When heart rates are slow enough, the profiles display the two phases of left ventricular filling. When heart rates exceed approximately 125, the two phases begin to overlap, and rates greater than 200 beats per minute show no separation of filling phases (75).

The E peak corresponding to rapid ventricular filling should have a higher velocity than the A peak in the normal heart. The E:A ratio is always greater than 1 in the dog, but both slow heart rates and high heart rates bring the E:A ratio closer to 1 (74,75,84). Increased flow associated with atrial contraction in animals with slow heart rates increases the A flow velocity, minimizing the difference in E and A velocities. Rapid heart rates decrease the E velocity secondary to decreased ventricular filling and increase flow associated with atrial contraction because of increased volume remaining within the atrium after the rapid filling phase. As opposed to dogs, the normal E:A ratio in sheep may be less than 1 with a mean value of 0.96 (86).

Tricuspid Valve Flow.   Tricuspid flow profiles are similar to mitral flow profiles in that there are two phases to ventricular filling and the profiles are always positive in the planes used for Doppler interrogation. However, tricuspid flow velocities are lower than mitral flow velocities probably because of the reduced pressure drop from right atrium to right ventricular when compared with the pressure drop from the left atrium to the left ventricular (74,75,80,86).

Peak tricuspid E velocities vary with respiration. Inspiration increases peak flow velocities and expiration decreases E flow velocities (75,86). The E:A ratio therefore increases with inspiration and decreases with expiration. The ratio can even be less than 1 under appropriate conditions in a normal heart, with ratios ranging from 0.69 to 3.08 in dogs, and from 0.75 to 1.91 in sheep (74,86). As with mitral inflow, rapid heart rates increase A velocities (75).

Evaluation of Color-Flow Doppler

Color-flow Doppler provides qualitative and semiquantitative flow information. Aliasing may not always be abnormal, and spectral Doppler usually is required to determine if flow velocity is truly high, turbulent, or reversed. Seeing insufficiencies at several valves is common. The leaks are trivial to mild and not hemodynamically significant. There are different opinions as to the definition of valvular insufficiency. The definitions vary from leaks that occupy the entire period of systole or diastole to reversed flow that occupies any amount of time during the time when the valve should be closed (80,87,88). The regurgitant jets in humans never extend more than 1 cm from the closed valves (89,90). These same insufficiencies are found in dogs; however, the timing and descriptions of the jets usually are not reported.

Pulmonic insufficiency is reported in 25 to 75% of normal dogs; aortic insufficiency is reported less often in approximately 10 to 11% of dogs; tricuspid insufficiency is reported in 50% of dogs; and mitral insufficiency is reported in 15% of dogs (Figs. 3.39, 3.40, 3.41, 3.42) (78,81,82,91). Combined aortic and pulmonic regurgitations are reported in only 4% of normal dogs; however, most studies have not looked for or reported combinations of insufficiencies (81). The incidence of these insignificant leaks varies greatly in humans and therefore probably also varies in animals (88,92). One study in beagles reported no dogs with tricuspid insufficiency (91). Kirberger found only insufficiency in mitral valves in a study of 50 beagles and German shepherds (74). Gaber found no incidence of mitral insufficiency in a study of 28 healthy normal dogs (78).

When spectral Doppler was used to interrogate the small regurgitant jets in beagles, the velocities were less than those seen with regurgitation secondary to

> Trivial to mild insufficiencies may be seen at all valves in normal animals.
> • The jets do not extend more than 1 cm past the annulus.

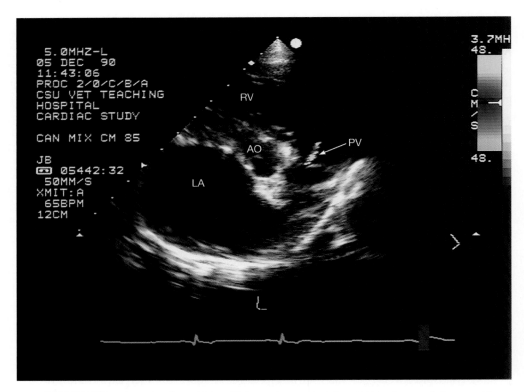

FIGURE 3.39   Trivial pulmonic insufficiency is seen in 25 to 75% of normal dogs and has a high incidence in horses as well. *RV,* right ventricle; *PV,* pulmonic valve; *AO,* aorta; *LA,* left atrium.

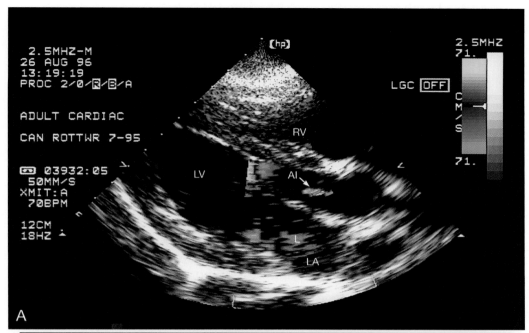

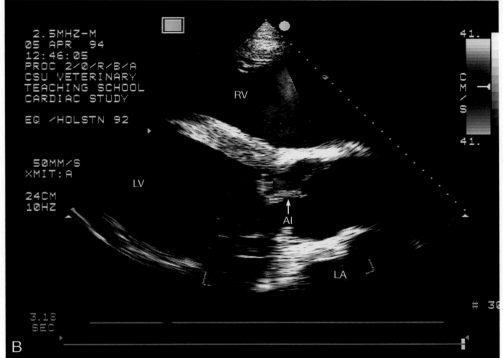

FIGURE 3.40   Trivial aortic insufficiencies are seen in 10 to 11% of dogs (**A**) and also are commonly seen in the horse (**B**). *RV*, right ventricle; *LV*, left ventricle; *AI*, aortic insufficiency; *LA*, left atrium.

pathology and less than would be expected from normal pressure gradients within the heart (91). Signal strength is also weak when interrogating these small jets (81,91). Usually no corresponding murmur exists to identify the presence of these clinically insignificant leaks (81,91). Pathologic regurgitation can be assessed semiquantitatively by measuring the size of the color-flow jet within the atria in the case of AV valvular insufficiency, or within the outflow tract or ventricle in the case of aortic or pulmonic insufficiency (93,94). Information on quantifying pathologic insufficiencies is presented in Chapter 4.

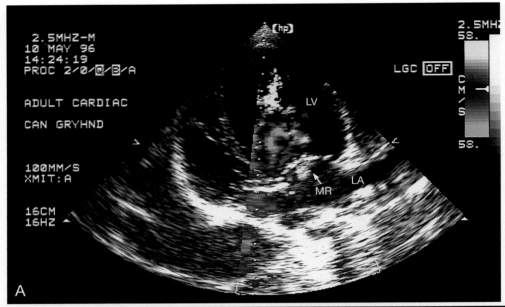

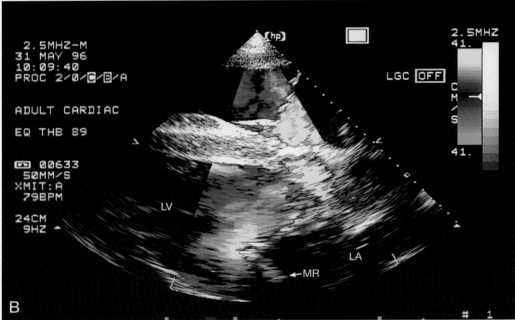

FIGURE 3.41   Fifteen percent of dogs (**A**) have trivial mitral regurgitation and a large number of horses (**B**) have these clinically insignificant leaks. *LV,* left ventricle; *LA,* left atrium; *MR,* mitral regurgitation.

Use color M-mode to help define the timing of color-flow patterns.

M-mode color can be performed during a color-flow examination. This helps separate the events of diastole and systole to time the color-flow information better. Figure 3.43 shows how color M-mode identifies both systolic and diastolic aliasing within the left ventricular outflow tract. This helps confirm the presence of a small amount of aortic insufficiency, which may have been missed otherwise.

LEFT VENTRICULAR FUNCTION

To understand the evaluation and application of function, a brief overview of systolic and diastolic function is included in the following sections. Many good resources exist for more in-depth information about systolic and diastolic cardiac

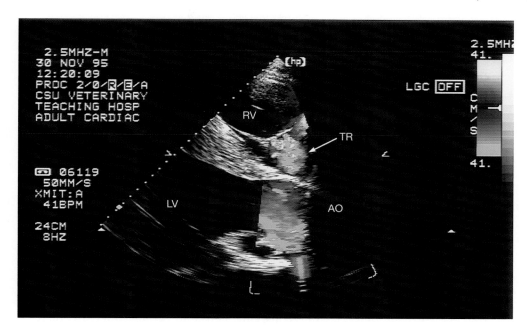

FIGURE 3.42   Tricuspid insufficiency is reported in as much as 50% of normal healthy dogs and also has a high incidence in normal horses as seen in this image. *RV*, right ventricle; *LV*, left ventricle; *AO*, aorta; *TR*, tricuspid regurgitation.

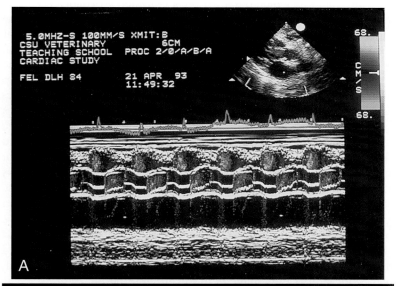

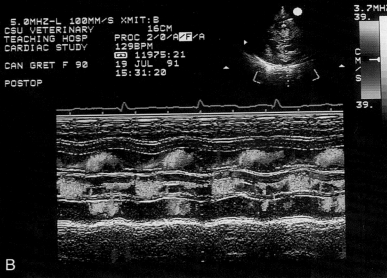

FIGURE 3.43   Timing of systolic and diastolic color-flow Doppler can be identified easily by using color-flow M-mode images. **A.** Normal color-flow M-mode shows a nonaliased red signal during systole within the aortic valve on this aortic M-mode image. **B.** Aortic insufficiency and aortic stenosis are displayed as aliased color mapping during systole and diastole on this aortic root M-mode image. *RA*, right atrium; *AO*, aorta; *LA*, left atrium.

function (64,95–102). The addition of Doppler echocardiography to the ultrasound examination allows assessment of cardiac hemodynamics and intracardiac pressures.

Systolic Function

An adequate amount of blood must be pumped out of the heart with every beat to perfuse the peripheral tissues and meet the metabolic needs of the body. The pumping ability or systolic function of the heart depends on several factors including the following: preload, afterload, contractility, distensibility, coordinated contraction, and heart rate. Systolic dysfunction is characterized by impaired pumping ability and reduced ejection fraction.

Abnormalities involving coordinated contraction are primarily the result of myocardial infarctions. Although myocardial infarctions are recognized more often in animals because echocardiography plays a more important role in the diagnostic work-up of potential cardiac patients, its effects on systolic function will not be considered in this discussion.

Preload is the force stretching the myocardium and depends on the amount of blood distending the left ventricle at end diastole. Starling's law states that the greater the stretch, the greater the force of contraction. Increases in left ventricular diastolic volume, with all other factors remaining constant, would therefore increase ventricular systolic function.

Afterload is the force against which the heart must contract. Normally, the heart will hypertrophy in response to increases in preload to normalize wall stress. The type of hypertrophy pattern seen in response to increased preload is eccentric, in that wall thickness or overall left ventricular mass increases in response to the volume increase. In the absence of hypertrophy, afterload is increased within the volume overloaded left ventricle. The peripheral pressure that the left ventricle must pump against also is afterload. Increased systemic pressure, vasoconstriction, and obstructions to left ventricular outflow therefore also will elevate afterload. These increases in afterload may be seen with hypertrophic obstructive cardiomyopathy, aortic stenosis, or systemic hypertension. The hypertrophy pattern seen with increased afterload secondary to outflow obstruction or systemic hypertension is concentric, in which wall thicknesses increase with no increase in volume, and if the afterload is severe, hypertrophy is at the expense of chamber size. Increases in afterload decrease the ability of the heart to contract effectively when all other factors are kept constant.

Contractility depends on mechanisms within the myocardial cell. These involve the contractile proteins (actin and myosin), transport mechanisms for calcium, and regulatory proteins (troponin and tropomyosin). Distinguishing between increased afterload and decreased contractility is difficult when cardiac function is impaired; however, Doppler echocardiography may aid in this differentiation.

Cardiac output can be calculated by multiplying heart rate and stroke volume. Increases in heart rate with no other changes will result in greater cardiac output. The body regulates heart rate to meet the metabolic demands of its tissues. Very high heart rates, however, can be detrimental to the heart itself and may induce myocardial failure.

M-mode Evaluation of Systolic Function

Fractional Shortening

Measurement.   Left ventricular fractional shortening (FS) is the most common measurement of left ventricular function. It is calculated by subtracting left ventricular systolic dimension from the diastolic dimension and dividing by the diastolic dimension to calculate a percent change in left ventricular size between filling and emptying. The equation is as follows:

Fractional shortening is NOT a measure of contractility.

$$FS = \frac{LVd - LVs}{LVd} \times 100$$

where LVd = left ventricular diastolic dimension and LVs = left ventricular systolic dimension. Once the points are identified on a frozen image on the ultrasound monitor, internal calculations automatically will display the FS.

Assessment.   It is important to remember that fractional shortening is not a measure of contractility but is a measure of function. The three conditions that affect fractional shortening the most are preload, afterload, and contractility. Each one of these may individually or together affect the FS.

When a low fractional shortening is calculated, it may be secondary to poor preload, increased afterload, or decreased contractility. Increased preload, on the other hand, tends to increase function as does decreased afterload (Fig. 3.44).

Although the preceding factors may be hard to differentiate, the M-mode size measurements and the Doppler flow analysis often aid in the determination. Increased left ventricular diastolic size suggests that decreased preload is not a factor when poor FS is seen, whereas decreased LV diastolic chamber size is either an indication of poor preload or increased afterload if wall and septal hypertrophy are present (Fig. 3.45). Hypertrophy that exceeds the normal ratio for chamber size to wall thickness is consistent with increased afterload or significantly decreased preload, which creates the appearance of hypertrophy simply due to a lack of distension.

Exercises involving measurements of size and function are found at the end of the chapter. The effects of preload, afterload, and contractility are evaluated in each of these cases.

Fractional shortening is not correlated to body surface area or weight; therefore, a range of values may be applied to all animals (14,15,17–19,21,28,31–33,35–51,53,57,59–62).

Volume, Ejection Fraction, and Cardiac Output.   The measurement of volume from M-mode echocardiographic images is not always applicable. Although many equations for volume measurement exist, all are reliable measures of volume in the

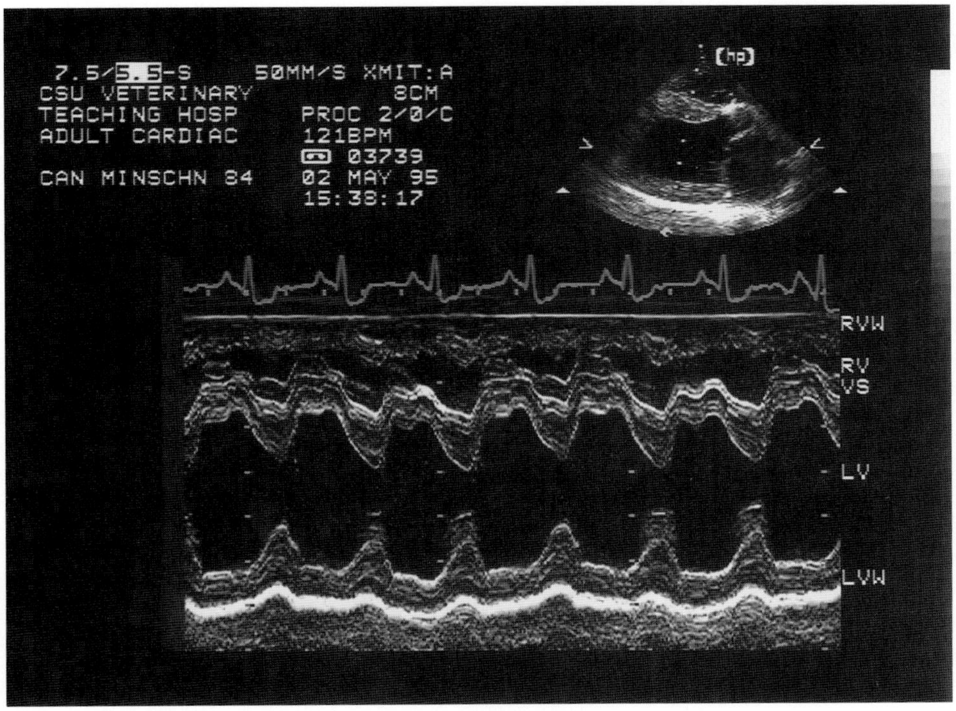

Factors Affecting FS
- Preload
- Afterload
- Contractility

- ↑ preload = ↑ FS
- ↓ preload = ↓ FS

- ↑ afterload = ↓ FS
- ↓ afterload = ↑ FS

FIGURE 3.44   Increased preload increases the fractional shortening in a heart that does not have myocardial dysfunction. *RVW*, right ventricular wall; *RV*, right ventricle; *VS*, ventricular septum; *LV*, left ventricle; *LVW*, left ventricular wall.

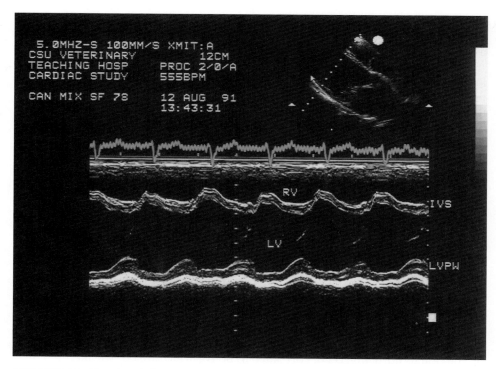

FIGURE 3.45 Fractional shortening in this heart is low normal, and in the presence of the volume overload, this suggests that the myocardium is failing. High afterload also may decrease fractional shortening. *RV*, right ventricle; *IVS*, interventricular septum; *LV*, left ventricle; *LVPW*, left ventricular wall.

normal heart in humans, and several have been shown to be valid in dogs and horses as well. The problem with most of these equations, however, is that they are not always applicable in the diseased heart. Two-dimensional assessment of volume and output is more accurate, but is also more time consuming. The ASE has listed recommendations for determining left ventricular volume and cardiac output in humans (103). Two-dimensional echocardiography is recommended because of the limited view of the heart in M-mode views. The one dimension may not be representative of the left ventricular chamber as a whole, which is clearly a more important factor in humans in which ischemic heart disease may distort the chamber configuration dramatically. Many studies in humans, however, have shown good comparisons between volume measured noninvasively and volume measured by applying the Teicholz equation to the LV M-mode image (104,105).

Several studies in dogs show a high correlation between M-mode–derived volumes and cardiac output when using the Teicholz method (106,107). The Teicholz equation is based on the assumption that the left ventricular chamber is an ellipse. The equation is as follows:

$$\text{LV diastolic volume (LVVd)} = \frac{(7 \times (\text{LVd})^3)}{(2.4 + \text{LVd})}$$

$$\text{LV systolic volume (LVVs)} = \frac{(7 \times (\text{LVs})^3)}{(2.4 + \text{LVs})}$$

$$\text{LV stroke volume (SV)} = \text{LVVd} - \text{LVVs}$$

$$\text{LV ejection fraction (EF)} = \frac{\text{LVVd} - \text{LVVs}}{\text{LVVd}} \times 100$$

Correlation coefficients for deriving volume with this formula from the M-mode left ventricular image were high at 0.93 and 0.87 (106,107). Uehara found a better correlation when using M-modes derived from transverse left ventricular real-time images as opposed to long-axis views. It is postulated that this view is easier to obtain and that the M-mode cursor also is easier to place correctly on this view. The inexperienced sonographer will undoubtedly find it easier and, therefore, more accurate to obtain the M-mode images from transverse planes.

These same results are not found in cats however (108). Although correlations using the Teicholz equation are not terrible under resting conditions with the cat under anesthesia (r = 0.89), when varying drugs were used to enhance or diminish cardiac output, the correlation diminished considerably to 0.71 and 0.84 respectively. The small dimensions of the feline heart provided little room for error and probably plays a role in these results.

M-mode volume calculations in the horse have shown that a cube method, which uses the M-mode measured diameter of the left ventricular chamber, is quite accurate (r^2 = 0.94) and easy to use in in vitro studies (109). When ventricular length was derived from a ratio as seen in the following equation, the correlation decreased slightly to 0.90. Values were just slightly less accurate than those that used two-dimensional methods. The equation used is as follows:

$$LVVd = \frac{\pi L \, (LVd)^3}{6}$$

$$LVVs = \frac{\pi L \, (LVs)^3}{6}$$

where L = ventricular length. Length may be obtained from the real-time long-axis image and measured from apex to mitral annulus. Or length may be calculated as a ratio of diameter to length developed from in vitro studies. The length is derived as follows:

$$Ld = 1.46 \, LVd$$

$$Ls = 1.46 \, LVs$$

where Ld and Ls = left ventricular length during diastole and systole respectively. Ejection fractions are calculated as shown previously for the dog.

Systolic Time Intervals

Measurement.   The images are not always easy to obtain; however, once a good aortic valve, left ventricular chamber, and associated electrocardiogram are obtained, systolic time intervals are easy to measure from M-mode images (78,81,82,91). Systolic time intervals reflect systolic function. M-mode systolic time intervals include the following: left ventricular ejection time (LVET); left ventricular pre-ejection period (PEP); velocity of circumferential shortening (Vcf); and left ventricular ejection time to pre-ejection time ratio (LVET/PEP).

The left ventricular ejection time requires measurement of the aortic valve from the time it opens to the time it closes (Fig. 3.34). A perfect aortic valve is not required, but clear definition of when it opens and when it closes is necessary.

Pre-ejection periods can only be measured when an electrocardiogram is used in conjunction with the echocardiogram. The measurement is made from the beginning of the QRS complex to where the aortic valve opens (Fig. 3.34). This period corresponds to isovolumic contraction where both the aortic and mitral valves are open and the ventricle is building up enough pressure to open the aortic valves.

A ratio of PEP to LVET often is calculated to reduce the effects of heart rate on LVET. This is a more accurate indicator of left ventricular function.

Velocity of circumferential fiber shortening is a calculation that incorporates the ejection time into the fractional shortening equation. This is a measure of how fast the left ventricle shortens and is calculated as follows:

$$Vcf = \frac{(LVd - LVs)}{(LVd \times LVET)}$$

where LVET is measured in seconds and chamber sizes are measured in centimeters.

Heart rate affects LVET, but the effect is minimized by normalizing the interval. The heart rate is multiplied by the slope of the regression line for heart rate versus the

LVET; this value is added to the measured LVET (110). This allows LVET to be extrapolated to a heart rate of zero. The slope for heart rate versus LVET is 0.55, and the resulting equation for heart-rate-corrected LVET, or left ventricular ejection time index (LVETI) is as follows:

$$LVETI = LVET + (0.55 \times HR)$$

Heart rate should be measured from the R to R interval on the beat preceding the measured LVET. Vcf may be divided by heart rate and multiplied by 100 to reduce the effects of rate on this systolic time interval. Because of the strong effect of heart rate on systolic time intervals, several beats should be measured and averaged. In animals with atrial fibrillation or marked sinus arrhythmia, many beats should be measured—more than 10 is recommended (110). Time intervals measured from the longest cardiac cycle are the most accurate indicators of left ventricular function when heart rates are variable (110,112). Avoid measuring during ventricular or supraventricular premature complexes or during the beats that follow them (110).

Evaluation.   Systolic time intervals (STI) are often better indicators of left ventricular systolic function than fractional shortening and are as accurate as invasive methodology in humans for assessing left ventricular performance (110,113,114). Just as with fractional shortening, the STI are not indicators of contractility, but rather function in general. STI are affected by preload, afterload, and contractility. In general, decreased preload will increase PEP, decrease LVET, and increase PEP/LVET (110,112–114). Increases in preload tend to shorten PEP, increase LVET, and decrease PEP/LVET (110,112–114). Afterload reduction will decrease PEP, increase LVET, decrease PEP/LVET, and increase Vcf (110,112–114). Increases in afterload tend to increase PEP, increase LVET, and decrease Vcf (110,112–114).

These do not need to be complicated to remember. When afterload is increased, the workload is increased on the heart, and as a result, the time that it takes to generate enough pressure within the left ventricle before the aortic valves can open will be longer. This time corresponds to the pre-ejection period. The rate at which the heart can contract in the face of high afterload also is reduced; this corresponds to Vcf, which is decreased when afterload is high. Decreases in afterload, however, allow the left ventricle to function with greater ease, and the force necessary to open the aortic valves is reached sooner, resulting in decreased PEP. The rate at which the heart can contract is also faster when the workload is reduced and Vcf is increased.

Changes in preload can be approached the same way. High preload or volume within the left ventricle allows the Frank Starling mechanism to come into play as fibers are elongated and function is enhanced. This shortens PEP, and increases LVET. Decreased preload, however, does not allow enough force to be generated by fibers that are not at optimum length and therefore PEP is increased. By the same token, volume within the left ventricle affects LVET, and a reduction in volume and force of contraction will decrease LVET. Table 3.1 summarizes this information.

Many applications exist for systolic time intervals within the diseased heart as listed in Table 3.2. There are limitations to their use, however, because heart rate and loading conditions do affect these applications significantly (110). Contractility can

TABLE 3.1
THE EFFECTS OF PRELOAD, AFTERLOAD, AND HEART RATE ON SYSTOLIC TIME INTERVALS

	PEP	LVET	PEP/LVET	Vcf
↑ Preload	↓	↑	↓	
↓ Preload	↑	↓	↑	
↑ Afterload	↑	↑		↓
↓ Afterload	↓	↑	↓	↑
↓ Heart rate		↑	↓	↓
↑ Heart rate		↓	↑	↑

↑, increase or lengthen; ↓, decrease or shorten.

Data from Atkins CE, Snyder PS. Systolic time intervals and their derivatives for evaluation of cardiac function. J Vet Intern Med 1992; 6:55.

TABLE 3.2
THE EFFECTS OF CARDIAC DISEASE ON SYSTOLIC TIME INTERVALS

	PEP	LVET	PEP/LVET	Vcf
Dilated cardiomyopathy	↑	↓	↑	↓
Mitral insufficiency	↑	↓	↑	–
Aortic stenosis	↓	↑	↓	–
Ventricular septal defect	↑	↓	↑	–
Right heart failure	↑	↓	↑	–

PEP, pre-ejection period; *LVET*, left ventricular ejection time; *Vcf*, velocity of circumferential shortening; ↑, increase or lengthen; ↓, decrease or shorten.

Data from Atkins CE, Snyder PS. Systolic time intervals and their derivatives for evaluation of cardiac function. J Vet Intern Med 1992; 6:55.

not be evaluated accurately without first analyzing the effects of preload and afterload on the individual heart. Doppler echocardiography has aided in this evaluation by allowing afterload assessment in some cases.

Two-Dimensional Measurement of Systolic Function

Volume, Ejection Fraction, and Cardiac Output.   Volume determination using two-dimensional echocardiography is a labor-intensive process that requires precise identification of left ventricular planes and evaluation through at least five cardiac cycles. Although volume determination is not a calculation that is done routinely during a clinical examination, it is used in research, and is briefly described here. Formulas are used that determine the ventricular volume at end diastole and end systole. A percent change is then calculated that equals the ejection fraction.

Whereas M-mode methods of volume determination sometimes have a poor correlation with more invasive methods of volume determination and may not be clinically useful in the setting of heart disease, volume determination using two-dimensional echocardiographic images is accurate in normal human hearts (103,108,115). These two-dimensional equations are based on the fact that the left ventricle forms an ellipse when normal. The modified Simpson's rule, which is recommended by the ASE, is the most commonly used formula for volume determination in humans (103). This formula shows the best correlation with actual left ventricular volumes in the diseased heart and appears relatively unaffected by changes in ventricular geometry. Even if volume is not accurate in some diseased hearts, the calculation may be used in an individual to follow progression or regression of left ventricular size. It should also be noted that ejection fraction does not imply forward stroke volume. Ejection fraction is a measure of volume leaving the left ventricle regardless of whether it flows through the aorta, a shunt, or the mitral valve. Planes used in volume calculations are frozen at end diastole and end systole. An end diastolic frame is defined as the frame just before the mitral valves close or the first frame that shows the QRS complex. An end systolic frame is identified as the frame just before the mitral valve opens.

The modified Simpson's rule involves tracing the left ventricular internal chamber, and computerized calculations treat the ventricle as a stack of discs (Fig. 3.46). A volume for each disc is calculated and summed for the total left ventricular volume. Other terms for this method of volume measurement are the method of discs or the disc summation method. Ideally, two long-axis apical planes should be used—the apical four-chamber and the apical two-chamber planes. Two imaging planes will account more accurately for any left ventricular chamber irregularities. The planes should maximize length and width. A true apex is difficult to obtain in both humans and animals, and in actuality, the lateral wall of the ventricle is really seen, as opposed to the apex. When ventricular size is maximized, the small amount of volume not accounted for is minimal and negligible. After tracing along the endocardial surface of the left ventricular chamber in both planes, following the mitral annulus at the

A

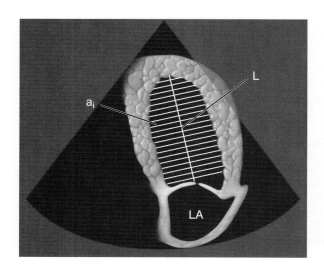
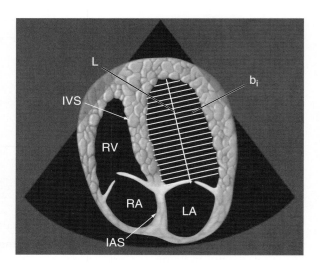

$$V = \frac{\pi}{4} \sum_{i=1}^{20} a_i b_i \cdot \frac{L}{20}$$

B

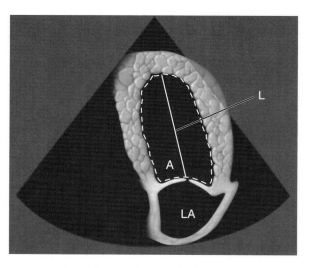

$$V = 0.85 \frac{(A)^2}{L}$$

FIGURE 3.46 **A.** Biplane volume calculations are performed on apical two- and four-chamber views. The endocardial surface of each view is traced, and volume is calculated by summating the areas of 20 or more discs. Internal software divides the length of the chamber (L) into the discs and applies the equation shown. **B.** Single plane volume calculation involves tracing the area of a single apical left ventricular plane as well as measuring its length (L) and applying the equation as shown. Adapted from Schiller NB, Shah PM, Crawford M, et al. Recommendations for quantitation of the left ventricle by two-dimensional echocardiography. American Society of Echocardiography Committee on Standards, Subcommittee on Quantitation of Two-Dimensional Echocardiograms. J Am Soc Echocardiogr 1989:2;358–367.

heart base, computation packages in the ultrasound equipment will divide the ventricle into discs and perform the volume calculation as shown in Figure 3.46.

When two views are not possible, a single apical plane may be used (Fig. 3.46). The use of one plane in veterinary medicine is potentially more accurate than in humans in which regional wall motion abnormalities secondary to coronary artery disease are common and affect volume calculations. An area length computation is used to calculate volume when one apical image is used. The area of the left ventricle is determined by tracing the endocardial surface, and the length is measured from the mitral annulus to the apex. The equation is as shown in Figure 3.46.

A study in dogs has used the Bullet formula for volume determination and found good correlation between echocardiographically determined ejection fractions in anesthetized dogs and gated equilibrium radionuclide ventriculography (107). This formula also has been used in dogs in which echocardiographically determined volumes were compared with post mortem values (116). There was a high correlation of 0.97. The Bullet method is so called because it assumes a bullet-shaped left ventricular chamber with a wider base and a chamber that tapers to a rounded apex. The Bullet method uses transverse left ventricular dimensions and left ventricular length. Transverse images at the level of the chordae are traced in diastole and systole to calculate areas (A)(Fig. 3.47). Left ventricular length (L) is measured on the right parasternal long axis, from the apex of the ventricle to the mitral aorta junction (Fig. 3.20). The Bullet formula is as follows:

$$LV = 5/6 \times area \times length = 5/6\ AL$$

Cross-sectional measurements of the horse's heart have been used to determine left ventricular volumes with high levels of correlation. These results were obtained in vitro; however, their accuracy in the living horse still needs to be determined (109,117).

An ellipsoid model of volume determination proved to be the simplest with no loss in accuracy(109). This involves tracing endocardial and epicardial boundaries of the left ventricular cross section at the level of the papillary muscles (Fig. 3.48). Volumes are calculated for systole and diastole using the ultrasound equipment. The equation is applied as follows:

$$LV\ vol = \frac{2AL}{3}$$

where A = area and L = length. Left ventricular length cannot be determined with any accuracy in the equine heart. An average ratio of length to diameter was determined and this value of 1.46 is applied to the diameter to determine length.

Left Ventricular Mass.   Cardiac hypertrophy usually involves an increase in left ventricular wall thickness and is not always visibly apparent because there may be wall thinning as the heart dilates. This increase in mass can be quantified by several methods, including angiography, M-mode echocardiography, and two-dimensional echocardiography. M-mode echocardiographic methods rely on accurate measurement of wall and septal thicknesses at specified locations. This assumes a hypertrophy pattern that remains consistent throughout the heart. Two-dimensional assessment of left ventricular mass is superior to M-mode measurement of mass because the entire geometry of the heart is taken into consideration. M-mode assessment of mass will not be discussed in this chapter, but references are available to investigate this method of mass quantification (26,118,119). Two-dimensional methods of determining mass have been tested in the dog and have proven to be accurate with a correlation coefficient of 0.98 between echocardiographically determined ventricular mass and necropsy-determined mass in dogs (103,120). The same formulas were applied to terminally ill humans with abnormal cardiac dimensions, and the formulas estimated mass accurately with an r value of 0.93. Only in vitro mass determination has been assessed in the horse, and the correlation was 0.96. In the appropriate hypertrophic conditions, two-dimensional methods are useful in clinical and research applications.

There is correlation between sex and ventricular mass, but there is a significant curvilinear or second order correlation between body weight and ventricular mass in dogs (121). Mass determination is an involved process that starts with two-dimensional volume determination, which is not routinely performed during a clinical examination. The basis of measuring cardiac mass is that external volumes and internal volumes of the heart are measured and the difference of the two should equate to myocardial volume. The myocardial volume is then multiplied by density to calculate ventricular mass.

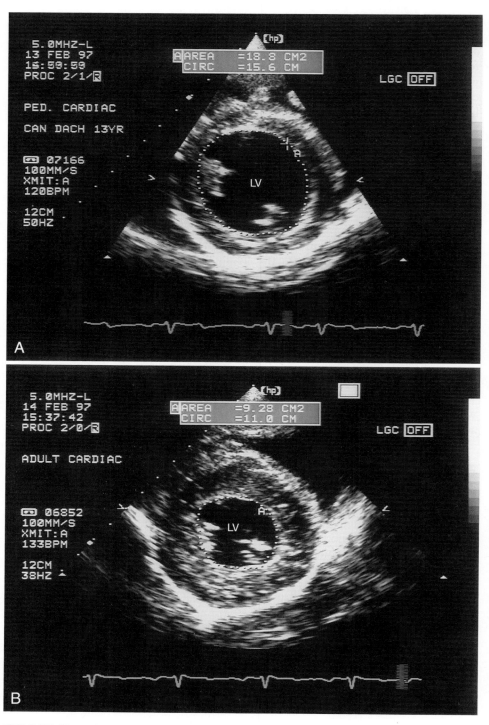

FIGURE 3.47   Volume determination based on the Bullet formula involves tracing the left ventricle endocardial surface on right parasternal transverse planes at the level of the chordae tendineae during diastole (**A**) and systole (**B**). *LV*, left ventricle.

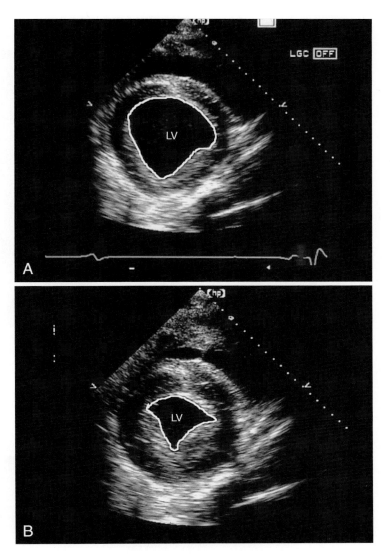

FIGURE 3.48   Volume in the equine heart involves tracing the left ventricular endocardial surface on right parasternal transverse planes at the level of the papillary muscles as opposed to the chordae during diastole (**A**) and systole (**B**). *LV*, left ventricle.

Mass should remain constant throughout the cardiac cycles and does so with a high correlation (0.92) between measurements taken in diastole and systole in the dog (120). Papillary muscles and trabeculae are easier to differentiate and eliminate in endocardial traces, however, when they are made during diastole. Measurements are taken in diastole just before atrial contraction. This creates the least amount of cardiac motion and the best visualization of muscle boundaries.

Only one method of mass determination will be described here, but two methods of measurement for mass determination have been studied in the dog. One is based on an assumption that the heart is shaped like a truncated ellipse (103,120). The other uses basically the same approach to mass determination but follows a simpler area length methodology (119). Neither is more accurate than the other.

The truncated ellipse is accurate in both normal and hypertrophied canine hearts and during both diastole and systole (Fig. 3.49)(103). Volume is determined from the longest possible apical four-chamber view of the heart. This method of analysis requires measurements of chamber size to be taken along three axes on the apical four-chamber view. The minor axis is located at the tip of the papillary muscles at the point of chordal attachment (B). The long axis of the heart is divided into both a semimajor (A) and a truncated semimajor axis (D). The minor axis is the dividing line between the semimajor axis and the truncated semimajor axis. The minor axis also

FIGURE 3.49 Short-axis (**A**) and long-axis (**B**) views of the heart are used to determine left ventricle mass based on the assumption that the heart is shaped like a truncated ellipse. Wall thickness (*t*) is derived from transverse sections at the level of the chordae tendineae by tracing epicardial and endocardial surfaces at end diastole and applying the equation as shown in **A**. A truncated semimajor axis (*d*) and a full semimajor axis (**A**) are determined from a long-axis plane (**B**). The semimajor axis is divided by b at the level of the papillary muscle—chordal junction. All values are inserted into the equation as shown in **B** to determine volume. Mass is then calculated by multiplying volume by the specific gravity of myocardium (1.05 g/mL). Adapted from Schiller NB, Skioldebrand CG, Schiller EJ, et al. Canine left ventricular mass estimation by two-dimensional echocardiography. Circulation 1983:68;210–216.

A

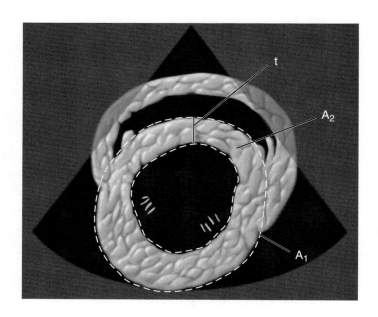

$$t = \sqrt{\frac{A_1}{\pi}} - \sqrt{\frac{A_2}{\pi}}$$

B

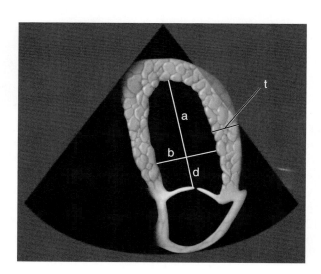

$$v = \pi \left\{ (b+t)^2 \int_0^{d+a+t} \left[1 - \frac{(x-d)^2}{(a+t)^2} \right] dx - b^2 \int_0^{d+a} \left[1 - \frac{(x-d)^2}{a^2} \right] dx \right\} =$$

$$\pi \left\{ (b+t)^2 \left[\frac{2}{3}(a+t) + d - \frac{d^3}{3(a+t)^2} \right] - b^2 \left[\frac{2}{3}a + d - \frac{d^3}{3a^2} \right] \right\}$$

is represented by the left ventricle diameter on both long-axis and short-axis views of the heart at the chordae level.

In addition to the left ventricular length and width measurements, wall thickness (t) is measured. On the transverse plane at the level of the tips of the papillary muscles, both the epicardial and endocardial surfaces are traced. The papillary muscles and any trabeculae are not included in the trace. Subtracting the systolic area from the diastolic area gives a mean wall thickness measurement. All the measurements are inserted into the equation shown in Figure 3.49 to calculate volume (V). The equation calculates the left ventricle volume when the epicardium is traced and the ventricle volume when the endocardium is traced. Subtracting the two volumes results in the ventricular myocardium volume. Mass is then calculated by multiplying the volume by myocardial specific gravity.

$$\text{Mass} = 1.05 \text{ V}$$

The echocardiographically derived mass has an excellent correlation with postmortem mass (r = 0.98) in dogs. Once echocardiographic mass is determined, the value is inserted into a regression equation that correlates echo-derived mass to actual postmortem mass as follows:

$$\text{echocardiographic mass} = 0.9 \text{ (actualweight)} + 4.2$$

Equine.   Cross-sectional images of the horse's heart have been used to determine left ventricular volumes with a high level of correlation (0.96), as discussed earlier. The volume is then multiplied by myocardial-specific gravity to calculate left ventricular mass. These results were obtained in vitro (109).

Doppler Evaluation of Systolic Function

Volumetric Flow.   Conservation of Mass is a physical principle used in Doppler to calculate volumetric flow. This principle states that mass in equals mass out. Because mass is equal to density times volume (V) times area (A), and density is constant, the equation can be modified to the following:

$$\text{Vi} \times \text{Ai} = \text{Vo} \times \text{Ao}$$

where Vi = volume in, Vo = volume out, Ai = area in, and Ao = area out.

The continuity equation is derived from this principle.

$$\text{Q1} = \text{ViAi} = \text{Q2} = \text{VoAo}$$

where Q = flow. In other words, flow into the heart equals flow out of the heart.

Flow Velocity Integral.   Flow volume is calculated by tracing the flow profile and determining the time velocity integral (area under the curve) (Fig. 3.36). The flow velocity integral (FVI) is also referred to as VTI (velocity time integral) or TVI (time velocity integral). FVI is multiplied by the area of the vessel or orifice through which flow volume is being calculated. The result is stroke volume through that part of the heart. This measurement can be done at any of the four valves (122–125). Flow velocity integrals should be traced from mitral inflow profiles, which maximize E and A peak velocities (Fig. 3.50).

VTI is directly proportional to stroke volume.

The FVI is directly proportional to stroke volume and its value is calculated internally once the flow profile is traced. The FVI can be measured manually by applying the following equation:

$$\text{FVI} = \frac{\text{V} \times \text{ET}}{2}$$

where V = peak velocity and ET = ejection time.

Area Measurement.   The other part of the continuity equation states that the area of the vessel or orifice must be calculated. Volumetric flow measurement assumes that the blood is flowing through a circular orifice because area calculations are based on a circle. Cross-sectional area (CSA) is calculated by the following:

$$\text{CSA} = \pi \, r^2$$

Cross-Sectional Areas

- Trace right parasternal aortic root cross sections.
- Use apical four-chamber view for mitral annulus.
- Use diameter of PA on transverse planes.

where r = radius and π = 3.14. The radius is obtained by measuring the diameter of the vessel or annulus involved in the flow calculation. Studies have tried to determine which locations are best for measuring valve areas and it remains the greatest source of error in this method of calculating stroke volume and cardiac output. Although aortic flow has been studied and validated in dogs, pulmonary, mitral, and tricuspid flows need more evaluation.

Studies in dogs have measured cardiac output by measuring aortic area from several imaging planes using both trace and diameter methods (81,106). Calculations based on the same TVI and areas calculated from the three views for aorta showed that the highest correlation (r = 0.93), when compared with thermodilution-derived cardiac output, was when aortic area was measured by tracing the lumen of the aorta on a right parasternal transverse plane of the heart base (Fig. 3.51)(106). This makes Doppler-derived left ventricular stroke volume calculations a fairly valid assessment of left ventricular function.

Measurement of output from the right side is variable and results in poor correlation (r = 0.31) with invasive measures of output in Uehara's study (81,106). This is primarily because of variability of the pulmonary artery diameter measurements (Fig. 3.52). Poor resolution of the lateral walls affect diameter measurements. Carefully obtaining the best images possible should increase the accuracy of this measure. Studies in humans show higher correlations with invasive measures of output, but these measures still are generally less accurate than flow measured at the aorta (126,127). The studies have shown that averaging several beats is important to account for the variation in flow caused by respiration.

Great variability exists in calculating mitral valve stroke volume, as with pulmonary flow, because of error introduced while measuring the mitral annular area. Two methods are used in humans and they have been studied in dogs (124,128). The annulus can be measured by either tracing the orifice from transverse views or by measuring the annulus diameter.

When tracing the orifice area, the largest mitral valve area is used on left ventricle transverse views at the level of the mitral valves (Fig. 3.53). Unfortunately, mitral flow is biphasic, and a mean flow area as opposed to maximal flow area needs to be calculated. This is done by tracing an M-mode mitral profile and determining a ratio of mean to maximal leaflet separation. The two-dimensional area is multiplied by

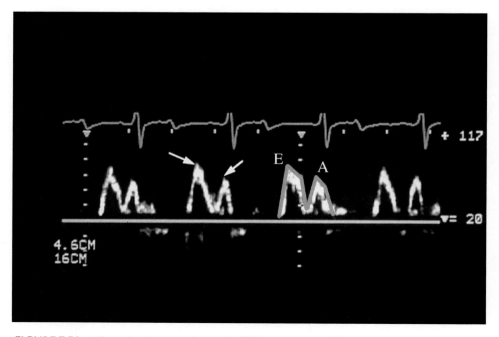

FIGURE 3.50   The velocity time integral (VTI) is measured by tracing the mitral inflow profile, which maximizes both the E and A peaks. Here, the E peak velocity (MAX V) is 87 cm/sec and the VTI is 12.0 cm. Patient is a canine.

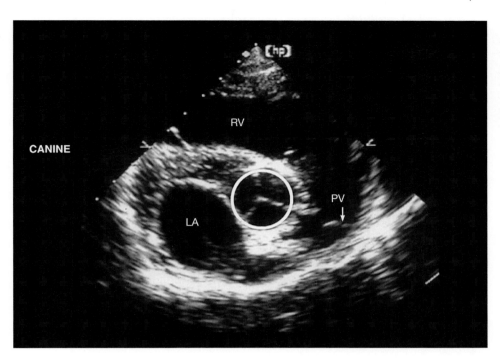

FIGURE 3.51 Although there are many places to measure the aorta, tracing the aortic lumen on right parasternal transverse views of the heart base shows the highest level of accuracy in assessing volumetric flow. *RV*, right ventricle; *LA*, left atrium; PV, pulmonic valve.

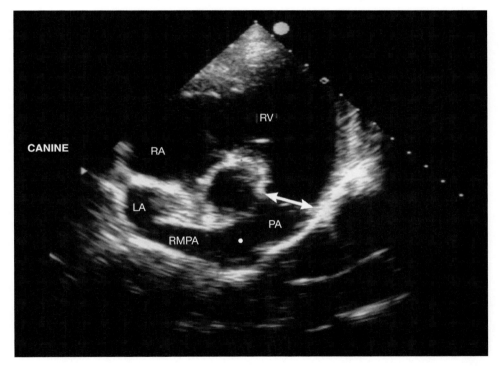

FIGURE 3.52 Pulmonary artery diameter is measured on right parasternal transverse images of the pulmonary artery at the level of the pulmonic valve. *RV*, right ventricle; *RA*, right atrium; *LA*, left atrium; *PA*, pulmonary artery; *RMPA*, right main pulmonary artery.

ratio area to obtain the mean mitral area for diastole. This was studied in open-chested dogs and found to have a high correlation to actual area (r = 0.97) (127). This method is difficult to apply, however, and results have varied in humans.

The mitral annulus can be measured from apical four-chamber views (Fig. 3.54). To account for changes in annular size during diastole, several frames should be measured and averaged after the valve opens. Both circular equations (πr^2) and elliptical equations ($\pi(d1/2) \times (d2/2)$) have been applied to area calculations (d = diameter) (124,129). Both show good correlations (r = 0.99 in circular method). At this time, the diameter measurement with circular equation appears to be the easiest and no less accurate than any other method, although more study is needed.

FIGURE 3.53 Mitral valve area may be measured from transverse images by tracing the largest area. Here, the area measurement is 6.52 cm². *RV,* right ventricle; *LV,* left ventricle.

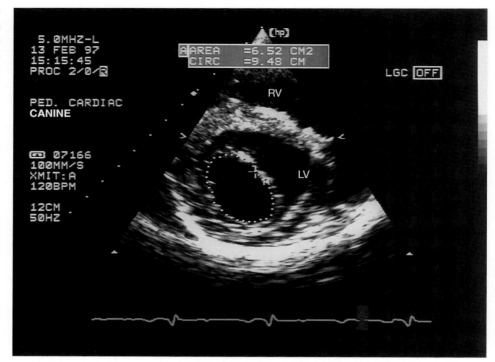

FIGURE 3.54 Mitral valve annular size also may be measured on left parasternal apical four-chamber views. *LV,* left ventricle; *RV,* right ventricle; *RA,* right atrium; *LA,* left atrium.

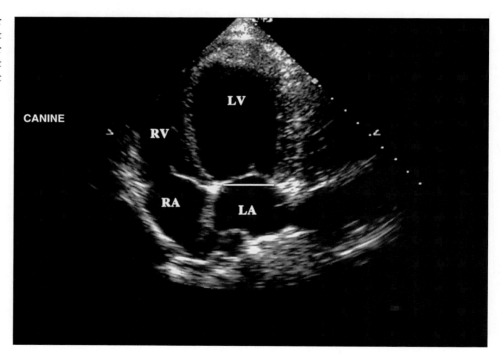

Flow measurements from the tricuspid valve have not been well studied, and results are variable enough that it is neither routinely used in humans nor reported in animals.

Stroke Volume.   Stroke volume is calculated by multiplying the FVI by the area of the vessel or annulus. Because small errors in diameter measurement result in large errors of area calculations once they are squared in the equation, using the FVI itself as an assessment of flow when diameter measurement is questionable, is valid. Increases in FVI may represent restriction to flow or increased volume as with a shunt, whereas decreases in FVI represent poor flow. Exercises can be found at the end of the chapter involving the application of flow velocity integrals.

Stroke Volume = CSA × VTI

Systolic Time Intervals. Research in animals has shown that the rate of acceleration during left ventricular ejection is an indicator of systolic function (Fig. 3.37). The force created within the left ventricle to open the aortic valves affects the rate at which maximum velocity is reached. This variable has been studied in dogs and in humans and is one of the better indicators of systolic function (130–132). It has been used to chart changes in left ventricular function; however, it depends on heart rate and systolic load. This value has been studied in dogs in which the mean aortic flow acceleration is 32 cm/sec^2 (75). Studies in veterinary medicine need to be performed to determine if this variable is applicable in the clinical setting.

Ejection time or flow time and pre-ejection period may be measured from aortic or pulmonary flow profiles, which has been described earlier (Fig. 3.38). The application is the same as when the values are derived from M-mode images.

Diastolic Function

Normal diastolic function is the ability of the heart to fill sufficiently at regular filling pressures. Diastolic failure is the result of increased resistance to filling and increased left ventricular filling pressures (100,133). Left ventricular failure may manifest itself as either systolic or diastolic dysfunction. Research in humans has shown that diastolic dysfunction often plays a large role in the clinical manifestation of heart failure. Systolic function actually may be normal in many patients with heart failure (134,135). Diastolic function of the heart is complex and involves many interactive components, which include myocardial relaxation, atrial contraction, rapid and slow filling phases, elastic properties, loading condition, pericardial sac, and elastic properties of the heart. An explanation of all these factors is beyond the scope of this text, but there are excellent reviews devoted to the subject (99,136–139). The echocardiographic assessment of diastolic function as it applies to the clinical situation will be presented here and will incorporate isovolumic relaxation, rapid ventricular filling, deceleration time, and atrial contraction.

Diastole extends from semilunar valve closure to atrioventricular valve closure. This roughly corresponds to the period from the T wave on an electrocardiogram to the beginning of the QRS complex. Isovolumic relaxation involves no change in ventricular volume when all valves are closed. In the left ventricle, isovolumic relaxation starts with aortic valve closure and stops with mitral valve opening.

Relaxation, however, does not end with mitral valve opening. After the mitral valve opens, there is a rapid ventricular filling phase, a slow ventricular filling phase, and atrial contraction. Diastolic filling abnormalities may be secondary to impaired relaxation or decreased compliance within the left ventricle. Diastolic function impairment can produce both backward and forward failure of the heart. Forward failure results from decreases in ventricular volumes because of restricted filling. Backward failure is the result of high left ventricular filling pressures reflected back into the left atrium.

Correlation of Doppler-derived mitral inflow velocities with more invasive techniques is good. Doppler may be more sensitive than noninvasive methods of measuring transmitral flow dynamics. Despite some inherent problems with Doppler echocardiography, mitral flow profiles do provide valuable information about the diastolic function.

The peak flow velocity between the left atrium and left ventricle is determined by the pressure gradient between the two chambers. The Bernoulli equation cannot be applied directly for flow across the mitral annulus because of various factors, including viscous forces, internal forces, and flow acceleration; however, the pressure differentials during the various phases of diastole are reflected in the mitral inflow profile. A basic understanding of the phasic flow associated with left ventricular filling is necessary to understand how alterations in myocardial relaxation and altered loading conditions can affect diastolic filling and function.

At end systole left ventricular pressures are lower than left atrial pressures, and there is a rapid inflow of blood into the left ventricle. This creates an increase in left ventricular pressure. As left ventricular pressures equal or even slightly exceed left

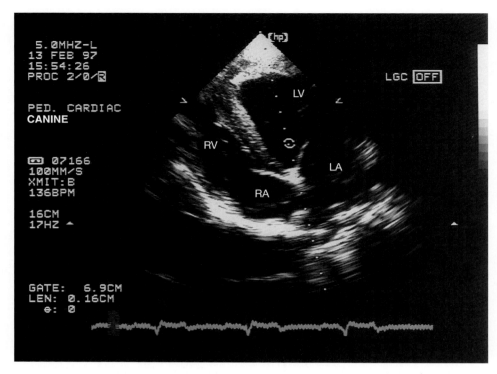

FIGURE 3.55   Isovolumic relaxation (IVRT) may be recorded by placing the Doppler cursor through the left ventricular outflow tract on left parasternal apical four-chamber views. *LV,* left ventricle; *RV,* right ventricle; *LA,* left atrium; *RA,* right atrium.

atrial pressures, flow velocity begins to decelerate. During mid diastole, blood passively flows into the left ventricle with very low velocities. No measurable change is in pressures is present during this phase of diastole. With the atrial contraction toward the end of diastole, a pressure differential occurs between the left atrium and left ventricle. Flow velocities accelerate, but not to the degree of the rapid ventricular filling phase of early diastole.

Measurement for Doppler Assessment of Diastolic Function

Measures of Diastolic Function

- Isovolumic relaxation time
- Pulmonary vein flow
- Mitral inflow appearance
- MV deceleration time

Isovolumic Relaxation Time.   The time that elapses from the end of ventricular ejection to the time the mitral valves open and diastolic flow into the left ventricle begins is the isovolumic relaxation period. No change in volume occurs, all valves are closed, pressures decrease, and the myocardium relaxes.

The isovolumic relaxation time (IVRT) can be measured by placing a CW or PW signal in the left ventricular outflow tract near the mitral valves and recording part of the aortic flow profile and the mitral inflow profile (Fig. 3.55). The time interval from cessation of aortic flow to the beginning of mitral inflow corresponds to the isovolumic relaxation period (Fig. 3.56).

Rapid Ventricular Filling.   This phase of ventricular relaxation extends from mitral valve opening to peak ventricular filling. Mitral inflow velocities are measured at the peak of both E and A points (Fig. 3.57). The rapid ventricular filling peak (E) is typically higher in normal hearts, and A peaks associated with atrial contraction are lower. An E:A ratio is therefore always greater than 1 in a normal heart.

Deceleration Time.   Deceleration times also are measured from mitral inflow profiles. This is measured by the slope of the line that extends from the point of maximal E velocity along its deceleration phase to the baseline (Fig. 3.57). The peak filling rate and flow deceleration are influenced by several factors, including isovolumic relaxation, pressure gradient from left atrium to left ventricle, and ventricular compliance.

Atrial Contraction.   Flow into the left ventricle during atrial contraction is represented by the A point of the mitral inflow profile. Peak velocity is measured (Fig. 3.57).

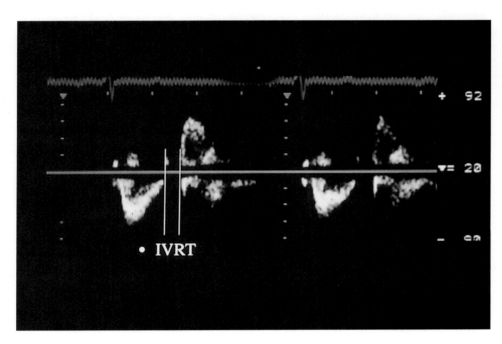

FIGURE 3.56 Doppler flow tracing of isovolumic relaxation time (IVRT) includes part of aortic systolic flow and part of diastolic mitral inflow. The period from the end of systolic flow to the start of mitral inflow corresponds to IVRT.

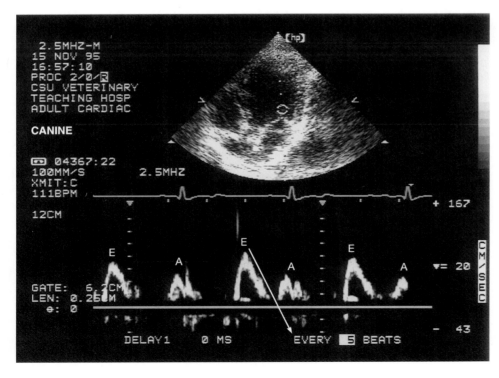

FIGURE 3.57   Peak E and A velocities are measured from mitral inflow profiles. Deceleration time also is measured by identifying peak E velocity and following the slope of the flow to the baseline. Calculations are performed automatically.

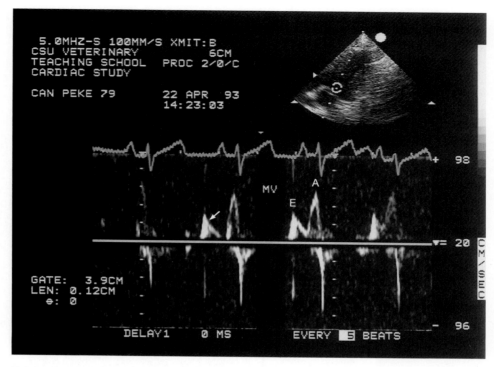

FIGURE 3.58 Abnormal myocardial relaxation in this dog results in decreased peak E velocity, increased A velocity, and longer deceleration time (*arrow*). *MV,* mitral valve.

Doppler Evaluation of Diastolic Function

Impaired Relaxation

- Reverse E:A ratio
- Slow deceleration
- Long IVRT

Impaired Relaxation.   Abnormal myocardial relaxation results in decreased peak velocities in early diastole (E peak); increased A velocities; a low E:A ratio; increased deceleration times; and increased isovolumic relaxation times (Figs. 3.58 and 3.59) (99,125,133,136). These changes in left ventricular filling secondary to impaired relaxation can be seen in patients with hypertrophic cardiomyopathy and hypertension.

Decreased peak E velocities occur because left ventricular diastolic pressures do not decrease as much as in normal hearts. The smaller pressure gradient between the left atrium and left ventricle results in a lower peak velocity. Deceleration times also are prolonged because the left ventricle takes longer to relax and allow filling. Because the ventricle may not relax completely until late in diastole, often the atrial contraction contributes more to ventricular filling than it normally would. This results in a high-peak A velocity and an E:A ratio less than 1. Prolonged isovolumic relaxation times also may be seen with impaired relaxation.

Restriction to Ventricular Filling

- Short IVRT
- High E:A ratio
- Rapid deceleration

Restriction to Ventricular Filling.   Restriction to left ventricular filling results in a short IVRT, increased E velocities, and decreased A velocities (Fig. 3.60) (99,125,133,136). Left ventricular filling in a stiff, noncompliant chamber produces a large increase in left ventricular pressure per unit volume. This kind of diastolic dysfunction is seen in patients with restrictive, dilated, hypertrophic, or ischemic cardiomyopathy in which high filling pressures are predominant. Most of the ventricular filling occurs early in diastole and less occurs with atrial systole because pressures within the left ventricle are so high, creating a high E:A ratio.

The IVRT may be reduced or normal in hearts with restriction to filling because atrial pressures are higher. Deceleration times typically are reduced in these hearts secondary to rapid equalization of atrial and ventricular pressures.

Low A velocities also may be seen if atrial function is compromised.

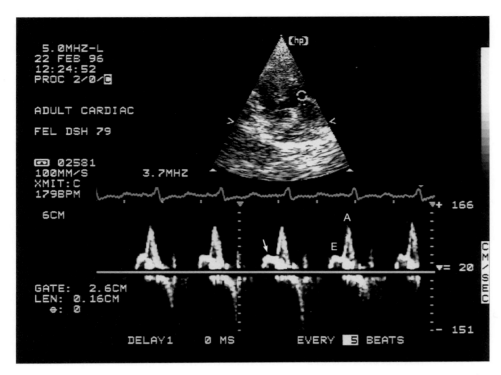

FIGURE 3.59 The heart rate in this cat is slow enough to separate the two phases of diastolic filling. The flow profile suggests impaired relaxation by the reduced E velocity, the high A velocity, and the slow deceleration time (*arrow*).

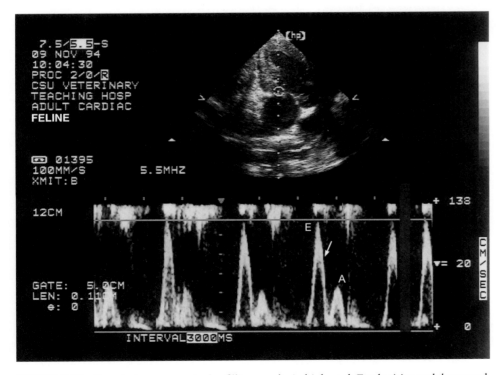

FIGURE 3.60 Restriction to ventricular filling results in high peak E velocities and decreased A velocities. Deceleration time is typically rapid in hearts with restrictive physiology because the atrial and ventricular pressures equalize rapidly (*arrow*).

Limitations. Diastolic function is not static, and various diseases create a continuum of changes in left ventricular preload and atrial pressures. Increased atrial pressures, for instance, would increase peak E inflow velocities by increasing the pressure gradient between the two chambers. A low left ventricular filling pressure can intensify the changes seen with impaired relation simply as a result of lack of volume. A mitral valve flow profile may appear normal despite impaired diastolic function, which is referred to as pseudonormalization.

Normal from abnormal diastolic function can sometimes be differentiated by looking at pulmonary vein flow. Reversal of flow within the pulmonary veins normally is seen during atrial contraction. High-velocity reversal, which encompasses the entire period of atrial contraction, is seen when left ventricular diastolic pressures increase abnormally during atrial contraction, regardless of mitral valve flow profiles (Figs. 3.61, 3.62). This may be used to evaluate diastolic pressures when heart rates are too high to separate the two phases of diastolic inflow. When left ventricular diastolic pressures are very elevated, diastolic mitral regurgitation may be seen as well.

Valvular insufficiencies will alter the mitral inflow profiles. Significant aortic insufficiency will elevate left ventricular diastolic pressures quickly during early diastole. The gradient from left atrium to ventricle will decrease rapidly, and deceleration time will decrease. Moderate to severe mitral insufficiency produces a large pressure gradient between the left atrium and ventricle. Peak E velocities will increase accordingly (Fig. 3.63). The presence of significant mitral insufficiency may affect the flow profiles of hearts with hypertrophic or dilated cardiomyopathy, altering the expected flow profile.

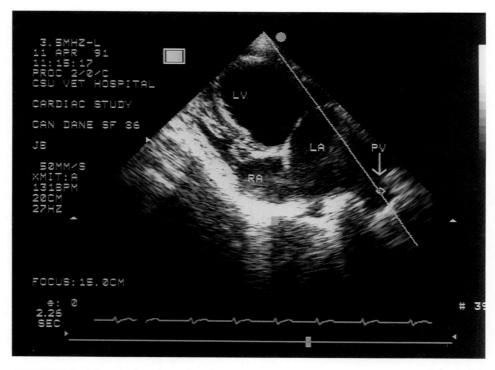

FIGURE 3.61   Flow within the pulmonary veins can be interrogated by placing the Doppler sample within any vein. *LV,* left ventricle; *RA,* right atrium; *LA,* left atrium; *PV,* pulmonary vein.

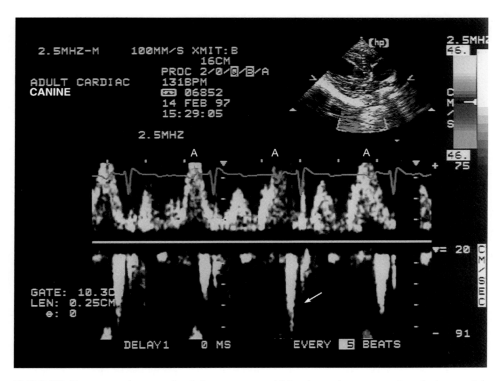

FIGURE 3.62   Normal reversal of flow occurs within the pulmonary veins during atrial contraction (*arrow*). The reversed flow velocity should not exceed forward flow velocity (**A**) during this period and its duration should be shorter than forward flow time.

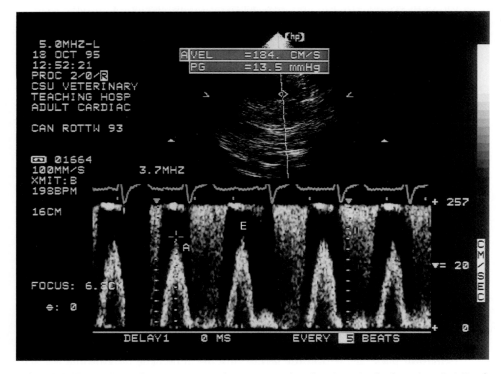

FIGURE 3.63   Peak E velocities increase for reasons other than impaired relaxation. **A.** Mitral insufficiency in this dog increases forward flow velocities to 184 cm/sec.

HEMODYNAMIC INFORMATION
Pressure Determination

Doppler echocardiography has created what is referred to as the noninvasive cardiac catheterization. The peak velocity of valvular regurgitations and shunts depend on the pressure difference between the two chambers involved. When a pressure gradient is calculated, it means that the pressure within the driving chamber is that much higher than the pressure within the receiving chamber. The pressure in the receiving chamber is estimated and added to the calculated gradient to determine pressure within the driving chamber. These are based on estimates of pressure within the receiving chamber, and some error is inherent within the application. As the following applications are described, methods of estimating atrial and ventricular pressures will be discussed.

Measurement of Pressure Gradients

Measuring pressure gradients is probably the most common application of Doppler echocardiography in veterinary medicine. The physical principle of Conservation of Energy is the basis of the Bernoulli equation that is used to calculate pressure gradients between two areas of the heart (80,125). The principle states that when a constant volume of blood flows through a narrowed area, its velocity must increase by an amount equal to the pressure drop (Fig. 3.64). When a constant volume of blood is moved through an orifice or vessel, the pressure increase proximal to the obstruction creates a proportional increase in blood velocity through the obstruction. The greater the degree of obstruction between the driving chamber and the receiving chamber or vessel, the greater the pressure differential and the higher the blood velocity. The Bernoulli Equation is as follows:

$$P_1 - P_2 = \frac{1}{2}\rho(V_2^2 - V_1^2) + \int_1^2 (dv/dt \times ds + R(v))$$

$$\underset{\text{gradient}}{\text{pressure}} = \underset{\text{acceleration}}{\text{convective}} + \underset{\text{acceleration}}{\text{flow}} + \underset{\text{friction}}{\text{viscous}}$$

The forces of viscous friction and flow acceleration are negligible in most cases of heart disease. The value of $\frac{1}{2}\rho$, the mass density of blood, is approximately 4; thus, the Bernoulli equation is simplified as follows:

$$\Delta P = 4(V_2^2 - V_1^2)$$

Modified Bernoulli Equation
$$PG = 4V^2$$

where ΔP = the pressure gradient, V_1 = blood velocity proximal to the obstruction or orifice, and V_2 = blood velocity distal to the obstruction or orifice. The velocities are measured in meters or centimeters per second and the pressure gradient is in mm Hg.

For example, if a PW sample just proximal to a subvalvular aortic stenosis within the left ventricular outflow tract records a velocity of 1.2 m/sec, and velocity distal to the obstruction in the aorta is 3 m/sec, the pressure gradient would be calculated as follows:

$$\Delta P = 4(V_2^2 - V_1^2)$$

$$\Delta P = 4(3^2 - 1.2^2)$$

$$\Delta P = 30.2 \text{ mm Hg}$$

Most normal flows within the heart are close to 1 m/sec; therefore, the effect of V_1 is negligible and an even more simplified form of the equation can be used as follows:

$$\Delta P = 4(V_2^2)$$

Mean pressure gradients calculated from Doppler flow profiles can be determined by calculation packages within the ultrasound machine. The flow profile is traced and digitized. An arithmetic mean gradient is calculated that has a high correlation with catheterization-derived mean gradients. A mean and peak pressure gradient calculation is shown in Figure 3.65.

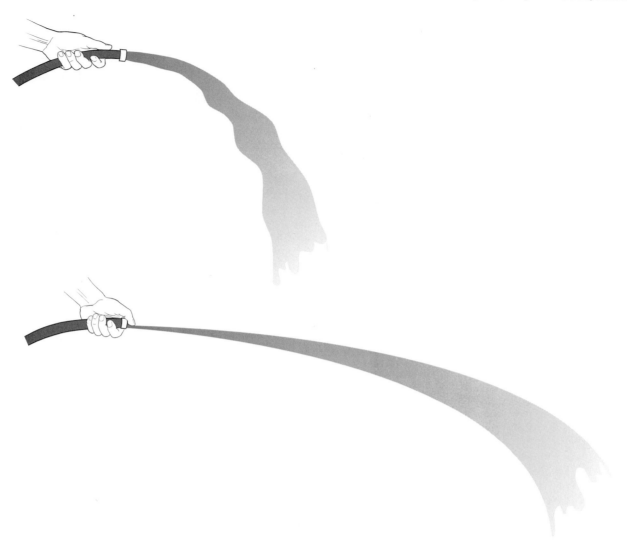

FIGURE 3.64   The velocity of a constant volume of fluid flowing through a narrowed vessel or tube must increase. This is seen in everyday life when a thumb is placed over the end of a hose to increase the velocity and pressure of the spray.

Limitations

Blood volume, tunnel lesions, and blood viscosity all place limitations on the application of the Bernoulli equation (80,125). Because flow velocity also depends on the volume of blood moving through a vessel or orifice, pressure gradient calculations will be inaccurate when a high flow state is present (V_1 will be elevated). Such conditions will exist when severe valvular insufficiency occurs through the stenotic area (i.e., aortic insufficiency and aortic stenosis, coexisting shunt, anemia, or sepsis). In the presence of conduit type of lesions, as in tunnel subvalvular aortic stenosis, the Bernoulli equation will overestimate the pressure gradient because the effects of friction are no longer insignificant. Pressure gradients also may be overestimated when the viscosity of blood is decreased, as with anemia. Increased blood viscosity may underestimate the pressure gradient. Because the sample site for measuring aortic flow velocity proximal to an aortic stenosis within the left ventricular outflow tract is often deep, the signal will alias even with low-frequency transducers. Therefore, determining the V_1 accurately would not be possible, and the calculated pressure gradient will be higher than it actually is.

Although there is a very good correlation between catheter and Doppler-derived pressure gradients, there is a difference in the way the gradients are measured that

Pressure gradients are not accurate when:

- The intercept angle is large
- Conduit-type obstruction is present
- Valvular insufficiency is present at the obstruction

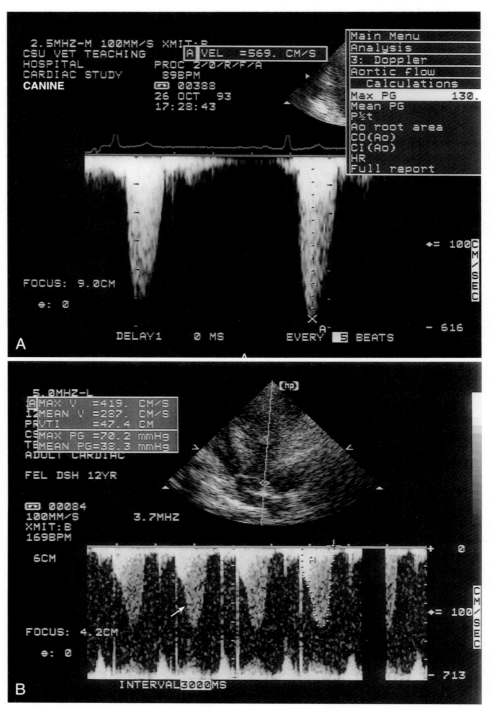

FIGURE 3.65 **A.** The peak velocity of 569 cm/sec is inserted into the modified Bernoulli equation, and a pressure gradient of 130 mm Hg is calculated. **B.** Tracing the flow velocity profile yields a 419 cm/sec maximum velocity (MAX V), a 287 cm/sec mean velocity (MEAN V), a 47.4 cm velocity time integral (VTI), a 70.2 mm Hg peak pressure gradient (MAX PG), and a 38.3 mm Hg mean pressure gradient (MEAN PG). Dynamic outflow obstruction is evident by the concave acceleration profile (*arrow*).

makes it appear that the Doppler-derived gradient often overestimates the gradient when compared with gradients derived during cardiac catheterization (80,125,140). Doppler-derived pressure gradients calculate maximal pressure differentials (instantaneous) across the stenotic lesion, whereas catheterization-derived pressure gradients calculate peak-to-peak differentials (Fig. 3.66). Peak-to-peak pressure gradients in aortic stenosis, for example, are determined by calculating the difference between maximal left ventricular pressure and maximal aortic pressure. These two pressures do not occur at the same time. Doppler-derived pressure gradients are calculated from the maximal instantaneous pressure difference between ventricular and aortic pressure. These two different methods of assessing pressure differentials create a discrepancy between invasive versus noninvasive derived gradients. Instantaneous gradients may be as much as 30 to 40% higher than peak-to-peak gradients. The more severe the stenosis, the closer peak-to-peak and instantaneous pressures are

A

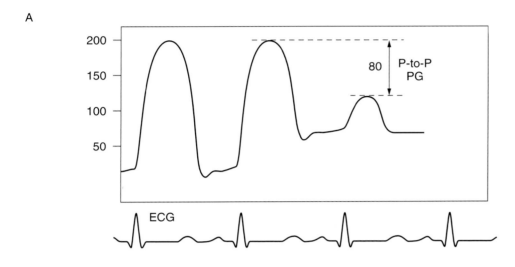

B

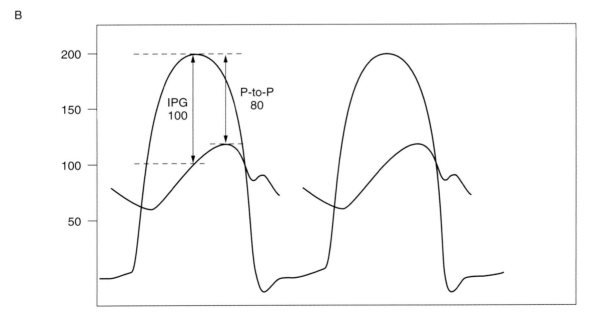

FIGURE 3.66 **A.** Pressure gradients (PG) derived from catheterization are peak-to-peak (P to P). Peak ventricular pressure is compared with peak aortic pressure, and the difference reflects the peak-to-peak pressure gradient. **B.** Doppler echocardiography derives instantaneous pressure gradients (IPG) by determining the maximum difference in pressure at any given instant during ejection. This is typically higher than peak-to-peak calculations.

because the highest left ventricular pressures will be generated later in systole. The arithmetic mean gradient calculated from Doppler flow profiles has a high correlation with catheterization-derived mean gradients.

Applications

To fully apply Doppler echocardiography, estimates of intracardiac pressures are necessary. Figure 3.67 shows typical pressures within the cardiac chambers and great vessels. Unless stated otherwise, these are the values that will be used in any exercises and examples presented in this book. Disease processes may change these pressures somewhat, but unless invasive procedures or reliable blood pressures are available, they are a good estimate. Using these representative pressures will not diminish the usefulness of Doppler-derived information in most applications.

Intracardiac pressure determination from Doppler flows and pressure gradients are based on estimates of pressure within the receiving chamber or vessel; some error is inherent within the application. The pressure gradient always can be used as an "at least" pressure. For example, if the pressure gradient from left ventricle to left atrium is calculated as 130 mm Hg, the left ventricular pressure is "at least 130 mm Hg" regardless of the left atrial pressures.

The simplified Bernoulli equation is used in many applications: stenotic lesions involving the great vessels or atrioventricular valves; ventricular and atrial septal defects; and intracardiac pressure determination by regurgitant jets. Mathematical packages within the ultrasound equipment will calculate pressure gradients after peak velocity through the stenosis, shunt, or leak is identified on the screen.

Aortic and Pulmonic Stenosis.   An example of a pressure gradient calculated from a dog with subvalvular aortic stenosis is seen in Figure 3.65. The pressure gradient indicates that pressure within the left ventricle is that many mm Hg higher

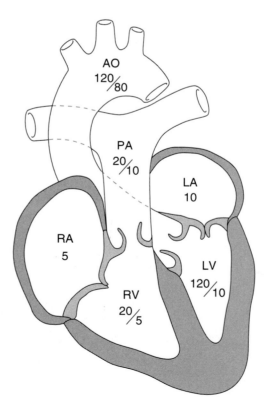

FIGURE 3.67   Typical intracardiac pressures are displayed in this diagram of the chambers and vessels of the heart. *AO,* aorta; *PA,* pulmonary artery; *LA,* left atrium; *RA,* right atrium; *RV,* right ventricle; *LV,* left ventricle.

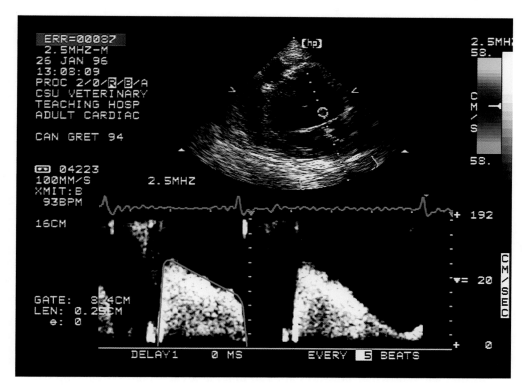

FIGURE 3.68 Pressure gradient calculation for mitral stenosis involves tracing the mitral inflow profile. Several beats should be measured to minimize the effects of heart rate.

than pressure beyond the obstruction in the aorta. Exercises involving pressure gradient calculations across stenotic lesions are found at the end of the chapter.

Mitral Stenosis.   Mean pressure gradients are considered accurate in assessing severity of mitral stenosis. The flow profile is traced and the equipment calculates mean gradients (Fig. 3.68). Studies have shown that Doppler-derived gradients for mitral stenosis are more accurate than invasive catheterization methods (141–143). Pressure half-times is another method of determining the severity of mitral stenosis, which will be discussed in later sections.

Systolic Left Ventricular and Systemic Pressures.   Systolic pressure within the left ventricle is fairly equal to peripheral systolic blood pressure in the absence of left ventricular outflow obstruction. The driving pressure of a mitral regurgitant jet therefore would equal both ventricular systolic pressures and systolic blood pressure. Because left ventricular pressures are typically at least 100 to 110 mm Hg, and left atrial pressures are usually less than 10 mm Hg, a pressure gradient close to 100 mm Hg is expected when the Bernoulli equation is applied to a mitral regurgitant jet peak velocity. This means that velocities of approximately 5 m/sec should be recorded from a mitral regurgitant jet ($4 \times 5^2 = 100$).

Left atrial pressure can be estimated and added to the pressure gradient to calculate left ventricular pressures; however, even if left atrial pressures are not estimated and assumed to be zero, left ventricular and systemic pressures are at least equal to the pressure gradient. As systemic pressures increase, the driving pressure from left ventricle to atrium will also increase, and peak velocities will increase accordingly (Fig. 3.69). An animal with a regurgitant jet velocity of 6.8 m/sec ($4 \times 6.8^2 = 185$) would have systolic systemic pressures of at least 185 mm Hg. Exercises at the end of the chapter apply this principle. Many cases of systemic hypertension have been found inadvertently by interrogating mitral regurgitant jets. Often, Doppler assessment of high blood pressure is easier to obtain than good peripheral

Use mitral or tricuspid insufficiencies to double-check a pulmonic or aortic pressure gradient.

measurements of blood pressure, especially in smaller animals. A "white coat" effect similar to that seen in humans may be seen in animals, and pressures may only be elevated secondary to the stress of the clinical environment.

Systolic Right Ventricular and Pulmonary Pressures.   These same principles are applied to the right side of the heart and have been studied in the dog (144). Right ventricular systolic pressures approximate pulmonary artery systolic pressures in the normal heart. Therefore, the driving pressure behind a tricuspid regurgitant jet will equal both right ventricular systolic pressures and pulmonary systolic pressures in the absence of pulmonic stenosis. Right ventricular and pulmonary systolic pressures are approximately 20 to 25 mm Hg, and right atrial pressures are normally less than 5 mm Hg. A normal pressure gradient between the right ventricle and atrium would be approximately 15 to 20 mm Hg. If a tricuspid insufficiency jet with a velocity of 2.3 is recorded, the calculated pressure gradient is 21 mm Hg, indicative of normal right ventricular and pulmonary systolic pressures. Regurgitant jets with higher velocities indicate elevated right ventricular and pulmonary artery systolic pressures (Fig. 3.70). Exercises applying the Bernoulli equation to tricuspid insufficiency may be found at the end of the chapter.

Mitral or Tricuspid Insufficiency and Stenosis.   When both aortic stenosis and mitral insufficiency are present, the left ventricular pressure affects both the aortic flow velocity and the mitral regurgitant velocity (Fig. 3.69). A pressure gradient of 100 mm Hg calculated from aortic flow profiles in the presence of aortic stenosis tells us that left ventricular pressures are 100 mm Hg greater than systemic pressures. Even if a blood pressure cannot be accurately measured, a systolic pressure of

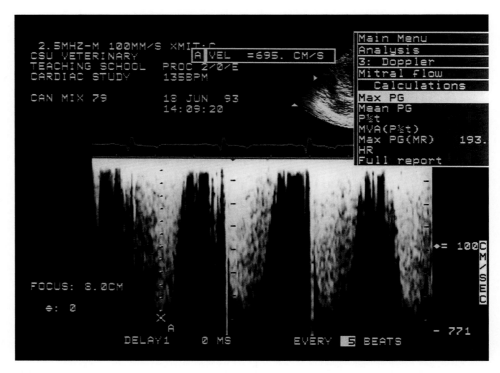

FIGURE 3.69   Peak velocities from mitral regurgitant jets can be used to determine the systolic driving pressure of the left ventricle. Here, a peak velocity of 695 cm/sec is inserted into the Bernoulli equation to yield a calculated pressure gradient of 193 mm Hg. Left ventricular pressures are at least 193 mm Hg. In the absence of aortic stenosis, this also is a reflection of systemic pressures. In the presence of aortic stenosis, it suggests a pressure gradient of approximately 73 mm Hg across the obstruction, because ventricular pressures are at least 193 mm Hg and aortic pressures are approximately 120 mm Hg.

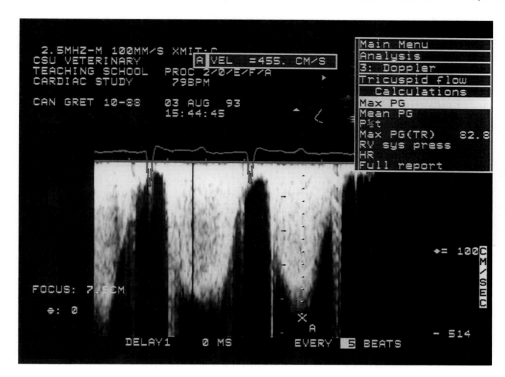

FIGURE 3.70 Peak velocities from tricuspid regurgitant jets are used to determine right ventricular systolic pressures. Here, a velocity of 455 cm/sec and a pressure gradient of 82.8 mm Hg suggests that right ventricular systolic pressures are at least 83 mm Hg. In the absence of pulmonic stenosis, this is a reflection of pulmonary systolic pressures. In the presence of pulmonic stenosis, it suggests a pressure gradient of approximately 63 mm Hg across the obstruction, because ventricular pressures are at least 83 mm Hg and pulmonary pressures are approximately 20 mm Hg.

approximately 100 mm Hg can be estimated and added to the gradient. Left ventricular pressures are therefore approximately 200 mm Hg. Doppler interrogation of mitral insufficiency should show a peak velocity of approximately 7 m/sec if aortic flow profiles were recorded accurately ($4 \times 7^2 = 196$). This can be used to double-check the Doppler results. Mitral regurgitation often can be used to verify or help determine a left ventricular to aorta pressure gradient in the presence of subvalvular or valvular aortic stenosis. If aortic flow velocities are difficult to align with the Doppler sound beam, mitral insufficiency, if present, can help determine the left ventricular pressures, and the pressure gradient across the stenosis can be estimated from that number. If a discrepancy exists between the two determinations of left ventricular pressure, the highest estimate should be used because Doppler rarely overestimates a pressure gradient but often underestimates a gradient when the interrogation angle with respect to flow becomes large. For example, with estimated blood pressure of 120/60, if a gradient of 60 is obtained for a subvalvular aortic stenosis (suggesting ventricular pressures of approximately 180 mm Hg), and a gradient of 200 mm Hg is obtained from a small mitral regurgitant jet (suggesting left ventricular pressures of approximately 210 mm Hg, 200 + 10), then the pressure gradient across the aortic valve is underestimated and should be closer to 90 mm Hg if systemic systolic pressures are estimated or measured at 120 mm Hg (210 − 120).

The same process can be applied to right-sided pressure calculations when both tricuspid insufficiency and pulmonic stenosis are present. The pressure gradient measured from the tricuspid regurgitant jet may be used to determine or verify the severity of the pulmonic stenosis. Applications of this can be found at the end of the chapter.

Diastolic Systemic Pressures.   Diastolic systemic pressures also can be determined noninvasively if aortic insufficiency is present. Peak velocity of the aortic insufficiency can be used to determine the pressure gradient between the aorta and left ventricle during diastole. A normal diastolic systemic pressure of 60 and a normal left ventricular end-diastolic pressure of 10 yields a pressure gradient of 50 mm Hg. A peak aortic insufficiency velocity of 3.5 m/sec would suggest normal systemic diastolic pressures ($4 \times 3.5^2 = 49$). When diastolic systemic pressure increases with hypertension, the driving pressure into the left ventricle becomes greater, and higher peak aortic regurgitant velocities are expected (Fig. 3.71). Aortic insufficiency with a peak velocity of 4.8 m/sec suggests diastolic blood pressure of at least 92 mm Hg $(4 \times 4.8^2 = 92)$. Exercises for pressure gradient calculation with aortic insufficiency are at the end of the chapter. As with systolic pressure estimation, animals do display a "white coat effect," and blood pressure may be only temporarily elevated because of the clinical environment.

Diastolic Pulmonary Pressures.   Pulmonary hypertension elevates both systolic and diastolic pressures. Because a large number of normal animals have pulmonic insufficiency, this jet may be used to determine pulmonary diastolic pressures if hypertension may be present. The presence of elevated diastolic pulmonary pressures confirms the presence of pulmonary hypertension even if systolic pulmonary pressures cannot be derived. Because normal pulmonary diastolic pressures are approximately 10 to 15 mm Hg, and right ventricular diastolic pressures are less than 5 mm Hg, a pressure gradient of approximately 10 to 15 mm Hg is expected in the normal heart from the pulmonary artery to the right ventricle. Pulmonic insufficiency jets should have velocities no greater than 2 m/sec in animals with normal pulmonary pressures $(4(2^2) = 16)$ (Fig. 3.72). See the exercises at the end of the chapter to apply these pressure calculations.

Other Hemodynamic Information

Regurgitant Fractions

Flow through the mitral annulus is equal to flow out of the aorta in a normal heart, as is flow through the mitral and tricuspid valves, flow through the aortic and pulmonic valves, and flow through the tricuspid and pulmonic valves. This is true over the course of several cardiac cycles because there are variations in stroke volume related to heart rate and respiration on a beat to beat basis. Only when insufficiencies or shunts exist will there be more volume flowing through one valve than another.

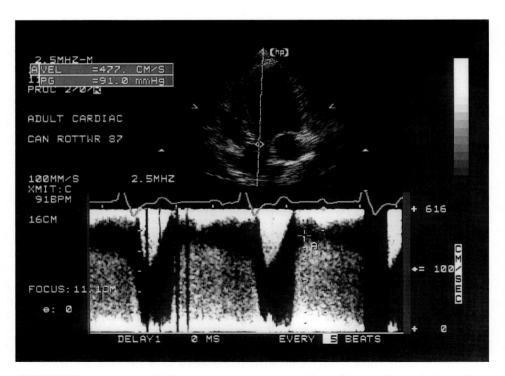

FIGURE 3.71   A velocity of 477 cm/sec and a pressure gradient of 91 mm Hg is calculated from this aortic insufficiency flow profile. This implies that diastolic systemic pressures are at least 91 mm Hg.

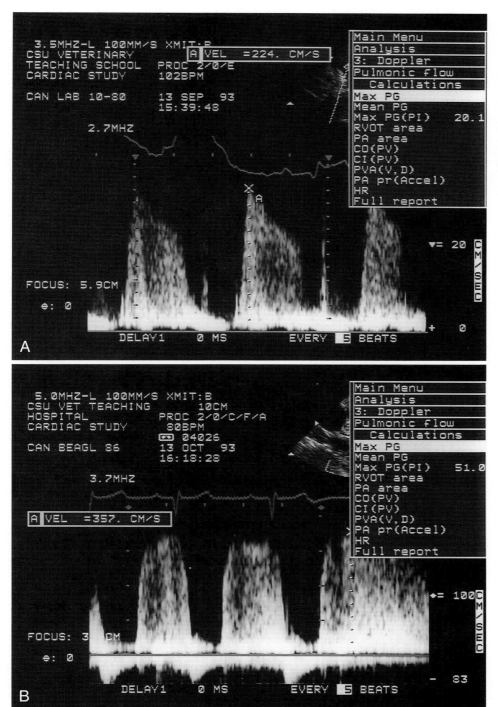

FIGURE 3.72 **A.** A velocity of 224 cm/sec and a pressure gradient of 20.1 mm Hg calculated from this pulmonic insufficiency flow profile suggests normal pulmonary diastolic pressures of approximately 25 mm Hg. (Add the estimated right ventricular diastolic pressures of approximately 5 mm Hg to the pressure gradient of 20 mm Hg.) **B.** A pressure gradient of 51 mm Hg on this pulmonic insufficiency flow profile is high and indicative of pulmonary hypertension.

With mitral insufficiency, flow through the mitral valve will be greater than flow through the aortic valve. The regurgitant volume plus the normal forward stroke volume moves past the mitral valve, and as the normal forward stroke volume goes through the aorta, the regurgitant volume flows back into the left atrium. Based on this flow pattern, regurgitant fractions (RF) can be calculated by applying the following equation:

$$\text{mitral RF} = \frac{\text{mitral SV} - \text{aortic SV}}{\text{mitral SV}}$$

where SV = stroke volume.

There are limitations to this application. Inaccuracies exist in area calculations for the aorta and mitral annuluses as well as the fact that the stroke volume at each valve also is not measured at the same time. Take care to measure five or more cardiac cycles for cross-sectional area measurements to eliminate as much technical error as possible and also to eliminate beat to beat flow differences. As with shunt ratios in the next section, no one piece of information should ever be used to assess the severity of a cardiac lesion. All the information available, including the degree of volume overload, function, flow velocities and profiles, as well as the clinical picture, should be evaluated. Regurgitant fractions are just one way of assessing regurgitation, and this area of echocardiography needs further investigation in veterinary medicine.

Shunt Ratios

Analysis of cardiac shunts should involve analysis of the shunt pathway. Only the chambers and vessels of the heart that are in the pathway will show enlargement or increased flow. A ventricular septal defect, therefore, has increased volume within the left ventricle, right ventricle, pulmonary artery, and left atrium. The right atrium and aorta never encounter the increased volume. With atrial septal defects, the increased volume flows through the left atrium, right atrium, right ventricle, and pulmonary artery. The left ventricle and aorta never encounter this increased volume. Patent ductus arteriosus volume overloads the pulmonary artery, the left atrium, the left ventricle, and ascending aorta. The right side of the heart never encounters the volume.

Based on the flow pathways, the severity of a ventricular septal defect, atrial septal defect, or patent ductus arteriosus (PDA) can be assessed by analyzing flow through an area that should not encounter the increased volume versus an area that does. This is done by determining Qp/Qs, where Qp = pulmonary flow and Qs = systemic flow. The greater the volume of blood shunting across a VSD, for instance, the greater the amount of flow out of the pulmonary artery versus the aorta, where the shunted blood never passes. Calculating a shunt ratio for VSD or ASD can be done by applying the following equation:

$$Qp/Qs = \frac{PAsv}{AOsv}$$

where PAsv = pulmonary artery stroke volume and AOsv = aortic stroke volume.

PDA is different in that the increased flow is seen in the ascending aorta and normal stroke volume is seen in the pulmonary artery. Its shunt ratio is therefore calculated as follows:

$$Qp/Qs = \frac{AOsv}{PAsv}$$

As with regurgitant fractions, this technique has limitations. The most limiting factor is, again, area calculation for the aorta and pulmonary artery. Shunt severity should never be assessed by one method alone. The entire examination should be considered, including cardiac size and flow velocities as well as the clinical picture.

Pressure Half-Times

Pressure Half-Times
= time for peak pressure gradient to decline by half

Right and Left Ventricular Diastolic Pressures. The effects of aortic insufficiency on left ventricular diastolic pressures can be assessed from the shape of the aortic regurgitant flow profile (80,125,145). At any point during aortic insufficiency, the instantaneous pressure difference between the aorta and left ventricle is reflected on the regurgitant jet flow profile. When aortic insufficiency is severe, the aortic diastolic pressure will decline rapidly because of runoff into the left ventricle, and left ventricular pressures will increase dramatically. Both of these factors will produce a rapid decline in regurgitant velocity as the driving pressure into the left ventricle declines, and the receiving pressure increases, creating less of a pressure gradient. The

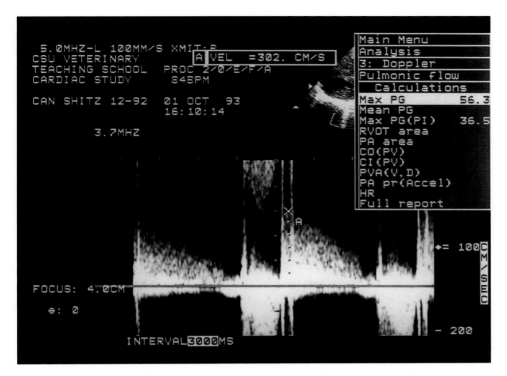

FIGURE 3.73   The rapid deceleration of this pulmonic insufficiency flow profile suggests that right ventricular diastolic pressures have elevated rapidly secondary to the back flow.

flow profile becomes more triangular as opposed to the flat plateau-shaped flow profiles seen in mild aortic insufficiency (Fig. 3.73). Mild aortic insufficiency does not elevate left ventricular diastolic pressure significantly or decrease aortic diastolic pressures dramatically. The result is a plateau-shaped flow profile because the pressure gradient remains similar throughout diastole (Fig. 3.74).

The rapid decline in aortic regurgitant velocity can be measured. This measurement is referred to as the diastolic half-time, which is the time it takes for the peak gradient to decrease by half. The measurement is taken by extending the deceleration slope to the baseline and measuring the deceleration time (Fig. 3.75). This deceleration time is multiplied by 0.29. The equipment automatically performs the calculations. No standards exist for measuring diastolic half-times in animals, and even in humans applying half-time measurements is problematic. Diastolic half-times less than 300 m/sec indicate severe aortic regurgitation (125,145). However, the measurement cannot separate groups of patients into mild, moderate, and severe insufficiency consistently, and there is much overlap. Part of the problem may be the fact that several flows affect aortic and ventricular pressures, including mitral inflow into the ventricle while the aortic valve is leaking, and forward aortic flow at the same time as the regurgitant flow. Nevertheless, a subjective assessment of flow profile is easy to apply, and significant aortic insufficiency as well as a rapid increase in left ventricular diastolic pressures can be assumed from a sharp decline in aortic regurgitant velocity during diastole.

The same theory is applied to pulmonic insufficiency. Half-times will be short in the presence of elevated right ventricular pressures, indicating a rapid equilibration of pulmonary and right ventricular pressures secondary to pulmonic insufficiency (Fig. 3.76). Figure 3.72B shows a plateau-shaped regurgitant flow profile indicative of an insufficiency that is not hemodynamically significant.

Right and Left Atrial Pressures.   The mitral and tricuspid regurgitant jet profiles also can provide some insight into atrial pressures (80,125). In the presence of high left or right atrial pressures and a noncompliant atrial chamber, there is often a

Pressure Half-Times
- Long ones are good for aortic and pulmonic insufficiencies
  = plateau-shaped profile
- Short ones are good for mitral stenosis
  = rapid deceleration

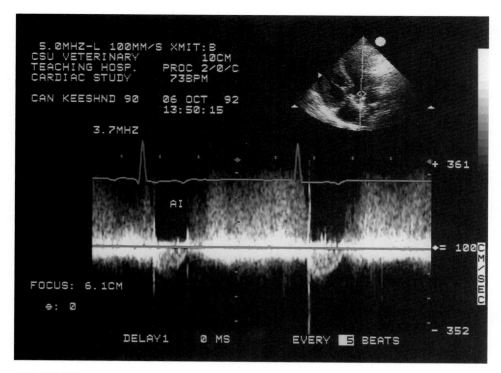

FIGURE 3.74   Mild to moderate pulmonary and aortic insufficiencies that do not increase ventricular diastolic pressures are plateau shaped.

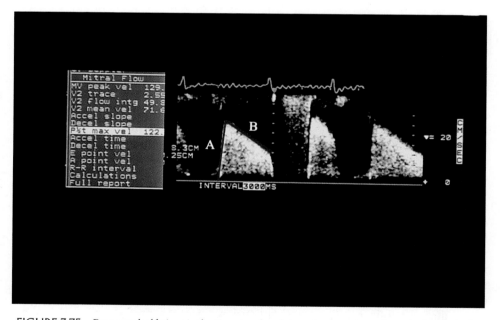

FIGURE 3.75   Pressure half-time is the time it takes for peak regurgitant jet velocity to decline by half. The deceleration slope is indicated on the flow profile, and the equipment calculates a pressure half-time. Here, a long half-time of 556 m/sec was calculated. Patient is a canine.

"cutoff sign" on the regurgitant jet flow profile (Figs. 3.77 and 3.78). This reflects a decrease in regurgitant flow in mid to late systole as atrial pressures elevate secondary to the large regurgitant volume. The flow profile is no longer symmetric as would be seen in patients without high atrial pressures and compliant atrial chambers. This type of flow profile often is seen in acute severe mitral insufficiency.

Elevated atrial pressures increase the driving pressure from left atrium to left ventricle during the rapid ventricular filling phase of diastole. Peak flow velocities for the E point of mitral valve inflow will increase accordingly (Fig. 3.63).

M-mode Hemodynamic Information

Doppler echocardiography provides direct assessment of blood flow within the heart and is the primary method used to assess the hemodynamics of flow within the ventricle and atria. This does not diminish the valuable hemodynamic information

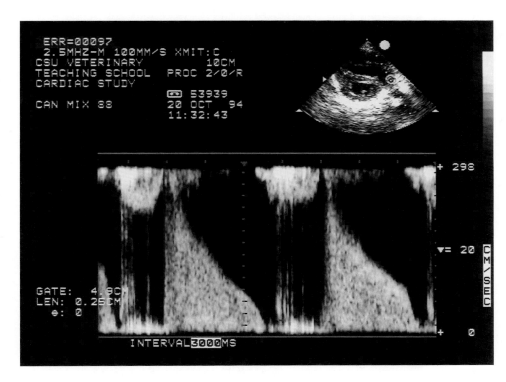

FIGURE 3.76   The half-time of this pulmonic insufficiency flow profile will be short, suggestive of significant regurgitation.

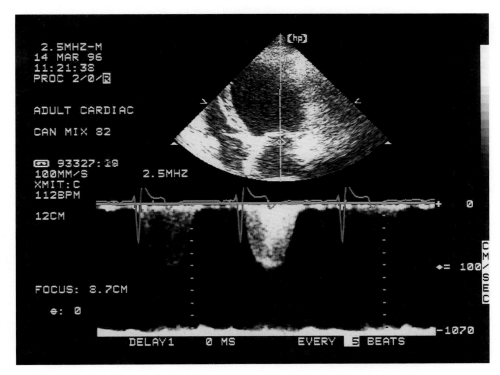

FIGURE 3.77   Mitral and tricuspid insufficiency flow profiles are typically symmetric as seen here in this profile of mitral insufficiency.

FIGURE 3.78 Flow profiles from AV valvular insufficiencies, which display a "cutoff" sign (*arrows*), are indicative of high pressures within the receiving atrial chamber. Examples **A**, **B**, and **C** show varying degrees of cutoff in mitral and tricuspid insufficiency flow profiles.

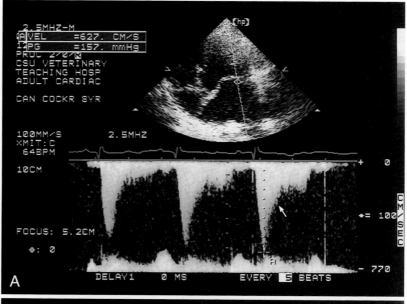

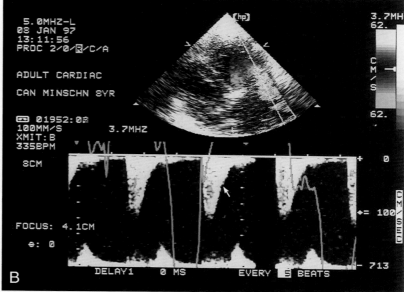

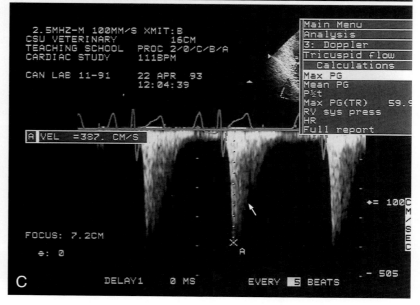

that can be derived from real-time and M-mode images. Even without the quantitative information available through Doppler, the following M-mode features can provide definite information about flow within the heart.

Aortic Valve Motion. Aortic valve motion on M-mode images also reflects cardiac output. Normally, the aortic valve opens rapidly and the leaflets parallel each other as they lie along the aortic wall during systole. The end of systole produces rapid closure of these cusps. M-mode images that show normal opening at the onset of systole but then show gradual closure of the cusps throughout systole, suggest that blood flowing through the aorta is decreasing as systole progresses (Fig. 3.79)(146). This is seen when systolic function is impaired and cardiac output cannot be maintained throughout systole. It is also a frequent finding in patients with severe mitral insufficiency in which blood flows into the low pressure left atrium as opposed to the higher pressure aorta.

Systolic aortic valve fluttering often is seen in diseases that create turbulent and rapid blood flow through the aorta as in subvalvular aortic stenosis or hypertrophic obstructive cardiomyopathy (Fig. 3.80). When the aortic valve exhibits midsystolic closure or notching, it is an indication that flow has been abruptly reduced at that point in time (Fig. 3.81) (147,148). This usually is seen with dynamic obstructions to left ventricular outflow. The subvalvular muscular obstruction increases with contraction of the ventricular septum, and the degree of obstruction increases. Discrete aortic stenosis also displays closure, which typically is seen earlier in the systolic time period (148). Systolic aortic valve closure is not specific to obstructive disease and is rarely seen with mitral insufficiency, ventricular septal defect, aortic root dilation, and dilated cardiomyopathy (148,149).

Mitral Valve Motion. As discussed previously, there are two phases to left ventricular filling—a rapid passive filling phase and a slower active phase secondary to atrial contraction. These two phases create the classic "M" shape of the mitral valve. A reduction in deceleration after peak E velocity has been reached is associated with a decrease in the filling rate secondary to decreased ventricular compliance or increased stiffness of the ventricular walls (Fig. 3.82). This is not a specific finding, and occasionally it may be seen in normal hearts and in patients with pulmonary hypertension.

Patients in which left ventricular filling pressures are high and exceed left atrial pressures earlier than usual will show early mitral valve closure (150–152). Typically, the valve closes after the beginning of the QRS complex. In early closure, the C point may occur before the QRS complex; however, this is a subtle and nonspecific finding. Mitral valve closure may also be delayed, producing what is called the "B" bump (Fig. 3.83) (51,153,154). This is also found with elevated left ventricular pressures and is thought to reflect diastolic mitral insufficiency secondary to the high filling pressures (155,156). The "B" bump is a normal finding in many horses and typically disappears after exercise.

The E point to septal separation (EPSS), as discussed earlier, correlates highly with left ventricular ejection fraction (Fig. 3.33) (65,65–67). The EPSS also may be affected by aortic insufficiency, however, because the regurgitant jet within the left ventricular outflow tract prevents the valve from moving completely up toward the septum (Fig. 3.84). Turbulence associated with aortic insufficiency also will create mitral valve vibration during diastole. This vibration sometimes may be seen on the interventricular septum. The worse the aortic insufficiency, the greater the EPSS, the coarser the mitral valve diastolic flutter, and the more abnormal the "M" appears.

Mitral valve motion also changes with left ventricular outflow obstruction. During systole, as flow velocities increase within the outflow tract secondary to narrowing of the tract, a Venturi effect is created, which pulls the mitral valve up with it toward the aorta. This creates systolic anterior motion (SAM) of the mitral valve (Fig. 3.85). The motion in itself adds to the obstruction to flow as the leaflet is pulled into the outflow tract (157–161). The greater the upward motion and the

FIGURE 3.79 Aortic valves that display gradual closure of the valve (*arrows*) imply a reduction in forward flow throughout systole. Three examples of gradual closure are shown. These animals had dilated cardiomyopathy (**A**), mitral insufficiency (**B**), and dilated cardiomyopathy (**C**). *AO*, aorta; *LA*, left atrium.

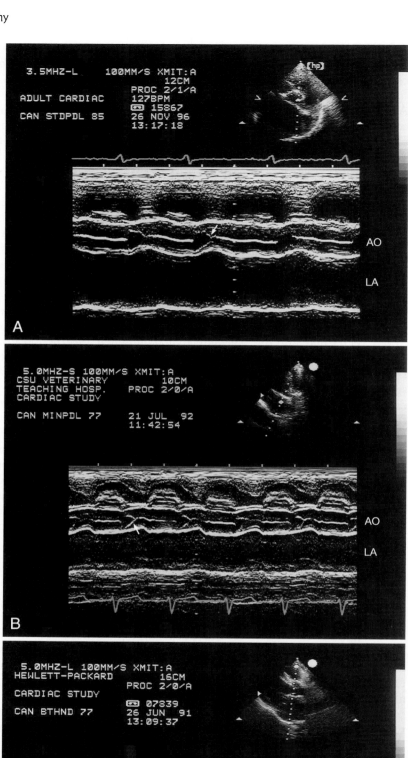

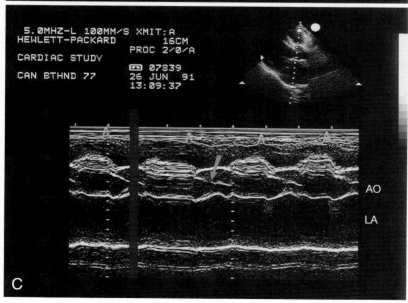

more apposition the mitral leaflet has with the septum during systole, the greater the degree of obstruction. This is a sensitive finding in moderate to severe dynamic left ventricular outflow obstruction, but may occasionally be seen in hearts with transposition of the great vessels, coronary artery disease, systemic hypertension, discrete aortic stenosis, tunnel aortic stenosis, and mitral stenosis (162–166). There are other less frequently reported incidences of SAM in patients with glycogen storage diseases and Friedreich's ataxia (167,168).

Left Ventricular Wall.   Restriction to ventricular filling as seen with restrictive pericarditis or restrictive cardiomyopathy is difficult to assess with M-mode or even two-dimensional images. In some cases, however, there are alterations in left ventricular wall motion. Normally, the left ventricle gradually fills and there is concomitant downward motion of the free wall during diastole. With restriction to filling, wall motion is flat with no increase in dimensions toward the latter part of diastole as filling is impaired (169). This is a subtle and nonsensitive finding; but it is specific when present.

Interventricular Septum.   Animals with right-sided pressure or volume overload show paradoxical or flattened septal motion (170–172), which appears specific to right sided-disease and is not seen in left-sided cardiac disease.

Normal septal motion involves downward motion during early systole with peak downward motion occurring just before peak upward motion of the left ventricular free wall. The septum then begins to move upward again at the end of systole and may show a diastolic dip (Fig. 3.86). The dip may be associated with early left ventricular filling or right ventricular filling that occurs slightly before left ventricular filling (170).

Paradoxical septal motion is characterized by peak downward septal motion occurring late in diastole (Fig. 3.87). This occurs because right-sided diastolic pressures exceed left ventricular pressures. The greater the difference in pressure between the two chambers, the more dramatic the septal motion becomes. As systole starts, left ventricular pressures exceed right ventricular pressures, and the septal

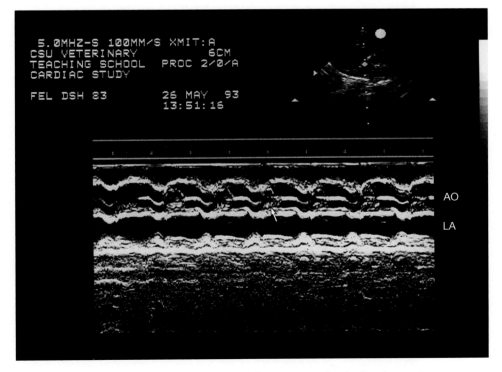

FIGURE 3.80   The rapid velocity of blood as it flows past a subvalvular obstruction can cause systolic flutter of the aortic valve (*arrow*). *AO*, aorta; *LA*, left atrium.

FIGURE 3.81 Varying degrees and displays of early or mid-systolic closure (*arrows*) of the aortic valve are seen in figures **A** through **E**. This motion usually is seen with subvalvular obstruction to aortic outflow as flow is disrupted in the dog and cat. *AO*, aorta; *LA*, left atrium.

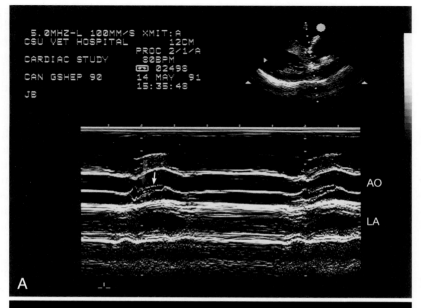

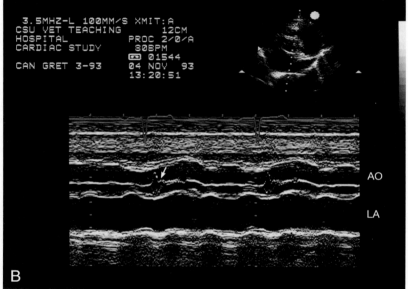

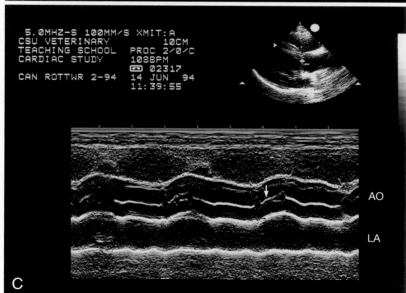

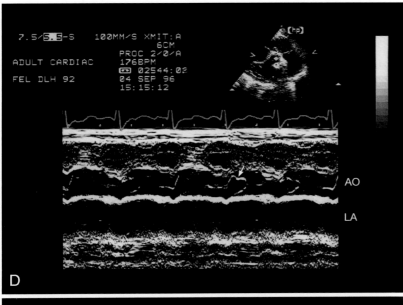

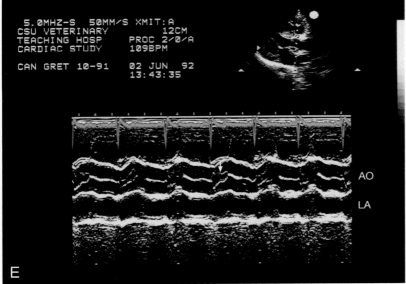

FIGURE 3.81 *(continued)*

motion will reverse and correct itself. This causes a sharp upward motion of the septum early in systole.

The right-sided volume overload must be moderate to severe before paradoxical septal motion is seen (170). Animals with right-sided volume overload which elevated RV diastolic pressures but did not exceed left side pressures did not show PSM but do exhibit flatter septal motion (170). When right ventricular pressure overload is present septal motion is flatter and there may be slight downward motion early in systole (170,173). In all cases of PSM, systolic thickening of the septum still occurs at the appropriate time in the cardiac cycle despite the abnormal motion.

Two-dimensional manifestation of paradoxical septal motion is seen as a flattened septum on transverse left ventricular planes (Fig. 3.12, 3.88). The normal circular left ventricular chamber appears as a triangular shape secondary to elevated right-sided pressures (170). Studies have shown that the degree of curvature of the septum correlates with the degree of right ventricular volume overload (173).

Paradoxical septal motion may be seen with left bundle branch block, pericarditis, mitral stenosis, aortic insufficiency, infarction, and after cardiac surgery (170,175,176).

FIGURE 3.82   A reduced deceleration slope (*arrow*) to the mitral valve on M-mode images usually is associated with reduced ventricular compliance. The downward mitral valve motion during systole is a sign of mitral valve prolapse.

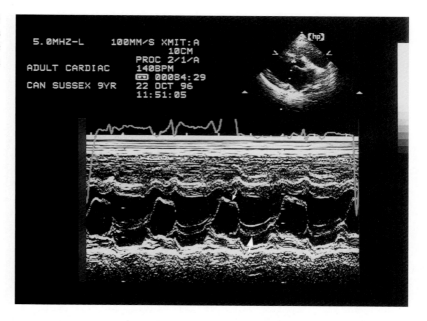

FIGURE 3.83   Delayed closure of the mitral valve (*arrows*) on these two figures indicates decreased ventricular compliance and increased stiffness to the ventricle. The delay is referred to as a B bump. *RV*, right ventricle; *LV*, left ventricle.

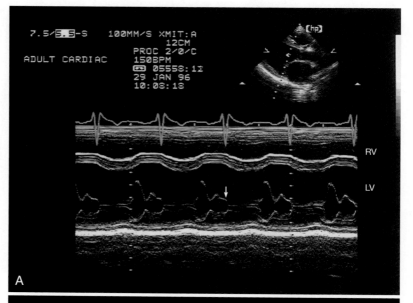

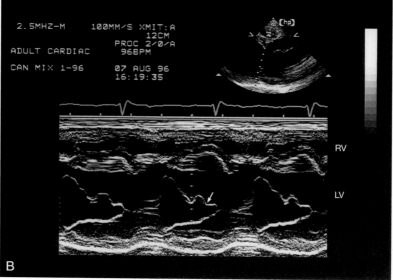

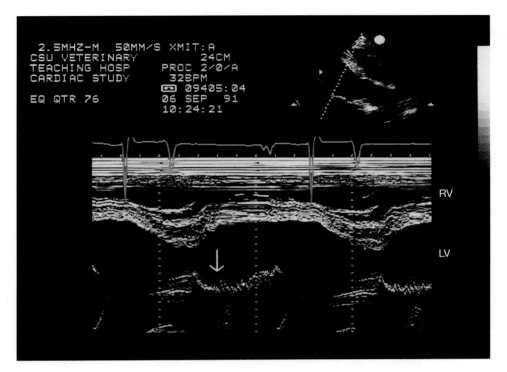

FIGURE 3.84 E point to septal separation (EPSS) may be larger than normal in animals with aortic insufficiency. Here, a horse with severe aortic regurgitation shows diastolic mitral valve flutter (*arrow*) and an increased EPSS. *RV,* right ventricle; *LV,* left ventricle.

FIGURE 3.85 Systolic anterior motion (SAM) of the mitral valve may be seen with increased flow velocity through the left ventricular outflow tract. **A.** Real-time images show the mitral valve pulled up into the outflow tract during systole (*arrow*). Figures **B** through **E** show varying degrees of SAM in a dog (**B** and **D**) and a cat (**C** and **E**). *RV,* right ventricle, *LV,* left ventricle, *AO,* aortic; *LA* left atrium.

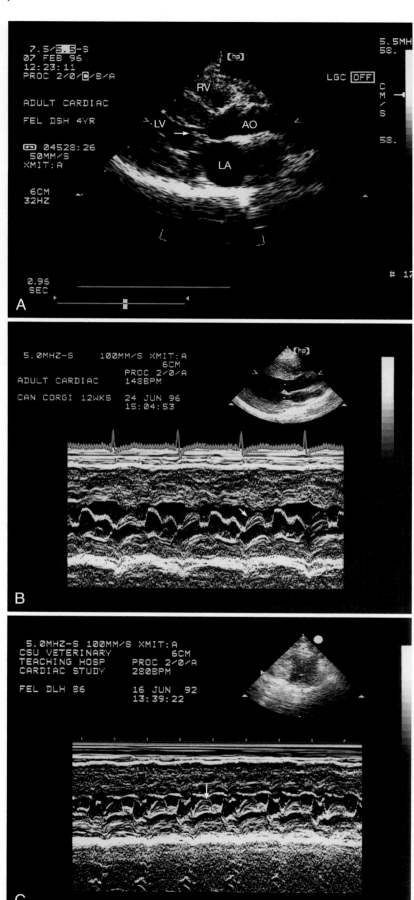

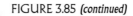

FIGURE 3.85 *(continued)*

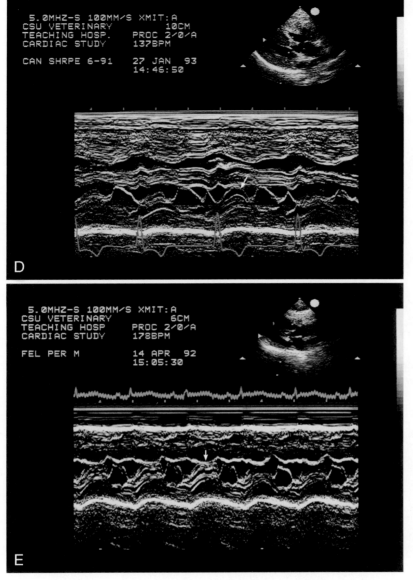

FIGURE 3.86   A diastolic dip (*arrow*) is seen on many left ventricle M-mode images. A diastolic dip is thought to be related to early diastolic filling. *RV*, right ventricle; *LV*, left ventricle.

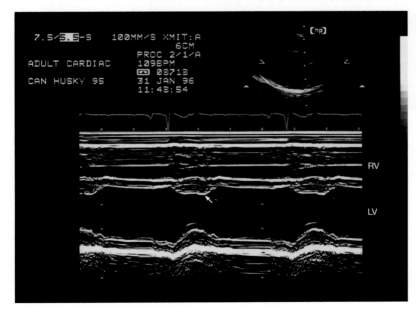

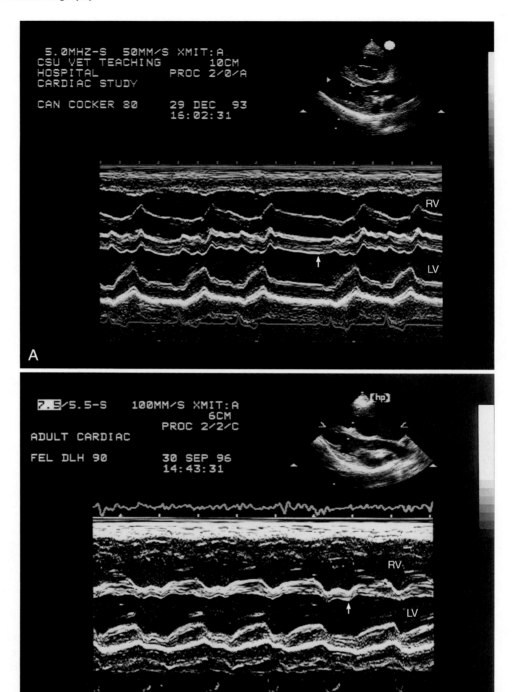

FIGURE 3.87   Paradoxical septal motion (PSM) is seen secondary to right ventricular volume overload. Figures **A** through **D** show varying degrees of PSM (*arrows*). *RV,* right ventricle; *LV,* left ventricle.

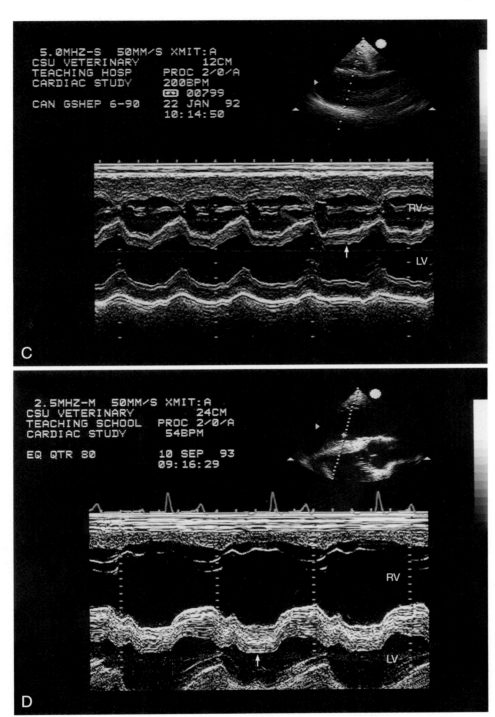

FIGURE 3.87 *(continued)*

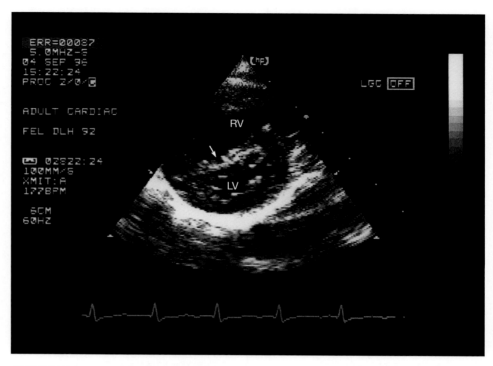

FIGURE 3.88   Two-dimensional manifestation of paradoxical septal motion (PSM) is seen as a flattened interventricular septum (*arrow*) on transverse left ventricular images. *RV,* right ventricle; *LV,* left ventricle.

▼   **EXERCISE 3-1**

Left ventricular measurements for a 15-lb dog are as follows.

		Normal
LVd	33.6	22.2–26.5
LVs	20.0	12.5–15.7
LVWd	7.5	5.1–6.4
LVWs	11.0	8.5–10.1
IVSd	9.0	6.4–8.0
IVSs	12.0	9.7–11.4
FS	40%	33–46
IVSd/LVd	0.26	0.22–0.34

a) What is the pattern of enlargement in this heart?

b) What can you say about this dog's ventricular function?

Answer Exercise 3-1

a) What is the pattern of enlargement in this heart?

This is eccentric hypertrophy—volume overload with compensatory hypertrophy.

b) What can you say about this dog's ventricular function?

Fractional shortening is within the normal range, but there is increased preload (large LVd) that should elevate fractional shortening. Systolic dimensions are increased, which suggests impaired myocardial function. Normal myocardium will allow even a severely dilated left ventricle to shorten down to normal systolic dimensions. Given these two facts, despite the normal fractional shortening, the findings in this heart imply myocardial systolic dysfunction. Blood pressure should be checked to rule out high afterload on the heart as a cause of the lower-than-expected functional parameters.

▼ EXERCISE 3-2

The following left ventricular measurements are obtained in a 30-lb dog.

		Normal
LVd	34.0	28.3–31.4
LVs	20.1	16.8–19.0
LVWd	8.5	6.2–7.1
LVWs	12.0	10.2–11.3
IVSd	11.9	7.8–8.9
IVSs	13.5	11.6–12.9
FS	41%	33–46
IVSd/LVd	0.35	0.22–0.34

a) What can you say about the pattern of left ventricular enlargement?

b) What can you say about left ventricular function?

Answer Exercise 3-2

a) What can you say about the pattern of left ventricular enlargement?

This represents eccentric hypertrophy—volume overload with compensatory hypertrophy. The hypertrophy appears excessive for the degree of volume overload because the ratio of septal thickness to chamber size is high.

b) What can you say about left ventricular function?

Volume overload (increased preload) should elevate fractional shortening. Fractional shortening, in this case, is only within the normal range. Excessive hypertrophy is present in this heart. High afterload should be suspected and ruled out as a cause of hypertrophy and depression in fractional shortening. If afterload can be ruled out as a factor in reducing function and preventing systolic dimensions from reaching normal values, then some degree of myocardial dysfunction may be present.

▼ EXERCISE 3-3

The following left ventricular dimensions are measured in a 23-lb poodle.

		Normal
LVd	22.5	25.7–29.3
LVs	15.1	14.9–17.5
LVWd	8.1	5.7–6.8
LVWs	12.0	9.5–10.8
IVSd	9.4	7.2–8.5
IVSs	13.9	10.8–12.2
FS	33%	33–46
IVSd/LVd	0.41	0.22–0.34

a) What kind of enlargement pattern is seen in this left ventricle?

b) What can be said of the function in this heart?

c) What kind of conditions would cause this pattern of hypertrophy to develop within the heart?

Answer Exercise 3-3

a) What kind of enlargement pattern is seen in this left ventricle?

This is representative of concentric hypertrophy—hypertrophy of the wall and septum at the expense of the chamber.

b) What can be said of the function in this heart?

Function is adequate. There is no increase in preload, and even if afterload is high, it has not depressed function to below acceptable levels.

c) What kind of conditions would cause this pattern of hypertrophy to develop within the heart?

–increased afterload such as hypertension or aortic stenosis
–hypertrophic cardiomyopathy
–decreased preload, creating the impression of hypertrophy as a result of a lack of stretch; causes would include dehydration or any other cause of volume contraction, severe pulmonary hypertension, and severe pulmonic stenosis

▼   EXERCISE 3-4

Give the intracardiac systolic and diastolic pressures for each of the following chambers and vessels (Fig. 3.89).

What is the normal pressure gradient between each of the following chambers?

a) Right atrium and right ventricle during systole:

b) Left atrium and left ventricle during systole:

c) Right ventricle and pulmonary artery during systole:

d) Right ventricle and pulmonary artery during diastole:

e) Left ventricle and aorta during systole:

f) Left ventricle and aorta during diastole:

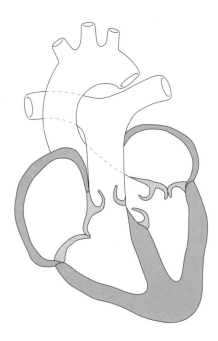

FIGURE 3.89

Answer Exercise 3-4

See Fig. 3.67 for chamber and vessel pressure.

What is the normal pressure gradient between each of the following chambers?
a) Right atrium and right ventricle during systole: 15
b) Left atrium and left ventricle during systole: 110
c) Right ventricle and pulmonary artery during systole: 0
d) Right ventricle and pulmonary artery during diastole: 5
e) Left ventricle and aorta during systole: 0
f) Left ventricle and aorta during diastole: 70

▼ EXERCISE 3-5

A golden retriever with aortic stenosis has a peak aortic flow velocity of 5.6 m/sec.

a) What is the pressure gradient across the obstruction?
b) If the dog's blood pressure is 120/75, what are pressures within the left ventricle?
c) Is the pressure gradient you calculated higher or lower than what would be measured during cardiac catheterization?

Answer Exercise 3-5

a) What is the pressure gradient across the obstruction?

$$4(5.6)^2 = 125 \text{ mm Hg}$$

b) If her blood pressure is 120/75, what are pressures within the left ventricle?

245 mm Hg—the pressure in the left ventricle is 125 mm Hg higher than systolic pressure within the aorta so left ventricular pressure equals 125 + 120.

c) Is the pressure gradient you calculated higher or lower than what would be measured during cardiac catheterization?

Doppler gradients are usually higher than gradients derived during catheterization because cardiac catheterization uses peak-to-peak gradients whereas Doppler calculates instantaneous gradients (see Fig. 3.66).

▼ EXERCISE 3-6

A terrier with pulmonic stenosis has a peak velocity of 4.0 m/sec within the pulmonary artery.

a) The pressure gradient is?
b) If systolic pressure within the pulmonary vasculature is estimated to be 20 mm Hg, what is the systolic pressure within the right ventricle?

Answer Exercise 3-6

a) The pressure gradient is?

$4(4)^2 = 64$ mm Hg

b) If systolic pressure within the pulmonary vasculature is estimated to be 20 mm Hg, what is the systolic pressure within the right ventricle?

84 mm Hg

Right ventricular pressure is 64 mm Hg higher than the pressure within the pulmonary artery; therefore, right ventricular pressure equals 64 + 20.

▼   EXERCISE 3-7

A dog has mild tricuspid insufficiency with no atrial dilation. Given the following information, calculate the right-sided pressures.

Tricuspid insufficiency velocity = 4.4 m/sec

Pulmonary flow velocity = 0.7 m/sec

Determine:

a) Pressure gradient from right ventricle to right atrium:

b) Estimate RA pressure:

c) RV systolic pressure:

d) PA systolic pressure:

e) Conclusions:

Answer Exercise 3-7

Determine:

a) Pressure gradient from right ventricle to right atrium:

$4(4.4)^2 = 77$ mm Hg

b) Estimate RA pressure:

5 mm Hg (see Fig. 3.67)

Regurgitation is mild and atrial size is not increased; therefore, pressures should be close to normal.

c) RV systolic pressure:

82 mm Hg

Right ventricular pressures are 77 mm Hg higher than right atrial pressures so right ventricular pressure equals 77 + 5.

d) PA systolic pressure:

Because pulmonary artery flow velocities show no evidence of pulmonic stenosis, right ventricular and pulmonary artery pressures are equal at 82 mm Hg.

e) Conclusions:

This dog has severe pulmonary hypertension.

▼   EXERCISE 3-8

A toy poodle presenting with mitral insufficiency has a mitral regurgitant jet velocity of 6.75 m/sec. Aortic flow velocity is 1.45 m/sec.

a) The pressure gradient from left ventricle to left atrium is:

b) Left ventricular pressures are at least:

c) Systemic systolic pressures are at least:

Answer Exercise 3-8

a) The pressure gradient from left ventricle to left atrium is:

$$4(6.75)^2 = 182 \text{ mm Hg}$$

b) Left ventricular pressures are at least:

182 mm Hg

In actuality, left ventricular pressures are 182 mm Hg higher than left atrial pressures, but they are at least 182.

c) Systemic systolic pressures are at least:

182 mm Hg

Because aortic flow velocity is normal without any evidence of aortic stenosis, left ventricular and aortic systolic pressures are equal. Systolic systemic pressures are at least 182 mm Hg, indicative of systemic hypertension.

▼ EXERCISE 3-9

A 12-month-old German shepherd puppy with subaortic stenosis has the following values on echocardiographic examination:

Aortic flow velocity of 4.5 m/sec
Mitral insufficiency with a velocity of 7.2 m/sec

a) What is the pressure gradient across the stenosis?

b) What is the pressure gradient from left ventricle to left atrium?

c) What are estimated left ventricular pressures based on the stenosis pressure gradient?

d) What are estimated left ventricular pressures based on the mitral regurgitant pressure gradient?

e) Comments.

Answer Exercise 3-9

a) What is the pressure gradient across the stenosis?

$$4(4.5)^2 = 81 \text{ mm Hg}$$

b) What is the pressure gradient from left ventricle to left atrium?

$$4(7.2)^2 = 207 \text{ mm Hg}$$

c) What are estimated left ventricular pressures based on the stenosis pressure gradient?

Ventricular pressures are 81 mm Hg higher than systemic pressures. Using 120 mm Hg as systemic systolic pressures, ventricular pressures would be

$$81 + 120 = 201 \text{ mm Hg}$$

d) What are estimated left ventricular pressures based on the mitral regurgitant pressure gradient?

Left ventricular pressures are 207 mm Hg higher than left atrial pressures. Using 10 mm Hg as estimated left atrial pressure, left ventricular pressures are equal to:

$$207 + 10 = 217 \text{ mm Hg}$$

e) Comments.

Both pressure gradients suggest left ventricular pressures just over 200 mm Hg. This means that velocities obtained across the stenosis and velocities of the regurgitant jet are probably accurate. When two different flows can be measured during the same time period, they can be used to double-check values.

▼   EXERCISE 3-10

A puppy with aortic stenosis is examined, and the following results are obtained.

Pulmonary flow velocities of 1.08 m/sec
Aortic flow velocities of 3.49 m/sec
Mitral regurgitant velocities of 3.57 m/sec

a) What is the gradient across the stenosis?

b) What is the pressure gradient across the mitral insufficiency?

c) Comments.

Answer Exercise 3-10

a) What is the gradient across the stenosis?

$$4(3.49)^2 = 49 \text{ mm Hg}$$

b) What is the pressure gradient across the mitral insufficiency?

$$4(3.57)^2 = 51 \text{ mm Hg}$$

c) Comments.

Estimated left ventricular pressures based on the stenotic pressure gradient are (49 + 120) 169 mm Hg. Estimated left ventricular pressure based on the mitral regurgitant jet are (10 + 51) 61 mm Hg. These two gradients do not support each other. Left ventricular pressures of 61 mm Hg are excessively low, even without aortic stenosis, and the gradient was not recorded accurately.

▼   EXERCISE 3-11

Signalment: canine, spaniel, 4 months old
M-mode findings:

		Normal
LVd	32.2	23.0–27.2
LVs	16.0	13.2–16.2
LVWd	6.9	5.3–6.5
LVWs	9.1	8.8–10.3
IVSd	8.9	6.6–8.1
IVSs	10.7	10.0–11.6
FS	50.3%	33–46

Two-dimensional findings:

–A VSD is seen high in the membranous septum

–All other structures appear normal –The right ventricle and the pulmonary artery are mildly dilated

Doppler findings:

–Color-flow Doppler shows the VSD (L to R)

–Color-flow Doppler also shows trivial aortic insufficiency

–Spectral Doppler records VSD velocities of 4.4 m/sec

–Pulmonary flow velocities are 3.2 m/sec

–Aortic flow velocities are 1.7 m/sec

Comments and conclusions:

What can be said about this VSD?

Answer Exercise 3-11

Comments and conclusions:

–VSD pressure gradient

$$4(4.4)^2 = 77 \text{ mm Hg}$$

–RV pressures if left ventricular pressures are 120

$$120 - 77 = 43 \text{ mm Hg}$$

The pressure gradient across the VSD is not high, suggesting either a) a large defect that doesn't restrict flow as much, resulting in velocities that are not high; b) elevated right-sided pressures; or c) both. Pulmonary artery flow velocity may be high, secondary to a large shunt volume, secondary to pulmonic stenosis, or both. Real-time images will need to be assessed for the presence of stenosis and hypertrophy. If no stenosis is suspected, then the PA velocities suggest a large shunt. Eccentric hypertrophy of the left ventricle exists with adequate compensatory hypertrophy.

▼ EXERCISE 3-12

Signalment: canine, small mix, 10 years old

M-mode findings:

		Normal
LVd dimension	35.6	27.0–30.3
LVs dimension	20.0	15.0–18.0
LVWd	7.3	5.9–6.9
LVWs	10.7	8.6–10.0
IVSd	9.1	7.5–8.7
IVSs	13.3	10.2–12.9
FS	43%	33–46
IVSd/LVd	0.26	0.22–0.34

Two-dimensional findings:

Small mitral valve lesions

All other structures visibly normal

Doppler findings:

Color flow shows mild mitral insufficiency

Aortic flow velocity of 113 cm/sec

Mitral insufficiency jet velocity of 707 cm/sec

Comments and conclusions:

a) What kind of enlargement pattern is seen based on M-mode measurements?

b) What is the pressure gradient between the left ventricle and left atrium?

c) Left ventricular pressures are at least:

d) What are the systemic pressures?

e) Conclusions?

Answer Exercise 3-12

Comments and conclusions:

a) What kind of enlargement pattern is seen based on M-mode measurements?

Eccentric hypertrophy, volume overload with compensatory wall and septal hypertrophy.

b) What is the pressure gradient between the left ventricle and left atrium?

$4(7.07)^2 = 200$ mm Hg

c) Left ventricular pressures are at least?

Because the gradient is 200, left ventricular pressures must be at least 200. Left atrial pressures can be added to the gradient to get a better estimate of LV pressure (200 + 10).

d) What are the systemic pressures?

Because aortic flow velocities are normal with no evidence of obstruction, systemic and ventricular pressures are the same at 210 mm Hg.

e) Conclusions?

Systemic hypertension is present with systolic pressures of about 210 mm Hg. Fractional shortening is typically higher than normal with volume overload; the high afterload may be depressing function. Repeating the echo to evaluate function after the hypertension is controlled is recommended to assess myocardial contractility.

▼ EXERCISE 3-13

Signalment: canine, Doberman, 6 years old

M-mode findings:

		Normal
LVd	58.2	41.8–45.4
LVs	55.1	26.0–28.6
LVWd	6.6	8.4–9.4
LVWs	7.1	13.6–14.9
IVSd	11.4	10.4–11.7
IVSs	11.9	15.9–17.3
IVSd/LVd	0.20	0.22–0.34
FS	5.3%	33–46

Two-dimensional findings:
  Generalized cardiomegaly
  No valvular lesions

Doppler findings:
  Color flow shows moderate mitral insufficiency
  Mitral regurgitant jet velocity of 4.8 m/sec

Determine:

a) What disease does this Doberman have?

b) What is the left ventricular to left atrial pressure gradient?

c) What does this pressure gradient suggest?

Answer Exercise 3-13

a) What disease does this Doberman have?

dilated cardiomyopathy

b) What is the left ventricular to left atrial pressure gradient?

$4(4.8)^2 = 92$ mm Hg

c) What does this pressure gradient suggest?

It implies low systemic pressures and/or high left atrial pressures.

▼ EXERCISE 3-14

Signalment: canine, Pomeranian, 1 year old
M-mode findings:

		Normal
LVd	8.6	17.6–23.0
LVs	2.5	9.6–13.5
LVWd	6.6	4.2–5.8
LVWs	10.5	7.4–9.4
IVSd	9.7	5.4–7.4
IVSs	12.2	8.3–10.4
IVSd/LVd	1.13	0.22–0.34
FS	71%	33–46

Two-dimensional findings:

Severe right ventricular hypertrophy
Valvular and subvalvular pulmonic stenosis

Doppler findings:
Color flow shows mild tricuspid insufficiency
Tricuspid regurgitant jet velocity of 6.2 m/sec
Could not obtain pulmonary flow velocities

Determine:
a) The RV to RA pressure gradient:
b) The RV to PA pressure gradient:
c) Comments and conclusions:

Answer Exercise 3-14

a) The RV to RA pressure gradient:

$4(6.2)^2 = 154$ mm Hg

Therefore, RV pressures are at least 154 mm Hg

b) The RV to PA pressure gradient:

If you assume the pulmonary artery systolic pressure is approximately 20 mm Hg, then the right ventricular to pulmonary artery pressure gradient is at least 134 mm Hg because RV pressures are at least 154 mm Hg (154 − 20).

c) Comments and conclusions:

This is an example of how other flows can help determine or support a pressure gradient calculation. This is severe pulmonic stenosis, and left ventricular dimensions are smaller than normal because of reduced volume entering the LV secondary to the stenosis. This creates a lack of LV distension and the appearance of left ventricular hypertrophy.

▼ EXERCISE 3-15

Signalment: canine, terrier cross, 6 months old
M-mode findings:

		Normal
LVd	34.4	35–38
LVs	20.5	21.7–23.5
LVWd	10.2	7.4–8.1
LVWs	14.7	12.0–13.0
IVSd	13.8	9.2–10.1
IVSs	16.7	13.9–14.9
FS	49%	33–46

Two-dimensional findings:
   Moderate right ventricular hypertrophy
   Valvular pulmonic stenosis
   Poststenotic dilation of pulmonary artery
   Ventricular septal defect
Doppler findings:
   Pulmonary flow velocity of 3.26 m/sec
   VSD left-to-right shunt velocity of 4.47 m/sec

Determine:

a) What is the pressure gradient across the pulmonic stenosis?

b) What are estimated right atrial pressures?

c) What are calculated right ventricular pressures?

d) What is the pressure gradient across the VSD?

e) What are calculated left ventricular pressures?

Answer Exercise 3-15

Determine:

a) What is the pressure gradient across the pulmonic stenosis?

$4(3.26)^2 = 43$ mm Hg

b) What are estimated right atrial pressures?

5 mm Hg (use Fig. 3.67)

c) What are calculated right ventricular pressures?

Right ventricular pressures are 43 mm Hg higher than pulmonary artery pressures; therefore, RV pressure = 43 + 20 = 63 mm Hg.

d) What is the pressure gradient across the VSD?

$4(4.47)^2 = 80$ mm Hg

e) What are calculated left ventricular pressures?

Because right ventricular pressures are approximately 63 mm Hg and the VSD gradient tells us that left ventricular pressures are 80 mm Hg higher than the right, left ventricular pressures are equal to 63 + 80 = 143 mm Hg.

▼ EXERCISE 3-16

Doppler echocardiography provides the following information from flow profiles in a puppy with aortic stenosis. The puppy's blood pressure is 120/80.

Moderate aortic insufficiency with a velocity of: 4.2 m/sec
Aortic flow velocity: 4.6 m/sec
Moderate mitral insufficiency with a velocity of: 6.9 m/sec

Determine:

a) Pressure gradient for flow from the aorta to the left ventricle:

b) Pressure gradient for flow from the left ventricle to the left atrium:

c) Pressure gradient for flow from the left ventricle to the aorta:

d) What is the pressure gradient of the aortic stenosis?

e) What are estimated left ventricular pressures?

f) What are calculated left atrial pressures?

Answer Exercise 3-16

a) Pressure gradient for flow from the aorta to the left ventricle:

$4(4.2)^2 = 71$ mm Hg

b) Pressure gradient for flow from the left ventricle to the left atrium:

$4(6.9)^2 = 190$ mm Hg

c) Pressure gradient for flow from the left ventricle to the aorta:

$4(4.6)^2 = 85$ mm Hg

d) What is the pressure gradient of the aortic stenosis?

85 mm Hg. The amount the aortic insufficiency volume adds to this gradient cannot be determined.

e) What are estimated left ventricular pressures?

Pressures in the left ventricle are 85 mm Hg higher than pressures in the aorta. Left ventricular pressures are approximately $85 + 120 = 205$ mm Hg.

f) What are calculated left atrial pressures?

Left ventricular pressures are 190 mm Hg higher than pressures in the left atrium; therefore, left atrial pressures are approximately 15 mm Hg $(205 - 190)$.

▼   EXERCISE 3-17

A cat presents with dyspnea and a murmur. Echocardiography reveals the presence of a VSD, mild pulmonic insufficiency, mild tricuspid insufficiency, mild aortic insufficiency, and moderate mitral insufficiency. No stenotic lesions were visualized on real-time images. The following velocities were derived:

Aortic flow velocity = 1.56 m/sec
Pulmonary flow velocity = 2.3 m/sec
Pulmonic insufficiency velocity = 3.4 m/sec
Tricuspid insufficiency velocity = 4.3 m/sec

Aortic insufficiency velocity = 4.2 m/sec
Mitral insufficiency velocity = 5.4 m/sec
VSD shunt velocity = not obtained

Determine the following:

a) Right ventricular to pulmonary artery pressure gradient:

b) Pulmonary artery to RV pressure gradient:

c) RV to RA pressure gradient:

d) Aorta to LV pressure gradient:

e) LV to LA pressure gradient:

f) Right ventricular systolic pressures:

g) Pulmonary artery diastolic pressures:

h) Left ventricular systolic pressures:

i) Aortic diastolic pressures:

j) Comments and conclusions based on Doppler:

Answer Exercise 3-17

a) Right ventricular to pulmonary artery pressure gradient: 21
b) Pulmonary artery to RV pressure gradient: 46
c) RV to RA pressure gradient: 74
d) Aorta to LV pressure gradient: 71
e) LV to LA pressure gradient: 117
f) Right ventricular systolic pressures: at least 74
g) Pulmonary artery diastolic pressures: at least 46
h) Left ventricular systolic pressures: at least 117
i) Aortic diastolic pressures: at least 71
j) Comments and conclusions based on Doppler:

Based on pressure gradients obtained from the right-sided insufficiencies, pulmonary hypertension is present with pressures of approximately 74/46. Pulmonary flow velocities are probably elevated secondary to the VSD flow because no visible stenosis is present. VSD flow is still left to right even though Doppler was not obtained on the shunt, because LV systolic pressures are still higher than RV systolic pressures. The gradient across the VSD is approximately 43 mm Hg (estimated LV pressure of 117 − estimated RV pressure of 74).

▼   EXERCISE 3-18

Left ventricular outflow area in the right parasternal long-axis with left ventricular outflow plane is 2.83 cm². Mitral annular area from apical four-chamber views is 6.6 cm². Pulmonary artery diameter at the right parasternal transverse plane is 2.40 cm². FVI for aortic flow is 12 cm, mitral inflow FVI is 25 cm, and pulmonic FVI is 11.4 cm. Calculate aortic, pulmonic, and mitral stroke volume (SV).

Answer Exercise 3-18

Aortic SV

$$SV = CSA \times FVI$$
$$= 2.83 \times 12$$
$$= 33.96 \text{ mL}$$

Pulmonic SV

$$SV = CSA \times FVI$$
$$= 2.40 \times 11.4$$
$$= 27.4 \text{ mL}$$

Mitral SV

$$SV = CSA \times FVI$$
$$= 6.6 \times 25$$
$$= 165 \text{ mL}$$

▼ EXERCISE 3-19

Mitral annulus cross-sectional area = 4.9 cm^2
Left ventricular outflow cross-sectional area = 3.14 cm^2
Mitral FVI = 17 cm
Aortic FVI = 15 cm

   a) Calculate mitral stroke volume

   b) Calculate aortic stroke volume

   c) Calculate regurgitant fraction

Answer Exercise 3-19

   a) Calculate mitral stroke volume

$$MV\ SV = CSA \times FVI$$
$$MV\ SV = 4.9 \times 17$$
$$MV\ SV = 83.3 \text{ mL}$$

   b) Calculate aortic stroke volume

$$AO\ SV = CSA \times FVI$$
$$AO\ SV = 3.14 \times 15$$
$$AO\ SV = 47.1 \text{ mL}$$

   c) Calculate regurgitant fraction

   In a normal heart with no leaking valves or shunts, the amount of blood flowing through each valve is equal. On a beat-to-beat basis, they may not be equal; however, over the course of several beats, volume will be similar. When mitral insufficiency is present, the extra volume flows through the mitral valve but not the aorta; therefore, the difference in volume between the two is equal to the regurgitant volume.

$$RF = \frac{MV\ SV - AO\ SV}{MV\ SV}$$
$$RF = \frac{83.3 - 47.1}{83.3}$$
$$RF = 43\%$$

▼   EXERCISE 3-20

Given the following information, calculate the mitral regurgitant fraction.

Mitral valve FVI = 18 cm
Aortic FVI = 17 cm
Mitral annulus area = 7.1 cm^2
Left ventricular outflow area = 4.15 cm^2

    a) Determine mitral stroke volume

    b) Determine aortic stroke volume

    c) Calculate regurgitant volume

    d) Calculate mitral regurgitant fraction

Answer Exercise 3-20

    a) Determine mitral stroke volume

$$MV\ SV = CSA \times FVI$$
$$= 7.1 \times 18$$
$$= 127.8\ mL$$

    b) Determine aortic stroke volume

$$AO\ SV = CSA \times FVI$$
$$= 4.15 \times 17$$
$$= 70.6\ mL$$

    c) Calculate regurgitant volume

$$RV = MV\ SV - AO\ SV$$
$$= 127.8 - 70.6$$
$$= 57.2\ mL$$

    d) Calculate mitral regurgitant fraction

$$RF = \frac{MV\ SV - AO\ SV}{MV\ SV}$$
$$= \frac{57.2}{127.8}$$
$$= 45\%$$

▼   EXERCISE 3-21

Given the following information, calculate the aortic regurgitant fraction.

Left ventricular outflow tract area = 5.72 cm^2
Mitral annulus area = 5.72 cm^2
MV FVI = 23 cm
AO FVI = 27 cm

    a) Determine mitral stroke volume

    b) Determine aortic stroke volume

    c) Calculate aortic regurgitant volume

    d) Calculate aortic regurgitant fraction

Answer Exercise 3-21

a) Determine mitral stroke volume

$$MV\ SV = CSA \times FVI$$
$$= 5.72 \times 23$$
$$= 131.6\ mL$$

b) Determine aortic stroke volume

$$AO\ SV = CSA \times FVI$$
$$= 5.72 \times 27$$
$$= 154\ mL$$

c) Calculate aortic regurgitant volume

$$RV = AO\ SV - MV\ SV$$
$$= 154 - 132$$
$$= 22\ mL$$

d) Calculate aortic regurgitant fraction

$$RF = \frac{AO\ SV - MV\ SV}{AO\ SV}$$
$$= \frac{22}{154}$$
$$= 14\%$$

▼ EXERCISE 3-22

A dog has a left-to-right ventricular septal defect. Given the following information, calculate the shunt ratio.

PA area = 4.15 cm^2
Left ventricular outflow area = 3.46 cm^2
PA velocity = 2.9 m/sec
PA FVI = 28 cm
AO velocity = 1.76 m/sec
AO FVI = 17 cm

a) Calculate pulmonary artery SV

b) Calculate aortic SV

c) Calculate Qp:Qs

d) Comments?

Answer Exercise 3-22

a) Calculate pulmonary artery SV

$$SV = CSA \times FVI$$
$$SV = 4.15\ cm^2 \times 28\ cm$$
$$SV = 116$$

b) Calculate aortic SV

$$SV = CSA \times FVI$$
$$SV = 3.46\ cm^2 \times 17\ cm$$
$$SV = 58.8\ mL$$

c) Calculate Qp:Qs

$$Qp:Qs = PA\ SV/\ AO\ SV$$
$$Qp:Qs = 116/59$$
$$Qp:Qs = 2.0{:}1$$

d) Comments:

Twice as much blood is flowing through the pulmonary circulation than in the systemic circulation because of the shunt. Because significant error can be built into the CSA measurements that can dramatically affect calculated shunt ratios, simply looking at peak flow velocities and flow integrals can provide information regarding the severity of the shunt. The higher the velocities and the larger the FVI, the greater the volume flowing through that vessel. Normal PA FVI ranges from 7 to 19 cm. Because this puppy had a PA FVI of 28, and a flow velocity of 2.9 m/sec, a significant shunt should be suspected. This only applies when no valvular insufficiencies are present at the interrogated flow sites.

▼   EXERCISE 3-23

A puppy has a left-to-right atrial septal defect. Given the following information, calculate the shunt ratio.

PA area = 1.13 cm²
Left ventricular outflow area = 0.63 cm²
PA velocity = 3.56 m/sec
PA FVI = 25 cm
AO velocity = 1.9 m/sec
AO FVI = 18 cm

a) Calculate pulmonary artery SV

b) Calculate aortic SV

c) Calculate Qp:Qs

d) Comments?

Answer Exercise 3-23

a) Calculate pulmonary artery SV

$$SV = CSA \times FVI$$
$$= 1.13 \times 25$$
$$= 28\ mL$$

b) Calculate aortic SV

$$SV = CSA \times FVI$$
$$= 0.63 \times 18$$
$$= 11.3\ mL$$

c) Calculate Qp:Qs

$$Qp:Qs = PA\ SV/\ AO\ SV$$
$$= 28/11$$
$$= 2.54{:}1$$

d) Comments:

A shunt ratio of greater than 2.5 is considered significant. FVI and peak velocities may be used to assess subjectively the severity of the shunt. Here, the high FVIs and peak velocities in the pulmonary artery suggest a hemodynamically significant shunt.

▼ EXERCISE 3-24

A puppy has a left-to-right patent ductus arteriosus. Given the following information, calculate the shunt ratio.

PA area = 1.13 cm^2
Left ventricular outflow area = 0.93 cm^2
PA velocity = 1.5 m/sec
PA FVI = 15 cm
AO velocity = 3.3 m/sec
AO FVI = 27 cm

a) Calculate pulmonary artery SV

b) Calculate aortic SV

c) Calculate Qp:Qs

d) Comments?

Answer Exercise 3-24

a) Calculate pulmonary artery SV

$$PA\ SV = CSA \times FVI$$
$$= 1.13 \times 15$$
$$= 17.0\ mL$$

b) Calculate aortic SV

$$AO\ SV = CSA \times FVI$$
$$= 0.93 \times 27$$
$$= 25.1\ mL$$

c) Calculate Qp:Qs

$$Qp:Qs = AO\ SV\ /\ PA\ SV$$
$$= 25.1\ /\ 17.0$$
$$= 1.5:1$$

d) Comments:

The extra volume flowing through the lungs is recorded in the aorta before shunting into the pulmonary artery. Flow in the pulmonary artery is not increased until after the ductus enters it, beyond where Doppler flow is normally recorded. Therefore, volume in the aorta is representative of flow that will go through the pulmonary circuit. Flow in the pulmonary artery is representative of flow that will enter the systemic circulation. The shunt ratio is calculated in reverse compared with the other intracardiac shunts.

REFERENCES

1. Reef VB. Advances in diagnostic ultrasonography. Vet Clin North Am Equine Pract 1991;7:451–466.
2. Reef VB. The use of diagnostic ultrasound in the horse. Ultrasound Quart 1991;9:1–33.
3. Reef VB. Echocardiographic examination in the horse: the basics. Comp Equine 1990;12:1312–1320.
4. Reimer J. Cardiac evaluation of the horse: using ultrasonography. Vet Med 1993;88:748–755.
5. Miller MW, Knauer KW, Herring DS. Echocardiography: Principles of interpretation. Semin Vet Med Surg 1989;4:58–76.
6. Bonagura JD. Echocardiography. JAVMA 1994;204:516–522.
7. Bonagura JD, Herring DS, Welker F. Echocardiography. Vet Clin North Am Equine Pract 1985;1:311–333.
8. Bonagura JD, O'Grady MR, Herring DS. Echocardiography. Vet Clin North Am Small Anim Pract 1985;15:1177–1194.
9. Bonagura JD, Miller MW. Veterinary echocardiography. Am J Cardiovasc Ultrasound Allied Tech 1989;6:229–264.
10. Bonagura JD. M-mode echocardiography: basic principles. Vet Clin North Am Small Anim Pract 1983;13:299–319.
11. Miles KG. Basic principles and clinical applications of diagnostic ultrasonography. Comp Small Anim 1989;11:609–622.
12. Ettinger SJ, Lusk RH. Echocardiographic techniques in the dog and cat. Proc 7th ACVIM 1989:229–236.
13. Kaplan PM. Instrumentation, principles, and pitfalls of ultrasonography. Probl Vet Med 1991;3:457–478.
14. Lombard CW, Evans M, Martin L, et al. Blood pressure, electrocardiogram and echocardiogram measurements in the growing pony foal. Equine Vet J 1984;16:342–347.
15. Stewart JH, Rose RJ, Barko AM. Echocardiography in foals from birth to three months old. Equine Vet J 1984;16:332–341.
16. Long KJ, Bonagura JD, Darke PGG. Standardized imaging technique for guided M-mode and Doppler echocardiography in the horse. Equine Vet J 1992;24:226–235.
17. Stadler P, Rewel A, Deegen E. M-mode echocardiography in dressage and show jumping horses of class "S" and in untrained horses. J Vet Med A 1993;40:292–306.
18. Jacobs G, Knight DH. M-mode echocardiographic measurements in nonanesthetized healthy cats: effects of body weight, heart rate, and other variables. Am J Vet Res 1985;46:1705–1711.
19. Fox PR, Bond BR, Peterson ME. Echocardiographic reference values in healthy cats sedated with ketamine hydrochloride. Am J Vet Res 1985;46:1479–1484.
20. DeMadron E, Bonagura JD, Herring DS. Two-dimensional echocardiography in the normal cat. Vet Radiol 1985;26:149–157.
21. O'Grady MR, Bonagura JD, Powers JD, et al. Quantitative cross-sectional echocardiography in the normal dog. Vet Radiol 1986;27:34–49.
22. Mahony C, Rantanen NW, DeMichael JA, et al. Spontaneous echocardiographic contrast in the thoroughbred: high prevalence in racehorses and a characteristic abnormality in bleeders. Equine Vet J 1992;24:129–133.
23. Garcia-Fernandez MA, Lopez-Sendon J, Coma-Canella I, et al. Echocardiographic detection of circulating blood in normal canine hearts. Am J Cardiol 1985;56:834–836.
24. Voros K, Holmes JR, Gibbs C. Anatomical validation of two-dimensional echocardiography in the horse. Equine Vet J 1990;22:392–397.
25. Voros K, Holmes JR, Gibbs C. Measurement of cardiac dimensions with two-dimensional echocardiography in the living horse. Equine Vet J 1991;23:461–465.
26. Sahn DJ, DeMaria A, Kisslo J, et al. Recommendations regarding quantitation in M-mode echocardiography: results of a survey of echocardiographic measurements. Circulation 1978;58:1072–1083, 1978.
27. O'Rourke RA, Hanrath P, Henry WN, et al. Report of the Joint International Society and Federation of Cardiology/World Health Organization task force on recommendations for standardization of measurements from M-mode echocardiograms. Circulation 1984;69(Suppl A):854–857, 1984.
28. Lusk RH, Ettinger SJ. Echocardiographic techniques in the dog and cat. J Am Anim Hosp Assoc 1990;26:473–488.

29. Mashiro I, Nelson RR, Cohn JH, et al. Ventricular dimensions measured noninvasively by echocardiography in the awake dog. J Appl Physiol 1976;41:953–961.

30. Jacobs G, Mahjoob K. Influence of alterations in heart rate on echocardiographic measurements in the dog. Am J Vet Res 1988; 49:548–552.

31. Jacobs G, Mahjoob K. Multiple regression analysis, using body size and cardiac cycle length, in predicting echocardiographic variables in dogs. Am J Vet Res 1988;49:1290–1294.

32. Lombard CW. Normal values of the canine M-mode echocardiogram. Am J Vet Res 1984;45:2015–2018.

33. Sisson D, Schaeffer D. Changes in linear dimensions of the heart, relative to body weight, as measured by M-mode echocardiography in growing dogs. Am J Vet Res 1991;52:1591–1596.

34. Snyder PS, Sato T, Atkins CE. A comparison of echocardiographic indices of the nonracing, healthy greyhound to reference values from other breeds. Vet Radiol Ultrasound 1995;36:387–392.

35. Page A, Edmunds G, Atwell RB. Echocardiographic values in the greyhound. Aust Vet J 1993;70:361–364.

36. Boon J, Wingfield WE, Miller CW. Echocardiographic indices in the normal dog. Vet Radiol 1983;24:214–221.

37. Bayón A, Fernández del Palacio J, Montes AM, et al. M-mode echocardiography study in growing Spanish mastiffs. J Small Anim Pract 1994;35:473–479.

38. Crippa L, Ferro E, Melloni E, et al. Echocardiographic parameters and indices in the normal beagle dog. Lab Anim 1992;26:190–195.

39. Gooding JP, Robinson WF, Mews GC. Echocardiographic assessment of left ventricular dimensions in clinically normal English cocker spaniels. Am J Vet Res 1986;47:296–300.

40. Morrison SA, Moise NS, Scarlett J, et al. Effect of breed and body weight on echocardiographic values in four breeds of dogs of differing somatype. J Vet Intern Med 1992;6:220–224.

41. Allen DG. Echocardiographic study of the anesthetized cat. Can J Comp Med 1982;46:115–122.

42. Jacobs G, Knight DH. Change in M-mode echocardiographic values in cats given ketamine. Am J Vet Res 1985;46:1712–1713.

42a. Allen DG, Downey RS. Echocardiographic assessment of cats anesthetized with xylazine-sodium pentobarbital. Can J Comp Med 1983;47:281–283.

43. Moise NS, Dietze A. Echocardiographic, electrocardiographic and radiographic detection of cardiomegaly in hyperthyroid cats. Am J Vet Res 1986;47:1487–1494.

44. Moise NS, Horne WA, Flanders JA, et al. Repeatability of the M-mode echocardiogram and the effects of acute changes in heart rate, cardiac contractility, and preload in healthy cats sedated with ketamine hydrochloride and acepromazine. Cornell Vet. 1986;76:241–258.

45. Moise NS, Dietze AE, Mezza LE, et al. Echocardiography, electrocardiography, and radiography of cats with dilation cardiomyopathy, hypertrophic cardiomyopathy, and hyperthyroidism. Am J Vet Res 1986;47:1476–1486.

46. Pipers FS, Reef V, Hamlin RL. Echocardiography in the domestic cat. Am J Vet Res 1979;40:882–886.

47. Pipers FS, Hamlin RL. Clinical use of echocardiography in the domestic cat. J Am Vet Med Assoc 1980;176:57–61.

48. Sisson DD, Knight DH, Helinski C, et al. Plasma taurine concentrations and M-mode echocardiographic measures in healthy cats and in cats with dilated cardiomyopathy. J Vet Intern Med 1991;5:232–238.

49. Soderberg SF, Boon JA, Wingfield WE, et al. M-mode echocardiography as a diagnostic aid for feline cardiomyopathy. Vet Radiol 1983;34:66–73.

50. Lescure F, Tamzali Y. Referring values in echocardiography TM in sport-horse. Revue Med Vet 1984;135:405–418.

51. Bertone JJ, Paull KS, Wingfield WE, et al. M-mode echocardiography of endurance horses in the recovery phase of long-distance competition. Am J Vet Res 1987;48:1708–1712.

52. O'Callaghan MW. Comparison of echocardiographic and autopsy measurements of cardiac dimensions in the horse. Equine Vet J 1985;17:361–368.

53. Paull KS, Wingfield WE, Bertone JJ, et al. Echocardiographic changes with endurance training. In: Gillespie JR, Robinson NE, eds. Equine exercise physiology 2. Davis: ICEEP Publications, 1987;34–40.

54. Pipers FS, Hamlin RL. Echocardiography in the horse. JAVMA 1977;170:815–819.

55. Moses BL, Ross JN. M-mode echocardiographic values in sheep. Am J Vet Res 1987;48:1313–1318.

56. Pipers FS, Muir WW, Hamlin RL. Echocardiography in swine. Am J Vet Res 1978;39:707–710.

57. Gwathmey JK, Nakao S, Come PC, et al. Echocardiographic assessment of cardiac chamber size and functional performance in swine. Am J Vet Res 1989;50:192–197.

58. Boon JA, Knight AP, Moore DH. Llama cardiology. Vet Clin North Am Food Anim Pract 1994;10:353–369.

59. Amory H, Kafidi N, Lekeux P. Echocardiographic evaluation of cardiac morphologic and functional variables in double-muscled calves. Am J Vet Res 1992;53:1540–1547.

60. Amory H, Jakovljevic S, Lekeux P. Quantitative M-mode and two-dimensional echocardiography in calves. Vet Rec 1991;128:25–31.

61. Amory H, Lekeux P. Effects of growth on functional and morphological echocardiographic variables in Friesian calves. Vet Rec 1991;128:349–354.

62. Pipers FS, Reef V, Hamlin RL, et al. Echocardiography in the bovine animal. Bov Pract 1978;13:114–118.

63. Gaasch WH. Left ventricular radius to wall thickness ratio. Am J Cardiol 1979;43:1189–1194.

64. Grossman W, Jones D, McLaurin LP. Wall stress and patterns of ventricular hypertrophy in the human left ventricle. J Clin Invest 1975;56:56–64.

65. Kirberger RM. Mitral valve E point to ventricular septal separation in the dog. J S Afr Vet Assoc 1991;62:163–166.

66. Child JS, Krivokapich J, Perloff JK. Effect of left ventricular size on mitral E point to ventricular septal separation in assessment of cardiac performance. Am Heart J 1981;101:797–805.

67. Ginzton LE, Kulick D. Mitral valve E-point septal separation as an indicator of ejection fraction in patients with reversed septal motion. Chest 1985;88:429–431.

68. Brown OR, Harrison DC, Popp RL. An improved method for detection of left atrial enlargement. Circulation 1974;50:58–64.

69. Colocousis JS, Huntsman IL, Curreri PW. Estimation of stroke volume changes by ultrasonic Doppler. Circulation 1977;56:914–917.

70. Bonagura JD, Darke PGG, Long K, et al. Doppler-echocardiographic estimation of heart function: comparison with invasive measurement in closed-chest dogs. Proc 8th ACVIM Forum 1990:863–866.

71. Darke PGG. An evaluation of transducer sites for measurement of aortic and pulmonary flows by Doppler echocardiography. Proc 9th ACVIM Forum 1991:703–705.

72. Darke PGG. Two-dimensional imaging for Doppler echocardiography in dogs. Proc 8th ACVIM Forum 1990;261–268.

73. Darke PGG, Bonagura JD, Miller M. Transducer orientation for Doppler echocardiography in dogs. J Small Anim Pract 1993;34:2–8.

74. Kirberger RM, Bland-Van Den Berg P, Darazs B. Doppler echocardiography in the normal dog. Part I. Velocity findings and flow patterns. Vet Radiol Ultrasound 1992;33:370–379.

75. Kirberger RM, Bland-Van Den Berg P, Grimbeek RJ. Doppler echocardiography in the normal dog. Part II. Factors influencing blood flow velocities and a comparison between left and right heart blood flow. Vet Radiol Ultrasound 1992;33:380–386.

76. Long KJ. Doppler echocardiography in the horse. Equine Vet Edu 1990;2:15–17.

77. Darke PGG. An evaluation of transducer sites for measurement of aortic and pulmonary flows by Doppler echocardiography. Proc 9th ACVIM 1991:703–705.

78. Gaber C. Doppler echocardiography. Prob Vet Med 1991;3:479–499.

79. Darke PGG. Doppler echocardiography. J Small Anim Pract 1992;33:104–112.

80. Hatle L, Angelsen B. Doppler ultrasound in cardiology. Physical principles and clinical applications. 2nd ed. Philadelphia: Lea & Febiger, 1985.

81. Brown DJ, Knight DH, King RR. Use of pulsed-wave Doppler echocardiography to determine aortic and pulmonary velocity and flow variables in clinically normal dogs. Am J Vet Res 1991;52:543–550.

82. Yuill CDM, O'Grady MR. Doppler-derived velocity of blood flow across the cardiac valves in the normal dog. Can J Vet Res 1991;55:185–192.

83. Reef VB, Lalezari K, De Boo J, et al. Pulsed-wave Doppler evaluation of intracardiac blood flow in 30 clinically normal standard bred horses. Am J Vet Res 1989;50:75–83.

84. Yamamoto K, Masuyama T, Tanouchi J, et al. Effects of heart rate on left ventricular filling dynamics: assessment from simultaneous recordings of pulsed Doppler transmi-

tral flow velocity pattern and hemodynamic variables. Cardiovasc Res 1993;27:935–941.

85. Gaber CE. Normal pulsed Doppler flow velocities in adult dogs. Proc 5th ACVIM 1987:923.

86. Kirberger RM. Pulsed wave Doppler echocardiographic evaluation of intracardiac blood flow in normal sheep. Res Vet Sci 1993;55:189–194.

87. Akasaka T, Yoshikawa J, Yoshida K, et al. Age-related valvular regurgitation: a study by pulsed Doppler echocardiography. Circulation 1987;76:262–265.

88. Kostucki W, Vandenbossche JL, Friart A, et al. Pulsed Doppler regurgitant flow patterns of normal valves. Am J Cardiol 1986;58:309–313.

89. Choong CY, Abascal VM, Weyman J, et al. Prevalence of valvular regurgitation by Doppler echocardiography in patients with structurally normal hearts by two-dimensional echocardiography. Am Heart J 1989;117:636–642.

90. Sahn DJ, Maciel BC. Physiological valvular regurgitation. Doppler echocardiography and the potential for iatrogenic heart disease. Circulation 1989;78:1075–1077.

91. Nakayama T, Wakao Y, Takiguchi S, et al. Prevalence of valvular regurgitation in normal beagle dogs detected by color Doppler echocardiography. J Vet Med Sci 1994;56:973–975.

92. Yock PG, Naasz C, Schnittger I, et al. Doppler tricuspid and pulmonic regurgitation in normals: is it real? Circulation 1984;70(Suppl II):40.

93. Helmcke F, Nanda NC, Hsiung MC, et al. Color Doppler assessment of mitral regurgitation with orthogonal planes. Circulation 1987;75:175–183.

94. Cooper JW, Nanda NC, Philpot EF, et al. Evaluation of valvular regurgitation by Doppler. J Am Soc Echocardiogr 1989;2:56–66.

95. Braunwald E. Pathophysiology of heart failure. In: Braunwald E, ed. Heart disease: a textbook of cardiovascular medicine. Philadelphia: WB Saunders, 1980:453–471.

96. Schlant RC, Sonnenblick EH. Pathophysiology of heart failure. In: Hurst JW, Schlant RC, Rackley CE, et al., eds. The heart. 7th ed. New York: McGraw Hill Book Co, 1990:387–418.

97. Hirota Y. A clinical study of left ventricular relaxation. Circulation 1980;62:756–763.

98. Atkins CE, Curtis MB, McGuirk SM, et al. The use of M-mode echocardiography in determining cardiac output in dogs with normal, low, and high output states: comparison to thermodilution method. Vet Radiol Ultrasound 1992;33:297–304.

99. Nishimura RA, Housmans PR, Hatle LK, et al. Assessment of diastolic function of the heart: background and current applications of Doppler echocardiography. Part I. Physiologic and pathophysiologic features. Mayo Clin Proc 1989;64:71–81.

100. Federman M, Hess OM. Differentiation between systolic and diastolic dysfunction. Eur J Cardiol 1994;15(Suppl D):2–6.

101. Kittleson MD. Left ventricular function and failure. Part I. Comp Small Anim 1994;16:287–308.

102. Kittleson MD. Left ventricular function and failure. Part II. Comp Small Anim 1994;16:1001–1017.

103. Schiller NB. Two-dimensional echocardiographic determination of left ventricular volume, systolic function, and mass. Summary and discussion of the 1989 recommendations of the American Society of Echocardiography. Circulation 1991;84:I280–I287.

104. Teicholz LE, Kreulen T, Herman MV, et al. Problems in echocardiographic volume determinations: echocardiographic–angiographic correlations in the presence or absence of asynergy. Am J Cardiol 1976;37:7–11.

105. Kronik G, Slany J, Mösslacher H. Comparative value of eight M-mode echocardiographic formulas for determining left ventricular stroke volume. A correlative study with thermodilution and left ventricular single plane cineangiography. Circulation 1979;60:1308–1316.

106. Uehara Y, Koga M, Takahashi M. Determination of cardiac output by echocardiography. J Vet Med Sci 1995;57:401–407.

107. Sisson DD, Daniel GB, Twardock AR. Comparison of left ventricular ejection fractions determined in healthy anesthetized dogs by echocardiography and gated equilibrium radionuclide ventriculography. Am J Vet Res 1989;50:1840–1847.

108. Dyson DH, Allen DG, McDonell WN. Comparison of three methods for cardiac output determination in cats. Am J Vet Res 1985;46:2546–2552.

109. Lord PF, Croft MA. Accuracy of formulae for calculating left ventricular volumes of the equine heart. Equine Vet J Suppl 1990;9:53–56.

110. Atkins CE, Snyder PS. Systolic time intervals and their derivatives for evaluation of cardiac function. J Vet Intern Med 1992;2:55–63.

111. Pipers FS, Andrysco RM, Hamlin RL. A totally noninvasive method for obtaining systolic time intervals in the dog. Am J Vet Res 1978;39:1822–1826.

112. Lewis RP, Rittgers SE, Forester WF, et al. A critical review of the systolic time intervals. Circulation 1977;56:146–158.

113. Hassan S, Turner P. Systolic time intervals: a review of the method in the noninvasive investigation of cardiac function in health, disease and clinical pharmacology. Postgrad Med J 1983;59:423–434.

114. Weissler AM. Current concepts in cardiology; systolic time intervals. N Eng J Med 1977;296:321–324.

115. Allen DG, Nymeyer D. A preliminary investigation on the use of thermodilution and echocardiography as an assessment of cardiac function in the cat. Can J Comp Med 1983;47:112–117.

116. Wyatt HL, Heng MK, Meerbaum S, et al. Cross sectional echocardiography II. Analysis of mathematical models for quantifying volume of the formalin fixed left ventricle. Circulation 1980;61:1119–1125.

117. Vörös K, Holmes JR, Gibbs C. Left ventricular volume determination in the horse by two-dimensional echocardiography: an in vitro study. Equine Vet J 1990;22: 398–401.

118. Troy BL, Pombo J, Rackley CE. Measurements of left ventricular wall thickness and mass by echocardiography. Circulation 1972;45:602–611.

119. Wyatt HL, Heng K, Weerbaum S, et al. Cross sectional echocardiography. Analysis of models for quantifying mass in the left ventricle in dogs. Circulation 1983;60:348–358.

120. Schiller NB, Skiôldebrand CG, Schiller EJ, et al. Canine left ventricular mass estimation by two-dimensional echocardiography. Circulation 1983;68:210–216.

121. Bienvenu JG, Drolet R. A quantitative study of cardiac mass in dogs. Can J Vet Res 1991;55:305–309.

122. Zogbbi WA, Quinones MA. Determination of cardiac output by Doppler echocardiography: a critical appraisal. Herz 1986;11:258–268.

123. Huntsman LL, Stewart DK, Barnes SR, et al. Noninvasive Doppler determination of cardiac output in man: clinical validation. Circulation 1983;67:593–602.

124. Fisher DC, Sahn DJ, Friedman MJ, et al. The mitral valve orifice method for noninvasive two-dimensional echo Doppler determination of cardiac output. Circulation 1983;67: 872–877.

125. Nishimura RA, Tajik AJ. Quantitative hemodynamics by Doppler echocardiography: a noninvasive alternative to cardiac catheterization. Prog Cardiovasc Dis 1994;36:309–342.

126. Labovitz AJ, Buckingham TA, Habermehl K, et al. The effects of sampling site on the two-dimensional echo-Doppler determination of cardiac output. Am Heart J 1985;109: 327–332.

127. Stewart WJ, Jiang L, Mick R, et al. Variable effects of change in flow rate through the aortic, pulmonary and mitral valves on valve area and flow velocity: impact on quantitative Doppler flow calculations. J Am Coll Cardiol 1985;6:653–662.

128. Valdes-Cruz LM, Horowitz S, Mesel E, et al. A pulsed Doppler method for calculation of pulmonary and systemic flow: accuracy in a canine model with ventricular septal defect. Circulation 1983;68:597–602.

129. Ascah KJ, Stewart WJ, Gillam LD, et al. Calculation of transmitral flow by Doppler echocardiography: a comparison of methods in a canine model. Am Heart J 1989;117: 402–411.

130. Bennett ED, Barclay SA, Davis AL, et al. Ascending aortic blood velocity and acceleration using Doppler ultrasound in the assessment of left ventricular function. Cardiovasc Res 1984;18:632–638.

131. Sabbath HN, Khaja F, Brymer JP, et al. Noninvasive evaluation of left ventricular performance based peak aortic blood acceleration measured with a continuous wave Doppler velocity meter. Circulation 1986;74:323–329.

132. Sabbath HN, Gheorghiade M, Smith ST, et al. Serial evaluation of left ventricular function in congestive heart failure by measurement of peak aortic blood acceleration. Am J Cardiol 1988;57:367–370.

133. DeMaria AN, Wisenbaugh TW, Smith MD, et al. Doppler Echocardiographic evaluation of diastolic function. Circulation 1991;84(Suppl I):288–295.

134. Dougherty AH, Naccarelli GV, Gray EL, et al. Congestive heart failure with normal systolic function. Am J Cardiol 1984;54:778–782.

135. Soufer R, Wohlgelernter D, Vita NA, et al. Intact systolic left ventricular function in clinical congestive heart failure. Am J Cardiol 1984;53:567–571.

136. Nishimura RA, Abel MD, Hatle LK, et al. Assessment of diastolic function of the heart: background and current applications of Doppler echocardiography. Part II. Clinical studies. Mayo Clin Proc 1989;64:181–204.

137. Brutsaert DL, Rademakers FE, Sys SU, et al. Analysis of relaxation in the evaluation of ventricular function of the heart. Prog Cardiovasc Dis 1985;28:143–163.

138. Hirota Y. A clinical study of left ventricular relaxation. Circulation 1980;62:756–763.

139. Yellin EL, Nikolic S, Frater RW. Left ventricular filling dynamics and diastolic function. Prog Cardiovasc Dis 1990;32:242–271.

140. Callahan MJ, Tajik AJ, Su-Fan Q, et al. Validation of instantaneous pressure gradients measured by continuous wave Doppler in experimentally induced aortic stenosis. Am J Cardiol 1995;56:989–993.

141. Holen J, Aaslid R, Landmark K, et al. Determination of pressure gradients in mitral stenosis with noninvasive ultrasound Doppler technique. Acta Med Scand 1976;199: 455–460.

142. Stamm RB, Martin RP. Quantification of pressure gradients across stenotic mitral valves by Doppler ultrasound. Am Coll Cardiol 1983;2:707–718.

143. Hatle L, Brubakk A, Tromsdal A, et al. Noninvasive assessment of pressure drop in mitral stenosis by Doppler ultrasound. Br Heart J 1978;40:131–140.

144. Uehara Y. An attempt to estimate the pulmonary artery pressure in dogs by means of pulsed Doppler echocardiography. J Vet Med Sci 1993;55:307–312.

145. Teague SM, Heinsimer JA, Anderson JL, et al. Quantification of aortic regurgitation utilizing continuous wave Doppler ultrasound. J Am Coll Cardiol 1986;8:592–599.

146. Lewis BS, Hasin Y, Pasternak R, et al. Echocardiographic aortic root motion in ventricular volume overload and the effect of mitral incompetence. Eur J Cardiol 1979;10:375–384.

147. Gilbert BW, Pollick C, Adelman AG, et al. Hypertrophic cardiomyopathy: subclassification by M-mode echocardiography. Am J Cardiol 1980;45:861–872.

148. Krajcer Z, et al. Early systolic closure of the aortic valve in patients with hypertrophic subaortic stenosis and discrete subaortic stenosis. Am J Cardiol 1978;41:823–829.

149. Gardin JM, Tommaso CL, Talano JV. Echocardiographic early systolic partial closure (notching) of the aortic valve in congestive cardiomyopathy. Am Heart J 1984;107: 135–142.

150. Botvinick EH, Schiller NB, Wickramasekaran R, et al. Echocardiographic demonstration of early mitral valve closure in severe aortic insufficiency: its clinical implications. Circulation 1975;51:836–847.

151. Pridie RB, Beham R, Oakley CM. Echocardiography of the mitral valve in aortic valve disease. Br Heart J 1971;33:296–304.

152. Johnson AD, Gosink BB. Oscillation of left ventricular structures in aortic regurgitation. J Clin Ultrasound 1977;5:21–24.

153. Konecke LL, Feigenbaum H, Chang S, et al. Abnormal mitral valve motion in patients with elevated left ventricular diastolic pressures. Circulation 1973;47:989–996.

154. Ohte N, Nakano S Mizutani Y, et al. Relation of mitral valve motion to left ventricular end-diastolic pressure assessed by M-mode echocardiography. J Cardiogr 1986;16:115–120.

155. Downee TR, Nomeir AM, Hackshaw BT, et al. Diastolic mitral regurgitation in acute but not chronic aortic regurgitation: implications regarding the mechanism of mitral closure. Am Heart J 1989;117:1105–1112.

156. Otsuji Y, Toda H, Ishigami T, et al. Mitral regurgitation during B bump of mitral valve studied by Doppler echocardiography. Am J Cardiol 1991;67:778–780.

157. Maron BJ, Gottendiener JS, Perry LW. Specificity of systolic anterior motion of anterior mitral leaflet for hypertrophic cardiomyopathy. Prevalence in a large population of patients with other cardiac diseases. Br Heart J 1981;45:206–212.

158. Shah PM Gramiak R, Kramer DH. Ultrasound localization of left ventricular outflow obstruction in hypertrophic obstructive cardiomyopathy. Circulation 1969;40:3–11.

159. Shah PM, Gramiak R, Adelman AG, et al. Role of echocardiography in diagnostic and hemodynamic assessment of hypertrophic subaortic stenosis. Circulation 1971; 44:891–898.

160. Popp RL, Harrison DC. Ultrasound in the diagnosis of idiopathic hypertrophic subaortic stenosis. Circulation 1969;40: 905–914.

161. Pridie RB, Oakley CM. Mechanism of mitral regurgitation in hypertrophic obstructive cardiomyopathy. Br Heart J 1970;32:203–208.

162. Park SC, Neches WH, Zuberbuhler JR, et al. Echocardiographic and hemodynamic correlation in transposition of the great arteries. Circulation 1978;57:291–298.

163. Sahn DJ, Terry R, O'Rourke R, et al. Multiple crystal cross sectional echocardiography in the diagnosis of cyanotic congenital heart disease. Circulation 1974;50:230–238.

164. Mintz GS, Kotler MN, Segal BL, et al. Systolic anterior motion of the mitral valve in the absence of asymmetric septal hypertrophy. Circulation 1978;57:256–263.

165. Maron BJ, Redwood DR, Roberts WC. Tunnel subaortic stenosis. Left ventricular outflow obstruction produced by fibromuscular tubular narrowing. Circulation 54: 404–416.

166. Davis RH, Feigenbaum H, Chang S, et al. Echocardiographic manifestations of discrete subaortic stenosis. Am J Cardiol 1984;33:277–280.

167. Rees A, Elbl F, Minhas K, et al. Echocardiographic evidence of outflow tract obstruction in Pompe's disease (glycogen storage disease of the heart). Am J Cardiol 1976;37:1103–1106.

168. Gattiker HF, Davignon A, Bozio A, et al. Echocardiographic findings in Friedreich's ataxia. Can J Neurol Sci 1976;3:329–332.

169. Voelkel AG, Pietro DA, Folland ED, et al. Echocardiographic features of constrictive pericarditis. Circulation 1978;58:871–875.

170. DeMadron E, Bonagura JD, O'Grady MR. Normal and abnormal paradoxical septal motion in the dog. Am J Vet Res 1985;46:1832–1841.

171. Kerber RE, Dippel WF, Abboud FM. Abnormal motion of the IVS in right ventricle volume overload: experimental and clinical echocardiographic studies. Circulation 1973;48:86–96.

172. Tanaka H, Tei CH, Nakao S, et al. Diastolic bulging of the interventricular septum toward the left ventricle: an echocardiographic manifestation of negative interventricular pressure gradient between right and left ventricles during diastole. Circulation 1980;62:558–563.

173. Kingma I, Tyberg JV, Smith ER. Effects of diastolic transseptal pressure gradient on ventricular septal position and motion. Circulation 1983;68:1304–1314.

174. Chandell-Riera J, Del Castilla GH, Permayer-Miralda G, et al. Echocardiographic features of the interventricular septum in chronic constrictive pericarditis. Circulation 1976;54:174–178.

175. Weyman AE, Heger JJ, Kronik TG, et al. Mechanism of paradoxical septal motion in patients with mitral stenosis: a cross-sectional echocardiographic study. Am J Cardiol 1977;40:691–699.

176. Dillon JC, Chang S, Feigenbaum H. Echocardiographic manifestations of left bundle branch block. Circulation 1974;49:876–880.

4

ACQUIRED HEART DISEASE

▼

MITRAL INSUFFICIENCY

Many clinically normal animals have small physiologic or clinically insignificant regurgitant jets at one or more valves. Physiologic mitral valvular insufficiency is seen less often than the insufficiencies at the other valves in most animals in which it has been studied. Both the size and duration of valvular leaks help differentiate between physiologic and pathologic regurgitation. Physiologic regurgitation has low velocity, occupies a small area behind the valve, and rarely encompasses the entire portion of systole or diastole (1). These small leaks often are associated with valve closure (1–4). Studies have shown that between 26 and 68% of horses have insignificant mitral insufficiencies (2–5). In the horse, clinically insignificant mitral leaks were described as elliptical in shape on color-flow examinations, with a length of 34 ± 13 mm and a width of 1.9 ± 1.3 mm. These jets only were seen on left parasternal long-axis views (2). This may be because less depth is required, and the angle can be manipulated better to optimize color-flow imaging in the horse from the left side.

Valvular Appearance and Motion

Degenerative Lesions

Acquired mitral valvular insufficiency is usually secondary to degenerative valvular disease. The characteristics of endocardiosis include the following: left ventricular and atrial dilation, wall and septal hypertrophy, thickening of the mitral valve leaflets, elevated parameters of function, and hyperdynamic wall and septal motion. Less common features include pericardial effusion, lack of hypertrophy, decreases in function, ruptured chordae, and leaflet prolapse. These are all discussed in the following sections.

Degenerative mitral valve disease causes the valve leaflets to thicken with eventual lack of proper leaflet alignment and closure. The lesions are generally smooth and small and create a small club-shaped appearance to the leaflet tips during early stages of the disease, but the lesions may become large and irregular as the disease progresses (6) (Figs. 4.1, 4.2, and 4.3). Larger lesions generally are associated with more severe insufficiency, but this is not always the case.

Lesions are identified by gain and depth, which are transducer dependent. It may be best to compare the leaflets with other structures that are at that approximate depth. Normal anterior mitral valve leaflets are comparable to the thickness of aortic valve cusps. The thickness of the endocardial echoes have been used to assess leaflet

Physiologic Regurgitation

- Low velocity
- Trivial
- Occurs during only a portion of systole or diastole

Take care not to identify chordal attachments as lesions.

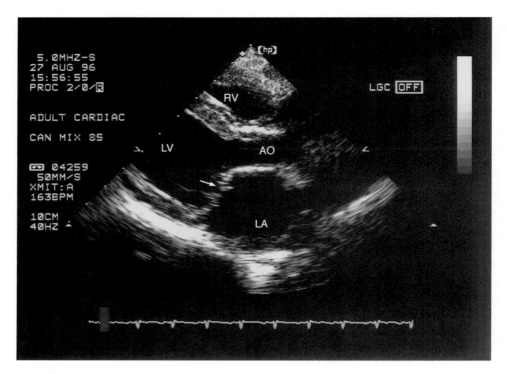

FIGURE 4.1   Mitral valve lesions associated with endocardiosis start out as small, smooth nodules on the valves (*arrow*). This right parasternal left ventricular outflow view of the heart also shows left atrial dilation. *RV*, right ventricle; *LV*, left ventricle; *LA*, left atrium; *AO*, aorta.

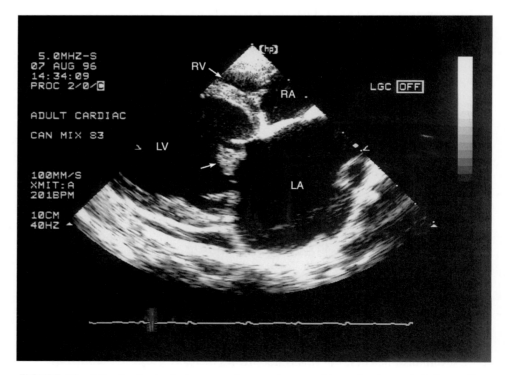

FIGURE 4.2   Mitral valvular lesions may become large and irregular (*arrow*). Echocardiography cannot differentiate between degenerative and vegetative lesions. Bowing of the interventricular and atrial septums toward the right indicates dilation of both chambers. *RV*, right ventricle; *RA*, right atrium; *LV*, left ventricle; *LA*, left atrium.

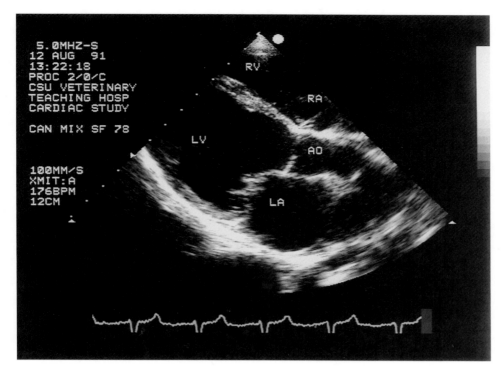

FIGURE 4.3   Thick irregular mitral valves are seen in this right parasternal long-axis left ventricular outflow view of the heart. Left atrial enlargement is present based on a large left atrial to aortic root ratio. The left ventricle also is dilated. *RV*, right ventricle; *RA*, right atrium; *LV*, left ventricle; *LA*, left atrium; *AO*, aorta.

thickness in humans; therefore, they should be similar (7). When mitral lesions are small, be careful to interrogate several planes because chordal attachments to the leaflets are difficult to distinguish from lesions (8). Right parasternal four-chamber views of the heart are excellent for imaging the mitral valves (Fig. 4.2). Left ventricular outflow views are also good, but the valves may appear thicker than they truly are if the transducer is not held properly (Fig. 3.9). The sound beam should be directed through the center of the annulus, and to do so, the probe should be lifted up toward the examination table, creating a clean left atrium and valves that move and open well into the left ventricle. Transverse images of the valves are useful for identifying large lesions but they can be misleading when looking for small ones (Fig. 4.4).

Shaggy, irregular lines define mitral valve motion on M-mode images when the valve is thickened (Fig. 4.5). Although it is not common, systolic fluttering of the mitral valve may occur on M-mode images as the regurgitant jet flows through it (6). When lesions are large, however, the thickness of the mitral valve on the image masks the fluttering.

Mitral Valve Prolapse

Mitral valve prolapse (MVP) may be primary or secondary. Primary MVP results from intrinsic abnormalities of the mitral valve leaflets, usually myomatous degeneration. Secondary MVP is present without inherent pathologic valvular abnormalities. This is typically secondary to hemodynamic causes such as volume contraction and reduced left ventricular size or myocardial disease resulting in akinetic muscle. Flail leaflets also are referred to as prolapsed, but chordae rupture is present (7). In dogs, prolapse of the mitral valve may be secondary to myxomatous degeneration of the valves, chronic stretch of the chordae tendinea, and redundancy into the atrium during systole in these hyperdynamic hearts. MVP may be seen without any evidence of insufficiency and seems to be genetically predisposed in

FIGURE 4.4 Transverse images may show mitral lesions well (*arrow*), but care must be taken because artifactual thickening may be seen in these planes. *LV*, left ventricle.

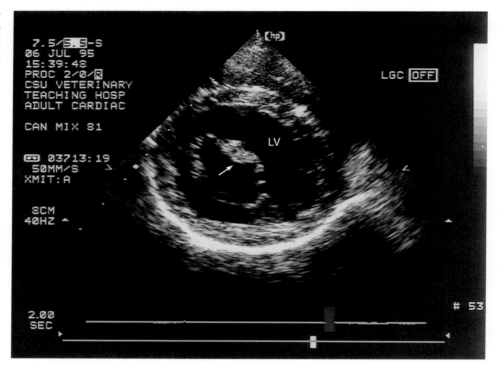

FIGURE 4.5 M-mode images of mitral valve lesions show irregular shaggy lines (*arrow*). *RV*, right ventricle; *VS*, interventricular septum; *LV*, left ventricle.

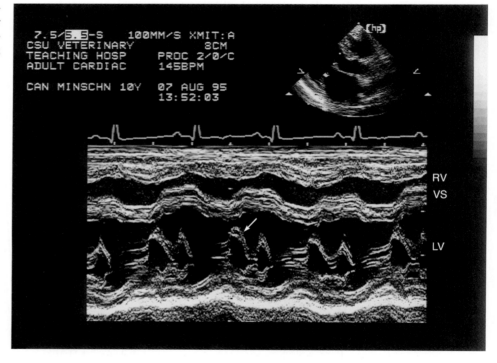

Cavalier King Charles Spaniels (CKCS) and Dachshunds (9–11). These dogs tend to show prolapse as early as 3 years of age without any clinical signs or murmurs and have a high incidence of mitral valvular insufficiency later in life. Of 19 CKCS dogs with mitral valvular insufficiency in one study, 84% had MVP. Three-year-old Dachshunds without heart murmurs had a 47% incidence of MVP. The course of MVP in humans is usually benign, but may not be benign in dogs in which there is a greater incidence of degenerative valvular disease (12,13). More severe insufficiency exists and a higher class of heart failure occurs with more severe prolapse (9,11).

MVP also may be secondary to rupture of minor chordae. The rupture creates only billowing of the leaflet body as opposed to a completely flail leaflet when a major chordae ruptures. MVP associated with chordae rupture has been described in the horse. No obvious flailing leaflet was seen, and the prolapse was not visualized in all planes (14).

The diagnosis of MVP is made when one or both leaflets buckle back toward the left atrium during systole. The mitral valve annulus is identified by either a line drawn from the aortic valve base to the point of attachment of the posterior mitral valve leaflet on right parasternal long-axis left ventricular outflow views or by a line joining the attachment points of both mitral leaflets on four-chamber views (15) (Figs. 4.6 and 4.7). On the four-chamber view in normal dogs, the body of the mitral valve leaflets does not extend beyond the line into the left atrium (8). Buckling of either leaflet into the atrium beyond this line indicates mild MVP. A line drawn further back into the atrium from the dense echogenic area at the lower part of the atrial septum to the atrioventricular junction behind the posterior mitral valve leaflet represents the border between mild and severe prolapse (8,9,15) (Figs. 4.8 and 4.9). One study has shown that the diagnostic accuracy of detecting MVP increases with experience (14). Apical four-chamber views are not recommended diagnosing MVP in humans, because this plane through the mitral annulus shows normal buckling of the anterior leaflet into the left atrium. Only when the leaflets billow greater than 1 cm into the left atrium on apical four-chamber views is it considered abnormal. However, posterior leaflet buckling in the apical four-chamber view is always abnormal. Parasternal left ventricular outflow views are recommended in humans (7). The accuracy of diagnosing MVP on apical four-chamber views has not been studied in animals.

MVP has been seen and described in the horse (2). There is a bent or curved configuration to the body of the leaflet when closed (2). No associated valvular lesions or regurgitation was present with the valvular prolapse.

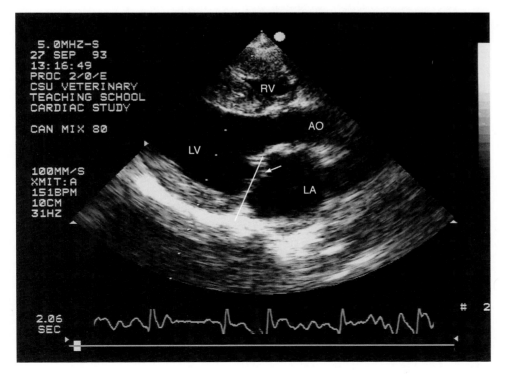

FIGURE 4.6   Mitral valve prolapse is diagnosed when one or both leaflets buckle back into the atrium beyond a line defined by the attachment points of each leaflet. The prolapse here is mild (*arrow*). RV, right ventricle; LV, left ventricle; AO, aorta; LA, left atrium.

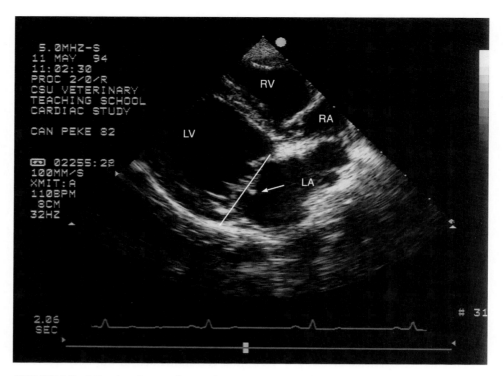

FIGURE 4.7   Mitral valve prolapse also may be identified on parasternal four-chamber images. The leaflets must buckle into the atrium beyond a line connecting the attachment points of both leaflets. This prolapse is mild (*arrow*). *RV*, right ventricle; *LV*, left ventricle; *RA*, right atrium; *LA*, left atrium.

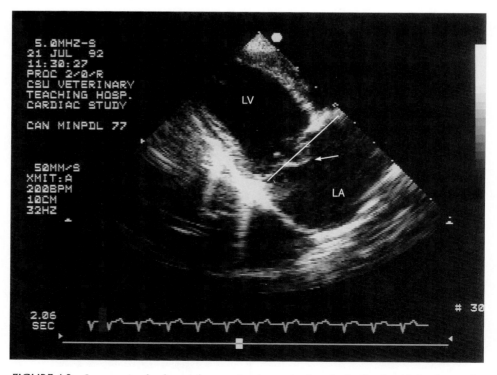

FIGURE 4.8   Severe mitral valve prolapse exists (*arrow*) when the leaflets buckle back into the atrium beyond a line drawn from the echodense area at the lower part of the septum to the atrioventricular junction. *LV*, left ventricle; *LA*, left atrium.

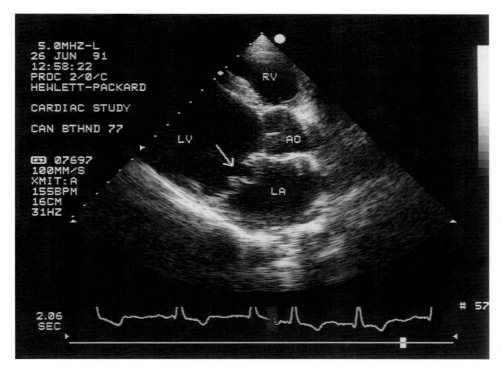

FIGURE 4.9   Here, severe mitral valve prolapse is seen on a right parasternal left ventricular outflow view (*arrow*). *RV,* right ventricle; *LV,* left ventricle; *AO,* aorta; *LA,* left atrium.

Ruptured Chordae Tendineae

Rupture of a chordae tendineae resulting in a flail leaflet is diagnosed on echocardiographic images when the leaflet tip or tips are pointing back into the left atrial chamber during systole (16,17) (Fig. 4.10). During diastole, the leaflet may sometimes be seen thrashing within the left ventricular outflow tract (17) (Figs. 4.11 and 4.12). The mitral valve also shows, on both M-mode and real-time images, chaotic motion during diastole and systole after a chorda has ruptured (6,17–19) (Fig. 4.13). These findings are seen on both parasternal and apical images (17) (Figs. 4.14 and 4.15) Localized rupture may be seen in only one echocardiographic plane, whereas major chordal rupture tends to be seen in several imaging planes (7). The jet of mitral regurgitation when seen by Doppler is often eccentric when it is secondary to chordae rupture (7). When Doppler confirms the presence of severe mitral insufficiency without the concurrent left ventricular and atrial dilation seen in a chronic process, one should look for a ruptured chorda (Fig. 4.16).

> Look for ruptured chordae when regurgitation is severe but volume overload is not significant.

Acute left ventricular congestive heart failure can occur secondary to papillary muscle rupture; this is usually a sequela of trauma (20). M-mode echocardiography shows the abnormal mass moving within the left ventricular chamber, but two-dimensional images provide clear visualization of the torn muscle and its movement within the chamber. The two-dimensional echocardiographic features of papillary muscle rupture include visualization of a portion of the papillary muscle attached to the chordae tendineae, severe MVP or flail leaflets, and the abnormal appearance of the papillary muscle in which the tip of it has torn off. The papillary muscle attached to the chordae appears as a highly mobile echoic mass within the ventricular chamber (21).

Left Ventricular Size and Function

Chamber Size and Valve Motion

Volume overload of the left atrium and ventricle is seen with hemodynamically significant chronic mitral valvular insufficiency (6) (Figs. 4.1, 4.2, 4.3, and 4.17). The degree of left atrial enlargement is often used to indicate the stage of heart

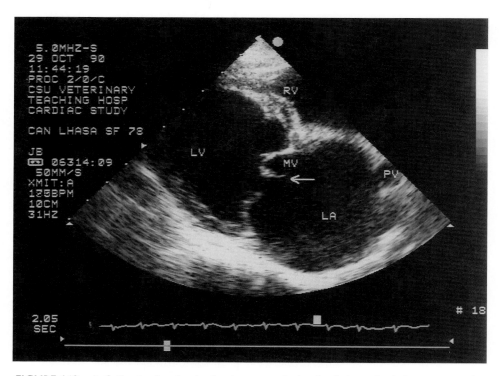

FIGURE 4.10   A flail mitral valve leaflet is seen pointing back into the left atrium in this parasternal four-chamber view of the heart (*arrow*). *RV*, right ventricle; *LV*, left ventricle; *LA*, left atrium; *PV*, pulmonary vein; *MV*, mitral valve.

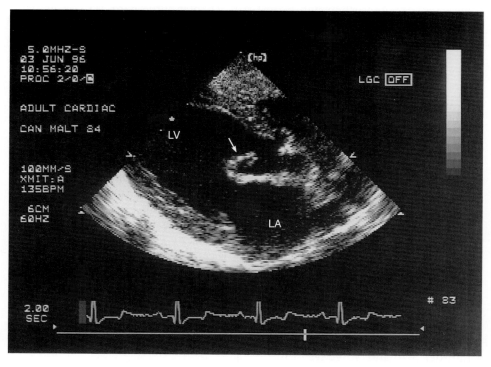

FIGURE 4.11   The anterior mitral valve leaflet and chordae are seen bent back into the left ventricular outflow tract during diastole in this image of ruptured chordae tendineae (*arrow*). *LV*, left ventricle; *LA*, left atrium.

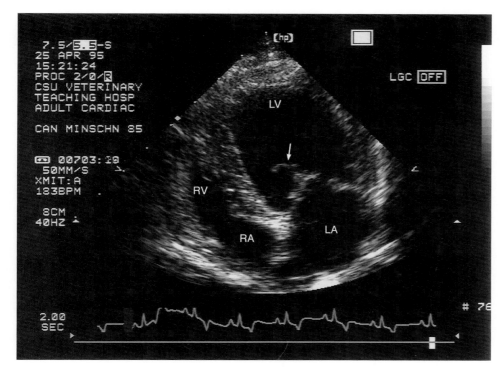

FIGURE 4.12   A chorda is seen flailing within the left ventricular chamber on this apical four-chamber view (*arrow*). *LV*, left ventricle; *LA*, left atrium; *RV*, right ventricle; *RA*, right atrium.

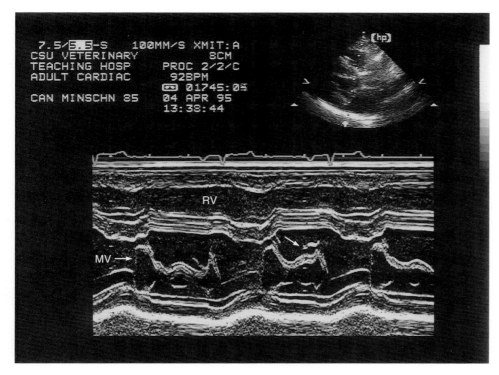

FIGURE 4.13   Mitral valve motion varies from beat to beat when a major chorda is ruptured. At times, the ruptured chorda may be seen within the left ventricular outflow tract above the leaflets (*arrow*). *RV*, right ventricle; *MV*, mitral valve.

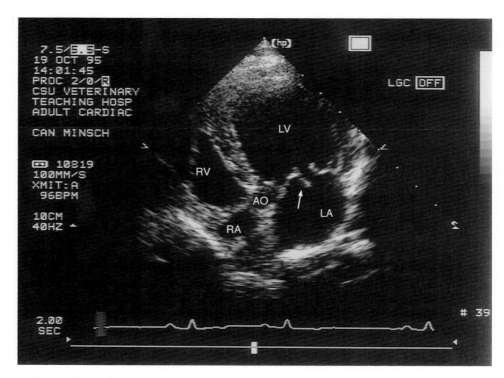

FIGURE 4.14   The anterior mitral valve leaflet is seen pointing back toward the left atrial chamber on this apical five-chamber view, a sign that a major chorda has ruptured (*arrow*). *LV*, left ventricle; *LA*, left atrium; *RV*, right ventricle; *AO*, aorta; *RA*, right atrium.

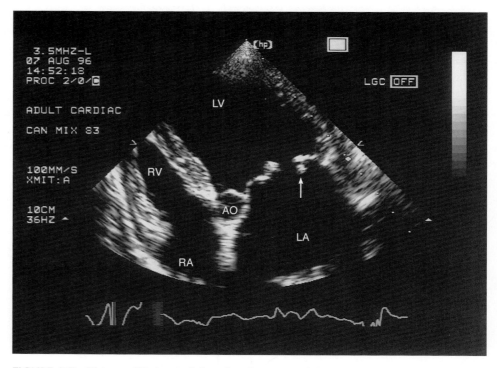

FIGURE 4.15   This modified apical five-chamber view of the heart shows a flail posterior leaflet (*arrow*). *LV*, left ventricle; *RV*, right ventricle; *AO*, aorta; *LA*, left atrium; *RA*, right atrium; *AO*, aorta.

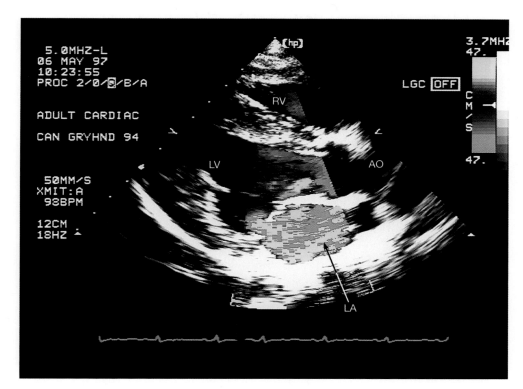

FIGURE 4.16   When Doppler examination reveals severe mitral insufficiency without concurrent ventricular and atrial dilation, a ruptured chorda should be suspected. Here, a color jet of severe mitral insufficiency fills the left atrial chamber of a dog with a ruptured chorda. Notice the normal left ventricular and atrial sizes. *RV*, right ventricle; *LV*, left ventricle; *AO*, aorta; *LA*, left atrium.

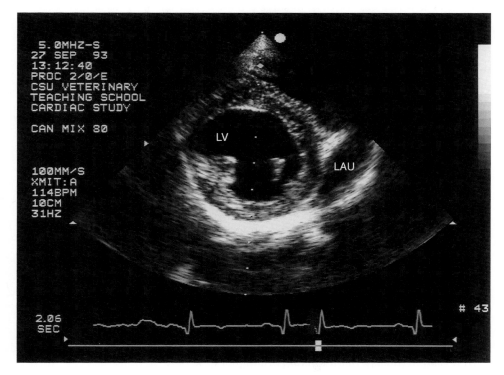

FIGURE 4.17   The left auricle is seen next to the left ventricular chamber on parasternal transverse images of the left ventricle when significant atrial dilation exists. *LV*, left ventricle; *LAU*, left auricle.

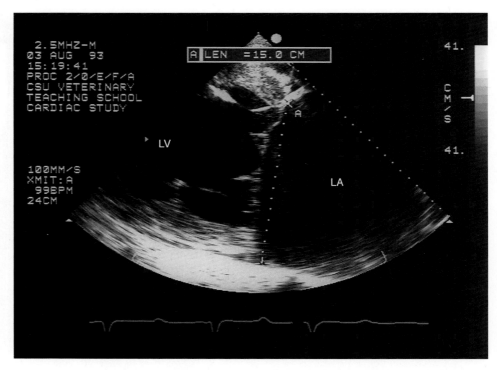

FIGURE 4.18   The size of the mitral valve annulus in this left parasternal two-chamber view of the heart is larger than 13.5 cm, implying left atrial enlargement in this horse. *LV,* left ventricle; *LA,* left atrium.

failure based on New York Heart Association (NYHA) criteria. The atrial sizes of dogs in stage 3 and 4 of the NYHA criteria are significantly larger than the atria of stage 2. The atrial sizes of dogs in stage 2 failure were significantly larger than the atria of dogs with no heart failure or stage 1 heart failure. There is no difference between the atrial sizes of dogs with stage 1 heart failure and dogs with no heart failure (22). Significant insufficiencies without the concurrent chamber enlargement is suggestive of an acute process and ruptured chordae (Fig. 4.16). As discussed, many horses have clinically insignificant insufficiencies. When the insufficiency in horses results in ventricular and atrial chamber enlargement or atrial dilation without ventricular enlargement, the prognosis is poor (23). Mild to moderate left atrial dilation without ventricular changes in the presence of regurgitation suggests a wary but less ominous prognosis in the horse (23). Atrial size in horses may be assessed from two-dimensional images because M-mode images often do not display the entire chamber. Left parasternal planes are used, and an atrial size of greater than 13.5 cm at its widest point is considered abnormal (24) (Fig. 4.18).

Mild left atrial enlargement may be seen in dogs with early mitral insufficiency before there is any measurable ventricular dilation. As discussed in Chapter 3, enlargement may not be apparent on the M-mode image, and real-time images should be used in various planes to determine if enlargement is present. Echocardiographic evidence of mild left atrial dilation may be more accurate than radiographic assessment because of the objective versus the subjective measuring involved (25). The left atrial to aortic root ratio also has been used to evaluate atrial size (26,27). As the severity of mitral insufficiency increases, however, this ratio may not reflect increases in atrial size accurately. Aortic root size decreases as forward flow decreases secondary to the severe regurgitation. This decrease in aortic root size also is seen in low circulating blood volume (25,28).

Severe left atrial enlargement and concurrent high left atrial pressures in dogs with mitral valvular disease can on rare occasions result in rupture of the left atrial wall (29,30). The tear may occur within the atrial septum, creating an atrial septal defect.

Mitral Insufficiency Features

- Mitral valve lesions
- Dilated atrium and ventricle
- Excessive VS and LVW motion
- Possible delayed mitral closure
- Gradual closure of aortic valve with significant leaks

Or, the left atrial wall may tear in the lateral wall of the atrium or auricular appendage, resulting in fluid accumulation within the pericardial sac (31). Echocardiographic evidence of fluid accumulation within the sac secondary to the rupture will be seen (30,32). Pericardial effusion secondary to congestive heart failure also can exist, but the presence of a clot within the fluid space can help confirm the diagnosis of atrial splitting because pericardial effusions secondary to neoplasia, pericarditis, or heart failure do not tend to clot (29) (Fig. 4.19). The clot appears as a disc-shaped, laminated hyperechoic structure adjacent to the heart within the sac (Fig. 4.20) (30,33). Tumors within the pericardial sac are more rounded and not laminated in appearance. Neoplasms also usually are found near the heart base or within the cardiac chambers (30).

Mitral valve motion may reflect elevated left ventricular diastolic pressures. Mitral valve closure is delayed after atrial contraction and a "B" bump, or shoulder, is described in animals and humans (34,36) (Figs. 3.83 and 4.21). This motion reportedly occurs in animals in which left ventricular diastolic pressures exceed 30 mm Hg (34).

Motion of the interventricular septum and free wall are exaggerated in animals with mitral valve insufficiency, volume overload, and preserved myocardial function. This is secondary to the increased volume flowing into and out of the left ventricular chamber relative to the volume filling the right ventricular chamber (37,38). Septal motion may be greater than free-wall motion because it is affected to a greater degree by volume changes in the right and left ventricles (Fig. 4.22).

Aortic valve motion may be abnormal in animals with significant mitral regurgitation. Blood will flow into the lower pressure left atrium instead of the higher pressure systemic circulation as systole progresses and gradual closure of the aortic valves is seen. A triangular-shaped aortic valve is seen on M-mode images as opposed to a rectangular shape during systole (39) (Fig. 4.23).

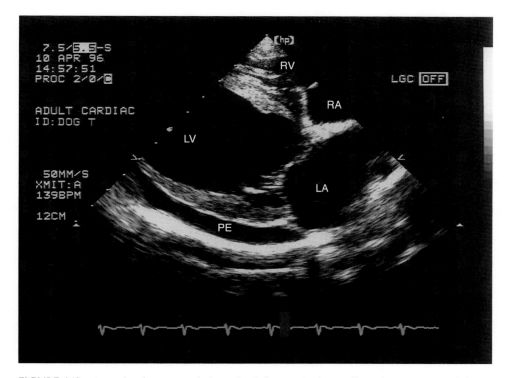

FIGURE 4.19 An echo-free space below the left ventricular wall in this parasternal four-chamber view representative of pericardial effusion is seen in this dog with congestive heart failure. Notice that the pericardial fluid is not seen at the heart base and stops just beyond the atrial and ventricular junction. *RV,* right ventricle; *RA,* right atrium; *LV,* left ventricle; *LA,* left atrium; *PE,* pericardial effusion.

FIGURE 4.20   Blood clots within the pericardial sac appear as disc-shaped or laminar echoes (*arrow*). *LV*, left ventricle; *RV*, right ventricle; *RA*, right atrium; *LA*, left atrium; *PE*, pericardial effusion.

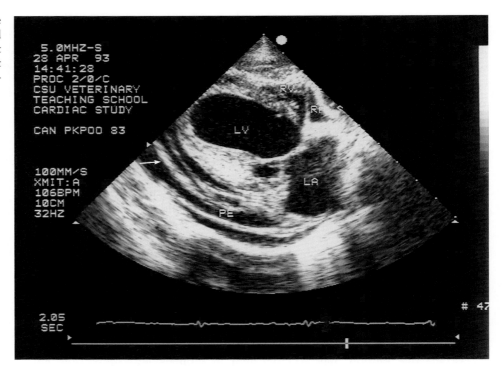

FIGURE 4.21   Significantly elevated left ventricular diastolic pressures may delay mitral valve closure and a "B" bump is seen (*arrow*). *RV*, right ventricle; *LV*, left ventricle.

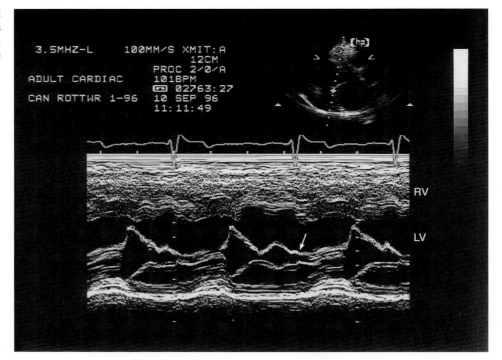

Left Ventricular Function

Fractional shortening (FS) as an index of myocardial function in dogs with chronic degenerative mitral valvular insufficiency should be elevated because of the presence of increased preload, decreased afterload, and increased contractile elements (6,40)(Fig. 4.24). These were discussed in Chapter 3. No correlation exists between the stage of heart failure, based on American Heart Association criteria, and the FS. Congestive heart failure in dogs with chronic mitral insufficiency is secondary to severe regurgitation and volume overload of the left atrium and ventricle, not myocardial failure in most cases (40,41) (Fig. 4.24).

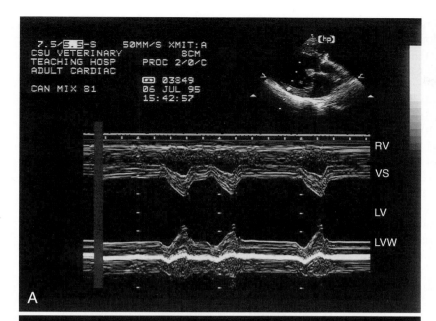

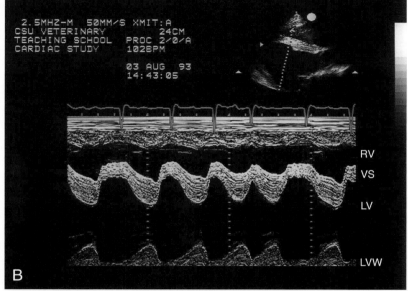

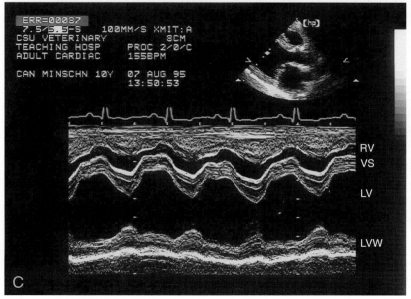

FIGURE 4.22   Motion of the interventricular septum and free wall are exaggerated in this dog (**A**) and this horse (**B**) with left ventricular volume overload and preserved myocardial function. **C.** Septal motion is often greater than free-wall motion with volume overload and preserved function because septal motion is affected to a greater degree by volume and pressure relationships between the right and left ventricles. *RV,* right ventricle; *LV,* left ventricle; *VS,* interventricular septum; *LVW,* left ventricular wall.

Normal myocardium will allow the left ventricle to contract down to normal size no matter how dilated the ventricle becomes.

Mitral Insufficiency—Assessment of Function

Normal myocardial function
• Systolic index = < 30 mL/m²
Severe myocardial failure
• Systolic index > 100 mL/m²
Moderate myocardial failure
• Systolic index ~ 70–100 mL/m²
Mild myocardial failure
• Systolic index ~ 34–70 mL/m²

Studies have shown, however, that using FS and systolic dimensions or systolic index in dogs can distinguish dogs with abnormal myocardial function from those with normal myocardial function (40). Hearts with normal myocardial contractility will shorten to normal systolic dimensions regardless of how dilated the heart becomes (40,42). Only when the intrinsic contractility of the myocardium starts to fail will systolic dimensions become larger than normal (Figs. 3.44, 3.45, and 4.25). Using this as an indicator, Kittleson found that dogs have a normal systolic index of less than 30 mL/m². Dogs with an index of greater than 100 mL/m² have severe myocardial failure; dogs with systolic indexes ranging from 52 ± 6 mL/m² have mild myocardial impairment; and dogs between these two ranges with a mean of 73 mL/m² have moderately reduced myocardial contractility. Systolic index is calculated by dividing the end-systolic volume by body surface area. The volume equation used in this study was Teichholz (40).

FS instead of systolic index also may be used to distinguish dogs with chronic mitral valve insufficiency and various degrees of impaired contractility (40). Dogs with any degree of mitral insufficiency from mild to severe, whether or not they are in congestive heart failure, will have FSs greater than 50% if they have no myocardial dysfunction. Dogs with mild to moderately impaired myocardial contractility will have FS within the normal range of 33 to 45%. Severe myocardial failure is present when FS is below the normal range (Fig. 4.25).

Color-Flow Doppler

Pathologic regurgitation can be assessed semiquantitatively by measuring the size of the color-flow jet within the atria in the case of AV valvular insufficiency or within the outflow tract or ventricle in the case of aortic or pulmonic insufficiency (43,44). In the case of mitral or tricuspid insufficiencies, a jet that occupies less than 20% of the atrium is considered to represent mild insufficiency (Figs. 4.26, 4.27, and 4.28). A jet that occupies 20 to 50% of the atrial area is considered to represent moderate

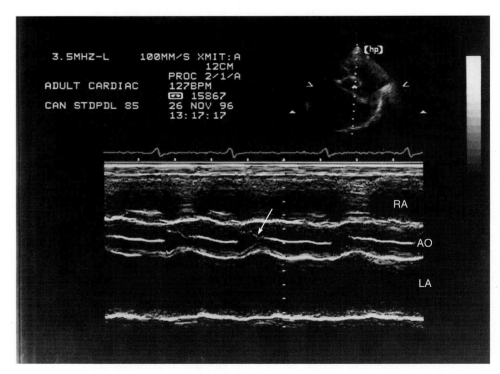

FIGURE 4.23   Gradual closure of the aortic valve is seen when cardiac output declines throughout systole (*arrow*). Blood will flow into the lower pressure left atrium with mitral insufficiency, and forward flow decreases. *RA*, right atrium; *AO*, aorta; *LA*, left atrium.

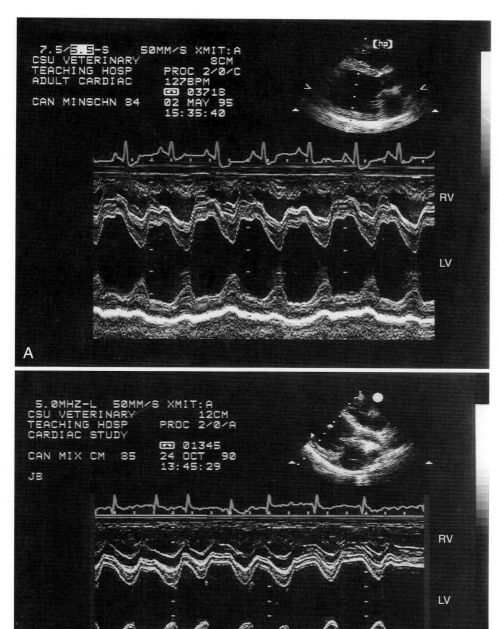

FIGURE 4.24   **A.** When myocardial function is preserved in volume-overloaded hearts, fractional shortening is elevated and systolic dimensions are normal. **B.** Although myocardial function is good in this volume-overloaded heart with mitral insufficiency, a small pericardial effusion seen below the left ventricular wall (*arrow*) is evidence of congestive heart failure. *RV,* right ventricle; *LV,* left ventricle.

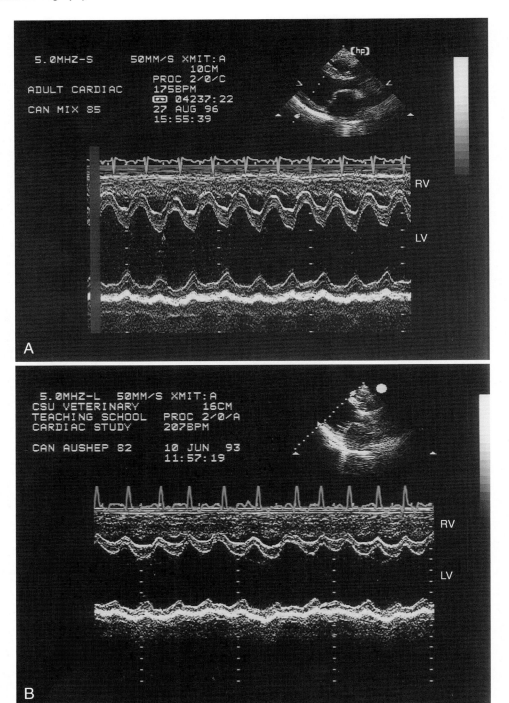

FIGURE 4.25 **A.** As myocardial failure develops, fractional shortening will fall within the normal range as opposed to being elevated, and systolic dimensions will become larger than normal. The fractional shortening in this left ventricle is just at the high end of normal. Notice that wall and septal motion are still excessive at this point. **B.** This dog with mitral insufficiency and left ventricular volume overload has fractional shortening below the normal range at approximately 26%. Systolic dimensions also are increased in this animal. Both of these factors imply severely impaired myocardial function. *LV,* left ventricle; *RV,* right ventricle.

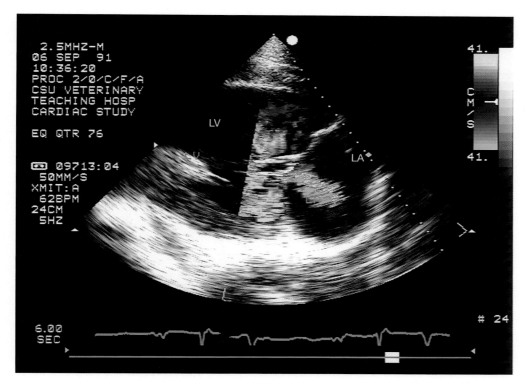

FIGURE 4.26 The color-flow jet of mitral insufficiency in this horse involves less than 20% of the left atrial chamber and is consistent with mild mitral regurgitation. *View,* left parasternal two chamber; *LV,* left ventricle; *LA,* left atrium.

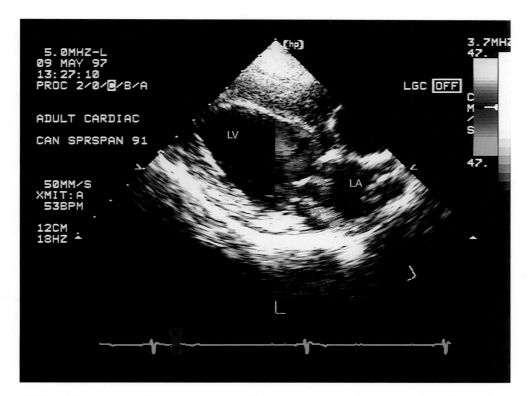

FIGURE 4.27 Two small jets of mitral insufficiency are seen in this heart with mild mitral insufficiency. *View,* right parasternal four chamber; *LV,* left ventricle; *LA,* left atrium.

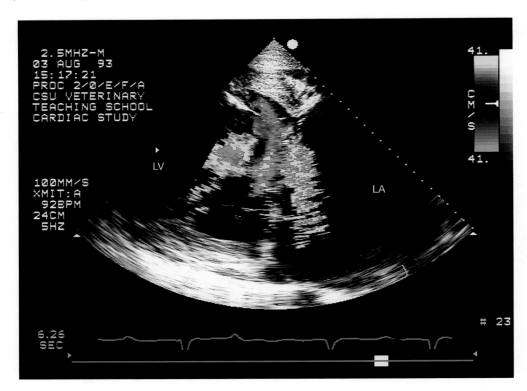

FIGURE 4.28   Mild mitral insufficiency is seen in this horse with an eccentric color-flow jet that fills less than 20% of the atrial chamber. *View*, left parasternal two-chamber; *LV*, left ventricle; *LA*, left atrium.

Use spectral or color Doppler to assess severity by determining the area of regurgitation compared with total left atrial size.
- < 20% = mild
- 20–50% = moderate
- > 50% = severe

When the mitral regurgitant jet is large with very little atrial dilation check for systemic hypertension.

insufficiency. When greater than 50% of the atrium is filled by the aliased regurgitation flow, it is considered to represent severe insufficiency (Figs. 4.16, 4.29, 4.30, and 4.31). This method uses the largest regurgitant jet found in any plane (43). Studies that average the jet size over several planes do not show any significant improvement in predicting severity (45). The correlation between regurgitant jet area with respect to total atrial area in the plane that shows maximal jet size is high, with predictive values of 100% for mild jets, 85% for moderate jets, and 93% for severe mitral regurgitation (43). This also can be assessed by spectral Doppler if the time is taken to place a PW gate at various points in the atrium to assess the extent of the jet (46,47).

When the systemic pressures driving the regurgitant jet are abnormal, the preceding percentages are no longer accurate. The driving pressure affects the velocity of the color-flow jet and the area that it encompasses. One in vitro study showed that an equal volume of regurgitant blood displayed varying sizes of color-flow jets based on the velocity of the regurgitant jet (48,49). Heart rate also affects regurgitant jet size. Fast heart rates tend to result in underestimation of the degree of insufficiency when assessed by Doppler (50). However, regardless of these limitations, when the regurgitant jet is centrally located and there is a fairly normal sinus rhythm, then the assessment of severity using color-flow Doppler is usually reliable (49,51).

Concern with the effects of gain, pulse repetition frequency, size of the dog, and heart rate in assessing color-flow evaluation of severity of regurgitation has led to studies that use other methods of assessing color-flow regurgitant jets. One study in dogs uses ratios of regurgitant to forward flow (52). Frames displaying the largest color-flow areas were used in this study. Regurgitant jets were traced, and a mitral regurgitant jet mapping area (MRMA) was determined as well as the color-flow area representing aortic forward flow (AFMA). The ratio of these two areas (MRMA/AFMA) correlated well to the New York Heart Association's classification of heart

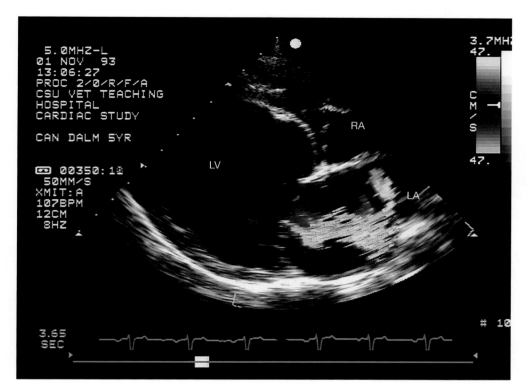

FIGURE 4.29   The color-flow jet of mitral insufficiency in the left atrium of this dog with dilated cardiomyopathy involves between 20 and 50% of the left atrial area consistent with a moderate amount of regurgitation. *View,* right parasternal four chamber; *LV,* left ventricle; *LA,* left atrium; *RA,* right atrium.

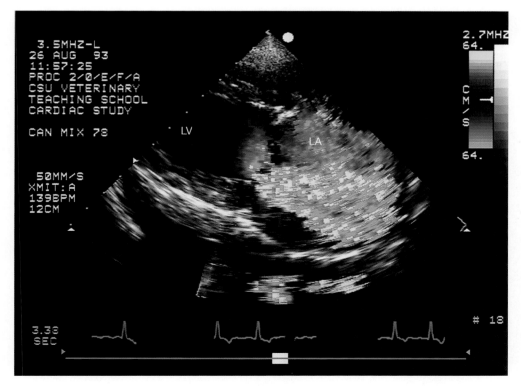

FIGURE 4.30   The color-flow jet of mitral insufficiency fills up approximately half of the left atrial chamber and implies moderate to severe mitral insufficiency in this dog with degenerative valvular disease. *View,* right parasternal four chamber; *LV,* left ventricle; *LA,* left atrium.

failure. Stage 1 heart failure with no clinical signs had an average ratio of 0.501 with a range of 0.273 to 0.875. Stage 2 had an average ratio of 0.779 with a range of 0.441 to 1.117. The stage 3 average value was 2.183 and ranged from 1.586 to 2.793. Stage 4 had an average ratio of 4.449 and a range of 4.025 to 4.873. This method is thought to eliminate machine and user variation. Additionally, it may help stage heart failure more appropriately by helping to differentiate the clinical signs of heart failure from other causes such as exercise intolerance as a result aging and joint disease (52).

Measuring the proximal jet height as it emerges into the left atrium through the mitral valve also has been studied in an effort to eliminate the other limitations of color-flow assessment. The smallest regurgitant color-flow jet at the mitral regurgitant orifice is identified by carefully angling the sound beam in various directions (Fig. 4.32). The height of this jet had a 0.85 correlation coefficient to angiographic data. Mild regurgitation in humans corresponded to a jet height of less than 0.55 cm; moderate insufficiency had a jet height of 0.55 to 0.8 cm; and severe insufficiency displayed proximal jet heights greater than 0.8 cm. Parasternal long-axis images were used in this study (53). Whether this study is applicable in dogs has not been determined.

Several limitations exist in assessing severity using color-flow mapping. When an insufficient jet flows along the wall of the atrium, the severity can no longer be assessed with any confidence. The Coanda effect plays a role in the size of these jets. This simply means that the flow is dampened by the wall, and the turbulence is no longer as apparent as if it was flowing into the middle of the chamber (54) (Fig. 4.33). Additionally, jet size is influenced by gain, depth, transducer frequency, and pulse repetition frequency.

Color-flow Doppler assessment of mitral insufficiency in horses is often limited by the size and depth of the left atrium. Often, spectral Doppler can document the

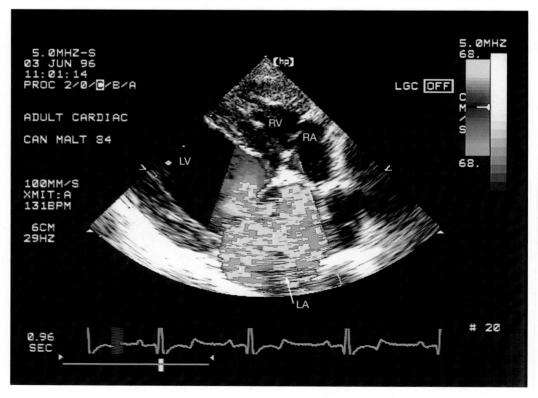

FIGURE 4.31   Greater than 50% filling of the left atrial chamber with a color-flow jet of mitral regurgitation (*arrow*) indicates severe mitral insufficiency. *View,* right parasternal four chamber; *RV,* right ventricle; *RA,* right atrium; *LV,* left ventricle; *LA,* left atrium.

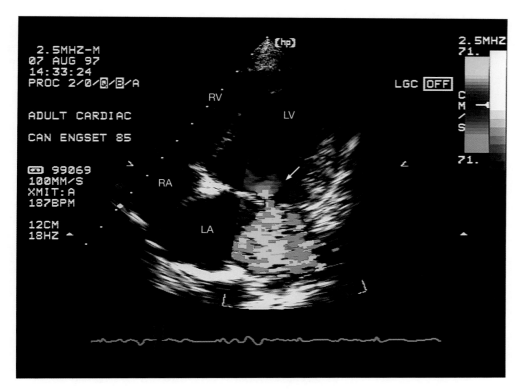

FIGURE 4.32   Measuring the height of the mitral regurgitant jet as it enters the left atrium can be used to assess the degree of insufficiency. See the text for details. *Plane*, left parasternal apical four chamber; *LV*, left ventricle; *RV*, right ventricle; *LA*, left atrium; *RA*, right atrium; *species*, canine.

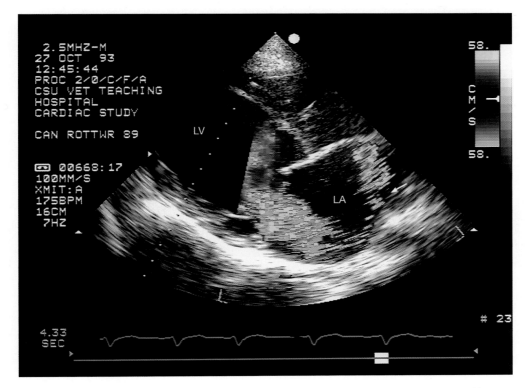

FIGURE 4.33   When regurgitant jets flow along the atrial wall, the turbulence is damped by the wall, and the severity of the insufficiency may be underestimated. The mitral insufficiency jet in this dog flows along the left atrial wall and up along the back wall (*arrow*). *View*, right parasternal four chamber; *LV*, left ventricle; *LA*, left atrium.

FIGURE 4.34 Interrogating the left atrial chamber with a pulsed-wave gate can identify the extent of the mitral insufficiency jet with an aliased signal. The severity can be determined by how much of the atrium contains an aliased signal. See the text for more details.

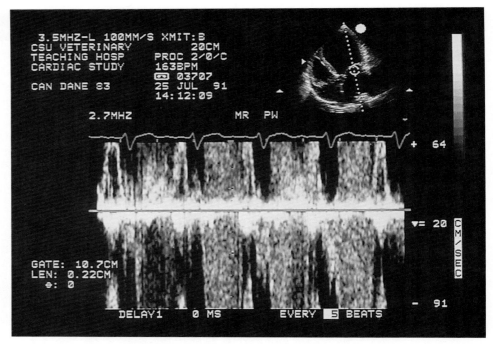

FIGURE 4.35 A cutoff in flow is seen on mitral regurgitant jets when left atrial pressures are significantly elevated (*arrow*).

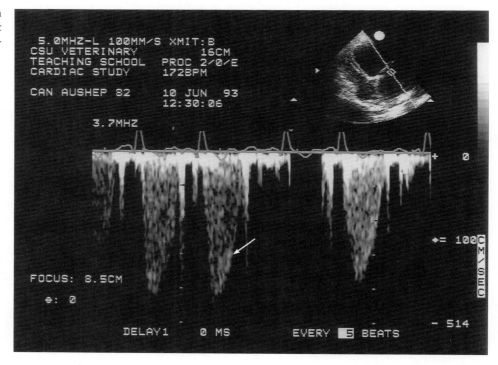

regurgitant jet, but color-flow Doppler cannot provide information on the extent of the leak (24). The best Doppler information in horses usually is found on left parasternal two- or four-chamber views where the left side of the heart is closer to the transducer.

Spectral Doppler

Spectral Doppler may be used to determine the severity of mitral insufficiency. Careful placement of the pulsed-wave Doppler gate at various depths within the left atrium can provide information on how wide and deep the regurgitant jet extends into the left atrium. An aliased signal will be seen at any point where the gate detects a regurgitant jet (Fig. 4.34). The area of the jet within the left atrium can be mapped. Increasing depth and width implies more severe regurgitation, and assessment is the same as with color-flow signals. The appearance of the spectral regurgitant display also provides some information. A flow profile with low or decreasing signal intensity throughout systole usually suggests mild mitral insufficiency. This is a time-consuming method, and it may not be possible to interrogate the entire left atrium in some unhappy patients.

Chapter 3 described how to measure regurgitant fractions. These methods show promise, and with experience and consistent measuring practices, they have high correlations with invasively measured outputs and regurgitant fractions. Using the mitral inflow velocity integral alone can provide a lot of information regarding volume flowing through the mitral valve without the potential error inherent in diameter measurements.

Regurgitant jet flow profiles provide some indication regarding the hemodynamic influence of the insufficient volume and left atrial pressures. A cutoff on the deceleration side of the flow profile suggests a rapid increase in left atrial pressures secondary to the regurgitant volume. This was discussed in more detail in Chapter 3 (Fig. 4.35).

Other than determining the presence and severity of regurgitation, the regurgitant flow velocity may be used to evaluate systemic pressures. Normally there is a pressure difference of 100 mm Hg or slightly higher between the left ventricle and left atrium. A pressure gradient of 100 to 160 mm Hg would reflect normal systolic driving pressure from the left ventricle to atrium, which is reflected in the regurgitant jet velocity (55) (Figs. 3.69 and 4.36). When systemic hypertension is

High pressure gradients derived from a mitral regurgitant jet imply systemic hypertension.

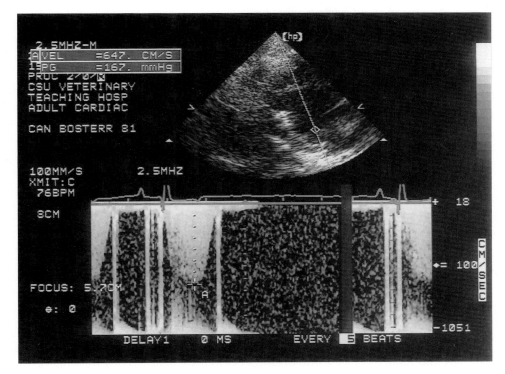

FIGURE 4.36   The mitral regurgitant jet pressure gradient reflects systemic pressures in the absence of aortic outflow obstruction. Here, a gradient of 167 mm Hg implies that systemic pressures are at least 167 mm Hg. A left atrial pressure estimate can be added to this value for greater accuracy.

present, ventricular systolic pressures will be elevated to the same degree; that pressure will drive the regurgitant jet velocity. Application of the Bernoulli equation will reflect the high left ventricular and systemic pressures. This pressure may be used as an estimate of systemic blood pressure when peripheral blood pressure is difficult to obtain. As with peripheral blood pressure readings, repeated measures should be made, and indirect peripheral pressures should be recorded if possible to validate the measures.

Diastolic Mitral Insufficiency

Diastolic mitral insufficiency may be seen in animals with atrioventricular (AV) conduction abnormalities. It is reported with first, second, and third degree AV block as well as retrograde P waves. The regurgitation typically is seen during late diastole when the atrial contraction is not followed by an appropriate ventricular contraction that normally would close the valve. The insufficiency is hemodynamically insignificant but should be differentiated from pathologic systolic leaking of the valve (56,57).

AORTIC INSUFFICIENCY

Aortic insufficiency may result from degeneration, vegetative lesions, torn or flail cusps, or congenital malformation of the leaflets. Differentiating between these causes of insufficiency echocardiographically may not be possible. All lesions do not create insufficiencies, but when they do the effects of the valvular insufficiency include the following: left ventricular volume overload, valvular lesions, diastolic flutter of the mitral and aortic valves, and an increased E point to septal separation (EPSS). Large increases in ventricular dimension also may result in dilation of the aortic root (58–60).

Valve Appearance and Motion

Lesions

Valvular lesions are not always visible on the echocardiogram, and the absence of lesions does not suggest the absence of disease (61,62). The resolving capabilities of low-frequency transducers often is not sensitive enough to show nodules and irregularities smaller than 2 mm on aortic valves (63,64). Even in small animals resolution of small lesions is sometimes difficult.

Degenerative lesions of the aortic valve will be smooth, small, and rounded (Figs. 4.37 and 4.38). Large irregular hyperechoic masses associated with the leaflets are more suggestive of vegetative endocarditis, but this does not mean that small thickenings are not endocarditis lesions (61,65,66) (Figs. 4.39, 4.40, and 4.41). Large vegetations are often floppy and prolapse into the outflow tract (58,67). Prolapsed aortic valve cusps with or without lesions bow into the outflow tract and are easily visible on real-time images (Fig. 4.42). This is seen more frequently in horses as a cause of aortic insufficiency (Fig. 4.43). M-mode images sometimes show multiple linear echoes representing the lesions during diastole or systole on aortic root images instead of the normal, fine single line associated with the closed aortic valve (58,59,67–69) (Fig. 4.44).

Effects on the Mitral and Aortic Valves

Diastolic fluttering of the mitral valve is probably the most common finding in humans and animals with aortic insufficiency. This is seen even if the volume of regurgitation is not severe or has not been chronic enough to produce left ventricular volume overload. The diastolic fluttering occurs secondary to turbulence associated with the regurgitant jet as it flows into the outflow tract. Real-time images may show

Aortic Insufficiency
Features

• Valvular lesions
  – may not be seen if small
• LV volume overload
  – if the leak is significant
• Diastolic mitral valve flutter
• Increased EPSS

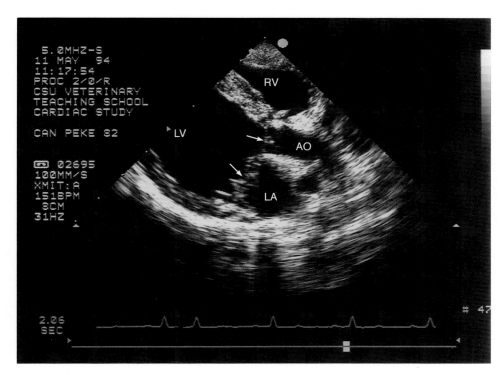

FIGURE 4.37   This dog has both mitral valve and small aortic valve lesions (*arrows*). Whether these are degenerative or vegetative cannot be determined echocardiographically. *View,* right parasternal left ventricular outflow view; *RV,* right ventricle; *LV,* left ventricle; *LA,* left atrium; *AO,* aorta.

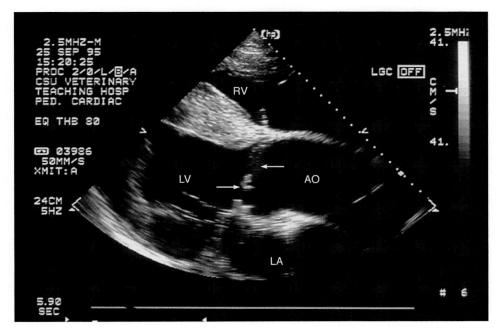

FIGURE 4.38   Small lesions are seen on the aortic valves of this horse. *RV,* right ventricle; *LV,* left ventricle; *AO,* aorta; *LA,* left atrium.

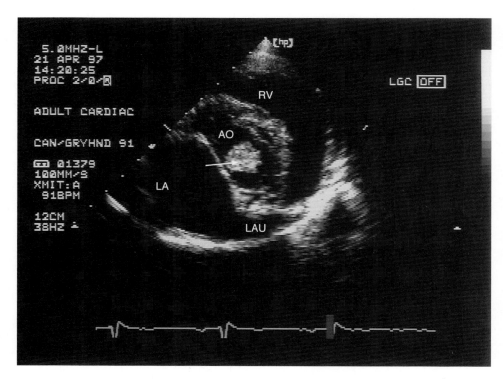

FIGURE 4.39   A large vegetative lesion is seen on the aortic valves of this dog (*arrow*). *View*, right parasternal transverse heart base; *RV*, right ventricle; *LA*, left atrium; *AO*, aorta; *LAU*, left auricle.

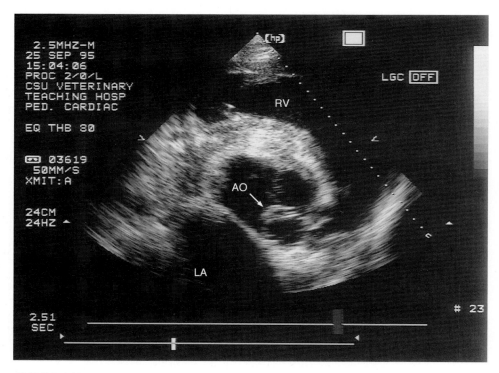

FIGURE 4.40   At least two aortic valve cusps are thickened in this horse (*arrow*). *View*, right parasternal transverse heart base; *RV*, right ventricle; *AO*, aorta; *LA*, left atrium.

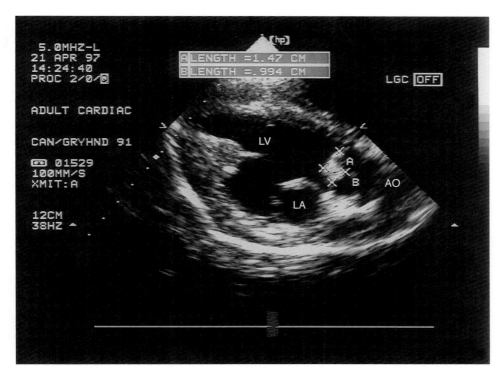

FIGURE 4.41   A large growth is seen on this dog's aortic valve. Lesions of this size have a greater chance of embolization and may create both insufficiency and obstruction. *View,* right parasternal long-axis left ventricular outflow view; *LV,* left ventricle; *AO,* aorta; *LA,* left atrium.

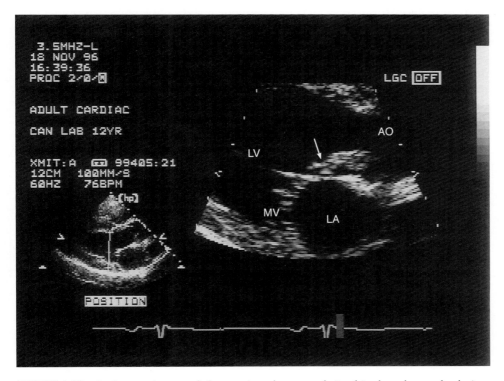

FIGURE 4.42   A closeup image of the aortic valve growth in this dog shows the lesion prolapsing into the outflow tract (*arrow*). *View,* right parasternal left ventricular outflow view; *LV,* left ventricle; *AO,* aorta; *LA,* left atrium; *MV,* mitral valve.

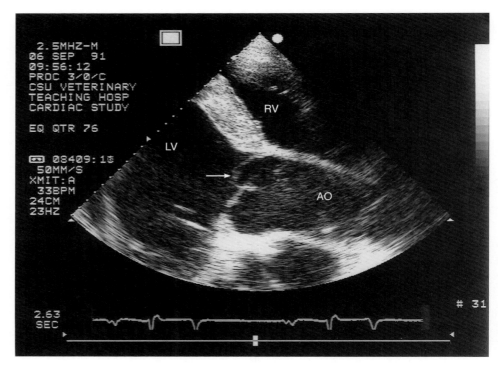

FIGURE 4.43   The aortic valve in this horse has no obvious lesions but does prolapse into the outflow tract and is the cause of aortic insufficiency in this animal (*arrow*). *View*, right parasternal left ventricular outflow view; *RV*, right ventricle; *LV*, left ventricle; *AO*, aorta.

dramatic mitral valve fluttering during diastole when the leaflet is wide open. Slower heart rates allow this to be seen better. M-mode images show fine sawtooth motion on the anterior mitral leaflet (58–60,65,70–73) (Figs. 3.84, 4.45, and 4.46). This fine vibration may encompass the entire diastolic period or any portion of it. The regurgitant jet does not have to directly strike the leaflet to create this fluttering. Jets directed away from the mitral valves create the vibration simply because of the turbulence within the left ventricular outflow tract. Regurgitant jets directed toward the ventricular septum may cause diastolic vibration of the septum during diastole and is seen at the end of systole on the up slope of septal motion on M-mode images.

The EPSS in animals with significant aortic insufficiency increases as the regurgitant jet restricts motion of the mitral valve (Figs. 3.84 and 4.46). A large EPSS in this case does not correlate with decreased ejection fraction and does not necessarily correlate with severity of the valvular insufficiency (74). Mitral valve motion may be altered dramatically and reduced with significant aortic insufficiency.

Along with diastolic mitral valve flutter and an increased EPSS, the mitral valve also may close earlier than usual, before the QRS complex. This is secondary to elevated left ventricular diastolic filling pressures and is usually only seen in animals that are already in congestive heart failure (58,59,75,76).

Diastolic flutter of the aortic valve also is reported with aortic insufficiency (Fig. 4.47). This is seen rarely in the small animal but is seen commonly in horses with aortic valve insufficiency (58,73,77). The vibration occurs secondary to flow through the cusps when they should be closed during diastole. Aortic valve diastolic flutter has been reported with fenestration of the aortic cusps, torn cusps, and endocarditis involving the cusps in horses (58,78,79).

Left Ventricular Size and Function

Volume overload occurs with chronic moderate to severe aortic insufficiency. Aortic insufficiency often has a greater impact on myocardial function than mitral insufficiency. Afterload is higher in animals with aortic insufficiency versus mitral

Acute insufficiency secondary to rapid vegetative growth will not show volume overload.

regurgitation because there is no pressure release into a low pressure left atrium early during systole. All the volume within the left ventricle must be dealt with when only the aortic valve is insufficient. Volume overload should cause compensatory eccentric hypertrophy, and function should elevate secondary to stretch of the myocardial fibers (58,73,80). Failure to see an elevation in FS and a normal systolic dimension suggests the presence of myocardial failure (62,65,80,81).

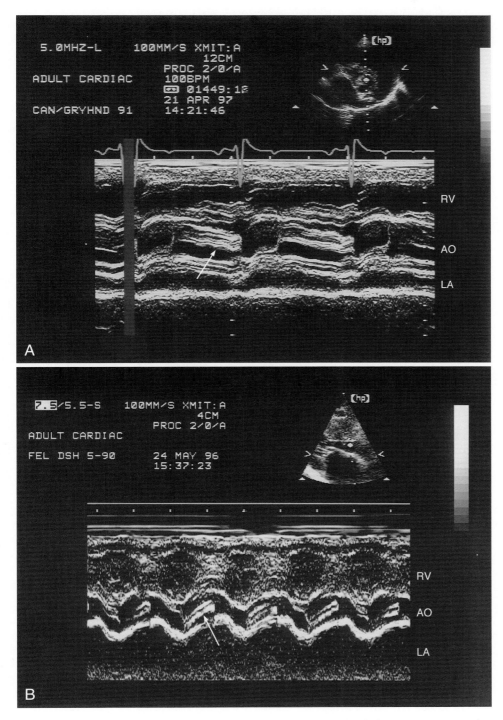

FIGURE 4.44   M-mode images of aortic valve lesions show multiple lines, representing the thickened cusps during diastole (**A**) (*arrow*) or systole (**B**) (*arrow*). *RV*, right ventricle; *AO*, aorta; *LA*, left atrium.

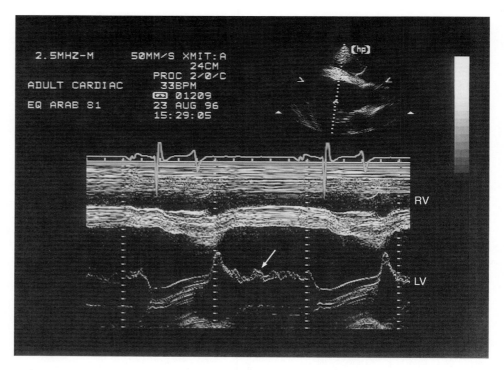

FIGURE 4.45   Fine vibrations on the mitral valve during diastole are a sign of aortic insufficiency (*arrow*) in this horse. *RV*, right ventricle; *LV*, left ventricle.

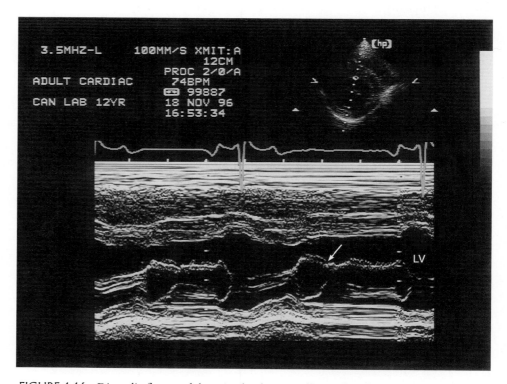

FIGURE 4.46   Diastolic flutter of the mitral valve as well as reduced excursion of the mitral valve (*arrow*) are signs of aortic insufficiency in this dog with bacterial endocarditis. *LV*, left ventricle.

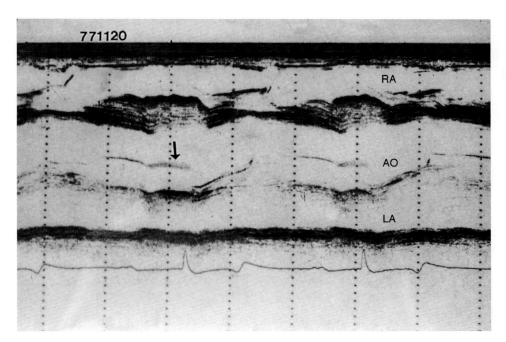

FIGURE 4.47 Diastolic flutter of the aortic valve occurs when an aortic regurgitant jet causes the leaflets to vibrate (*arrow*). *RA*, right atrium; *AO*, aorta; *LA*, left atrium.

The severity of aortic insufficiency is best evaluated with Doppler ultrasound but the effect of aortic insufficiency on the left ventricle must be assessed as well. Hemodynamically insignificant insufficiencies will not cause the ventricle to dilate. Mild to moderate leaks with time will cause an increase in left ventricular diastolic dimension, compensatory hypertrophy, and elevated FS. A heart that is affected by acute severe insufficiency will not have developed these compensatory changes.

Color-Flow Doppler

The Doppler assessment of the severity of aortic insufficiency is based on the width of the jet and its extent into the left ventricular chamber. An insufficiency that extends just beyond the valve and dissipates quickly to an unaliased signal is considered mild. A jet that extends to the tips of the mitral valves is considered moderate. A jet extending beyond the mitral leaflets into the left ventricular chamber is severe (Figs. 4.48, 4.49, 4.50, 4.51, and 4.52). The correlation here with actual severity is less than that for mitral insufficiency, partly because the volume of the left ventricular chamber as well as the velocity of the jet play large roles in this assessment (82,83). Jet width compared with left ventricular outflow tract diameter also is used (r = 0.91). Jet width to outflow tract ratio of > 65% correlates highly with severe insufficiency; a jet width to outflow tract ratio of < 46% represents mild insufficiency; and those in between represent moderate insufficiency (84).

Doppler Assessment of Aortic Insufficiency Severity

Mild
- Jet extends just beyond aortic valve
- Jet width < 45% of LVOT

Moderate
- Jet extends to mitral valve tips
- Jet width 45–65% of LVOT

Severe
- Jet extends well into LV chamber
- Jet width > 65% of LVOT

Spectral Doppler

Using slopes and pressure half-times, spectral Doppler provides additional hemodynamic information concerning the severity and hemodynamic significance of aortic regurgitation. The slope and half-time (see Chapter 3) of an aortic insufficiency jet depends on how fast the aortic and ventricular pressures equilibrate during diastole. A large regurgitant orifice allows the pressure to equilibrate rapidly, resulting in a steep slope and short half-time (Fig. 4.53). A small regurgitant orifice delays the equilibration, and a plateau-shaped profile is seen with a decreased slope

Large leaks allow LV and AO diastolic pressures to equilibrate quickly, and pressure half-times are short.

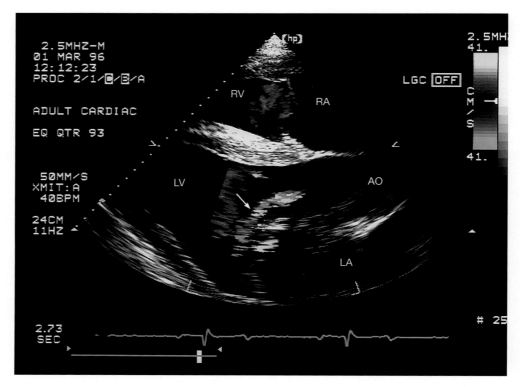

FIGURE 4.48   This small jet of aortic insufficiency would be graded as mild insufficiency (*arrow*). It has a small point of origin and quickly dissipates to an unaliased signal. *Plane*, right parasternal left ventricular outflow view; *RV*, right ventricle; *RA*, right atrium; *LV*, left ventricle; *AO*, aorta; *LA*, left atrium.

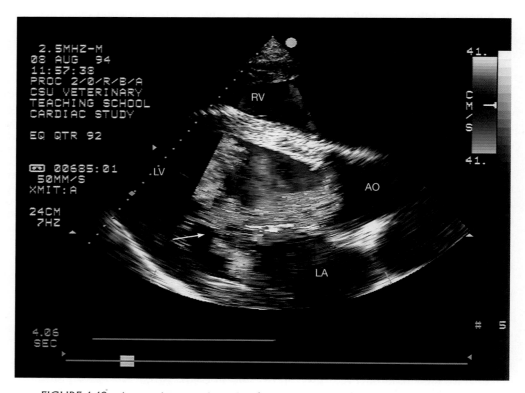

FIGURE 4.49   An aortic regurgitant jet that encompasses less than half the width of the outflow tract and extends to the tips of the mitral valve leaflets is considered moderate in severity (*arrow*). *Plane*, right parasternal left ventricular outflow view; *RV*, right ventricle; *LV*, left ventricle; *AO*, aorta; *LA*, left atrium.

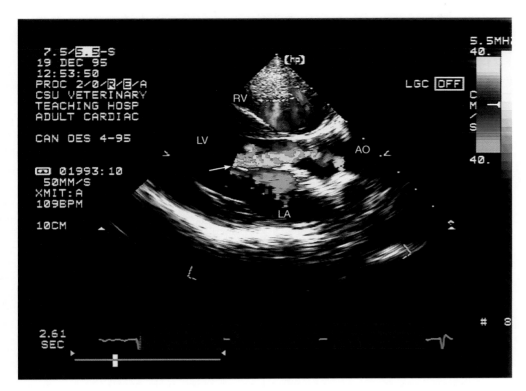

FIGURE 4.50   The severity of the aortic insufficiency in this dog is moderate based on its size within the outflow tract and its extent into the left ventricular chamber (*arrow*). *Plane*, right parasternal long-axis left ventricular outflow view. *RV*, right ventricle; *LV*, left ventricle; *LA*, left atrium; *AO*, aorta.

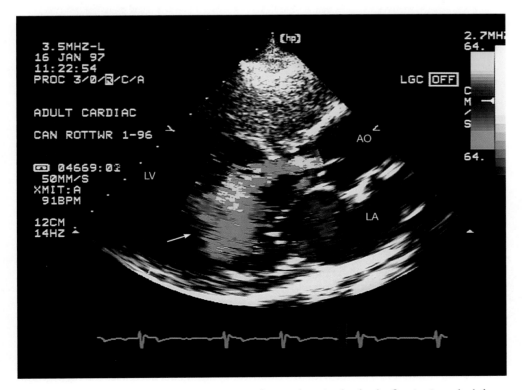

FIGURE 4.51   Severe aortic regurgitation extends past the mitral valve leaflet tips into the left ventricular chamber in this dog (*arrow*). *Plane*, right parasternal left ventricular outflow view. *LV*, left ventricle; *AO*, aorta; *LA*, left atrium.

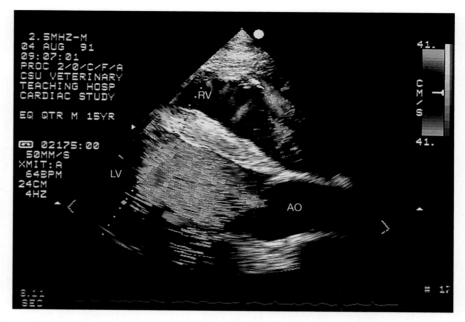

FIGURE 4.52   This severe aortic regurgitant jet fills up the outflow tact and extends significantly beyond the mitral valve leaflets. *RV,* right ventricle; *AO,* aorta; *LV,* left ventricle.

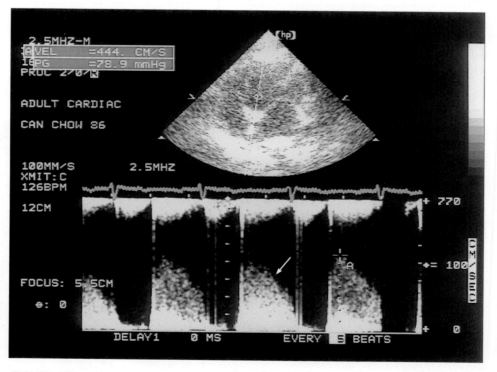

FIGURE 4.53   A large aortic regurgitant orifice allows aortic and left ventricular pressures to equilibrate rapidly, resulting in a rapid decline in velocity (*arrow*).

and a long pressure half-time (Fig. 4.54). These two parameters, slope and half-time, depend on several different factors, however, including the size of the regurgitant hole, left ventricular compliance, and systemic vascular resistance. Decreasing systemic vascular resistance with afterload-reducing agents decreases the regurgitant fraction but also increases aortic compliance, which allows the pressures between the left ventricle and aorta to equilibrate faster. This increases the slope (making the profile less plateau shaped) and decreases the pressure half-time of the regurgitant jet flow profile, giving the false impression that the regurgitant fraction has worsened. (Figs. 3.73, 3.74, 3.75, and 3.76). Increased afterload increases the regurgitant fraction, but slope and pressure half-times are not affected to any great degree because both ventricular and aortic compliance decrease to relatively the same degree (85).

When the amount of regurgitation is related directly to a change in the orifice size, slopes and pressure half-times are related directly to the regurgitant fraction. However, when changes in afterload occur secondary to drug therapy or other disease processes, slope and half-time variables are no longer related directly to regurgitant volume. Clinical relief of symptoms is a better indicator of reduction in regurgitant volume than slopes and pressure half-times after afterload reduction has been initiated (85).

Studies in humans have shown that the errors inherent in deriving regurgitant fraction by measuring cross-sectional areas and flow velocity integrals may be avoided by simply using flow velocity integrals (86). Normal human individuals have a ratio of 0.77 of mitral valve flow integral to left ventricular outflow tract flow integral. Regurgitant fractions (RF) may then be estimated by applying the following equation (86).

> Comparing pressure half-times before and after afterload reduction usually is not a valid comparison.

$$\%RF = \left(1 - \frac{1}{0.77} \times \frac{FVI_{MV}}{FVI_{LVOT}}\right) \times 100$$

This has not been studied in animals but it lends support to the fact that simply measuring flow velocity integral may be accurate enough to assess volume.

Aortic valve lesions also may create an obstruction to outflow (Fig. 4.55). When this occurs, the effects on the heart will include hypertrophy of the wall and septum. A pressure gradient can be derived by applying the Bernoulli equation to the flow velocity through the stenotic area.

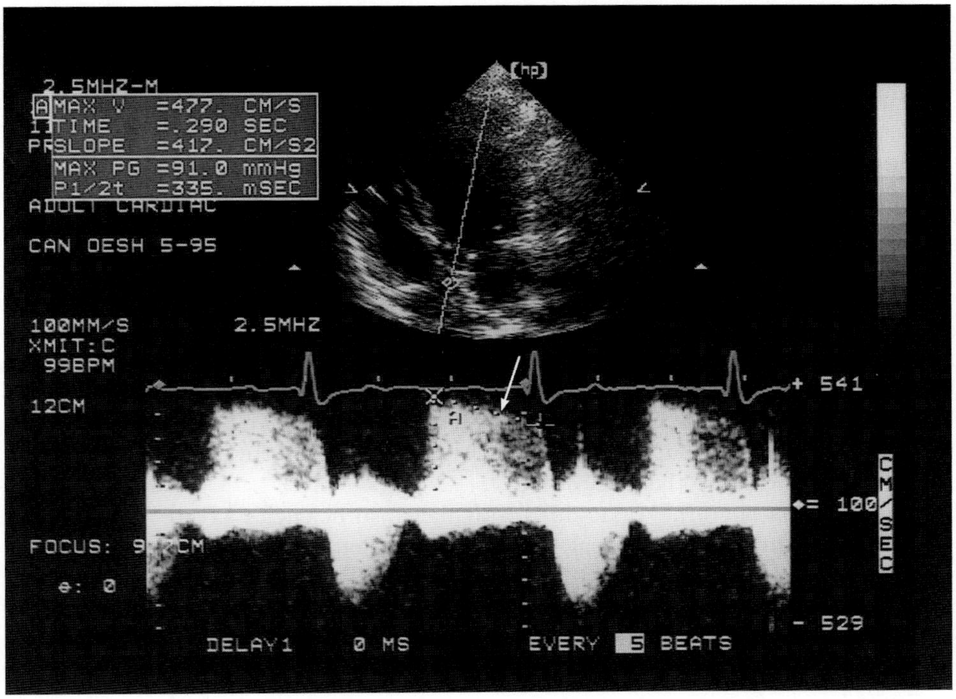

FIGURE 4.54   A small aortic regurgitant orifice prevents equilibration of pressures between the aorta and left ventricle, and the flow profile is plateau shaped (*arrow*).

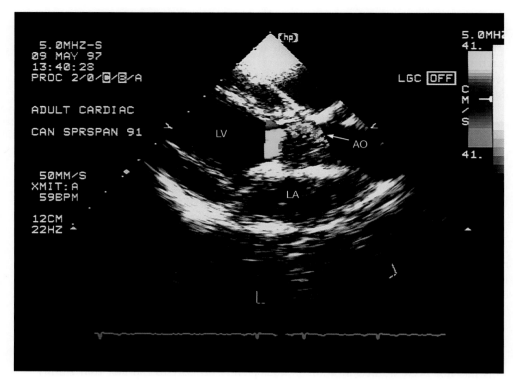

FIGURE 4.55   Aortic valve lesions may cause obstruction to flow as well as insufficiency. Here, color-flow evidence of obstruction to flow (*arrow*) is seen above a large aortic valvular lesion. *Plane*, right parasternal left ventricular outflow view; *LV*, left ventricle; *AO*, aorta; *LA*, left atrium.

TRICUSPID AND PULMONIC INSUFFICIENCIES

Degenerative valvular disease involving the tricuspid valve occurs less commonly than endocardiosis of the mitral valve. Degenerative valvular disease usually occurs in addition to the left-sided valvular diseases. A high percentage of animals have trivial to mild tricuspid insufficiency normally, which should not be mistaken for tricuspid valve disease. Chapter 3 shows some examples of normal tricuspid insufficiency in various species. Small amounts of pulmonic insufficiency are also a normal finding in most species. Generally, pulmonic insufficiency occurs secondary to infective lesions or in association with another disease such as patent ductus arteriosus, pulmonic stenosis, pulmonary hypertension, or significant volume overload of the right side of the heart where the pulmonic annulus may be dilated.

The appearance of the tricuspid valve is best seen on four-chamber parasternal or apical views. Long-axis left ventricular outflow views of the heart with part of the tricuspid valve showing are not clear enough to assess the tricuspid valve. It often appears thick when it actually is not. This is true in the small and large animal. The tricuspid valve may prolapse just as the MVPs secondary to stretch of the chordae or minor chordal rupture (Fig. 4.56).

The changes that the right-sided valvular insufficiencies create in the right ventricle and atrium are of greater importance when assessing the hemodynamic significance of the leaks (Figs. 4.57 and 4.58). The normal right ventricle is approximately one-third the size of the left ventricular chamber on long-axis left ventricular outflow views. Once this relationship changes, tricuspid insufficiency, pulmonic insufficiency, pulmonary hypertension, or all of the above should be suspected.

Once diastolic pressures within the right ventricle increase and exceed left ventricular diastolic pressures, paradoxical septal motion will be seen. The motion

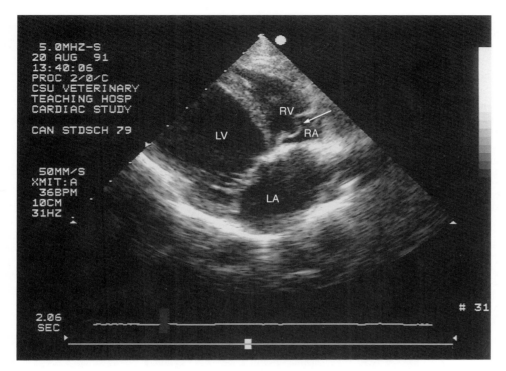

FIGURE 4.56   The tricuspid valve may prolapse (*arrow*) with tricuspid insufficiency second-ary to chronic stretch or, possibly, ruptured minor chordae as does the mitral valve. *Plane*, right parasternal four-chamber view; *RV*, right ventricle; *LV*, left ventricle; *RA*, right atrium; *LA*, left atrium.

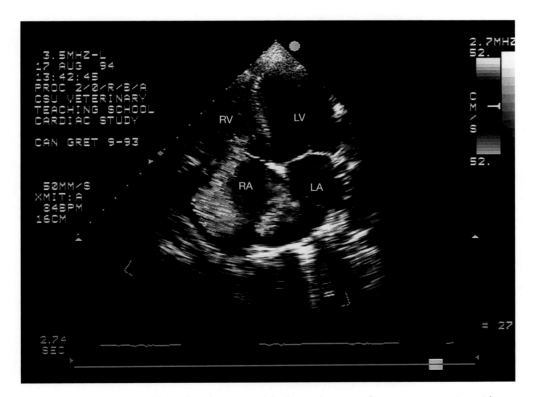

FIGURE 4.57   This apical four-chamber view of the heart shows moderate to severe tricuspid insufficiency. The right atrium is very dilated when compared with the left atrium. *RV*, right ventricle; *LV*, left ventricle; *RA*, right atrium; *LA*, left atrium.

FIGURE 4.58 The following images are all obtained from a horse in right heart failure secondary to tricuspid valve disease. Severe right atrial dilation (**A**) and severe tricuspid insufficiency (**B**) are documented with color-flow Doppler in this horse with right ventricular cardiomyopathy. **C.** Significant tricuspid insufficiency results in paradoxical septal motion caused by elevated right ventricular diastolic pressures. The septum is flattened as a result of this motion (*arrow*). This horse also has pericardial effusion. *RV,* right ventricle; *RA,* right atrium; *AO,* aorta; *LA,* left atrium; *LV,* left ventricle; *PE,* pericardial effusion.

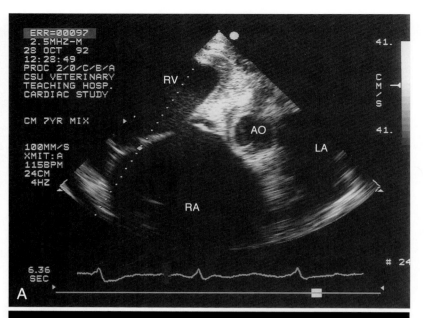

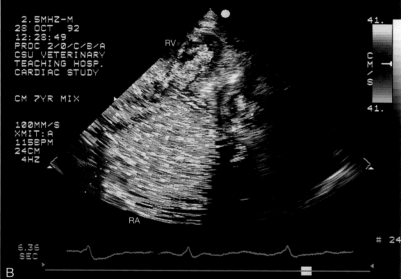

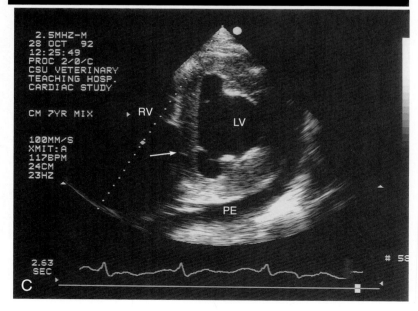

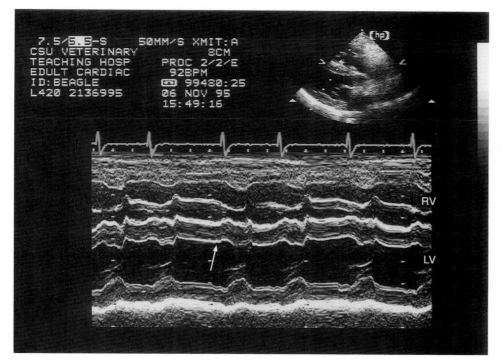

FIGURE 4.59   Mild paradoxical septal motion (*arrow*) is seen on this M-mode secondary to mildly elevated right ventricular diastolic pressures. *RV*, right ventricle; *LV*, left ventricle.

may be subtle when pressures are fairly equal or it may be dramatic when right ventricular pressure elevation is severe (Figs. 3.87 and 4.59). If concurrent left-sided disease is present, which would elevate left ventricular diastolic pressure as in mitral or aortic insufficiencies, then paradoxical motion will not be seen until right-sided pressure exceeds left ventricular pressure despite a very large right ventricle.

Right heart enlargement secondary to primary tricuspid insufficiency as opposed to pulmonary disease can be differentiated. Tricuspid insufficiency will create right atrium and ventricle volume overload but will not enlarge the pulmonary artery. Pulmonary hypertension causes the pulmonary artery and right ventricle to dilate and hypertrophy. Right atrial dilation only is seen with pulmonary hypertension when the tricuspid valve becomes incompetent. Paradoxical septal motion may be seen with tricuspid insufficiency or pulmonary hypertension because diastolic pressure elevate with both pulmonary hypertension and tricuspid regurgitation. Spectral Doppler can be used to determine regurgitant jet velocity and estimated pressure of the pulmonary system (87,88). This is discussed further when pulmonary hypertension is covered later in this chapter.

ENDOCARDITIS

The aortic valve is the most common site of vegetative endocarditis in the horse, with the mitral and tricuspid valves following in frequency of occurrence (60,63,89). (Figs. 4.38 and 4.40). In the dog, the mitral valve is the most susceptible valve for vegetative growth followed by the aortic, pulmonic, and tricuspid valves (90,91) (Figs. 4.2, 4.3, 4.39, 4.41, 4.42, and 4.60). Cows develop endocarditis lesions more frequently on the tricuspid and pulmonic valves (92–95) (Fig. 4.61).

The lesions of bacterial endocarditis are usually smooth and nodular when small but become irregular as they grow (65,94).

Large vegetative lesions often have a heterogeneous appearance with hypoechoic areas within the lesion (Fig. 4.62). When the growths involve the AV valves the growths may extend onto the chordae tendineae. The lesions may cause valvular

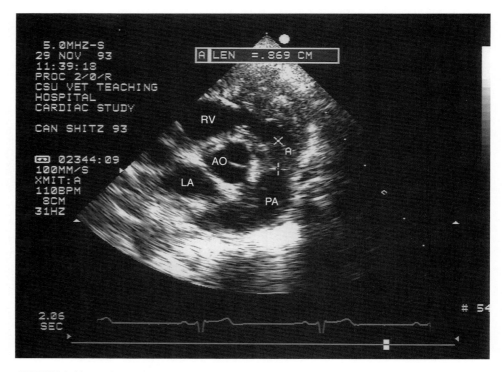

FIGURE 4.60   Pulmonic valve vegetative lesions are uncommon in a dog, but here, a large growth is seen on right parasternal transverse images of the heart base (*cursors*). *RV,* right ventricle; *PA,* pulmonary artery; *AO,* aorta; *LA,* left atrium.

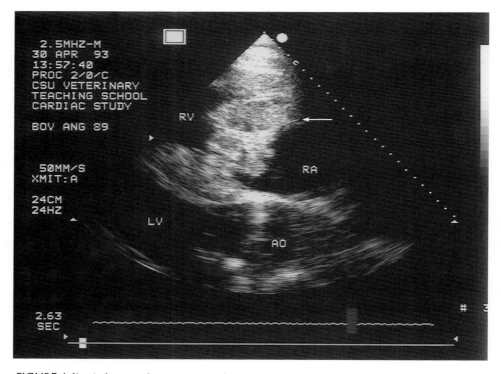

FIGURE 4.61   A large echogenic irregular mass on the tricuspid valve of this cow is a vegetative growth (*arrow*). The right-sided valves are the most common places for endocarditis in the bovine. The right side of the heart is dilated secondary to tricuspid insufficiency. The septum bows downward as a result of the right ventricular volume overload. *Plane,* right parasternal left ventricular outflow view. *RV,* right ventricle; *RA,* right atrium; *AO,* aorta; *LV,* left ventricle.

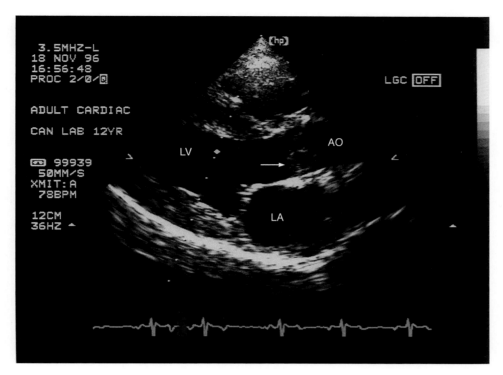

FIGURE 4.62   The hypoechoic area within this aortic valve growth is common in endocarditis lesions (*arrow*). *View*, right parasternal left ventricular outflow view; *LV*, left ventricle; *AO*, aorta; *LA*, left atrium.

insufficiency when the growth prevents proper closure of the cusps. However, even large lesions may only create small insufficiencies. The lesions will become somewhat smaller when the infective process resolves and only scar tissue remains. However, the lesions will never completely disappear, and insufficiencies, when present, often remain and may worsen (63,66). Although the lesions most commonly cause insufficiencies, they may also cause obstruction to flow (67). This can be determined with Doppler echocardiography and by applying the Bernoulli equation to the velocity of inflow or outflow through the affected valve.

Cardiac chamber sizes will be normal unless hemodynamically significant insufficiencies develop (63,66). Acute endocarditis results in rapid development of heart failure, whereas chronic endocarditis may take months to progress before signs of failure occur (96–98). Chamber enlargement will be accompanied by compensatory hypertrophy, increased cardiac function, and excessive wall motion secondary to the volume overload, unless myocardial failure is present (65,67,94,95). Tricuspid and pulmonic insufficiencies will create right-sided volume overload, whereas mitral and aortic insufficiencies will cause left-sided changes. The hemodynamic effects on the heart with chronic endocarditis are the same as those seen with chronic degenerative lesions that result in insufficiency.

Endocarditis may cause abscesses and secondary rupture of the ventricular, atrial, or great vessel wall adjacent to the infective lesion (66,67). Other complications of infective endocarditis include myocardial infarction secondary to embolism into the coronary arteries, pulmonary thromboembolism secondary to right-sided lesions, or congestive heart failure secondary to significant valvular insufficiency. Studies in humans have shown that aortic valve endocarditis embolizes less often than mitral valve endocarditis, but aortic valve lesions are more often associated with abscess formation (99). Myocardial infarction will create localized or widespread myocardial dysfunction visible on real-time images. M-mode images obtained over the infarcted area show hypokinetic or akinetic

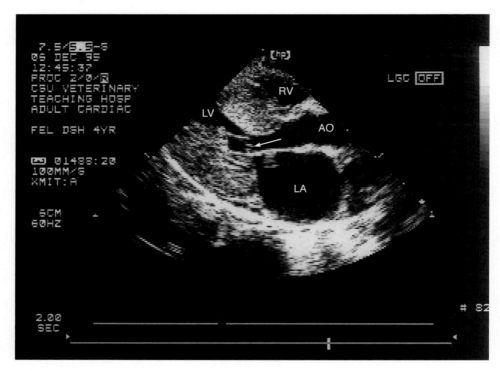

FIGURE 4.63   Symmetric concentric left ventricular hypertrophy is the most common form of hypertrophy pattern in cats with hypertrophic cardiomyopathy. Here, the septum and free wall are of similar thickness. The hypertrophy is severe. This image also shows systolic anterior motion of the mitral valve (*arrow*) and a dilated left atrium. *Plane,* right parasternal long-axis left ventricular outflow view; *RV,* right ventricle; *LV,* left ventricle; *AO,* aorta; *LA,* left atrium.

myocardium (63,100–102). The heart failure may be right or left depending on the location of the lesion (63,71). Lesions approaching 1 cm in size are associated with high complication and mortality rates (99).

Many cases of vegetative endocarditis are undetected until necropsy examination or until an echocardiogram is obtained for other unrelated reasons. The lesions are small and create no significant hemodynamic alterations.

HYPERTROPHIC CARDIOMYOPATHY

Hypertrophic cardiomyopathy (HCM) is a disease that primarily affects cats. Rarely do other species develop this disease (103,104). HCM is characterized by unexplained left ventricular hypertrophy. The left ventricular chamber is not dilated and is often smaller than normal (105–108).

Left Ventricular Size

The hypertrophy in cats may present with varying morphology. Most cats present with symmetric hypertrophy in which both the ventricular septum and the free wall are affected to a similar degree (Figs. 4.63 and 4.64). However, about as many cats present with asymmetric hypertrophy affecting primarily the septum (Figs. 4.65 and 4.66). Fewer cats (17%) present with asymmetric hypertrophy affecting primarily the left ventricular free wall (Figs. 4.67 and 4.68). In rare cases, only the apex, midventricular areas, or the very base of the septum are hypertrophied (109) (Fig. 4.69). Asymmetric septal hypertrophy was the most common form of hypertrophy in one study in dogs with HCM, with 80% of 20 dogs in one study displaying this asymmetry (103).

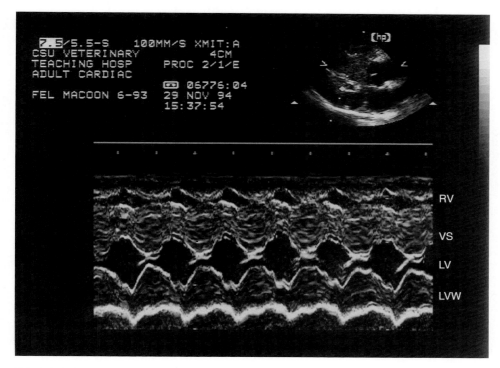

FIGURE 4.64   This M-mode of the left ventricular chamber in a cat with hypertrophic cardiomyopathy shows severe symmetric hypertrophy with elevated fractional shortening. *RV*, right ventricle; *LV*, left ventricle; *VS*, ventricular septum; *LVW*, left ventricular wall.

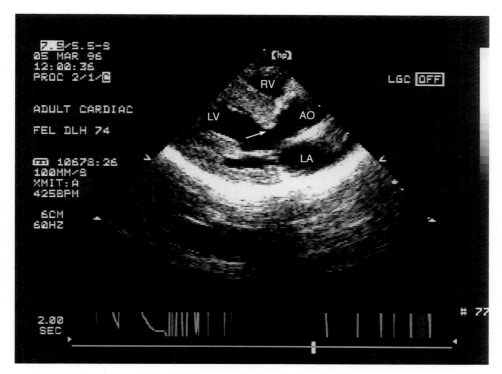

FIGURE 4.65   Asymmetric hypertrophy is seen almost as often as symmetric hypertrophy. This cat has a thicker septum than free wall, and the septum bulges into the outflow tract (*arrows*), creating outflow obstruction despite mild hypertrophy. *Plane*, right parasternal left ventricular outflow view; *RV*, right ventricle; *LV*, left ventricle; *LA*, left atrium; *AO*, aorta.

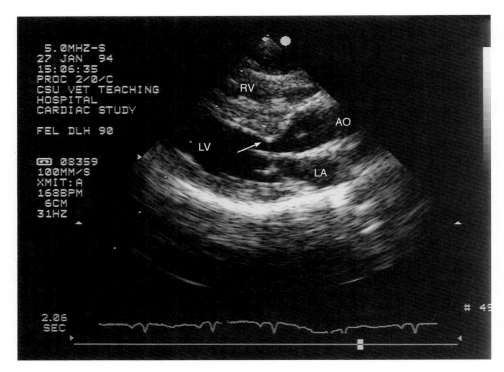

FIGURE 4.66   Primarily mild to moderate septal hypertrophy with outflow obstruction (*arrow*) is seen in this cat with hypertrophic cardiomyopathy. *Plane*, right parasternal long-axis left ventricular outflow view; *RV*, right ventricle; *LV*, left ventricle; *AO*, aorta; *LA*, left atrium.

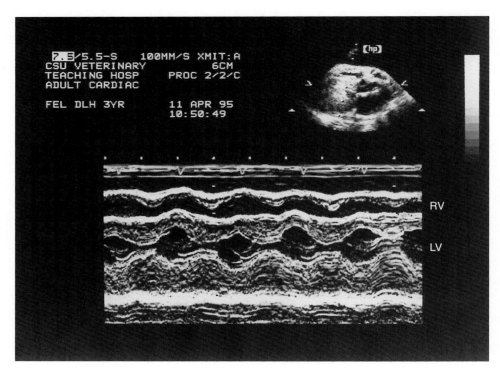

FIGURE 4.67   Asymmetric hypertrophy affecting the left ventricular free wall in this M-mode is seen infrequently with hypertrophic cardiomyopathy. *RV*, right ventricle; *LV*, left ventricle.

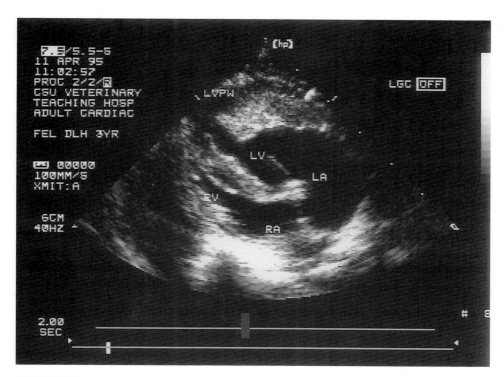

FIGURE 4.68   Severe hypertrophy of the left ventricular free wall is seen in this cat. The septum is normal. *Plane*, left parasternal four-chamber view; *LVPW*, left ventricular free wall; *LV*, left ventricle; *LA*, left atrium; *RV*, right ventricle; *RA*, right atrium.

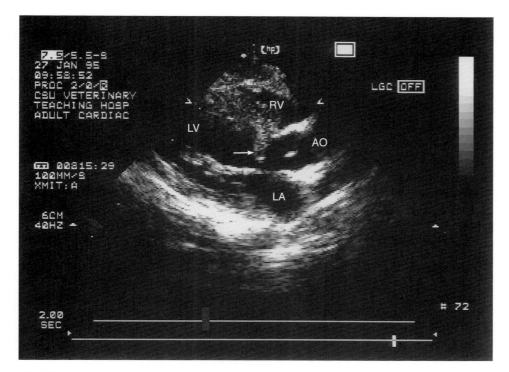

FIGURE 4.69   In this cat, atypical hypertrophy of the very base of the interventricular septum is seen, creating obstruction to outflow (*arrow*). *Plane*, right parasternal long-axis left ventricular outflow view; *RV*, right ventricle; *LV*, left ventricle; *AO*, aorta; *LA*, left atrium.

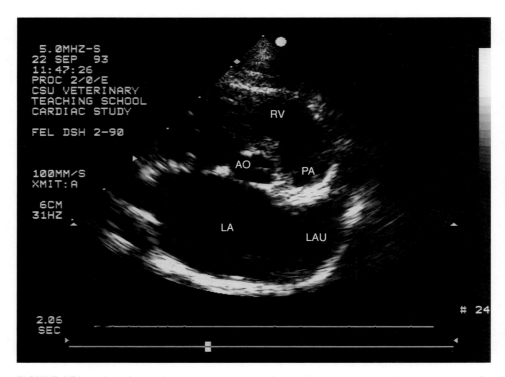

FIGURE 4.70   The left atrial dilation present on this real-time image may be seen in animals with hypertrophic cardiomyopathy secondary to diastolic or systolic dysfunction. *Plane*, right parasternal transverse heart base; *RV*, right ventricle; *AO*, aorta; *LA*, left atrium; *LAU*, left auricle; *PA*, pulmonary artery.

The hypertrophy may obstruct flow within the left ventricular outflow tract. This occurs primarily when the ventricular septum base impinges on the outflow tract, but occasionally may occur when extensive free-wall thickening displaces the mitral valve upward into the outflow tract. Cats with symmetric hypertrophy or hypertrophy primarily affecting the septum tend to have a significantly higher incidence of murmurs, probably associated with outflow tract obstruction (109). Hearts with midventricular hypertrophy may have midcavity obstruction associated with contraction (105,106,108,109). Significant right ventricular hypertrophy in addition to left ventricular hypertrophy has been seen in several cats (108).

Left atrial size may or may not be enlarged in animals with HCM (Fig. 4.70). The larger the left atrium, however, the worse the prognosis. The cause of left atrial enlargement may be secondary to diastolic dysfunction, systolic dysfunction, or abnormal mitral valve function (109). Clots may form within the left atrium (Figs. 4.71, 4.72, and 4.73). The size of the left atrium does not appear to correlate with the incidence of thrombus formation.

Hemodynamic and Functional Information

Systolic anterior motion (SAM) of the mitral valve is infrequently reported in cats with HCM (105,106). However, the incidence of SAM probably would be higher if the mitral valve is interrogated by M-mode at a midpoint along the length of the valve as opposed to the leaflet tips. The midpoint is often where the body of the leaflet is pulled up into the outflow tract. Systolic anterior motion of the mitral valve occurs in the presence of moderate to severe left ventricular outflow tract obstruction. High-velocity flow within a narrowed outflow tract creates a Venturi effect and tends to pull one or both mitral valve leaflets along with it toward the septum. An experienced eye can detect this motion on real-time two-dimensional images, but the

Hypertrophic Cardiomyopathy Features

- Concentric LV hypertrophy
  - Most have symmetric or just VS hypertrophy
- LA does not have to be dilated
- Most have obstruction to outflow
  - SAM seen
  - Systolic aortic valve closure seen
- Elevated fractional shortening

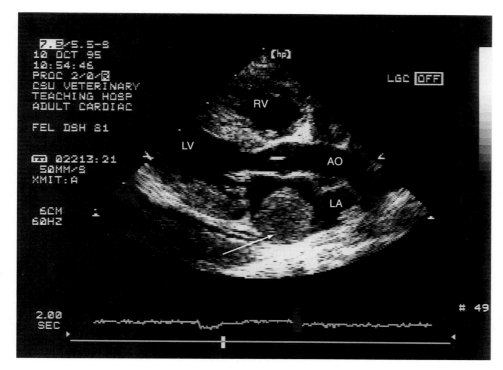

FIGURE 4.71   A thrombus may form within the left atrial chamber of cats with hypertrophic cardiomyopathy. The thrombus (*arrow*) may be attached to the wall and is immobile or it may freely move within the chamber. *Plane*, right parasternal left ventricular outflow view; *RV*, right ventricle; *LV*, left ventricle; *LA*, left atrium; *AO*, aorta.

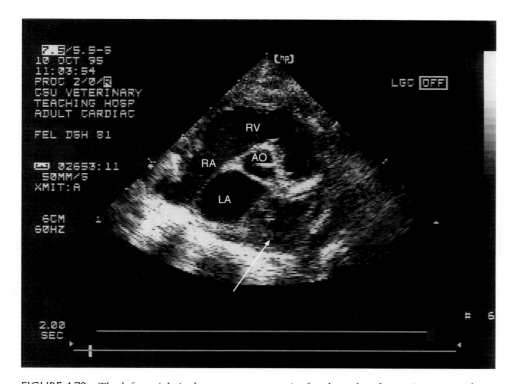

FIGURE 4.72   The left auricle is the most common site for thrombus formation as seen here on this transverse view of the heart base (*arrow*). *RA*, right atrium; *RV*, right ventricle; *AO*, aorta; *LA*, left atrium.

The degree and duration of septal contact correlate with severity of dynamic outflow obstruction.

motion is easier to detect and document on M-mode images of the mitral valve (Figs. 3.85, 4.63, 4.74, 4.75, and 4.76). The duration of mitral valve septal contact directly correlates to severity of the outflow tract gradient (106,110,111). Longer apposition with the septum indicates more severe obstruction. Late-peaking SAM with little if any contact suggests mild obstruction to flow. Small gradients will not create any SAM (106,112–114).

The obstruction to outflow seen in many cases of HCM occurs primarily during late systole. Spectral Doppler displays show this clearly with a concave indentation during late acceleration on left ventricular outflow tract flow profiles (106,113) (Fig. 4.77). This indentation occurs when flow velocities increase as the septum contracts, creating the dynamic obstruction. The indentation also correlates to the systolic anterior motion that may also aggravate the obstruction. As the obstruction to left ventricular outflow becomes more severe and holosystolic, the aortic flow profile will not show the late-peaking appearance but will become more symmetric in shape. Pressure gradients can be measured using the Bernoulli equation.

Mitral insufficiency is almost always present in cats with obstructive HCM. In most cases, the regurgitation is secondary to the abnormal mitral valve motion present with outflow obstruction (Figs. 4.78, 4.79). The presence and degree of regurgitation is directly related to SAM. The greater the obstruction and the greater the degree of SAM, the greater the degree of insufficiency. Alleviating the outflow tact obstruction reduces or eliminates the SAM and mitral insufficiency (112,114). However, some patients have mitral insufficiency unrelated to their hypertrophic disease.

Aortic valve motion is altered in humans and cats with hypertrophic obstructive cardiomyopathy. Ejection time increases in direct proportion to the degree of subvalvular dynamic obstruction. Evidence exists of early or mid-systolic partial closure of the aortic valve corresponding to the decrease in forward flow as the dynamic obstruction occurs (106,112,115,116) (Figs. 3.80, 3.81, and 4.80). This motion usually involves only one or two aortic valve cusps, and M-mode images of the aortic valve taken from parasternal long-axis views may not show early or mid-systolic partial closure of the aortic valve, whereas M-modes obtained from transverse views may.

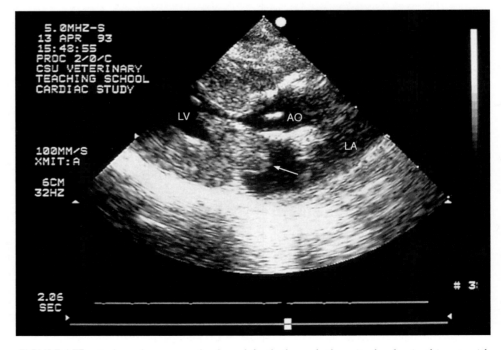

FIGURE 4.73 A thrombus moves back and forth through the mitral valve in this cat with hypertrophic cardiomyopathy (*arrow*). *LV,* left ventricle; *LA,* left atrium; *AO,* aorta.

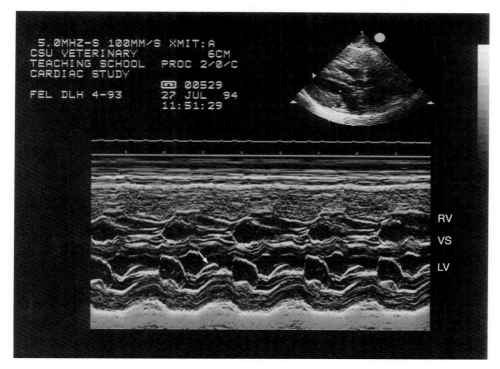

FIGURE 4.74 Mild systolic anterior motion associated with increased velocity of blood flow in the left ventricular outflow tract is seen on the M-mode of this cat (*arrow*). The amplitude and duration of SAM is related to the degree of obstruction. Obstruction here is mild. Severe right ventricular hypertrophy also is present. *RV*, right ventricle; *LV*, left ventricle; *VS*, ventricular septum.

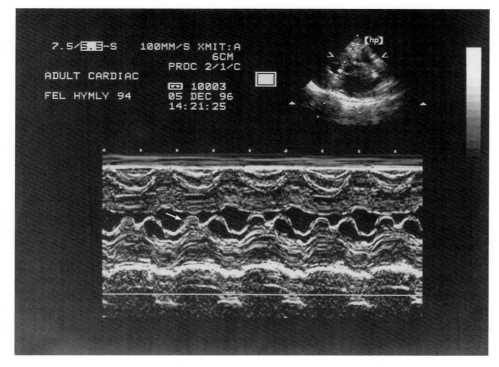

FIGURE 4.75 The systolic anterior motion barely touches the septum in this cat but its duration is fairly long. This probably correlates with a moderate degree of outflow tract obstruction (*arrow*).

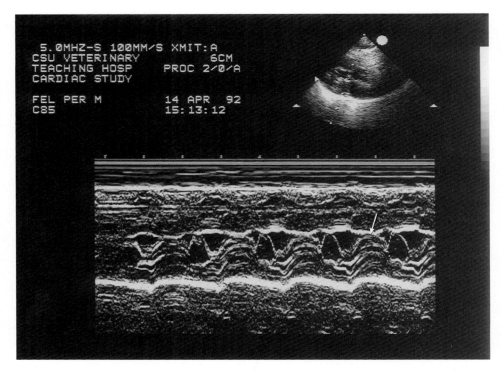

FIGURE 4.76   Significant systolic anterior motion is seen on this M-mode, implying significant obstruction to left ventricular outflow (*arrow*).

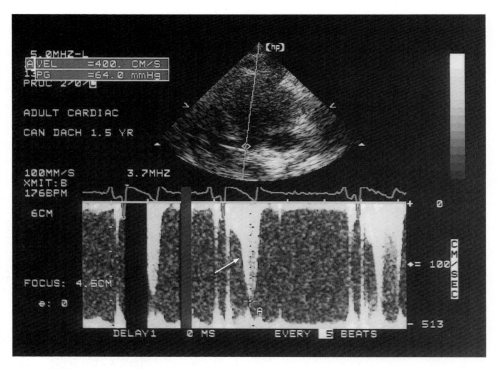

FIGURE 4.77   Dynamic left ventricular outflow obstruction in cats with hypertrophic cardiomyopathy results in increased aortic flow velocities and a concave dagger shape during acceleration associated with reduction in flow (*arrow*). The pressure gradient of 64 mm Hg is calculated by applying the Bernoulli equation to the velocity of 400 cm/sec.

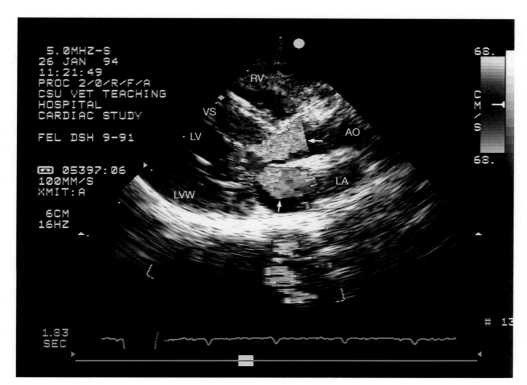

FIGURE 4.78 Aliased color-flow signals within the left ventricular outflow tract (*large arrow*) and left atrium (*small arrow*) reveal the presence of obstruction to flow and mitral insufficiency respectively in this cat with hypertrophic cardiomyopathy. The hypertrophy in this heart is symmetric. *Plane*, right parasternal left ventricular outflow view; *RV*, right ventricle; *VS*, ventricular septum; *LV*, left ventricle; *AO*, aorta; *LA*, left atrium; *LVW*, left ventricular wall.

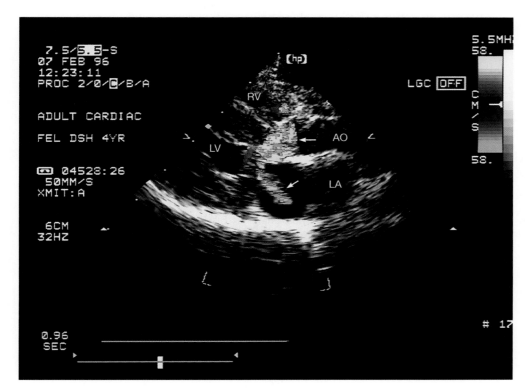

FIGURE 4.79 A small jet of mitral insufficiency (*small arrow*) is seen secondary to left ventricular outflow obstruction (*large arrow*) and systolic anterior motion in this cat with hypertrophic cardiomyopathy. This cat has symmetric hypertrophy. *Plane*, right parasternal left ventricular outflow view; *RV*, right ventricle; *LV*, left ventricle; *AO*, aorta; *LA*, left atrium.

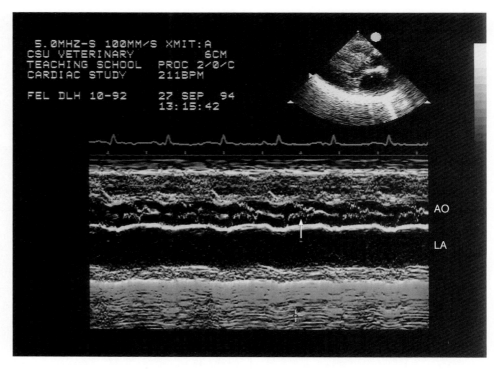

FIGURE 4.80 Systolic closure of the aortic valve (*arrow*) on M-mode images occurs when dynamic obstruction reduces flow abruptly through the valve in this cat with hypertrophic cardiomyopathy. *AO*, aorta; *LA*, left atrium.

When color-flow or an imaging Doppler probe is not used, mitral regurgitation flow must be differentiated from left ventricular outflow on left apical five-chamber views of the heart. Mitral regurgitation starts earlier in the cardiac cycle near the beginning of the QRS complex. Aortic flow starts later during the latter part of the QRS complex. When the late-peaking flow profile is seen, you know it is the outflow tract and not mitral insufficiency. With a very dynamic heart, recording both at the same time is possible with superimposed tracings (Fig. 4.81).

Right ventricular outflow tract obstruction occasionally is seen in humans and has been reported in cats (106,117,118). The cause of the obstruction is not well defined and may simply be secondary to excessive hypertrophy of the right ventricular wall or septum within the right ventricular outflow tract or cavity. The gradients associated with RV outflow or midventricular obstruction are low with velocities ranging from 1.7 to 4 m/sec in cats and humans (106,117) (Fig. 4.82). This is sometimes the only detectable abnormality in some cats with murmurs and clinical signs related to cardiac disease are not present. RV outflow obstruction in the cat is associated with HCM, chronic renal failure, hyperthyroidism, anemia, neoplasia, and inflammatory processes (117).

FS in HCM increases and the hearts are visibly hyperdynamic (Fig. 4.64). This is not necessarily indicative of increased intrinsic contractility, but may be only secondary to altered loading conditions in the heart. Paradoxically, this increase in function often impedes cardiac output, and dynamic obstruction is aggravated by the hypercontractile septum. Only in rare cases, as end-stage HCM is reached does function of the septum or free wall decrease. In one study, 72% of cats with FSs less than 30% died 3 months after their initial examination (109) (Figs. 4.83 and 4.84). Whether these cats had reduced FSs because of systolic dysfunction alone or diastolic disease that had progressed to include systolic dysfunction is not known.

Although systolic function is not impaired in patients with HCM, diastolic dysfunction is a common abnormality. Diastolic dysfunction is the result of impaired

Severe long-standing HCM may result in depressed function and areas of myocardial ischemia and infarction.

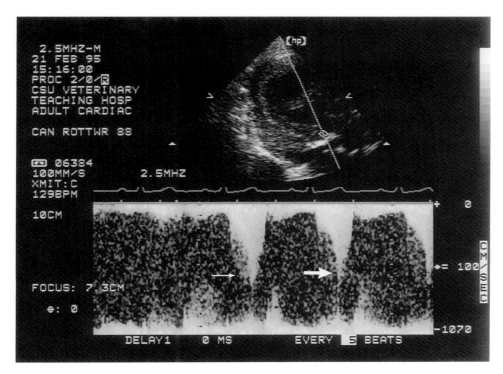

FIGURE 4.81 It is possible to record both dynamic obstruction and mitral regurgitation in one image because both jets are in close proximity. The dagger shape identifies the outflow tract flow (*large arrow*), whereas the lighter flow information is mitral (*small arrow*).

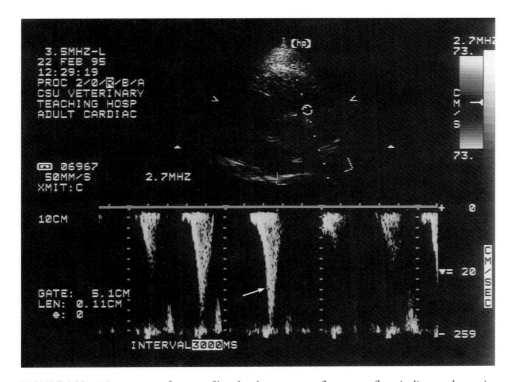

FIGURE 4.82 The concave flow profile of pulmonary outflow tract flow indicates dynamic obstruction (*arrow*). Velocities here are just above 200 cm/sec.

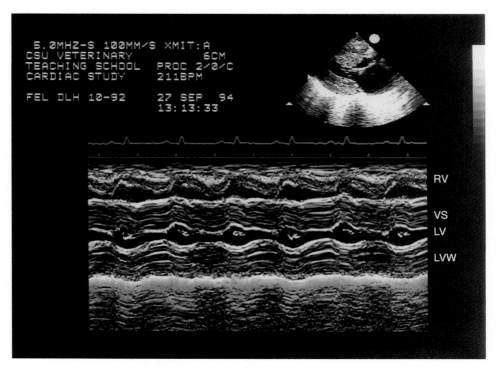

FIGURE 4.83 Left ventricular function in this cat with hypertrophic cardiomyopathy is decreased as seen by poor septal and free-wall thickening during systole. *RV*, right ventricle; *VS*, ventricular septum; *LV*, left ventricle; *LVW*, left ventricular wall.

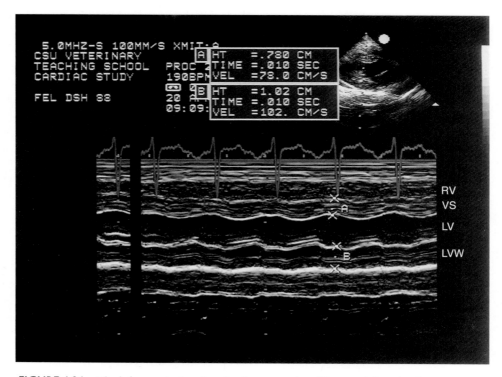

FIGURE 4.84 The left ventricular chamber has started to dilate, and function is very poor in this cat with hypertrophic cardiomyopathy. *RV*, right ventricle; *LV*, left ventricle; *VS*, ventricular septum; *LVW*, left ventricular wall.

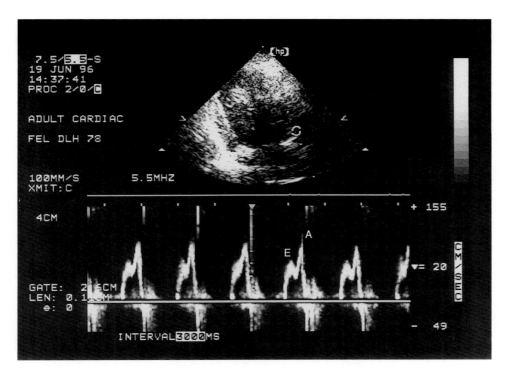

FIGURE 4.85   Reversed E:A ratios on Doppler examination of mitral inflow suggest impaired ventricular relaxation in this cat with hypertrophic cardiomyopathy.

myocardial relaxation, restriction to left ventricular filling, and increased left ventricular filling pressures (119). Impaired myocardial relaxation affects the rate of relaxation, and isovolumic relaxation time will be increased (108). Myocardial relaxation time may be measured from M-mode images run at 100 mm/sec. The measurement is made from the point of smallest left ventricular dimension to the point of mitral valve opening. In one study, cats with HCM had relaxation times of 102 ± 9 msec, which decreased to 47 ± 4 msec by 3 months of treatment with calcium channel blockers (120). The measurement of isovolumic relaxation time from Doppler images was discussed in Chapter 3. The left ventricular filling pattern of most patients, both animals and humans, is abnormal. Mitral inflow profiles recorded by Doppler echocardiography show decreased early filling and a larger late diastolic filling component after the atrial contraction (Figs. 3.58, 4.85, and 4.86). The overall peak velocity is not different from normal. This reflects the impaired left ventricular filling associated with delayed relaxation and a larger atrial contribution to left ventricular volume (106,119,121). As discussed in Chapter 3, diastolic dysfunction is a continuum of events, and the flow profiles typical of decreased compliance may also be seen. Mitral inflow profiles are difficult to record in cats when heart rates are very high. Relaxation times may be all that can be assessed in the cat to confirm impaired diastolic function.

Complications

Myocardial ischemia occasionally may be seen in cats with HCM. Initially, only depressed systolic thickening of either the septum or left ventricular free wall is seen (Fig. 4.87). Chronic ischemia may cause infarction, and a regional area of hypokinesis with thin walls and potentially an aneurysmal dilatation may be seen (Fig. 4.88). FS may be reduced in these cats if the M-mode measurement incorporated the ischemic portion of the ventricle. Infarction typically is seen as a sequela to severe, long-standing disease (108).

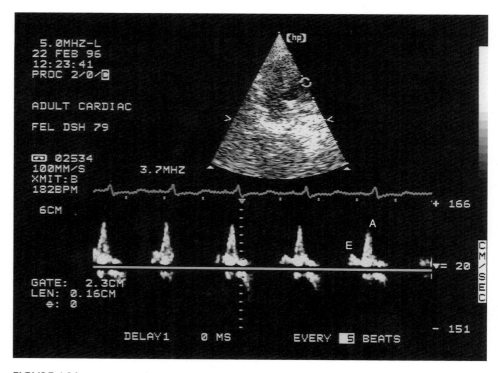

FIGURE 4.86   Dramatically reduced E-wave velocity, slow E-wave deceleration, and an E:A ratio less than 1 imply diastolic dysfunction and abnormal relaxation in this cat with hypertrophic cardiomyopathy. This pattern of flow also may be seen with other forms of cardiomyopathy.

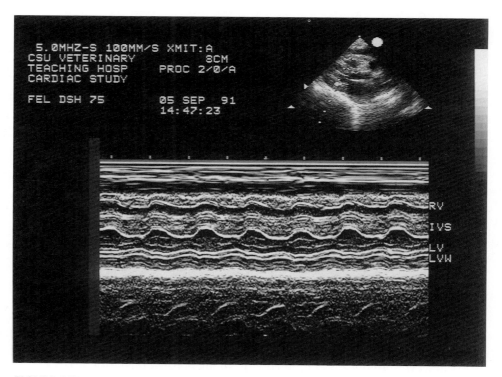

FIGURE 4.87   Depressed systolic thickening of the free wall is indicative of myocardial ischemia in this heart with hypertrophic cardiomyopathy. *RV*, right ventricle; *VS*, ventricular septum; *LV*, left ventricle; *LVW*, left ventricular wall.

Pericardial effusion may be seen in cats with severe HCM and clinical signs of heart failure (108). Pleural effusion and dyspnea also are often seen as a presenting complaint in cats with HCM (107,108) (Figs. 4.89 and 4.90).

Other Causes of Hypertrophy

True HCM is idiopathic, and the presence of other diseases that may lead to potentially reversible left ventricular hypertrophy should be ruled out. These other diseases include systemic hypertension, a common sequela of chronic renal failure seen often in older cats, and hyperthyroidism (122–124). Hyperthyroidism is reported to cause hypertrophy of the septum and wall. One study showed free-wall hypertrophy in 72% of cats with hyperthyroidism, whereas only 40% of them had septal hypertrophy. Seventy percent of these same cats also had left atrial dilation. Almost 50% of these cats are reported to have had an increase in ventricular diastolic chamber size. The vast majority of cats have hyperdynamic wall and septal motion and increased FSs (123,125,126). Although there appears to be some differences between idiopathic and nonidiopathic left ventricular hypertrophy in the cat, there is no way to differentiate between these causes of hypertrophy echocardiographically; they may even coexist (106,122,127,128). The degree of hypertrophy, the incidence of SAM, and the degree of outflow obstruction are similar in both hypertension and idiopathic HCM in human patients. The presence of hypertension as well as HCM will create a greater degree of hypertrophy, however (129). There are also irreversible causes of left ventricular hypertrophy that can mimic HCM, including hypertrophic feline muscular dystrophy and other infiltrative disorders (130,131).

An unusual presentation for cats with hyperthyroidism is left and right ventricular chamber dilation with normal wall and septal thickness and poor FS. This may occur

Rule out reversible causes of hypertrophy such as hypertension and hyperthyroidism; they cannot be differentiated echocardiographically from HCM.

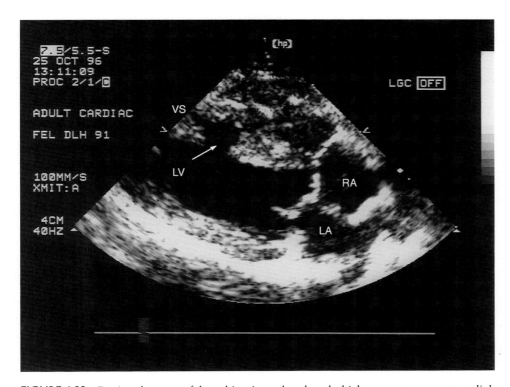

FIGURE 4.88 Regional areas of hypokinesis and reduced thickness suggest myocardial ischemia and, possibly, infarction in some cats with severe long-standing hypertrophic cardiomyopathy. Here, a thin area of the ventricular septum is seen with a slight aneurysmal dilation (*arrow*). The area was hypokinetic, but the areas next to it were hyperdynamic. *Plane*, right parasternal four chamber; *VS*, ventricular septum; *RA*, right atrium; *LV*, left ventricle; *LA*, left atrium.

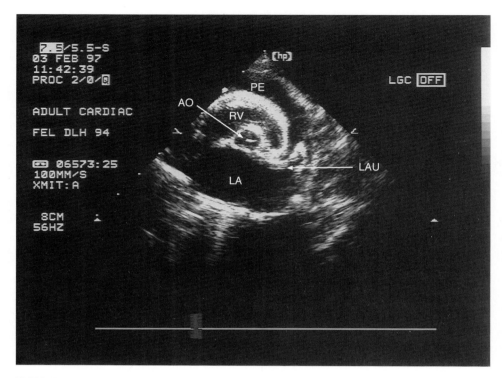

FIGURE 4.89   Pericardial effusion may be seen at times in cats with congestive heart failure secondary to hypertrophic cardiomyopathy. Notice that the effusion is not seen behind the left atrium but only around the right ventricular wall. This helps differentiate pleural from pericardial effusion. This image also shows a very large left atrial chamber. *Plane*, right parasternal transverse heart base; *PE*, pericardial effusion; *RV*, right ventricle; *AO*, aorta; *LA*, left atrium; *LAU*, left auricle.

secondary to increased systolic wall stress and myocardial dysfunction after chronic hyperthyroidism, leading to congestive heart failure. Even these changes are reversible to a certain degree when the hyperthyroid state is corrected (132).

Left Ventricular False Tendons

False tendons, or moderator bands, may be a normal finding in many animals and are common in the right side of the heart (Figs. 4.91 and 4.92). Occasionally, they may restrict left ventricular filling. These tendons cross the ventricular cavity, connecting the septum and free wall or papillary muscles (133). Echocardiographic abnormalities include a rounded left ventricular apex, irregular contours to the chamber, and a narrowed ventricular chamber. Cats with false tendons may present with symptoms very similar to cats with cardiomyopathy of any form (134). However, not all moderator bands create problems, and identifying a false tendon by echocardiography should not be immediately associated with cardiac malfunction (87,133,135).

DILATED CARDIOMYOPATHY

Idiopathic dilated cardiomyopathy (DCM) is a myocardial disease of unknown etiology. In humans, some known causes of dilated cardiomyopathy exist, including toxins, such as ethanol and lead; metabolic abnormalities, such as nutritional and endocrine disorders; inflammatory and infectious processes; and neuromuscular diseases, such as several dystrophies. There is a definite familial component with

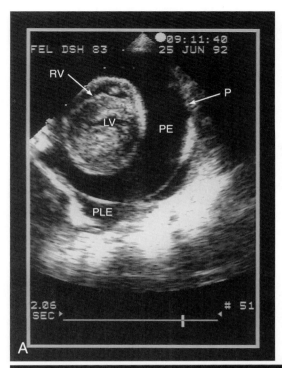

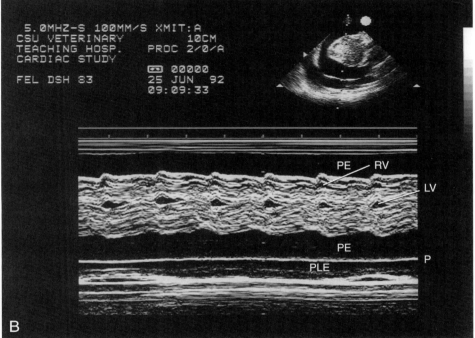

FIGURE 4.90   Severe pericardial effusion and some pleural effusion is seen in and around this cat's heart. Left ventricular hypertrophy appears severe, but this amount of fluid may restrict ventricular filling, creating the appearance of more significant hypertrophy than would be present without the effusion. **A.** Transverse real-time image of the left ventricle showing the effusions. **B.** M-mode of the same heart showing tamponade with total collapse of the ventricular chambers. *PE*, pericardial effusion; *P*, pericardial sac; *RV*, right ventricle; *LV*, left ventricle; *PLE*, pleural effusion.

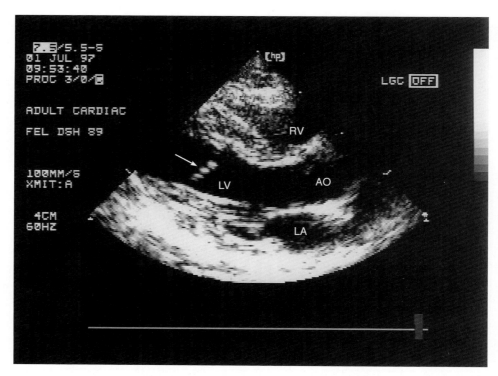

FIGURE 4.91   Left ventricular false tendons or moderator bands may or may not create restriction to filling within the left ventricle (*arrow*). *Plane*, right parasternal left ventricular outflow view; *RV*, right ventricle; *LV*, left ventricle; *AO*, aorta; *LA*, left atrium.

dilated cardiomyopathy (136–138). The cause of most dilated cardiomyopathies in animals remains unknown, but several potential underlying causes are being studied, which include carnitine deficiencies, metabolic abnormalities including hypothyroidism, and myocarditis (136–145). Taurine deficiency was established as a cause of dilated cardiomyopathy in cats and the disease is now rare in the feline (146–149). Plasma taurine levels are not low in dogs with DCM except for possibly the Cocker spaniel (150).

The prominent features of DCM are similar in dogs, cats, and horses and include ventricular dilation, atrial dilation, normal or thin wall and septal thicknesses, depressed systolic thickening of the wall and septum, poor FS, large EPSS, reduced aortic wall motion, and global hypokinesis (136,138,151–158). The dilation generally involves the left side of the heart. The right ventricle may be normal or also affected (157–159). Dobermans display less right-sided involvement than other breeds with DCM (155). The dysfunction is diffuse and involves the entire ventricle, but some areas of the ventricle may exhibit better function than others. This is thought to be secondary to variable areas of abnormal wall stress (136,142,151,159).

Chamber Sizes

Ventricular dilation and poor function are the hallmarks of DCM (Figs. 4.93 and 4.94). Several breeds including the boxer, Doberman pinscher, and the Dalmatian display either a lack of dilation or severe dilation as a consequence of the myocardial disease (160–162). The Dalmatian and Doberman appear to exhibit the most severe ventricular and atrial dilation of any breeds with DCM. Boxer DCM may manifest itself with normal ventricular chamber size. The impaired function is still present, and all other features of DCM are present. Early DCM

Dilated Cardiomyopathy Features
_____

- Dilated left ventricle
  – Boxers may not show this
- Atrial dilation
- Normal to thin LVW and VS
- Poor fractional shortening
- Large EPSS

may exhibit only increased systolic left ventricular dimensions and normal diastolic dimensions as FS decreases. Diastolic chamber size will increase as function deteriorates and as forward flow is compromised (156,158,162). A study in cats with taurine deficiency showed only increased systolic left ventricular dimensions and decreased FS with no dilation of the ventricle during diastole (146).

Left atrial and sometimes right atrial dilation develops as myocardial failure progresses. Elevated left ventricular end-systolic pressure creates less of a pressure gradient from the atrium into the ventricle, resulting in less atrial emptying, high left atrial pressures, and atrial dilation (138,155–157). Many cats display normal left atrial size on echocardiographic examinations but do have parameters that are at the high end of the normal range (157). Echocardiographic evidence of atrial enlargement may be present before radiographic indication of atrial dilation. As with HCM, a thrombus may form within the left atrial or auricular chamber (Fig. 4.95). Mitral insufficiency is common in animals with DCM secondary to dilation of the mitral annulus. The insufficiency may vary from mild to severe when DCM is present and may aggravate the clinical signs of congestive heart failure. Valvular lesions will not be evident if the insufficiency is truly secondary to the dilation.

With DCM, septal and free-wall thicknesses are typically thinner than normal but may be normal in early DCM (156–158). No measurable hypertrophy is present even though heart size and weight are increased. A decrease in wall thickness to chamber size ratio implies inadequate hypertrophy, myocardial abnormalities, and dilated cardiomyopathy. The prognosis is considered poorer in human patients with lower ratios (163,164). The wall and septum also have reduced systolic thickening and excursions as myocardial function deteriorates. The lack of compensatory hypertrophy as the ventricle dilates increases left ventricular afterload and wall stress, further decreasing FS and velocity of circumference shortening.

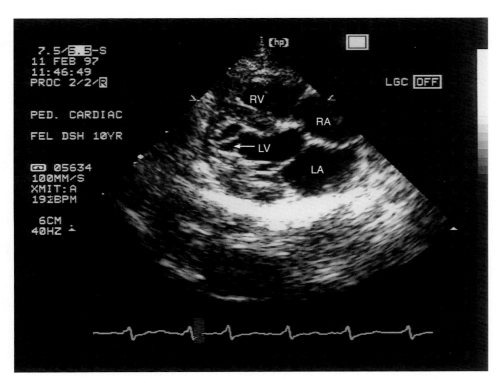

FIGURE 4.92   Moderator bands are seen within the apex of this cat's heart (*arrow*). The moderator bands created no problems for this animal. *Plane,* right parasternal four chamber. *RV,* right ventricle; *LV,* left ventricle; *RA,* right atrium; *LA,* left atrium.

Hemodynamic and Functional Information

The EPSS is always increased in dogs and cats with DCM (Figs. 3.84 and 4.96). The degree of mitral valve motion toward the interventricular septum depends on flow from the atrium into the ventricle. As end-systolic volume remains large secondary to poor contraction, elevated end-systolic left ventricular pressures limit the amount of blood flowing from the atrium into the ventricle. EPSS increases as a result because mitral excursion is reduced. This is a sensitive and specific sign of early DCM even in asymptomatic dogs and in dogs with equivocal values for all other parameters of size and function (156).

A "B" bump at the end of mitral valve diastolic motion signifying delayed closure is a sign of increased end-diastolic left ventricular pressures. This may or may not be found in dogs with DCM (153,156) (Figs. 3.83 and 4.21). It has routinely only been seen in dogs with severe heart failure.

Parameters of systolic function are always altered in DCM. FS, and velocity of circumferential shortening (Vcf) decrease while pre-ejection period (PEP) increases (Fig. 4.97). The ratio of PEP to left ventricular ejection time (LVET) increases in DCM secondary to slow rate of pressure rise during isovolumic contraction. This value is not sensitive, however, because PEP/LVET ratios still may be normal even in dogs with overt heart signs of heart failure (156). LVET does not appear to be affected on a consistent basis in cats treated for DCM (165). Although these values are still abnormal after the initiation of therapy, they improve and move toward the normal range. Even when LVET is normal, gradual closure of the aortic valve may be seen as ventricular systolic pressures decline throughout systole and forward flow declines (Fig. 3.79).

The total systolic time, QAVC, measured from the onset of the QRS complex to closure of the aortic valve increases in cats with systolic dysfunction and dilated cardiomyopathy. This parameter consistently reflects increases in systolic function as cats with DCM are treated with inotropic drugs (165).

Poor Fractional Shortening

- Rule out poor preload as a cause
- Rule out increased afterload as a cause
- Should be a global dysfunction

Early Diagnosis

Early DCM is a challenge to diagnose. The first signs of DCM may be cardiac arrhythmias, which include ventricular premature contractions and tachycardia, supraventricular tachycardia, or brady-arrhythmias (166). The disease in these dogs may be subclinical, or the animals may have exercise intolerance, weakness, collapse, or syncope. Echocardiographic examinations in these dogs typically reveal normal cardiac dimensions but very mild to moderately depressed FS (158,167)(Fig. 4.98). Diastolic left ventricular chamber size of greater than 46 mm, or a systolic chamber size of greater than 38 mm, or even one premature ventricular contraction suggests occult DCM in Doberman pinschers (167). The progression of the disease is slow in most cases, and heart failure may not manifest itself for several years. Left ventricular chamber size will increase over the years as FS continues to deteriorate (138,158,166–168). Repeat echocardiographic examinations usually are necessary to verify the diagnosis of DCM. Reevaluation in which there is no increase in ventricular chamber size or decrease in FS indicates that the equivocal parameters of size and function may be normal for that specific animal. FS has increased dramatically, by as much as 10% in some human patients, but it is generally transient (136). The same occurs in many dogs. FS may fluctuate from study to study.

Predictors of Outcome

The clinical course of these animals is variable and there are no useful echocardiographic indices that can predict outcome and survival (161,169). Although 50% of dogs in one study survived past 3 months, echocardiography could not predict which dogs would be long-term survivors and which would not. The degree of dilation or FS does not provide an indication as to the length of survival. Only the presence of pleural effusion and pulmonary edema was found to suggest poorer survival

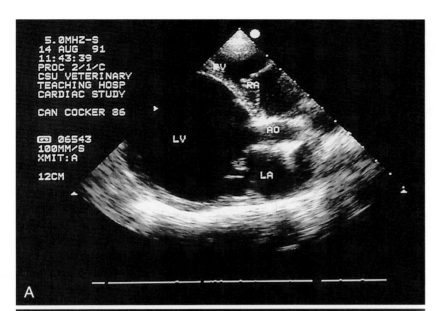

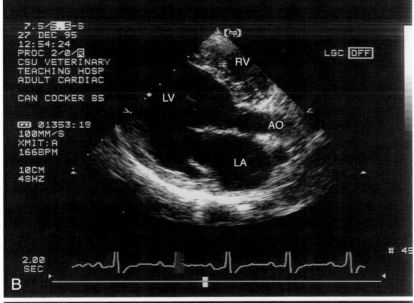

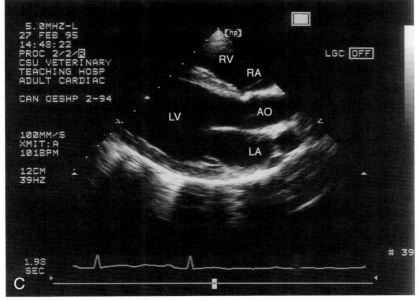

FIGURE 4.93 These images display severe (**A**), moderate (**B**), and mild (**C**) left ventricular and atrial dilation in dogs with dilated cardiomyopathy. The wall and septum are thin for the volumes in these hearts. *Plane*, right parasternal left ventricular outflow view; *RV*, right ventricle; *LV*, left ventricle; *RA*, right atrium; *LA*, left atrium; *AO*, aorta.

FIGURE 4.94 Left ventricular function is depressed to varying degrees in these animals with dilated cardiomyopathy. **A.** A horse showing virtually no contraction of the septum or wall. **B.** A cat with poor function and pleural effusion. **C.** Some contraction is still evident in the septum of this dog, but the free wall is akinetic.

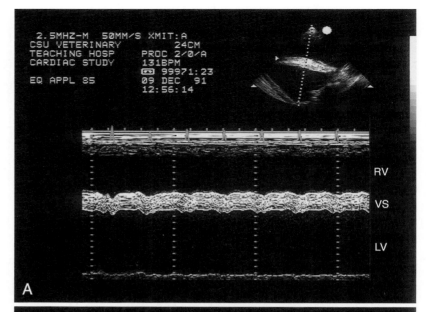

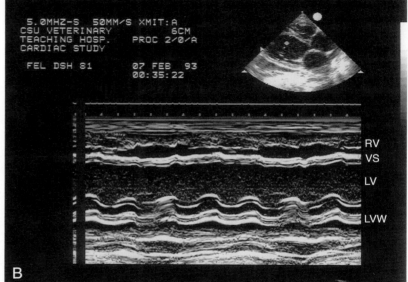

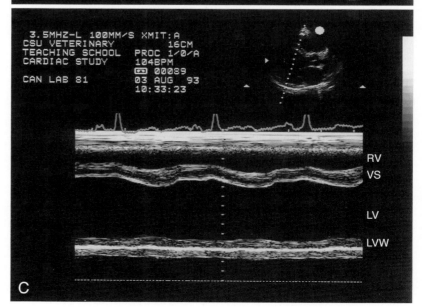

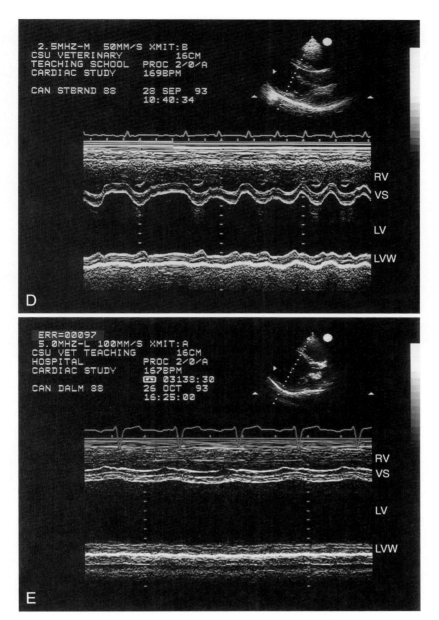

FIGURE 4.94 *(continued)*   **D.** The wall and septum still thicken slightly in this dog's heart. **E.** No visible contractions are present on this M-mode. *RV*, right ventricle; *VS*, ventricular septum; *LV*, left ventricle; *LVW*, left ventricular wall.

times (169). The presence of pulmonary hypertension is associated with a poorer prognosis for human patients with dilated cardiomyopathy. This is measured echocardiographically by Doppler evaluation of tricuspid regurgitation. Eighty-nine percent of human patients with hypertension died or were hospitalized after 2 years compared with 32% of patients with cardiomyopathy without pulmonary hypertension (170).

When taurine deficiency was considered the underlying cause of DCM in cats, improvement in cardiac size and function occurs 3 to 16 weeks after supplementation (171). These cats had essentially normal echocardiograms 6 months to 1 year after initial presentation (171).

The usually reversible systolic dysfunction found in dogs with hypothyroidism does not manifest itself with any significant dilation of the left ventricular chamber during diastole. Echocardiographic features in these hypothyroid dogs include

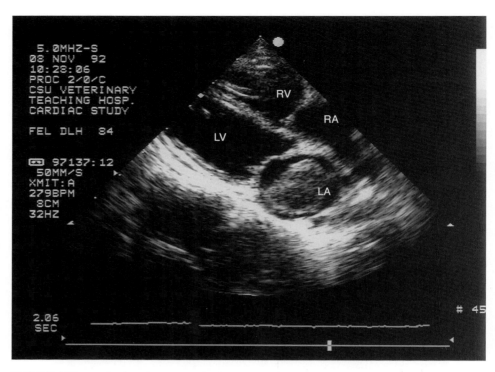

FIGURE 4.95   A clot has formed in the left atrium of this cat with dilated cardiomyopathy. Left ventricular chamber size was still within the normal range but fractional shortening was very poor. The right side of the heart appears dilated. *Plane,* right parasternal four chamber; *RV,* right ventricle; *LV,* left ventricle; *RA,* right atrium; *LA,* left atrium.

increased systolic dimensions, decreased FS and Vcf, as well as increased PEP. Dogs with hypothyroidism and impaired function typically do not show signs of heart failure unless preexisting myocardial failure exists (141,172).

Right Ventricular Cardiomyopathy

Right Ventricular Cardiomyopathy Features

- RV dilation
- RA dilation
- Paradoxical septal motion
- Irregular endocardial surface

Right ventricular dilated cardiomyopathy occurs as an entity that typically spares the left side of the heart (159,173,174). This entity also is referred to as right ventricular dysplasia. Severe right ventricular and atrial dilation is present with poor right ventricular systolic function and paradoxical septal motion secondary to the elevated right-sided diastolic pressures (Fig. 4.99). Other signs of right heart failure, such as pleural and pericardial effusion, may be seen both radiographically and echocardiographically. Tricuspid insufficiency may be present, and if so, spectral Doppler should be used if possible to rule out pulmonary hypertension as a cause of right heart failure instead of cardiomyopathy. The foramen ovale may become patent when right atrial pressures become excessive (173). In humans, right ventricular cardiomyopathy is associated with highly irregular endocardial surfaces appearing as prominent bulges and deep fissures (159,174).

Spectral Doppler

Doppler can provide additional information regarding systolic and possibly diastolic function of the heart. Maximal aortic flow velocity is reduced in animals with DCM (154,175) (Fig. 4.100). Aortic flow velocities that remain within the normal range suggest maintenance of adequate cardiac output. Acceleration rate (dv/dt) may be a better indicator, but this parameter varies tremendously in both healthy dogs and dogs with DCM (154,176). Systolic time intervals may be measured from Doppler flow studies instead of M-mode images because Doppler may provide better images for measuring.

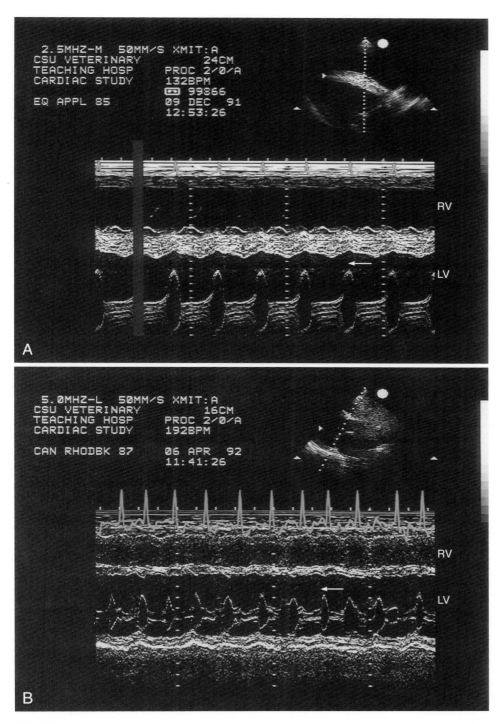

FIGURE 4.96   **A.** A large EPSS (*arrow*) in this horse is present secondary to poor ventricular function. The right ventricle also is dilated. **B.** A large EPSS correlates inversely with ejection fraction in animals with dilated cardiomyopathy. This dog has atrial fibrillation with no A wave to the mitral trace and a large EPSS (*arrow*). There is also right ventricular dilation. *RV,* right ventricle; *LV,* left ventricle.

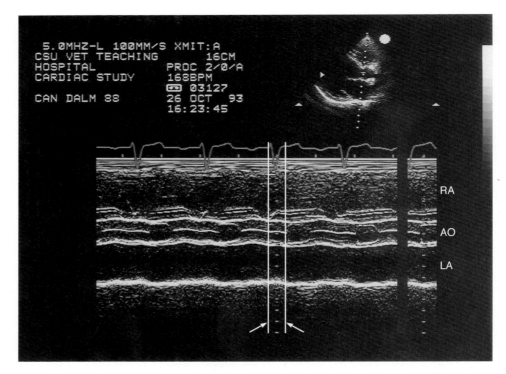

FIGURE 4.97   Pre-ejection periods are longer in hearts with dilated cardiomyopathy because systolic pressure takes longer to rise during isovolumic contraction (*arrows*). *RA*, right atrium; *AO*, aorta; *LA*, left atrium.

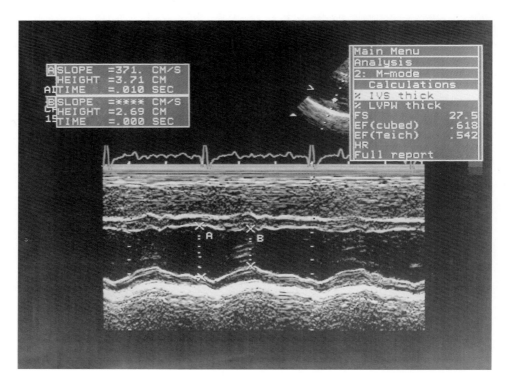

FIGURE 4.98   This Doberman dog has normal diastolic dimensions and increased systolic dimensions, resulting in poor fractional shortening. These are signs of early dilated cardiomyopathy. *RV*, right ventricle; *LV*, left ventricle.

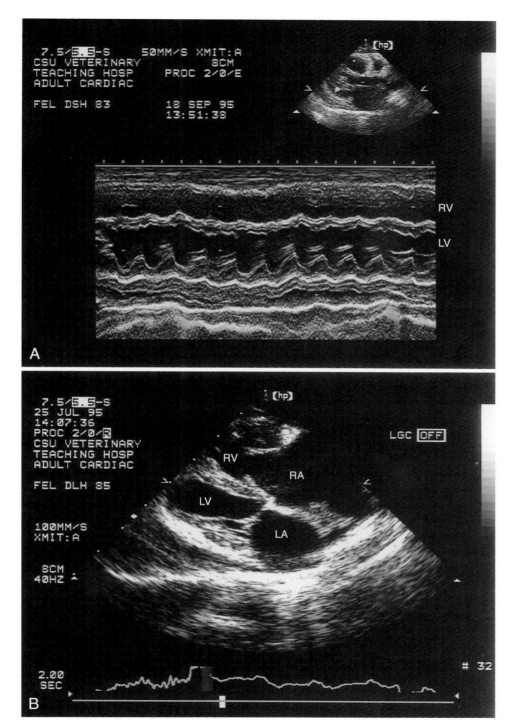

FIGURE 4.99   Right ventricular cardiomyopathy spares the left side of the heart. The right ventricle in both the M-mode image (**A**) and the right parasternal four-chamber image (**B**) is dilated and functions poorly. *RV,* right ventricle; *RA,* right atrium; *LV,* left ventricle; *LA,* left atrium.

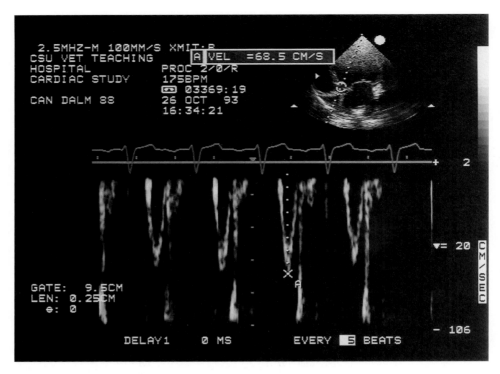

FIGURE 4.100   Aortic flow velocities are reduced in animals with poor cardiac output. This flow velocity of 68 cm/sec was recorded in a dog with dilated cardiomyopathy.

Mitral inflow studies in dogs with DCM show increased E wave velocities, no change in A wave velocities, increased E wave durations, and increased E:A ratios. (Figs. 3.60 and 4.101). The increased E velocity and E duration may be secondary to increased atrial pressure or volume associated with mitral insufficiency. Moderate to severe mitral insufficiency will increase E velocities also and must be considered when evaluating diastolic function and atrial pressures (Fig. 3.63).

Changes in mitral inflow profiles in humans are closely correlated with the improvement or deterioration of clinical status. An increase in E:A ratio signifies deterioration of clinical status, whereas a decrease in E:A ratio signifies resolving heart failure. These changes correlated with changes in capillary wedge pressure (177). Diastolic function may have a more significant impact on clinical signs than systolic function. Humans and dogs with extremely poor systolic function often do not show significant clinical symptoms. Congestive heart failure may develop as diastolic pressures increase and ventricular filling is reduced, causing dilation of the left atrium and increased left atrial pressures (154,177–180).

Rapid mitral valve inflow deceleration times (< 180 msec) correlate with high LA pressures in humans.

Rapid deceleration times (< 180 msec) after peak E velocity are highly sensitive and specific for high mean left atrial pressures in humans. Rapid deceleration times are apparently more sensitive than E:A ratios but has not been studied in animals (181).

Spectral Doppler may be used to measure the pressure gradient between the left ventricle and atrium when mitral insufficiency is present. Low pressure gradients are seen when systemic pressures are low secondary to poor cardiac output (Fig. 4.102). Low pressure gradients also are affected by high left atrial pressure. A cutoff sign may be seen when left atrial pressures are significantly elevated and ventricular pressures are low (Fig. 4.35). High pressures have been recorded, and systemic hypertension has been documented as a cause of poor function.

RESTRICTIVE CARDIOMYOPATHY

Restrictive cardiomyopathy (RCM), found primarily in cats, is poorly characterized and is sometimes called intermediate cardiomyopathy. However, restrictive

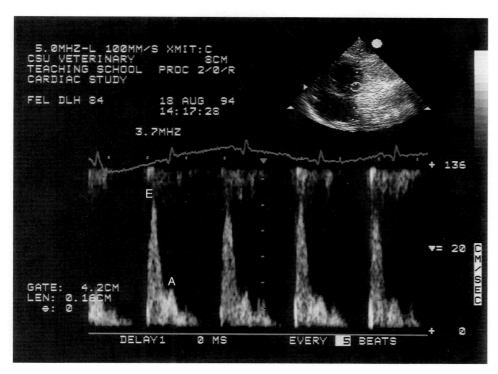

FIGURE 4.101   Doppler evaluation of mitral inflow in hearts with dilated cardiomyopathy may show increased E velocities, normal A velocities, and an increased E:A ratio secondary to increased atrial pressures and reduced ventricular compliance.

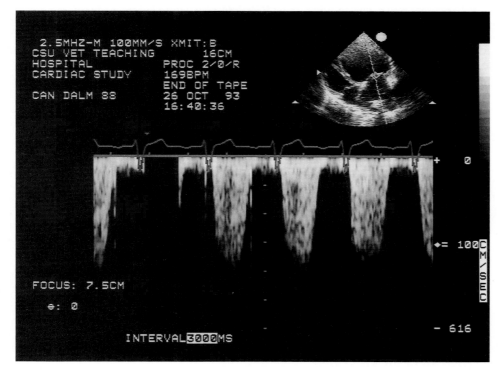

FIGURE 4.102   Low pressure gradients are seen on mitral regurgitant jets in dilated cardiomyopathy when systemic pressures are low and atrial pressures are high, reducing the gradient between the two chambers. Here, the gradient is approximately 64 mm Hg.

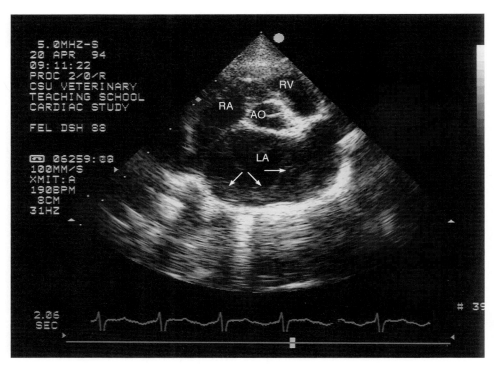

FIGURE 4.103   Very large atria classically are seen with restrictive cardiomyopathy. This atrium contains smokelike echoes, indicating sluggish blood flow through the chamber (*arrows*). *Plane*, right parasternal transverse heart base; *RA*, right atrium; *RV*, right ventricle; *LA*, left atrium; *AO*, aorta.

cardiomyopathy is the preferred term. Intergrade cardiomyopathy should be reserved for cases in which features of more than one type of cardiomyopathy exist and differentiation is not possible (182,183). Primary RCM is idiopathic. A less common form of RCM is endomyocardial fibrosis, which is an obliterative process. Secondary processes that may result in restrictive physiology include amyloid heart disease, hypertension, HCM, and DCM. Restrictive physiology is characterized by reduced ventricular compliance in which diastolic filling is completed early in the diastolic period (159,183–185).

Chamber Size

Restrictive Cardiomyopathy Features

- Left atrial dilation
  - Usually severe
  - Often with mild or no mitral insufficiency
- Hypertrophy only mild if present
- Echogenic areas in myocardium
- Function is normal or mildly depressed

Echocardiographic features are not well documented and restrictive cardiomyopathy does not have uniformly accepted diagnostic criteria. However, moderate to severe left atrial enlargement is one consistently accepted criteria for RCM. Atrial enlargement may be seen only on the left, but both atria are involved. Atrial dilation occurs secondary to the high left ventricular filling pressures and reduced ventricular compliance. Mild mitral insufficiency may be present, but often regurgitation does not occur at all (87,183,186). At times a thrombus is seen within the left atrial or auricular cavity (183,186). More often, however, the smokelike echoes of sluggish blood may be seen within the atrial chamber (Fig. 4.103).

Hypertrophy, if present, is mild, and left ventricular chamber size usually is normal but may be slightly dilated. The endocardial surface is irregular; areas of the septum or free wall may be visibly thicker than other areas. There may be echogenic areas within the myocardium representing fibrosis, but this is not a consistent finding (87,159,183,186) (Fig. 4.104).

When cats decompensate, right heart changes become evident on the echocardiographic examination. These signs include right ventricular dilation with hypertrophy and pleural and pericardial effusions (183,186).

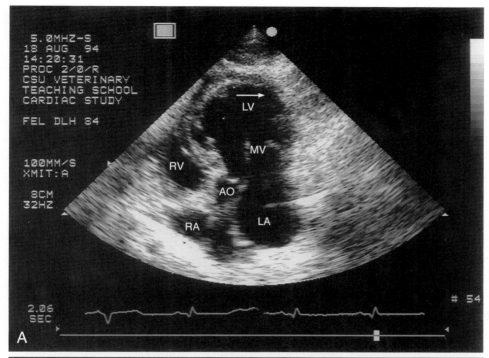

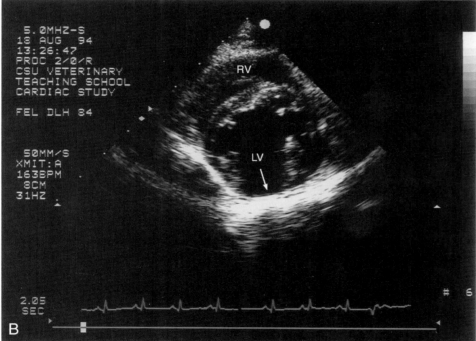

FIGURE 4.104   An irregular endocardial surface as well as small focal areas of fibrosis seen as bright hyperechoic areas are found in restrictive cardiomyopathies. Here, an area of infarcted muscle is present with aneurysmal dilation along the free wall (*arrow*) where the myocardium is almost nonexistent. **A.** Apical five-chamber view of a heart with restrictive cardiomyopathy. **B.** Transverse left ventricular plane in a restrictive cardiomyopathy heart. *RV*, right ventricle; *LV*, left ventricle; *RA*, right atrium; *AO*, aorta; *LA*, left atrium; *MV*, mitral valve.

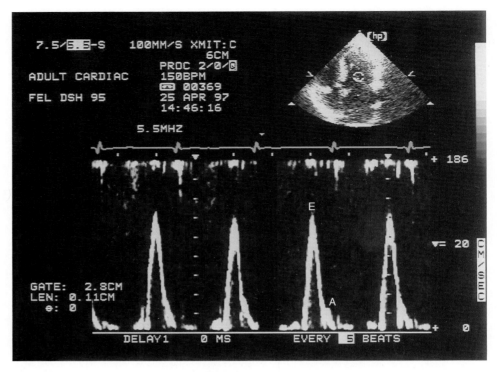

FIGURE 4.105   Restrictive physiology results in high atrial pressures and large E-wave velocities with little if any filling secondary to atrial contraction (A).

Function

Systolic left ventricular function in RCM is normal to mildly depressed, with FSs above 22%. Areas of hypokinesis or dyskinesia may be present associated with the myocardial fibrosis (87,183,186). Diastolic dysfunction is the predominant feature of RCM, however (87,183,186,187). Doppler evaluation of mitral inflow may show increased E velocities, rapid early deceleration, and little if any filling late in diastole, resulting in reduced or absent A waves on the inflow profile (Figs. 3.60 and 4.105). Early RCM may not show the restrictive pattern of filling but instead shows evidence of impaired relaxation. This mitral inflow pattern shows reduced early filling with a strong atrial component to filling, resulting in an E:A ratio less than 1. In the cat, this is a very difficult pattern to record. Not only are apical four-chamber and five-chamber images difficult to obtain in some cats, but heart rates are usually too rapid to differentiate the two phases of left ventricular filling (87,159,185).

Differentiation from Other Disease

Differentiation of RCM from other heart disease is often difficult. HCM and constrictive pericarditis are the two most common differentials (186). Constrictive pericarditis is associated with respiratory variation in peak mitral and tricuspid inflow velocities as well as respiratory variation in isovolumic relaxation times. RCM does not show this respiratory variation (159,188).

RCM is often diagnosed in humans when all other causes of heart failure are ruled out, even though RCM features are absent.

HCM may show the restrictive inflow pattern associated with RCM. In humans when restrictive physiology is present in the absence of outflow obstruction, and only mild or moderate myocardial hypertrophy as well as a disproportionately large atrium compared with ventricular changes, then the diagnosis of RCM is made versus HCM (159). Differentiating between RCM and HCM is still a challenge, but the therapeutic approach is often the same and so the distinction often is not critical (186).

Endocardial Fibroelastosis

Endocardial fibrosis in the dog has been described with features including a dilated left ventricular chamber with decreased wall and septal motion; depressed FS; dilated left atrium and auricle; and abnormal mitral valve morphology and motion. Endocardial fibrosis was not described as an echocardiographic finding because these studies were obtained with M-modes; however, necropsy findings showed extensive endocardial and myocardial fibrosis with variable areas of hypertrophy (184). The mitral apparatus is involved in this disease process, with thickening of the leaflets and chordae. This disease is differentiated from degenerative mitral valve disease by the excellent systolic function present in most hearts with mitral insufficiency secondary to endocardiosis (184). Endocardial fibrosis is only reported in young dogs and its status as an acquired defect is debatable.

MYOCARDIAL INFARCTION

Myocardial infarction does not occur frequently in animals; however, when it does occur it is typically secondary to other cardiac disease such as aortic stenosis, cardiomyopathy, neoplasia, or endocarditis (189). The features of acute myocardial ischemia on echocardiograms include reduced wall or septal systolic thickening, dyskinetic wall motion, and systolic thinning as opposed to thickening of the wall or septum (100–102,190–193). The infarcted myocardium will become thinner and appear echodense as the affected areas become fibrotic (194–196) (Figs. 4.106, 4.107, 4.108, 4.109, and 4.110).

Myocardial Infarction

Acutely
- Regional areas of decreased systolic LVW or VS thickening
  or
- VS systolic thinning

Chronically
- Fibrosis and thin areas of muscle are seen with old infarctions

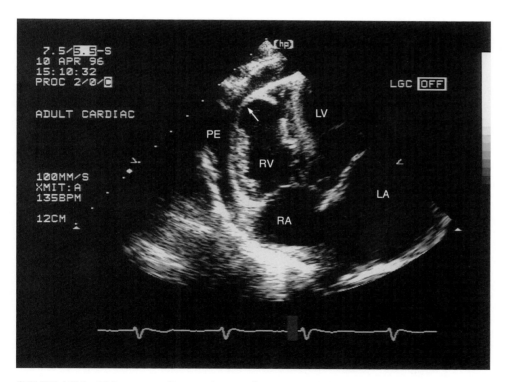

FIGURE 4.106   Thin myocardium with a small aneurysmal dilation in the apex of the right ventricle indicates infarcted muscle (*arrow*). This dog also has a small pericardial effusion. *Plane*, modified apical four chamber; *RV*, right ventricle; *LV*, left ventricle; *RA*, right atrium; *LA*, left atrium; *PE*, pericardial effusion.

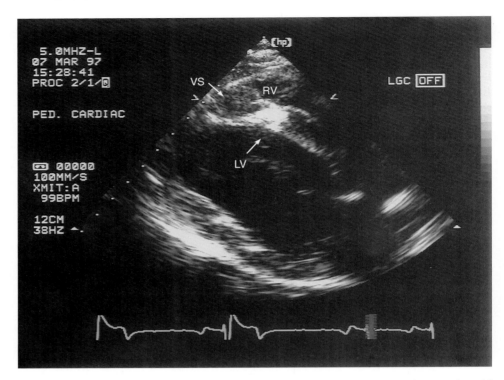

FIGURE 4.107   An area of fibrosis and thinning in this ventricular septum is the site of an old myocardial infarction (*arrow*). *Plane*, right parasternal four chamber; *RV*, right ventricle; *LV*, left ventricle; *VS*, ventricular septum; *species*, dog.

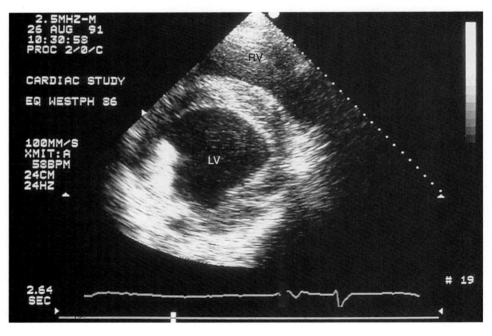

FIGURE 4.108   A dense echogenic area within the myocardium of this horse was found to be an area of infarcted myocardium at necropsy. *Plane*, right parasternal transverse left ventricle; *RV*, right ventricle; *LV*, left ventricle.

Features

When an area of muscle becomes infarcted, the percent systolic thickening decreases (101,190,191) (Fig. 4.87). This is evident on real-time and M-mode images if imaged carefully. The decrease in systolic thickening is not gradual from infarcted areas to adjacent normal areas. The decrease in thickening is sudden. The appearance of reduced motion toward the center of the ventricular chamber during systole on transverse or long-axis real-time images reveals infarcted areas of myocardium but usually overestimates the extent of the affected area. M-mode analysis of systolic thickening in the region will define the extent of the affected segment more accurately. Percent systolic thickening is an abrupt change between affected and nonaffected myocardium, whereas wall motion abnormalities overlap between affected and adjacent areas of myocardium. These areas may display paradoxical motion and are called dyskinetic.

When an area of muscle displays systolic thinning it is always associated with infarcted muscle (99,102,192,193) (Fig. 4.111). The extent of the infarction is less than 20% when there is any evidence of systolic thickening in the segment of wall or septum that is being evaluated (100).

Not all abnormally moving or thickening myocardium is indicative of permanent damage. Myocardial muscle simply may be stunned or hibernating and therefore function will spontaneously return to normal on its own if this is the cause of poor muscle contraction (102,197–200).

Myocardial Contusions

Myocardial contusions resulting from trauma may also impair myocardial function. Features seen echocardiographically on two-dimensional images include increased diastolic wall or septal thickness in the affected segment, increased echogenicity of

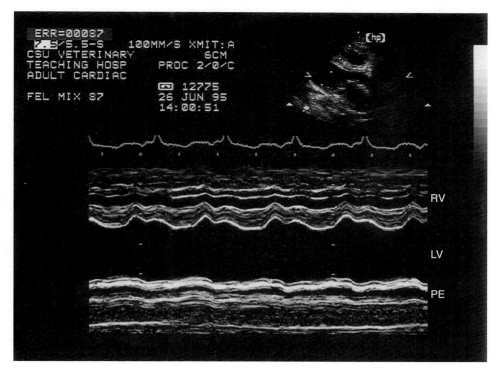

FIGURE 4.109   This thin free wall with no systolic thickening is consistent with an old myocardial infarction on this M-mode image of the left ventricle. *RV*, right ventricle; *LV*, left ventricle; *PE*, pericardial effusion.

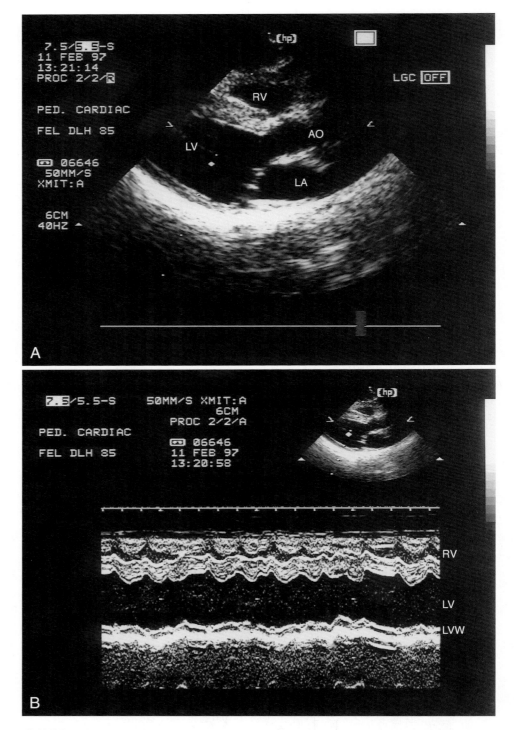

FIGURE 4.110   The real-time (**A**) and M-mode (**B**) images of this cat's heart show a thin left ventricular wall with poor function. Septal function is normal. *Plane,* right parasternal left ventricular outflow view; *RV,* right ventricle; *LV,* left ventricle; *AO,* aorta; *LA,* left atrium; *LVW,* left ventricular wall.

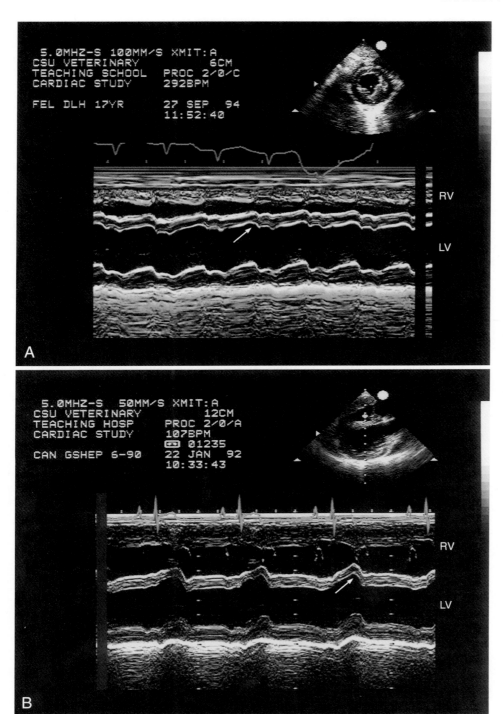

FIGURE 4.III   Systolic thinning of the septum or free wall on M-mode images always is associated with infarcted myocardium. **A.** This cat's M-mode shows mild systolic thinning of the septum associated with myocardial infarction. **B.** The M-mode in this dog shows dramatic systolic thinning after an ischemic episode. Paradoxical septal motion secondary to right-sided volume overload would still show systolic thickening at the appropriate time. *RV*, right ventricle; *LV*, left ventricle.

the affected myocardium, decreased systolic thickening in the affected area, and occasionally pericardial effusion. Hypoechoic areas also may be present as a result of hematomas within the myocardium (201). The increased wall thickness is associated with edema of the injured muscle, and the increased echogenicity is the result of hemorrhage and altered tissue structure. Studies show that myocardial perfusion remains normal or may actually increase, and that ischemia is not responsible for the decrease in thickening of the affected area. The effect is similar to that of stunned myocardium in which function will spontaneously return given time. The poor function may be related to edema and hemorrhage in the area, creating less myocardial compliance within the affected segment (201).

PULMONARY HYPERTENSION

Pulmonary hypertension may be caused by primary disorders of the pulmonary vasculature and lungs, including heartworm disease, chronic obstructive pulmonary disease, or secondarily to left heart failure. The term cor pulmonale traditionally is reserved for pulmonary hypertension related to pulmonary disease and excludes all left heart disease as an underlying cause (202). The echocardiographic effects on the right heart regardless of underlying cause are similar.

The prominent features of pulmonary hypertension include the following: right ventricular dilation, right ventricular hypertrophy, tricuspid insufficiency, paradoxical septal motion, enlarged pulmonary artery, decreased left ventricular chamber size, prolapse of the tricuspid valve and pulmonic valves, and increased left ventricular wall and septal thicknesses (203–205). Echocardiographic measurements reflecting left ventricular function are typically normal even though cardiac output is compromised (204).

Pulmonary Hypertension Features

- Dilated right ventricle and pulmonary artery
- RV hypertrophy
- Paradoxical septal motion
- Decreased LV chamber size
- Prolapse of pulmonic or tricuspid valves

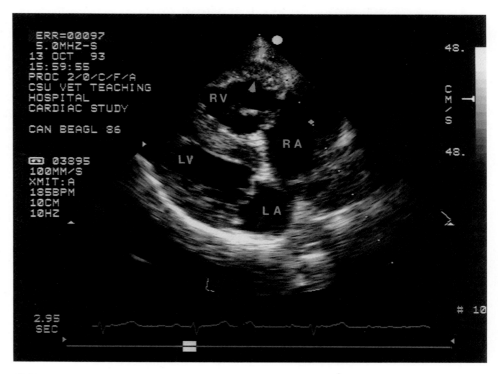

FIGURE 4.112 Right ventricular dilation as well as hypertrophy are characteristic of hearts with pulmonary hypertension. This dog's heart also shows bowing of the ventricular septum towards the left, secondary to the elevated right ventricular diastolic pressures. *Plane,* right parasternal four chamber; *RV,* right ventricle; *RA,* right atrium; *LV,* left ventricle; *LA,* left atrium.

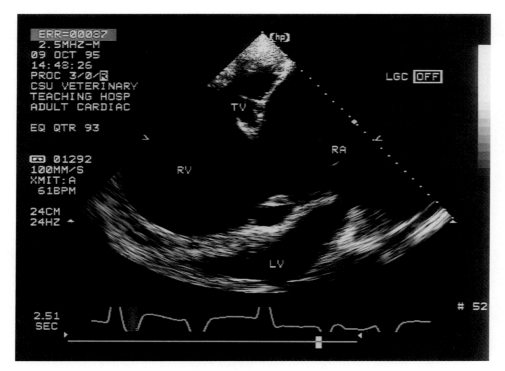

FIGURE 4.113   Chronic obstructive pulmonary disease with pulmonary hypertension caused severe right ventricular and atrial dilation in this horse's heart. The ventricular septum bows toward the left ventricle, which is a sign of paradoxical septal motion. Left ventricular chamber size is very small secondary to poor preload flowing from the right heart. *RV*, right ventricle; *TV*, tricuspid valve; *RA*, right atrium; *LV*, left ventricle.

Chamber Sizes

Right-sided volume overload and hypertrophy are secondary to the increased afterload on the heart created by the pulmonary hypertension (Figs. 4.112, 4.113, 4.114, and 4.115). Volume overload occurs as diastolic pressures increase and as tricuspid insufficiency develops.

Paradoxical septal motion (PSM) is present to some degree if right-sided volume overload is present (Figs. 3.87, 3.88, 4.116, and 4.117). The motion may be mild to significantly paradoxical. As the ratio of left to right ventricular chamber size in dogs with pulmonary hypertension becomes less than 1.5, some degree of PSM is present and will progressively increase as the right ventricular volume overload increases (204). The motion is created when right-sided diastolic pressures exceed left-sided diastolic pressures. This causes the septum to bulge downward during diastole and then correct itself with an exaggerated upward or rightward motion during systole (204,206).

The development of tricuspid regurgitation precedes the finding of right-sided volume overload. The tricuspid insufficiency is aggravated by the pulmonary hypertension (204). Even when caval syndrome is present with heartworm disease, the presence of worms occluding inflow into the right ventricle does not decrease right-sided volume overload. The volume overload is still present secondary to the hypertension and tricuspid insufficiency (204).

The right atrium is not dilated with pulmonary hypertension unless the tricuspid valve is insufficient.

High pulmonary artery pressures cause the pulmonary artery to dilate and may cause the pulmonic valve to prolapse and arc back toward the right ventricular chamber (Figs. 4.118 and 4.119). The prolapse is not specific for pulmonary hypertension, however, and also may be seen with patent ductus arteriosus and pulmonic stenosis. Dilation of the pulmonary artery helps differentiate right heart enlargement secondary to tricuspid valve disease from pulmonary disease. Tricuspid insufficiency

RA and RV enlargement without pulmonary artery dilation is not consistent with pulmonary hypertension.

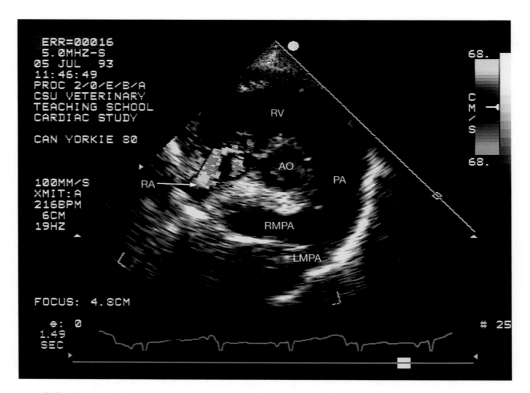

FIGURE 4.114   The pulmonary artery is dilated when pulmonary pressures are dilated. Both branches of the pulmonary artery are easily visible. Note that the artery is dilated even at the level of the pulmonic valve, which helps distinguish this dilation from that seen with pulmonic stenosis. A color jet of tricuspid insufficiency is seen. *AO*, aorta; *RV*, right ventricle; *RA*, right atrium; *PA*, pulmonary artery; *RMPA*, right main pulmonary artery; *LMPA*, left main pulmonary artery.

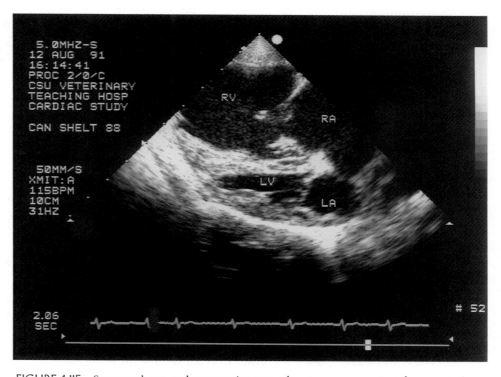

FIGURE 4.115   Severe pulmonary hypertension secondary to a reverse patent ductus arteriosus causes severe dilation of the right side of the heart, while the left ventricle and atrium become volume contracted. *RV*, right ventricle; *LV*, left ventricle; *RA*, right atrium; *LA*, left atrium.

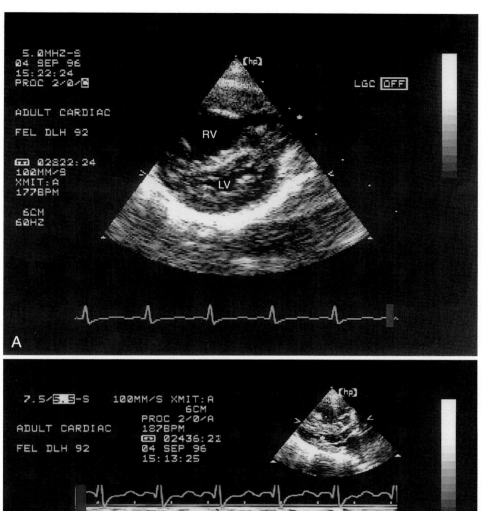

FIGURE 4.116   Paradoxical septal motion secondary to right ventricular volume overload and elevated right ventricular diastolic pressure is seen with severe pulmonary hypertension. **A.** Real-time images show a flattened septum. **B.** M-mode images show downward motion of the septum during diastole. *Plane*, right parasternal transverse left ventricle; *RV*, right ventricle; *LV*, left ventricle; *VS*, ventricular septum.

without hypertension will not cause the pulmonary artery to dilate and may even cause it to be smaller than normal if the regurgitation is severe and forward flow is compromised. Prolapse of the tricuspid valve also occurs frequently in the presence of pulmonary hypertension. When this is seen in small breed dogs presenting with left-sided congestive heart failure, pulmonary hypertension should be ruled out as a cause of cough even without obvious right heart enlargement (Fig. 4.120).

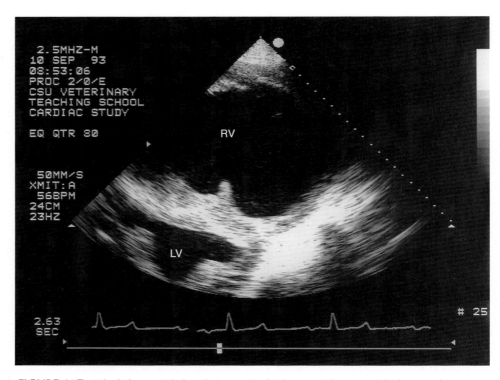

FIGURE 4.117   The left ventricle barely is seen in this horse with severe right heart enlargement secondary to pulmonary hypertension. The septum is flattened, which is a sign of paradoxical septal motion. *Plane,* right parasternal transverse left ventricle *RV,* right ventricle; *LV,* left ventricle.

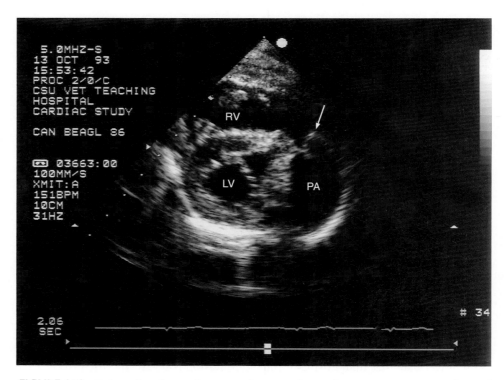

FIGURE 4.118   Pulmonic valve prolapse may be seen when pulmonary pressures are elevated (*arrow*). The right ventricle is dilated and hypertrophied. *Plane,* right parasternal modified transverse view of the pulmonary artery; *RV,* right ventricle; *LV,* left ventricle; *PA,* pulmonary artery.

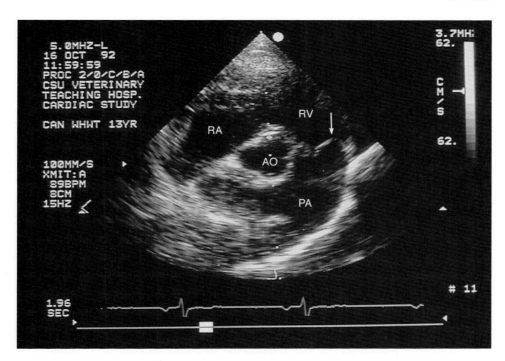

FIGURE 4.119 The dilated right ventricle, atrium, and pulmonary artery are all signs of pulmonary hypertension. The pulmonic valves prolapse during diastole from the pulmonary artery pressure (*arrow*). Notice the dilation involves the entire artery from the valves to the bifurcation, which helps differentiate this from pulmonic stenosis. *RA*, right atrium; *RV*, right ventricle; *AO*, aorta; *PA*, pulmonary artery.

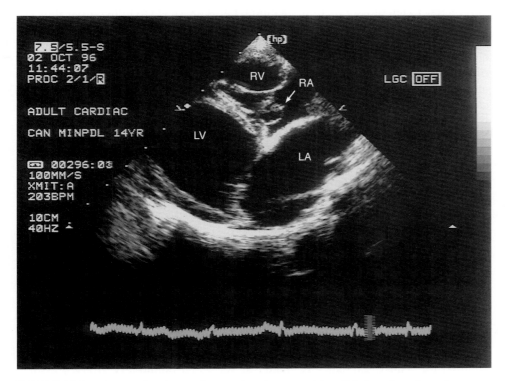

FIGURE 4.120 Tricuspid valve prolapse often is seen with mild elevations in pulmonary pressure. This dog also has left-sided heart disease. *Plane*, right parasternal four chamber; *RV*, right ventricle; *LV*, left ventricle; *RA*, right atrium; *LA*, left atrium.

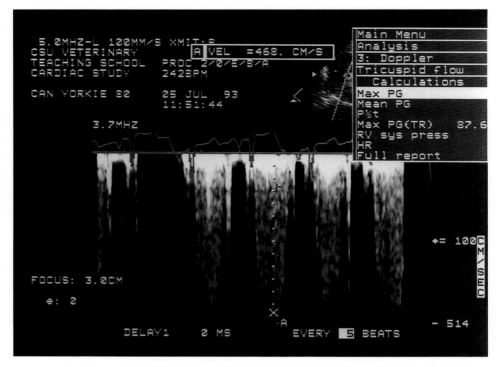

FIGURE 4.121   Pulmonary artery systolic pressure can be measured if tricuspid insufficiency is present. The Bernoulli equation is applied to the tricuspid regurgitant flow velocity to derive a pressure gradient of 87 mm Hg in this dog. Pulmonary artery systolic pressures are at least 87 mm Hg in the absence of pulmonic stenosis.

Function

Parameters of left-sided function, including FS, velocity of circumferential shortening, ejection fraction, and pre-ejection period, are all normal and are sometimes elevated in dogs with heartworm disease and pulmonary hypertension (204). This elevation in function occurs despite documented reduced cardiac output. The finding of normal echocardiographic parameters of function may be related to decreased afterload secondary to decreased preload, poor output, and hypotension. Volume cannot move into the left side of the heart when significant pulmonary hypertension is present, which is why the left ventricular chamber is smaller than normal with thicker wall and septal measurements (204).

Spectral Doppler

Use tricuspid insufficiency flow velocities to determine the pressure within the right ventricle and pulmonary artery. This value will be inflated when the insufficiency is moderate to severe.

Moderate to severe pulmonary hypertension can be documented with Doppler echocardiography when tricuspid or pulmonic insufficiency is present. The pressure gradient across the tricuspid valve can be used to estimate pulmonary artery pressure in the absence of pulmonary outflow obstruction. The velocity of the regurgitant jet is inserted into the Bernoulli equation and a pressure gradient is calculated. The pressure gradient is then added to estimated right atrial pressures and the value is an estimate of systolic pulmonary artery pressures (Fig. 4.121). See Chapter 3 for more information on this application. The same principles apply to pulmonic insufficiency. The velocity is inserted into the Bernoulli equation and pulmonary diastolic pressures are estimated from this application (207,208) (Fig. 4.122). This application is useful but sometimes the gradient underestimates true pulmonary pressures by as much as 20 mm Hg even when right atrial pressures are accounted for. This discrepancy is greater at very high pulmonary artery pressures (209). However, this discrepancy does not diminish the applicability of Doppler-derived pulmonary artery pressure because true pressure will be at least as high as the Doppler-derived value.

When tricuspid insufficiency is moderate to severe, the derived pressure gradient will overestimate pulmonary pressures. If the pulmonary artery is not dilated, but velocities suggest elevated pressure, the pressure gradient is probably a consequence of a large regurgitant tricuspid volume.

Pulmonary hypertension changes the pulmonary flow profile and velocity. Normal pulmonary flow profiles are symmetric with peak velocities close to the middle of the ejection phase, and the peak itself is rounded (Fig. 4.123). As pressures increase, the peak becomes sharper, acceleration becomes more rapid, acceleration time is decreased, and peak velocity is reached earlier during ejection. At very higher pressures, notching of the profile may occur during deceleration. Even higher pressures result in decreased velocities, and flow is either not discernable or a reversal of flow may be seen at end-systole. These changes in the pulmonary flow profile are not highly sensitive, however. Although there is a relationship between the flow profile and degrees of pressure elevation, correlation between flow profile appearance and specific pulmonary artery pressures is poor (207).

In dogs, there appears to be good correlation between the ratio of acceleration time to ejection time (AT/ET) and pulmonary artery pressures (207). Simply using acceleration time alone did not yield as good a correlation with pulmonary pressures, even though the time decreases with increasing pressures. The correlation coefficient between AT/ET and systolic pulmonary artery pressures is 0.84. The equation is as follows:

$$y = 102.71 + -2.07x$$

where y = systolic pulmonary pressure, and x = AT/ET.

Abnormalities of left ventricular diastolic function exist when pulmonary hypertension is present, which include increased isovolumic relaxation times and abnormal mitral inflow profiles. These changes are secondary to increased right

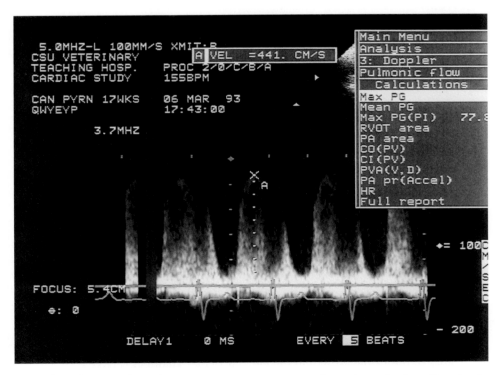

FIGURE 4.122   Diastolic pulmonary artery pressures can be estimated when Doppler is applied to a pulmonic insufficiency jet. A velocity of 441 cm/sec results in a pressure gradient of 77 mm Hg when the Bernoulli equation is applied. Pulmonary artery diastolic pressures are at least 77 mm Hg in this dog.

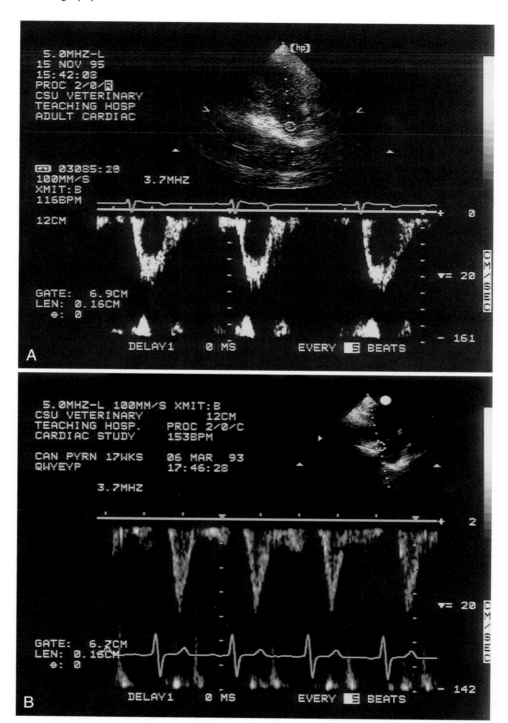

FIGURE 4.123 **A.** Normal pulmonary flow profiles are symmetric with a rounded peak. **B.** As pulmonary artery pressures increase, the flow profile has a sharper peak.

ventricular diastolic pressures, resulting in paradoxical septal motion and impaired left ventricular filling (209). Reversed E:A ratios for mitral valve inflow profiles may be related to poor preload within the left ventricular chamber (Fig. 4.124).

Heartworms

When heartworms are the underlying cause of pulmonary hypertension, they sometimes can be detected on two-dimensional echocardiographic images. Although

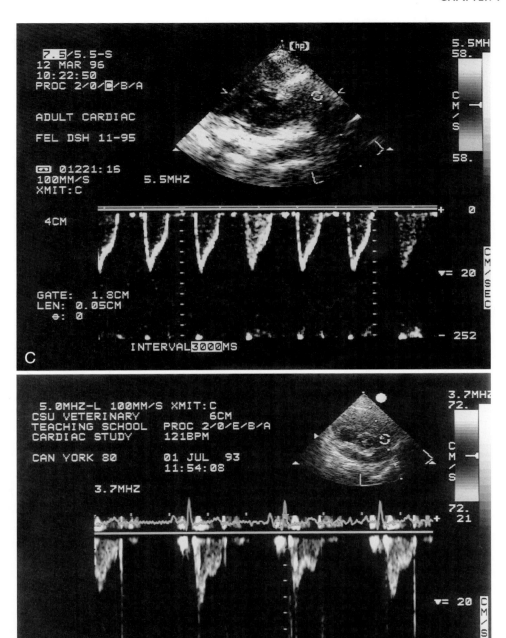

FIGURE 4.123 *(continued)*   C. With higher pressures, the acceleration time becomes faster and the symmetric shape is lost, with peak velocity occurring earlier during systole. **D.** Very high pulmonary artery pressures create a notched or concave shape during deceleration on the pulmonary flow profile.

M-mode images can document the presence of heartworms within the right side of the heart, two-dimensional images are more sensitive (205). Linear echoes representing the worms can be seen within the chambers of the right heart. The linear echoes are typically seen as two parallel lines separated by a very thin hypoechoic area (205). When the heartworm infestation is massive, the worms may be displayed as an echogenic mass within the chambers. This mass may be seen moving back and

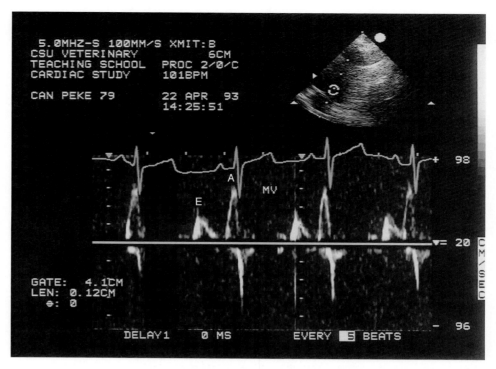

FIGURE 4.124   Reduced preload within the left ventricle secondary to pulmonary hypertension will cause the mitral valve E:A ratio to reverse.

forth within the chambers or through the tricuspid annulus as flow varies during systole and diastole. The absence of echocardiographically displayed heartworms does not support the absence worms. If the ultrasound beam is not directed perpendicularly to the worms, the worms may not be detected. Additionally, if the heartworms are within the pulmonary arteries beyond the bifurcation, they will not be seen (205).

SYSTEMIC HYPERTENSION

The definition of what constitutes systemic hypertension is variable. Pressures ranging from 150/90 to 180/100 and up are all defined as hypertensive in various canine studies (210–212). Systolic blood pressure above 160 and diastolic above 100 have been established as upper limits of normal in cats (213–215).

Patterns of Hypertrophy

Concentric or eccentric hypertrophy may be seen with systemic hypertension.

Chronic increases in afterload, as is seen with systemic hypertension, leads to compensatory myocardial hypertrophy to normalize wall stress (212,216–218) (Fig. 4.125). Although logic would suggest that the degree of left ventricular hypertrophy would be directly related to the degree of hypertension, studies have shown that the development of hypertrophy does not correlate linearly to the development of pressure (219,220). Other factors including neural and humoral influences play a role in the development of wall thickness to compensate for the elevation in pressure (218,221). Studies also have shown that pressure elevation during daily normal activities in patients with eccentric hypertrophy is less than the pressure elevation in patients with concentric hypertrophy (222).

There are patients in which echocardiographically measurable increases in wall or septal thickness does not develop, but overall cardiac mass and chamber size increases (218,221). Hypertensive patients may respond by developing either concentric or eccentric hypertrophy of the left ventricular chamber. Eccentric hypertrophy with increased left ventricular mass may exist. The following also may be present: normal wall thickness to chamber ratio, concentric hypertrophy with normal left ventricular mass and high wall thickness to chamber size ratio, and concentric hypertrophy with increased left ventricular mass and increased wall thickness to chamber size ratio (221,222). Studies in humans have shown a poorer

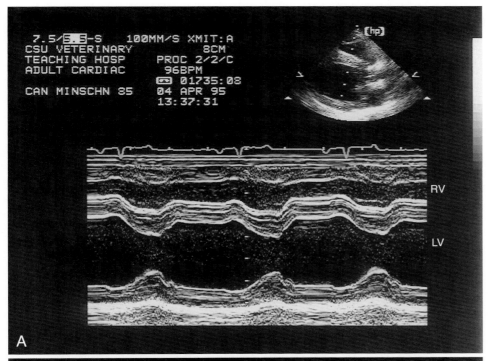

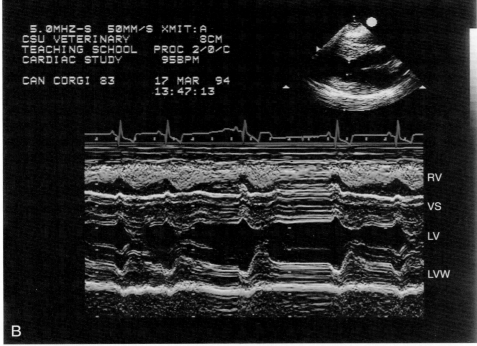

FIGURE 4.125   Chronic systemic hypertension leads to compensatory left ventricular hypertrophy. **A.** A dog with mitral insufficiency has excessive hypertrophy for the degree of dilation and was found to be hypertensive. **B.** Concentric hypertrophy without dilation is seen in this dog with systemic hypertension. *RV*, right ventricle; *LV*, left ventricle; *VS*, ventricular septum; *LVW*, left ventricular wall.

prognosis with cardiovascular complications in hypertensive patients who have concentric hypertrophy with normal left ventricular mass but increased wall thickness and decreased chamber size (222).

Hypertrophy has two basic manifestations. Symmetric hypertrophy is the most common pattern in humans and probably in dogs and cats. In the cat, symmetric hypertrophy may mimic hypertrophic obstructive cardiomyopathy and often cannot be differentiated based on echocardiographic features. The increased wall thickness involves both the free wall and septum to a similar degree. Asymmetric hypertrophy involving primarily the septum is a less common presentation in humans and animals. Asymmetric hypertrophy may involve only the basal part of the septum near the outflow tract, the entire septum, or the entire septum and part of the apical portion of the free wall (218). It is important to check systemic pressures whenever echocardiography reveals unexplained hypertrophy.

Systolic Function

Fractional shortening may be normal, but systolic dysfunction is present if wall thickening is depressed.

Systolic dysfunction also is present in the hearts of humans and dogs with hypertension. Systolic dysfunction occurs after the onset of diastolic impairment (216). FS cannot be used as an indicator of systolic dysfunction in hypertensive hearts. Increases in systolic and, eventually, diastolic chamber sizes as well as decreased systolic thickening of the wall and septum indicate that systolic dysfunction is present, despite normal FSs. Congestive heart failure is the end result (212, 216, 217, 221, 223, 224). This systolic impairment may be secondary to impaired myocardial perfusion caused by changes in the small coronary vessels, increased afterload, and wall stress in patients without adequate compensatory hypertrophy (217,221). When hypertension is treated appropriately, hypertrophy will regress and diastolic function will improve. Part of the improvement in diastolic function with reduction in the degree of hypertrophy is secondary to the reduced afterload and the better rate of myocardial relaxation (216).

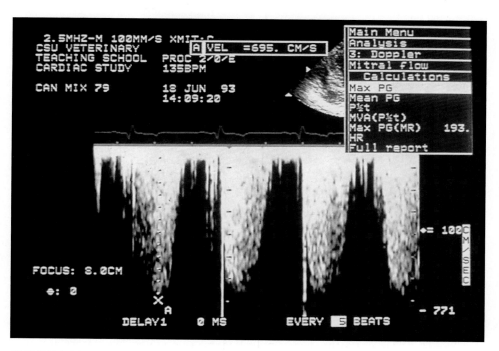

FIGURE 4.126   Spectral Doppler evaluation of a mitral regurgitant jet can provide systemic pressures information. The pressure gradient reflects left ventricular driving pressures and systolic systemic pressures when there is no obstruction to outflow. Here, the gradient suggests that systemic pressures are at least 193 mm Hg.

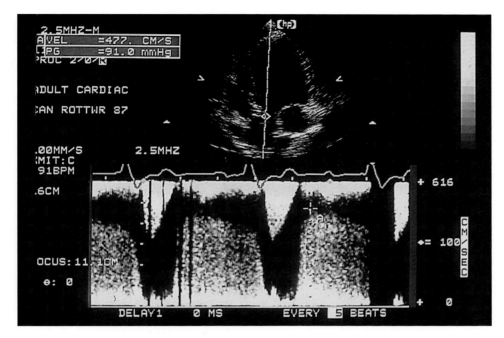

FIGURE 4.127   Aortic insufficiency jets may provide information about systemic diastolic pressures. Here, systemic diastolic pressures are at least 91 mm Hg.

Spectral Doppler

Doppler examination of patients with systemic hypertension shows left ventricular diastolic dysfunction. Impaired relaxation manifests itself by decreasing E velocities, except when elevated atrial pressures counteract this decrease. As diastolic failure progresses, the myocardium may become less compliant, and the E:A ratio will increase. Therefore, depending on the hemodynamic status of hypertensive heart disease, either of the abnormal left ventricular filling patterns may be present (225). Further manifestations of diastolic impairment include prolonged isovolumic relaxation time and prolonged deceleration time of the rapid ventricular filling phase. The exact cause of this diastolic impairment is not fully understood; however, the increased mass found in athletic hearts does not create this diastolic dysfunction (217,221,223). Left atrial enlargement may be seen secondary to the diastolic failure (225).

Systemic pressures can be estimated with spectral Doppler when mitral insufficiency or aortic insufficiency is present. The pressure gradient calculated from a mitral regurgitant jet reflects systemic pressures in the absence of aortic stenosis. The gradient should be added to an estimate of the left atrial pressure (Fig. 4.126). The same calculation can be done with aortic insufficiency, except this gradient reflects diastolic systemic pressures. These concepts are explained in more detail in Chapter 3 (Fig. 4.127).

PERICARDIAL EFFUSIONS, PERICARDIAL DISEASE, AND CARDIAC MASSES

The causes of pericardial effusion in animals include pericardioperitoneal hernias, congestive heart failure, left atrial rupture, infection, neoplasia, trauma, and benign idiopathic causes (226–230). The pericardial effusion may lead to tamponade (231).

Feline infectious peritonitis is the most common cause of pericardial effusion in the cat and is often accompanied by pleural effusion and ascites. Pericarditis with effusion also may occur secondary to systemic bacterial, fungal, and other viral infections and has been reported with leukemia (230).

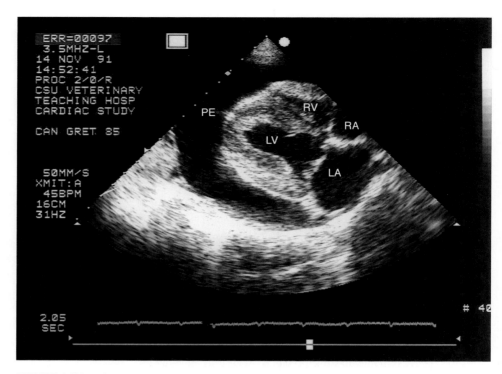

FIGURE 4.128   The large echo-free space of pericardial effusion surrounds the heart of this dog with idiopathic pericardial effusion. Notice that the fluid does not extend around the base of the heart and its boundaries are relatively smooth and circular. *Plane*, right parasternal four chamber; *PE*, pericardial effusion; *RV*, right ventricle; *LV*, left ventricle; *LA*, left atrium; *RA*, right atrium.

HCM is the most common form of heart disease leading to pericardial effusion in cats (230). Other less common forms of heart disease resulting in pericardial effusion in the cat include dilated and restrictive cardiomyopathies and mitral valve abnormalities (232,233).

Intracardiac and pericardial tumors are the primary causes of pericardial effusion in the dog. Of these tumors, hemangiosarcoma, chemodectoma, and mesothelioma lead the list for highest incidence (234). Pericardial disease may be secondary to metastatic disease involving the sac, with lymphosarcoma being the most common. Other cancers found to metastasize to the pericardial sac include melanomas, mammary and pulmonary adenomas, mesothelioma, and rarely, hemangiosarcoma (230).

Pericardial Effusion

Features

The echocardiographic features of pericardial effusion in all animals include the presence of an echo-free space between the epicardium and the pericardial sac, swinging motion of the heart when the amount of effusion is significant, and if tamponade is present, diastolic collapse of the right atrium or ventricle (228,230,235).

Pericardial effusion is not seen behind the left and right atrium on echocardiographic images because the pericardial sac is more adherent to the epicardium at the heart base (Figs. 4.19, 4.128, 4.129, 4.130, and 4.131). This helps differentiate pleural from pericardial effusions (236). The pericardial effusion boundaries are smooth and round around the heart, whereas pleural effusion is seen as more irregular with ill-defined boundaries. Large amounts of thoracic or mediastinal fat sometimes have been misdiagnosed as pericardial effusion; therefore, care should be taken to set the gain correctly and to image multiple cardiac planes (236). The

Pericardial effusion is not seen at the heart base below the atria, whereas pleural fluid is.

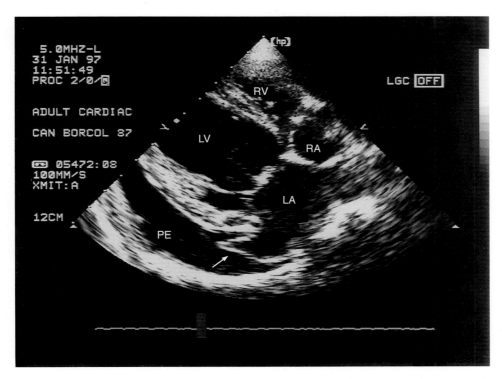

FIGURE 4.129   The left auricle can be seen within the pericardial space in this dog with effusion (*arrow*). *Plane*, right parasternal four chamber; *RV*, right ventricle; *LV*, left ventricle; *RA*, right atrium; *LA*, left atrium.

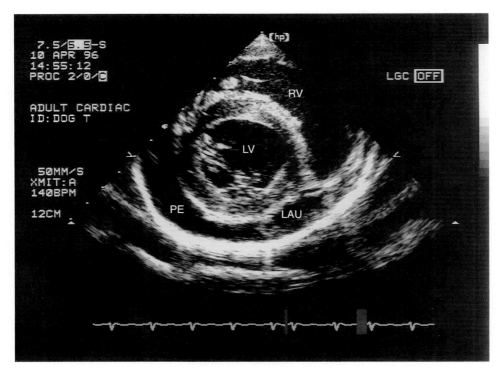

FIGURE 4.130   The left auricle may be seen within the pericardial fluid next to the left ventricle on transverse images. *Plane*, right parasternal transverse view at the level of the chordae; *LAU*, left auricle; *PE*, pericardial effusion; *RV*, right ventricle; *LV*, left ventricle.

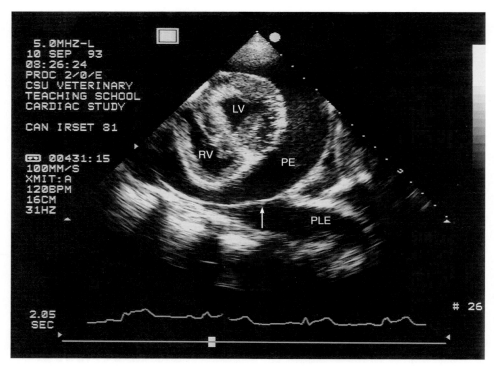

FIGURE 4.131 Pericardial and pleural effusion are seen surrounding this dog's heart. The sac (*arrow*) is smooth and round, whereas the pleural fluid space contains irregularities. *Plane*, left parasternal transverse left ventricle; *PE*, pericardial effusion; *PLE*, pleural effusion; *RV*, right ventricle; *LV*, left ventricle.

diagnosis of a thickened pericardium is sometimes possible on echocardiographic images, but there will be many false positives unless pleural effusion is present to help define both boundaries of the sac (236).

Large pericardial effusions create dyskinetic and paradoxical septal motion, which prevents adequate cardiac function assessment (236,237). Assessment of function should be made after resolution of the effusion.

Bleeding into the pericardial sac results in long layers of organized clot.

Organized thrombi may be seen as free-floating layers or bands of echogenic material within the pericardial space. This may be seen secondary to acute bleeding from hemangiosarcoma, ruptured atrium, idiopathic hemorrhagic effusion, or after a pericardiocentesis, if the heart was stuck (29,238) (Fig. 4.20).

Cardiac Tamponade

The amount of pericardial fluid does not determine whether tamponade is present. Large pericardial effusions do not always create a tamponade effect. The elasticity of the pericardial sac decreases with age, and smaller amounts of fluid are needed to generate a large amount of pressure on the cardiac chambers. Additionally, a chronic slow-developing effusion is less likely to develop tamponade (228,239,240).

The size of the effusion does not determine whether tamponade is present. Diastolic collapse of the right atrium and/or ventricle confirms the presence of tamponade.

Cardiac tamponade involves diastolic collapse of the right atrium and sometimes the right ventricle (Fig. 4.132). This collapse is seen on M-mode images as a very small or totally collapsed right ventricular chamber with parallel motion of the right ventricular wall and septum. The left ventricular free wall often moves in parallel with the septum and RV wall. Two-dimensional imaging is superior to M-mode in identifying both pericardial effusion and the presence of tamponade. Real-time images will show the collapse of the right side of the heart. Right parasternal long-axis images may be used to view the collapse because the heart is displaced from the thoracic wall, and right-sided structures are easier to visualize. However, multiple planes should be interrogated to obtain an accurate diagnosis and to identify an underlying cause (237).

Tapping the pericardial fluid results in visibly increased chamber sizes (241). A sudden increase in venous return and volume overload of the heart resulting in acute pulmonary edema has been associated with pericardiocentesis in several animals and humans (242,243).

Clinical signs related to cardiac tamponade can exist without echocardiographic evidence of diastolic collapse of the right-sided chambers. This is seen when there is increased right-sided pressure secondary to cardiac diseases such as pulmonary hypertension, tetralogy of Fallot, intracardiac tumors, and pulmonic stenosis (237,244).

Cardiac tamponade has been reported in humans secondary to large pleural effusion without the presence of pericardial effusion. Evidence of diastolic collapse on the right side of the heart is visible in these patients (245).

Cardiac Function with Pericardial Effusion

Pericardial fluid with or without tamponade reduces the amount of filling and output from the right side of the heart, which will reduce left-sided volume and output. Function is reduced when a significant volume of pericardial fluid is present; therefore, the diagnosis of myocardial failure should wait until after resolution of the effusion. Often, adequate assessment of function is not possible because the heart motion is too erratic as it swings within the pericardial sac (226,237,246). Chronic myocardial hypoxia may occur with large effusions, resulting in depressed function, which may persist for days or weeks after resolution of the effusion.

Idiopathic Effusion

Idiopathic benign pericardial effusion is a common occurrence in dogs, and the effusion is generally large (Figs. 4.108 and 4.114). The fluid accumulates slowly and signs of tamponade are a late sequela. Pleural effusion is usually present as well, which allows better imaging of the pericardial sac (Fig. 4.133). The sac is usually thickened and irregular because of the chronic fibrin accumulation on the pleural

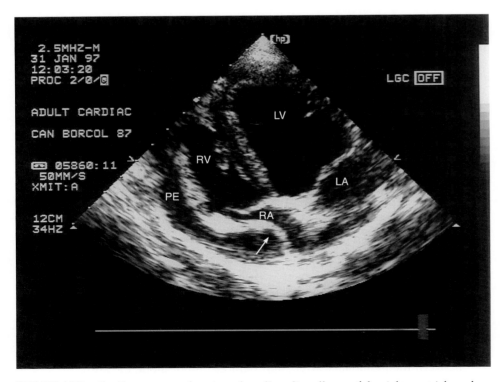

FIGURE 4.132   Cardiac tamponade exists when diastolic collapse of the right ventricle and or atrium occurs (*arrow*). *Plane*, left parasternal apical four chamber; *RV*, right ventricle; *LV*, left ventricle; *PE*, pericardial effusion; *LA*, left atrium; *RA*, right atrium.

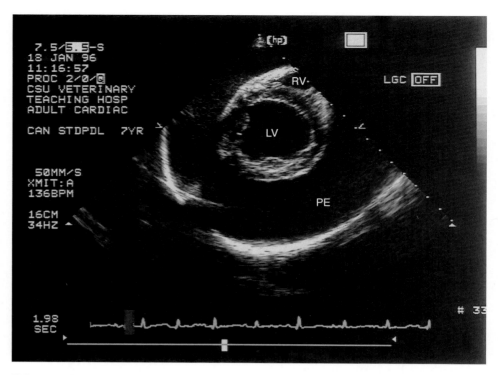

FIGURE 4.133   The effusion is very large in animals with idiopathic pericardial effusion. *RV,* right ventricle; *LV,* left ventricle; *PE,* pericardial effusion.

side of the sac. Undulating fibrin tags may be seen within the pleural space and adhere to the sac. At times, the fibrin accumulation may appear to be masses (Fig. 4.134). A thorough examination to rule out masses still does not lead to a definitive diagnosis of idiopathic effusion because small masses may not be seen. Massive effusions, however, make it easier to identify neoplasia. Surgical or necropsy examination is necessary for a definitive diagnosis of idiopathic effusion (234,239).

Neoplasia as a Cause of Pericardial Effusion

When searching for neoplasia, always examine the heart from both sides of the thorax while the animal is standing and lying down.

Searching for cardiac masses is easier when pericardial effusion is present. Diligently search in every possible cardiac plane for a potential mass. The animal should be scanned lying down and from both sides of the thorax. If a mass is not seen, continue the search with the animal standing and scan from both sides both sides of the thorax. Masses have been found by repositioning the animal into a standing position when no evidence of a mass was seen in lateral recumbency. Even then, the absence of a mass does not rule out its presence, especially when pericardial effusion is not present to highlight the auricular chambers and other structures at the heart base (226,227,247,248). Serial echocardiographic examinations are sometimes necessary in the event of recurrent pericardial effusion before some masses are large enough to be visualized (227,234,248–250).

Heart Base Tumors

Heart base tumors may or may not have associated pericardial effusion. When present, the effusion may be small or large in volume. The tumors typically are seen at the level of the aorta or pulmonary artery or on long-axis or transverse views. On transverse views the mass is seen around the aorta or pulmonary artery and between the pulmonary artery and right atrium or along the aortic arch. The presence of a large tumor along the aortic arch will allow visualization of the arch and, possibly, the brachycephalic trunk as the mass wraps around these structures

(234,247,251–254). Often, the tumor appears to invade the atria or the great vessels but may simply be in the field of view or may be compressing the atria (Figs. 4.135 and 4.136). Deciding whether a mass is within the cardiac chambers or compressing the chambers is sometimes not possible. Heart base tumors on long-axis views are seen at the heart base around the aorta pushing into either atrium.

Heart base tumors are homogeneous in appearance with no hypoechoic areas within them; however, there are exceptions (Fig. 4.137). Small masses are usually oval or circular and well defined and localized. Large heart base masses have irregular boundaries and may diffusely invade the adjacent atria and ventricles (189, 247). Some heart base tumors may be impossible to detect because they manifest themselves as thin, small masses that are spread out over the aorta surface (249). The entire mass is rarely seen because the mass beyond the immediate cardiac boundaries is usually obscured by lung. However, masses that are large enough to see are usually in a well-defined location and their accessibility for surgical removal can usually be determined (247).

Do not confuse collapsed lung with a mass at the heart base or mediastinum. Lung will maintain a wedge shape, float within the pleural fluid, and may contain small hyperechoic areas (Figs. 4.138 and 4.139).

Hemangiosarcoma

Hemangiosarcoma is a tumor that commonly is found within the right atrial wall or as an auricular mass extending into the pericardial space or into the auricular lumen (Figs. 4.140 and 4.141). Often, hemangiosarcoma involves the right ventricular wall, invades the pericardial sac, or is found within the left ventricular chamber (234,248,255) (Figs. 4.142 and 4.143). Hemangiosarcomas are usually smooth

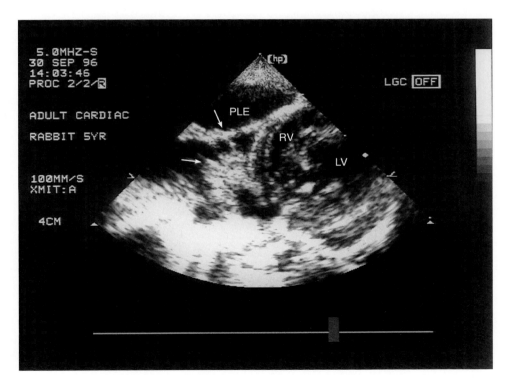

FIGURE 4.134   Fibrin deposition along the pericardial sac (*arrows*) is evident with chronic pleural effusion and should not be mistaken for neoplasia. *PLE,* pleural effusion; *LV,* left ventricle; *RV,* right ventricle.

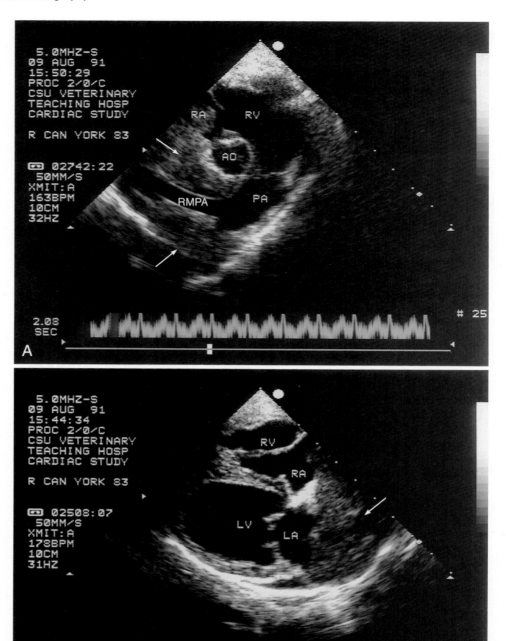

FIGURE 4.135 Here, base tumors are found along the aortic arch, pulmonary artery, and left atrium on real-time images. This large mass (*arrows*) grew around the pulmonary artery along each side of the right main pulmonary artery and appears to invade the right and left atrium. **A.** Right parasternal transverse image at the heart base. **B.** Right parasternal four chamber. *RV*, right ventricle; *RA*, right atrium; *AO*, aorta; *LA*, left atrium; *LV*, left ventricle; *RMPA*, right main pulmonary artery.

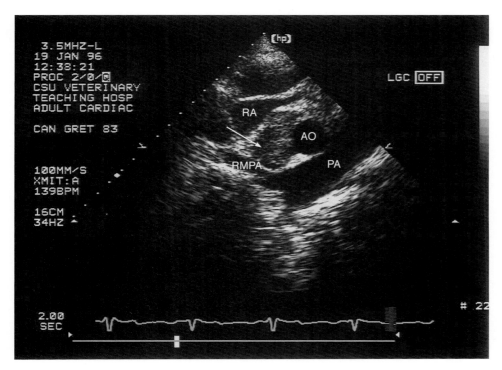

FIGURE 4.136   Heart base masses grow along the aortic wall above the right main pulmonary artery branch (*arrow*) as seen on echocardiographic images, but may be seen anywhere around the heart base. *Plane*, right parasternal transverse heart base; *AO*, aorta; *PA*, pulmonary artery; *RA*, right atrium; *RMPA*, right main pulmonary artery.

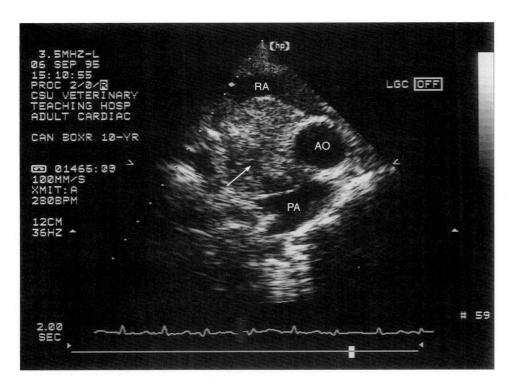

FIGURE 4.137   Although heart base masses are usually homogeneous in appearance, they may contain hypoechoic areas (*arrow*) similar to hemangiosarcoma. *Plane*, right parasternal transverse heart base; *AO*, aorta; *PA*, pulmonary artery; *RA*, right atrium.

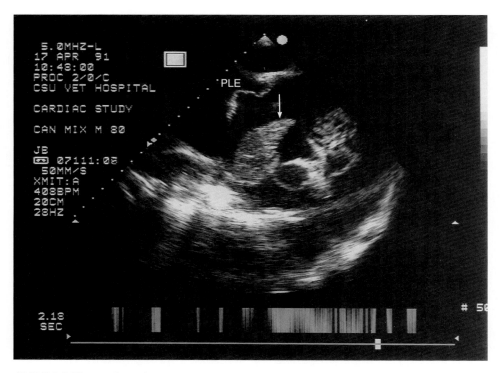

FIGURE 4.138 Collapsed lung (*arrow*) should not be mistaken for a mass at the heart base or mediastinum. The lung will maintain a wedge shape and may contain hyperechoic areas. *PLE,* pleural effusion.

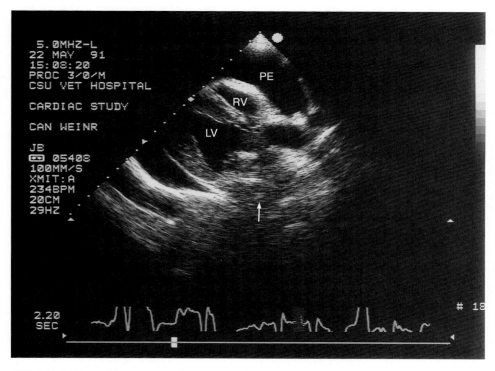

FIGURE 4.139 Diffuse areas of poor image at the heart base (*arrow*) should not be misinterpreted as a tumor. A mass should be examined and seen in several planes to confirm its presence. *Plane,* right parasternal four chamber; *PE,* pericardial effusion; *RV,* right ventricle; *LV,* left ventricle.

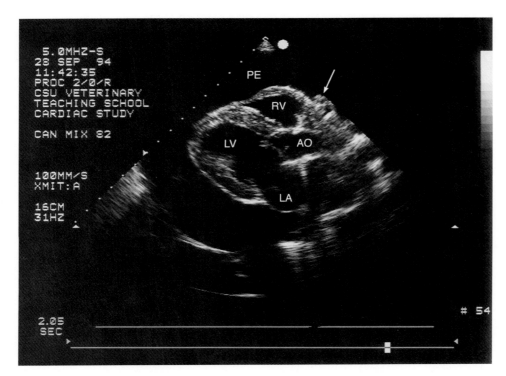

FIGURE 4.140   Hemangiosarcoma is found within the right auricle and atrium. When pericardial effusion is present, the right auricle and most masses can be seen on right parasternal images (*arrow*). The left parasternal view of the right auricle should also be examined. *PE*, pericardial effusion; *RV*, right ventricle; *AO*, aorta; *LV*, left ventricle; *LA*, left atrium.

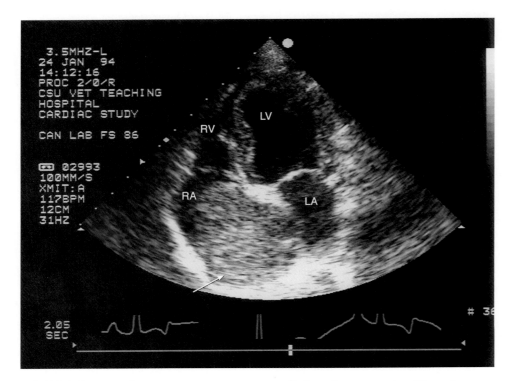

FIGURE 4.141   Large hemangiosarcomas are easy to find on almost any view. Here, the mass fills the right atrial chamber on an apical four-chamber plane (*arrow*). *RV*, right ventricle; *LV*, left ventricle; *RA*, right atrium; *LA*, left atrium.

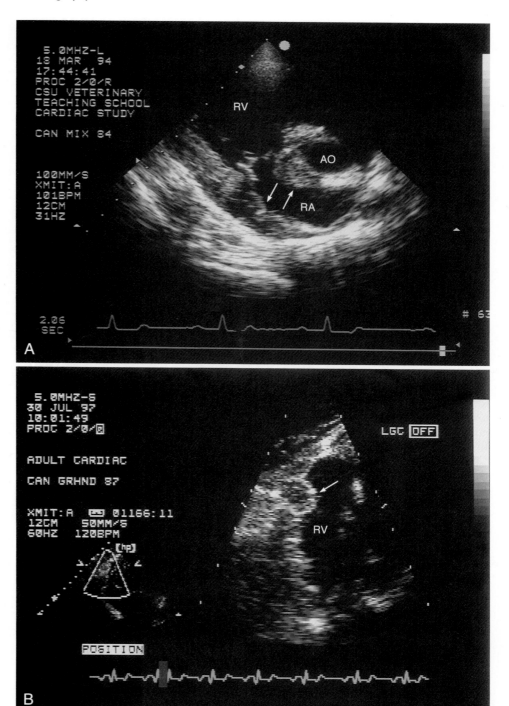

FIGURE 4.142   Less commonly, hemangiosarcoma may be seen within the right atrial and ventricular walls. **A.** Here, the irregular wall of the right atrial chamber is abnormal (*arrows*). **B.** A distinct mass (*arrow*) with characteristic hemangiosarcoma appearance is seen toward the right ventricular apex in this dog. *Plane,* left parasternal apical four chamber; *RV,* right ventricle; *RA,* right atrium.

circular or oval shapes with well-defined boundaries and are rarely an irregular mass. The appearance of the mass is heterogeneous, containing hypoechoic areas (Fig. 4.144). High-resolution transducers are necessary to resolve diffuse hemangiosarcoma involving just the wall of the ventricle or atrium. Although hemangiosarcoma may be found in many different imaging planes (each view should be interrogated), the left cranial long-axis view of the right auricular appendage is probably the most useful view for identifying cardiac hemangiosarcoma (247).

The most current report on the detection of hemangiosarcoma in the dog indicates a 69% sensitivity in detecting the mass (248). This report includes repeat examinations in several dogs when no mass was found on initial examinations. No fluid was present or fluid was tapped from the pericardial space before the initial negative examinations. Pericardial effusion was present when positive findings were reported on the repeat examinations. The authors report that effusion is not necessary to diagnose hemangiosarcoma, but effusion helps highlight the areas of interest, especially the right auricle. Right auricular tumors are the most difficult to visualize, and small tumors may be identified only when effusion is present and the right auricle floats within the pericardial fluid on left cranial long-axis views of the right atrium and auricle (232) (Fig. 4.145).

> Hemangiosarcomas are best seen on left parasternal cranial long-axis views of the right atrium and auricle.

Other Intracardiac Neoplasia

Masses may be found almost anywhere in the heart and can infiltrate the myocardium. Differentiating the tumor type usually is not possible (Fig. 4.146). When neoplasia occurs as an infiltrative process, the ventricular wall will appear hypertrophied. Increased areas of echogenicity may be present.

Right ventricular tumors associated with the pulmonic valve have been reported (Fig. 4.147). These tumors have been identified as myxomas, thyroid carcinoma, neurofibromas, and fibrosarcomas (240). When associated with the pulmonic valve

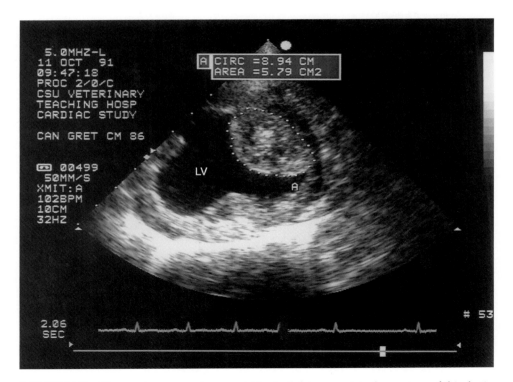

FIGURE 4.143   Hemangiosarcoma is seen within the left interventricular septum of this dog's heart. *Plane,* right parasternal transverse left ventricle; *LV,* left ventricle.

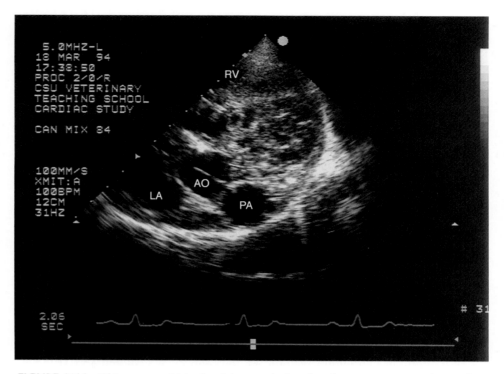

FIGURE 4.144   This tumor within the right ventricular chamber contains many hypoechoic areas within it, which is characteristic of hemangiosarcoma. *Plane*, right parasternal heart base; *AO*, aorta; *PA*, pulmonary artery; *LA*, left atrium; *RV*, right ventricle.

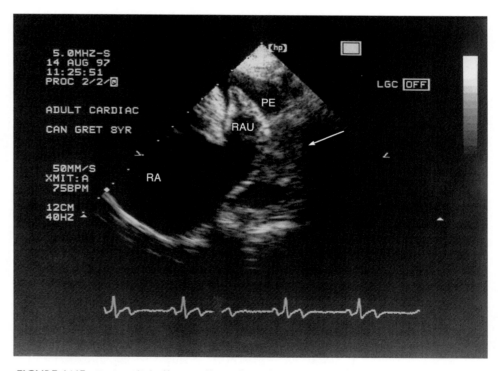

FIGURE 4.145   Pericardial effusion allows the right auricle boundaries to be seen better as it floats within the fluid. The mass (*arrow*) in this image may not have been detected if an effusion had not occurred. *Plane*, left parasternal cranial long-axis right auricle view; *RA*, right atrium; *RAU*, right auricle; *PE*, pericardial effusion.

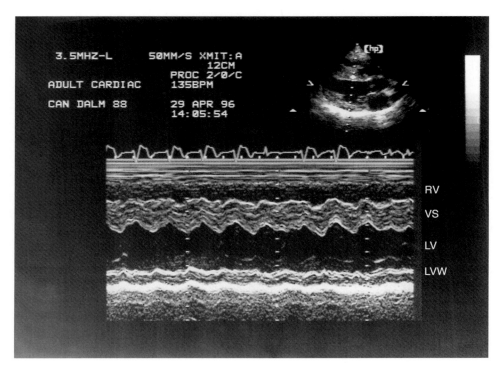

FIGURE 4.146   Lymphosarcoma infiltrated the septum of this dog and was seen as asymmetric hypertrophy involving the septum. Function of the heart was also compromised. *RV*, right ventricle; *VS*, ventricular septum; *LV*, left ventricle; *LVW*, left ventricular free wall.

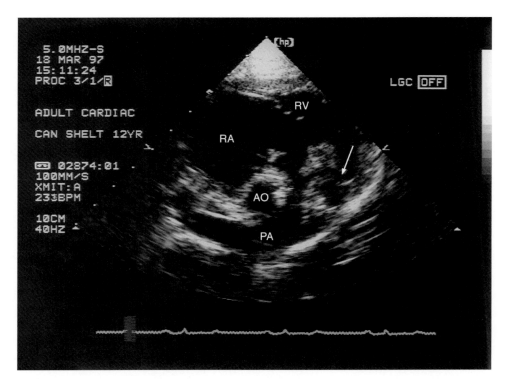

FIGURE 4.147   This tumor (*arrow*) attached to the pulmonic valve was fairly mobile and moved with the valve but obstructed flow from the right ventricle. The right heart was enlarged secondary to the obstruction, and tricuspid insufficiency was significant. *Plane*, right parasternal transverse heart base *RA*, right atrium; *RV*, right ventricle; *PA*, pulmonary artery; *AO*, aorta.

and right ventricular outflow tract, these tumors have created right ventricular outflow obstruction to varying degrees. Right heart failure as well as decreased preload to the left ventricle may develop if occlusion is severe. The masses may be fairly immobile and adherent to the wall of the outflow tract or may move freely with the pulmonic valve depending on the extent of adherence to the walls of the outflow tract (241,242).

Pericardial Disease as a Cause of Pericardial Effusion

Pericardial Tumors

Pericardial tumors are difficult to diagnose. When no effusion is present, the pericardial sac cannot be defined well. When pericardial effusion is present, the sac may still appear normal because the tumor is so diffuse in nature (218,233). Pericardial effusion is typically present with pericardial tumors and is usually a significant volume. When the sac is thick and irregular, pericardial neoplasms cannot be differentiated echocardiographically from other pericardial disease or fibrin deposition on the sac (Fig. 4.134).

Abscesses

Abscesses rarely involve the pericardial sac. The abscesses appear to have thin walls with large hypoechoic areas within them and adhere to the pericardial sac instead of the heart as do other cardiac masses. Large abscesses may compress the cardiac chamber that is next to the abscess (231).

Fibrinous Pericarditis

Traumatic fibrinous pericarditis is seen frequently in the bovine and less commonly in the small animal and horse. Differentiating fibrinous pericarditis from other forms of pericardial disease is easy because of the extensive amount of fibrin adhered to the epicardial surface and moving around within the pericardial space (Figs. 4.148 and

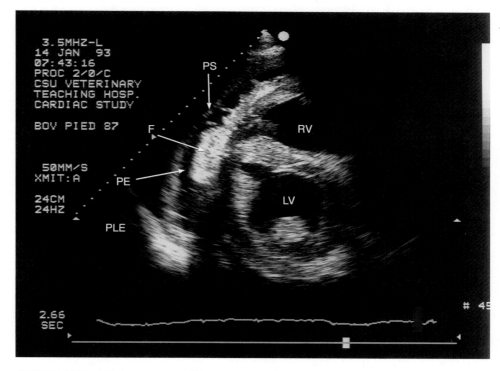

FIGURE 4.148   Fibrinous pericarditis presents with varying amounts of pericardial effusion. A small effusion is seen in this cow with traumatic pericarditis. The pericardial sac contains many echodensities, and the epicardium is also affected. *PS*, pericardial sac; *PE*, pericardial effusion; *F*, fibrinous adhesions; *RV*, right ventricle; *LV*, left ventricle; *PLE*, pleural effusion.

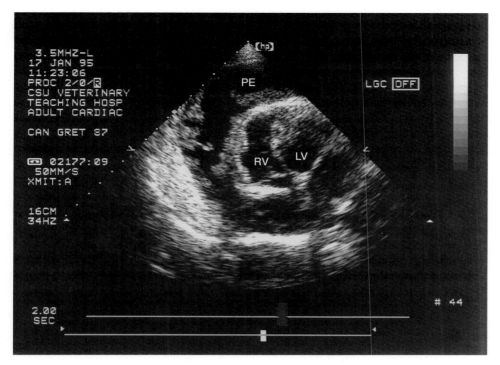

FIGURE 4.149   Fibrinous pericarditis in a dog showing many fibrinous strands attached to the pericardial sac and epicardium floating within the pericardial fluid. *PE*, pericardial effusion; *RV*, right ventricle; *LV*, left ventricle.

4.149). The epicardial surface appears irregular because of the fibrin buildup, and the sac is thick. The amount of pericardial fluid varies from a lot to very little. When pleural fluid is also present, the outside of the pericardial sac will also appear irregular, and the thickness of the sac can be determined with greater accuracy. Not all pericarditis is fibrinous in nature, and there are no specific echocardiographic changes to help differentiate idiopathic effusions from pericarditis.

Constrictive Pericarditis

Constrictive pericarditis may not be effusive, and there are usually no visible adhesions connecting the sac to the epicardium (243–245). When the pericarditis leads to constrictive physiology, the cardiac chambers are smaller than normal because the pericardial sac constricts the heart and prevents filling (Fig. 4.150). Both sides of the heart are affected equally by the increased pressures applied by the small amount of fluid and the thickened sac. Signs of right-sided heart failure predominate because of the thinner right ventricular wall (218,230,244). When constrictive pericarditis exists, the ventricles stop filling early in diastole. This filling sometimes is seen on M-mode images as a decrease in the gradual downward motion seen on the left ventricular free wall throughout diastole (244,245). Left atrial dilation is commonly seen with constrictive pericarditis secondary to increased left ventricular filling pressures (246).

Echogenic areas within the myocardium may be seen after resolution of the pericarditis on follow up examinations. These areas are thought to be fibrosis areas secondary to myocarditis, which was probably present in addition to the pericarditis (224).

MISCELLANEOUS CONDITIONS AFFECTING THE HEART

Anemia

Anemia causes volume overload within the heart. All chambers of the heart are affected (263). Afterload decreases in animals with anemia secondary to the reduced

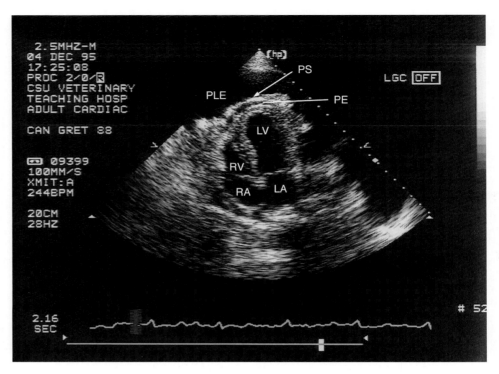

FIGURE 4.150   Constrictive pericarditis has little pericardial effusion. Fibrin is seen attached to the outside of the pericardial sac. The heart is small and volume contracted secondary to the constriction. *PLE*, pleural effusion; *PS*, pericardial sac; *PE*, pericardial effusion. *RV*, right ventricle; *LV*, left ventricle; *LA*, left atrium; *RA*, right atrium.

blood viscosity and reduced peripheral vascular resistance as the peripheral vessels vasodilate secondary to tissue hypoxia. This, in turn, increases venous return and preload, resulting in increased volume within the cardiac chambers (264). Both diastolic and systolic dimensions increase with a concurrent decrease in FS (263). Chronic effects on the heart include an increase in muscle mass as the heart hypertrophies in response to the additional wall stress created by the volume overload. An eccentrically hypertrophied heart develops. Function will return to normal as the compensatory hypertrophy develops. These changes are reversible with resolution of the anemia. It may take several weeks for the cardiac size and function to return to normal (263,264). Congestive heart failure can develop, however, if the myocardium becomes hypoxic (264).

Obesity

The effects of obesity on cardiac size and function have not been reported in animals but have been extensively studied in humans. Although hypertension results in concentric hypertrophy, patients who are obese with normal blood pressure display an eccentric hypertrophy pattern. The diastolic chamber size is larger with compensatory hypertrophy of the free wall and septum. This increase in volume enhances stroke volume and cardiac output, but ejection fraction remains the same in obese patients (265–267). The degree of eccentric enlargement correlates to the duration of obesity; enlargement is significantly greater in human patients who have been obese for longer periods (265).

Wall stress may be elevated in obese patients in which the degree of hypertrophy is inadequate and abnormal wall thickness to chamber size ratios exist (265). Systolic dysfunction is variable in obese patients, but there appears to be a correlation between inadequate hypertrophy and decreased FS (268). Early preclinical signs of systolic dysfunction are present if the PEPs are prolonged (a reflection of isovolumic contraction) and ejection times shorten, resulting in a higher PEP/LVET

ratio (267,269). These changes in systolic function are present long before the clinical manifestations of myocardial failure are present (267,270).

The degree of systolic dysfunction directly correlates to the degree of obesity (267,270). Systolic dysfunction may progress to clinically significant heart failure, especially if hypertrophy is inadequate for the degree of volume overload. This is referred to as obesity cardiomyopathy (268,270,271). Although there is no clear connection between hypertension and obesity in the dog or cat, in humans hypertension in addition to obesity adds to the potential of developing heart failure (268).

With obesity, diastolic dysfunction is impaired also. Prolonged isovolumic relaxation times suggesting impaired relaxation are found in obese patients. Flow velocity integrals for both E and A filling peaks are higher in obese patients, but the ratio remains the same (267).

REFERENCES

1. Yosida K, Yoshikawa J, Shakudo M, et al. Colour Doppler evaluation of valvular regurgitation in normal subjects. Circulation 1988;78:840–847.
2. Marr CM, Reef VB. Physiological valvular regurgitation in clinically normal young racehorses: prevalence and two dimensional colour flow Doppler echocardiographic characteristics. Equine Vet J Suppl 1995;19:56–62.
3. Blissitt KJ, Bonagura JD: Colour flow Doppler echocardiography in normal horses. Equine Vet J Suppl 1995;19:47–55.
4. Blissett KJ, Bonagura JD. Colour flow Doppler echocardiography in horses with cardiac murmurs. Equine Vet J Suppl 1995;19:82–85.
5. Blissitt KJ, Bonagura JD. Pulsed wave Doppler echocardiography in normal horses. Equine Vet J Suppl 1995;19:38–46.
6. Bonagura JD, Herring DS. Echocardiography—acquired heart disease. Vet Clin North Am Small Anim Pract 1985;15:1209–1224.
7. Shah PM. Echocardiographic diagnosis of mitral valve prolapse. J Am Soc Echocardiogr 1994;7:286–293.
8. Nakayama T, Wakao Y, Nemoto H, et al. Mitral valve protrusion assessed by use of B-mode echocardiography in dogs with mitral regurgitation. Am J Vet Res 1996;57:791–797.
9. Pederson HD, Kristensen BO, Lorentzen KA, et al. Mitral valve prolapse in 3-year old healthy Cavalier King Charles Spaniels. An echocardiographic study. Can J Vet Res 1995;59:294–298.
10. Beardow AW, Buchanan JW. Chronic mitral valve disease in Cavalier King Charles Spaniels: 95 cases (1987–1991). JAVMA 1993;203:1023–1029.
11. Pedersen HD, Kristensen BO, Norby B, et al. Echocardiographic study of mitral valve prolapse in Dachshunds. J Vet Med A 1996;43:103–110.
12. Kogure K. Pathology of chronic mitral valvular disease in the dog. Jpn J Vet Sci 1980;42:323–335.
13. Pomerance A, Whitney JC. Heart valve changes common to man and dog: a comparative study. Cardiovasc Res 1980;4:61–66.
14. Marr CM, Pirie HM, Northridge DB. Confirmation by Doppler echocardiography of valvular regurgitation in a horse with a ruptured chorda tendinea of the mitral valve. Vet Rec 1990;127:376–379.
15. Pedereson HD, Lorentzen KA, Kristensen BO. Observer variation in the two-dimensional echocardiographic evaluation of mitral valve prolapse in dogs. Vet Radiol Ultrasound 1996;37:367–372.
16. Olivier NB, Kittleson MD, Eyster G, et al. M-mode echocardiography in the diagnosis of ruptured mitral chordae tendineae in a dog. JAVMA 1984;184:588–589.
17. Jacobs GJ, Calvert CA, Mahaffey MB, et al. Echocardiographic detection of flail left atrioventricular valve cusp from ruptured chordae tendineae in 4 dogs. J Vet Intern Med 1995;9:341–346.
18. Mintz GS, Kotter MN, Segal BL, et al. Two-dimensional echocardiographic recognition of ruptured chordae tendinea. Circulation 1978;57:244–250.
19. Reef VB. Mitral valvular insufficiency associated with ruptured chordae in three foals. JAVMA 1987;191:329–331.

20. Harpster N, VanZwieten MJ, Bernstein M. Traumatic papillary muscle rupture in a dog. JAVMA 1974;165:1074–1079.

21. Kaplan PM, Fox PR, Garvey MS, et al. Acute mitral regurgitation with papillary muscle rupture in a dog. JAVMA 1987;191:1436–1438.

22. Häggstrom J, Hamlin RL, Hansson K, et al. Heart rate variability in relation to severity of mitral regurgitation in Cavalier King Charles spaniels. J Small Anim Pract 1996;37:69–75.

23. Stadler P, Weinberger T, Kinkel N, et al. B-mode, M-mode- and Doppler sonographic findings in mitral valvular insufficiency in horses. J Vet Med A 39:704–718.

24. Reef VB. Color flow mapping of horses with valvular insufficiency. Proc 8th ACVIM 1990:483–485.

25. Lombard CW, Spencer CP. Correlation of radiographic, echocardiographic, and electrocardiographic signs of left heart enlargement in dogs with mitral regurgitation. Vet Radiol 26:89–97.

26. Bonagura JD. M-mode echocardiography: basic principles. Vet Clinic North Am Small Anim Pract 1983;13:299–320.

27. Thomas WP, Gaber CE, Jacobs GJ, et al. Recommendations for standards in transthoracic two-dimensional echocardiography in the dog and cat. J Vet Intern Med 1993;7:247–252.

28. Feigenbaum H. Echocardiography. 5th ed. Philadelphia: Lea and Febiger, 1994:184–185.

29. Buchanan JW, Kelly AM. Endocardial splitting of the left atrium in the dog with hemorrhage and hemopericardium. J Am Vet Rd Soc 1964;5:28–39.

30. Sadanaga KK, MacDonald MJ, Buchanan JW. Echocardiography and surgery in a dog with left atrial rupture and hemopericardium. J Vet Intern Med 1990;4:216–221.

31. Buchanan JW. Spontaneous left atrial rupture in dogs: In Bloom CM, ed. Comparative pathophysiology of circulatory disturbances. New York: Plenum Press, Adv Exp Med Biol 1972;22:315–334.

32. Sisson D. Acquired valvular disease (endocardiosis) in dogs and cats. In: Bonagura JD, ed. Cardiology: contemporary issues in small animal practice. New York: Churchill Livingstone, 1987;59–116.

33. Berry CR, Lombard CW, Hager DA, et al. Pericardial effusion secondary to chronic endocardiosis and left atrial rupture in a dog. Comp Small Anim 1988;10:800–805.

34. Pipers FS, Bonagura JD, Hamlin RL, et al. Echocardiographic abnormalities of the mitral valve associated with left-sided heart diseases in the dog. JAVMA 1981;179:580–586.

35. Bertone JJ, Paull KS, Wingfield WE, et al. M-mode echocardiography of endurance horses in the recovery phase of long-distance competition. Am J Vet Res 1987;48:1708–1712.

36. Feigenbaum H. Echocardiography. 5th ed. Philadelphia: Lea and Febiger, 1994:151–155.

37. Fujino T, Ito M, Kanaya S, et al. Echocardiographic abnormal motion of interventricular septum in mitral insufficiency. J Cardiogr 1976;6:613.

38. Ajisaka R, Iesaka Y, Takamoto T, et al. Echocardiographic assessment of left ventricular volume overloading in aortic insufficiency and mitral insufficiency. J Cardiogr 1978;8:209.

39. Lewis BS, Hasin Y, Pasternak R, et al. Echocardiographic aortic root motion in ventricular volume overload and the effect of mitral incompetence. Eur J Cardiol 1979;10:375–384.

40. Kittleson MD, Eyster GE, Knowlen GG. Myocardial function in small dogs with chronic mitral regurgitation and severe congestive heart failure. JAVMA 1985;184:1253–1256.

41. Pouchelon JL. Study of the fractional shortening in 110 dogs suffering from mitral insufficiency through endocardiosis. Recueil de Med Vet 1989;165:801–806.

42. Crawford MH. Valvular heart disease. Curr Opin Cardiol 1994;9:143–145.

43. Helmcke F, Nanda NC, Hsiung MC, et al. Color Doppler assessment of mitral regurgitation with orthogonal planes. Circulation 1987;75:175–183.

44. Cooper JW, Nanda NC, Philpot EF, et al. Evaluation of valvular regurgitation by color Doppler. J Am Soc Echocardiogr 1989;2:56–66.

45. Spain MG, Smith MD, Grayburn PA, et al. Quantitative assessment of mitral regurgitation by Doppler color flow imaging: angiographic and hemodynamic correlations. J Am Coll Cardiol 1989;13:585–590.

46. Abbasi AS, Allen MW, DeCristofara D, et al. Detection and estimation of the degree of mitral regurgitation by range-gated Doppler echocardiography. Circulation 1980;61:143–147.

47. Quinones MA, Young JB, Waggoner AD, et al. Assessment of pulsed Doppler echocardiography in the detection and quantification of aortic and mitral regurgitation. Br Heart J 1980;44:612–620.

48. Losordo DW, Pastore JO, Coletta D, et al. Limitations of color flow Doppler imaging in the quantification of valvular regurgitation: velocity of regurgitant jet, rather than volume, determines size of color flow Doppler image. Am Heart J 1993; 126:168–176.

49. Krivokapich J. Echocardiography in valvular heart disease. Curr Opin Cardiol 1994; 9:159–163.

50. Cape EG, Yoganathan AP, Levine RA. Increased heart rate can cause underestimation of regurgitant jet size by Doppler color flow mapping. J Am Coll Cardiol 1993;21:1029–1037.

51. Enriquez-Sarano M, Tajik AJ, Bailey KR, et al. Color flow imaging compared with quantitative Doppler assessment of severity of mitral regurgitation: influence of eccentricity of jet and mechanism of regurgitation. J Am Coll Cardiol 1993;21:1211–1219.

52. Uehara Y, Takahashi M. Quantitative evaluation of the severity of mitral insufficiency in dogs by color Doppler method. J Vet Med Sci 1996;58:249–253.

53. Mele D, Vandervoort P, Palacios I, et al. Proximal jet size by Doppler color flow mapping predicts severity of mitral regurgitation. Circulation 1995;91:746–754.

54. Chao K, Moises VA, Shandas R, et al. Influence of the Coanda effect on color Doppler jet area and color encoding. Circulation 1992;85:333–341.

55. Bodey AR. Systemic hypertension in the dog—fact or fiction? 18th Annual Waltham/OSU Symposium, 1994:44–53.

56. Appleton CP, Basnight MA, Gonzales MS, et al. Diastolic mitral regurgitation with atrioventricular conduction abnormalities: relation of mitral flow velocity to transmitral pressure gradients in conscious dogs. J Am Coll Cardiol 1991;18:843–849.

57. Rosenthal SL, Fox PR. Diastolic mitral regurgitation detected by pulsed wave Doppler echocardiography and color flow Doppler mapping in five dogs and two cats with second- and third-degree atrioventricular block. Vet Radiol Ultrasound 1995;36:152–156.

58. Bonagura JD, Pipers FS. Echocardiographic features of aortic valve endocarditis in a dog, a cow, and a horse. JAVMA 1983;182:595–599.

59. Sisson D, Thomas WP. Endocarditis of the aortic valve in the dog. JAVMA 1984;184:570–577.

60. Bonagura JD, Herring DS, Welker F. Echocardiography. Vet Clin North Am Equine Pract 1985;1:311–334.

61. Elwood CM, Cobb MA, Stepien RL. Clinical and echocardiographic findings in 10 dogs with vegetative bacterial endocarditis. J Small Anim Pract 1993;34:420–427.

62. Clark ES, Reef VB, Sweeney CR, et al. Aortic valve insufficiency in a one-year old colt. JAVMA 1987;191:841–844.

63. Ball MA, Weldon AD. Vegetative endocarditis in an Appaloosa gelding. Cornell Vet 1992;82:301–309.

64. Popp RL. Echocardiography. N Engl J Med 1990;323:165–172.

65. Lombard CW, Buergelt CD. Vegetative bacterial endocarditis in dogs: echocardiographic diagnosis and clinical signs. J Small Anim Pract 1983;24:325–339.

66. Dedrick P, Reef VB, Sweeney RW, et al. Treatment of bacterial endocarditis in a horse. JAVMA 1988;193:339–342.

67. Lacuata AQ, Yamada H, Nakamura Y, et al. Electrocardiographic and echocardiographic findings in four cases of bovine endocarditis. JAVMA 1980;176:1355–1365.

68. Zanotti S, Kaplan P, Garlick D, et al. Endocarditis associated with urinary bladder foreign body in a dog. J Am Anim Hosp Assoc 1989;25:557–561.

69. Reef VB. The use of diagnostic ultrasound in the horse. Ultrasound Quart 1991;9:1–33.

70. Feigenbaum H. Echocardiography. 5th ed. Philadelphia: Lea and Febiger, 1994:287–290.

71. Pipers FS, Hamlin RL, Reef V. Echocardiographic detection of cardiovascular lesions in the horse. J Equine Med Surg 1979;3:68–77.

72. Winsberg F, Gabor GE, Hernberg JG, et al. Fluttering of the aortic valve in aortic insufficiency. Circulation 1970;41:225–229.

73. Reef VB, Spencer P. Echocardiographic evaluation of equine aortic insufficiency. Am J Vet Res 1987;48:904–908.

74. Nakao S, Tanaka H, Tahara M, et al. A regurgitant jet and echocardiographic abnormalities in aortic regurgitation: an experimental study. Circulation 1983;67:860–865.

75. Botvinik EH, Schiller NG, Wickeranase-Karan R, et al. Echocardiographic demonstration of early mitral valve closure in severe aortic insufficiency. Circulation 1975;51:836–847.

76. Mann T, McLautin L, Grossman CE. Assessing the hemodynamic severity of acute aortic regurgitation due to infective endocarditis. N Engl J Med 1975;293:108–112.

77. Reef VB. Clinical and echocardiographic evaluation of equine aortic insufficiency. Pract 4th ACVIM 1986;7:49–51.

78. Wray TM. The variable echocardiographic features in aortic valve endocarditis. Circulation 1975;52:658–663.

79. Lee CC, Das G, Weissler AM. Characteristic echocardiographic manifestations in ruptured aortic valve leaflet. Circulation 1974;50(Suppl III):144.

80. Kittleson MD, Eyster GE, Knowlen GG, et al. Myocardial function in small dogs with chronic mitral regurgitation and severe congestive heart failure. JAVMA 184:455–459.

81. Henik RA, Allen TA, Jones RL, et al. Endocarditis caused by Corynebacterium sp. in a dog. JAVMA 1986;1458–1461.

82. Krivokapich J. Echocardiography in valvular heart disease. Curr Opin Cardiol 1994;9:158–163.

83. Losordo DW, Pastore JO, Coletta D, et al. Limitations of color flow Doppler imaging in the quantification of valvular regurgitation: velocity of regurgitant jet rather than volume, determines size of color Doppler image. Am Heart J 1993;126:168–17.

84. Perry GJ, Helmke F, Nanda JC, et al. Evaluation of aortic insufficiency by Doppler color flow mapping. J Am Coll Cardiol 1987;9:952–959.

85. Griffin BP, Flachskampf FA, Reimold SC, et al. Relationship of aortic regurgitant velocity slope and pressure half-time to severity of aortic regurgitation under changing hemodynamic conditions. Eur Heart J 1994;15:681–685.

86. Xie G-Y, Berk MR, Smith MD, et al. A simplified method for determining regurgitant fraction by Doppler echocardiography in patients with aortic regurgitation. J Am Coll Cardiol 1994;24:1041–1045.

87. Bond BR. Problems in veterinary ultrasonographic analysis of acquired heart disease. Prob Vet Med 1991;3:520–554.

88. Takemura N, Koyama H, Motoyoshi S. Congestive heart failure due to bilateral atrioventricular valve insufficiency in two dogs. J Vet Med Sci 1996;58:381–384.

89. Tavers CW, Van Den Berg JS. Pseudomonas spp. associated vegetative endocarditis in two horses. Tydskr S Afr Vet Ver 1995;66:172–176.

90. Calvert C. Valvular bacterial endocarditis in the dog. JAVMA 1982;180:1080–1084.

91. Dear MG. Bacterial endocarditis. In: Kirk RW, ed. Current veterinary therapy VI. Philadelphia: WB Saunders, 1977:357–359.

92. Smith JA. Bacterial endocarditis in cattle. Bov Clin 1983;3:4–6.

93. Pipers FS, Rings DM, Hull BL, et al. Echocardiographic diagnosis of endocarditis in a bull. JAVMA 1978;172:1313–1316.

94. Yamaga Y, Too K. Diagnostic ultrasound imaging of vegetative endocarditis in cattle. Jpn J Vet Res 1987;35:49–63.

95. Ware WA, Bonagura JD, Rings DM, et al. Echocardiographic diagnosis of pulmonic valve vegetative endocarditis in a cow. JAVMA 1986;188:185–187.

96. Weinstein L, Schlesinger JJ. Pathoanatomic, pathophysiologic and clinical correlations in endocarditis. Part 2. N Engl J Med 1974;291:1122–1125.

97. Roussel AJ, Kasari TR. Bacterial endocarditis in large animals. Part II. Incidence, causes, clinical signs, and pathologic findings. Comp Cont Ed Pract Vet 1989;11:769–774.

98. Power HT, Rebhun WC. Bacterial endocarditis in adult dairy cattle. JAVMA 1983;181:806–808.

99. Baxley WA. Aortic valve disease. Curr Opin Cardiol 1994;9:152–157.

100. Lieberman AN, Weiss JL, Jugdutt BI, et al. Two-dimensional echocardiography and infarct size: relationship of regional wall motion and thickening to the extent of myocardial infarction in the dog. Circulation 1981;63:739–746.

101. Gallagher KP, Kumada T, Koziol JA, et al. Significance of regional wall thickening abnormalities relative to transmural myocardial perfusion in anesthetized dogs. Circulation 1980;62:1266–1274.

102. Charlat ML, O'Neill PG, Hartley CJ, et al. Prolonged abnormalities of left ventricular myocardium in conscious dogs. Time course and relation to systolic function. J Am Coll Cardiol 1989;13:185–194.

103. Liu SK, Maron BJ, Tilley LP. Canine hypertrophic cardiomyopathy. JAVMA 1979;174:708–713.

104. Marks CA. Hypertrophic cardiomyopathy in a dog. JAVMA 1993;203:1020–1022.

105. Liu S. Pathology of feline heart diseases. Vet Clin North Am 1977;7:323–339.

106. Louie EK, Edwards LC. Hypertrophic cardiomyopathy. Prog Cardiov Diseases 1994; 36:275–308.

107. Moise NS, Dietze AE, Mezza LE, et al. Echocardiography, electrocardiography, and radiography of cats with dilation cardiomyopathy, hypertrophic cardiomyopathy, and hyperthyroidism. Am J Vet Res 1986;47:1476–1486.

108. Bright JM, Golden AL, Daniel GB. Feline hypertrophic cardiomyopathy: variations on a theme. J Small Anim Pract 1992;33:266–274.

109. Peterson EN, Moise S, Brown CA, et al. Heterogeneity of hypertrophy in feline hypertrophic heart disease. J Vet Intern Med 1993;7:183–189.

110. Henry WL, Clark CE, Galncy PL, et al. Echocardiographic measurement of the left ventricular outflow gradient in idiopathic hypertrophic subaortic stenosis. N Engl J Med 1973;288:989–993.

111. Pollick C, Morgan CD, Gilbert BW, et al. Muscular subaortic stenosis: the temporal relationship between systolic anterior motion of the anterior mitral leaflet and the pressure gradient. Circulation 1982;66:1087–1094.

112. Wigle ED, Sasson Z, Henderson MA, et al. Hypertrophic cardiomyopathy. The importance of the site and the extent of the hypertrophy. A review. Prog Cardiovasc Dis 1985;28:1–83.

113. Yock PG, Hatle L, Popp RL. Patterns and timing of Doppler detected intracavity and aortic flow in hypertrophic cardiomyopathy. J Am Coll Cardiol 1986;8:1047–1058.

114. Rakowski H, Sasson Z, Wigle ED. Echocardiographic and Doppler assessment of hypertrophic cardiomyopathy. J Am Soc Echocardiogr 1988;1:31–47.

115. Sakurai S, Tanaka H. Temporal relationship between early systolic closure of the aortic valve and aortic flow: experimental study with and without systolic anterior motion of the mitral valve. Am Heart J 1986;112:113–121.

116. Krajcer Z, Orzan F, Pechacek LW, et al. Early systolic closure of the aortic valve in patients with hypertrophic subaortic stenosis and discrete subaortic stenosis. Am J Cardiol 1978;41:823–829.

117. Rishniw M, Thomas WP, Kienle RD, et al. Dynamic right mid-ventricular obstruction in 50 cats. J Vet Intern Med 1996;10:159.

118. VonDoenhoff LJ, Nanda NC. Obstruction within the right ventricular body: two dimensional echocardiographic features. Am J Cardiol 1983;51:1498–1501.

119. Federman M, Hess OM. Differentiation between systolic and diastolic dysfunction. Eur Heart J Suppl D 15:2–6.

120. Bright JM, Golden AL, Gompf RE, et al. Evaluation of the calcium channel blocking agents diltiazem and verapamil for treatment of feline hypertrophic cardiomyopathy. J Vet Intern Med 1991;5:272–282.

121. Nishamura RA, Abel MD, Hatle LK, et al. Assessment of diastolic function of the heart: background and current applications of Doppler echocardiography. Part II: clinical studies. Mayo CLin Proc 1989;64:181–204.

122. Lesser M, Fox PR, Bond BR. Assessment of hypertension in 40 cats with left ventricular hypertrophy by Doppler-shift sphygmomanometry. J Small Anim Pract 1992;33:55–58.

123. Moise NS, Dietze AE. Echocardiographic, electrocardiographic, and radiographic detection of cardiomegaly in hyperthyroid cats. Am J Vet Res 1986;47:1487–1494.

124. Skelton CL, Coleman HN, Wildenthal K, et al. Augmentation of myocardial oxygen consumption in hyperthyroid cats. Circ Res 1970;3:301–309.

125. Bond BR, Fox PR, Peterson ME, et al. Echocardiographic findings in 103 cats with hyperthyroidism. JAVMA 1988;192:1546–1549.

126. Atkins C. The role of noncardiac disease in the development and precipitation of heart failure. Vet Clin North Am 1991;21:1035–1080.

127. Dukes J. Hypertension: a review of the mechanisms, manifestations and management. J Small Anim Pract 1992;33:119–129.

128. Doi YL, Deanfield JE, McKenna WJ, et al. Echocardiographic differentiation of hypertensive heart disease and hypertrophic cardiomyopathy. Br Heart J 1980;44:395–400.

129. Karam R, Lever HM, Healy BP. Hypertensive hypertrophic cardiomyopathy or hypertrophic cardiomyopathy with hypertension? A study of 78 patients. JACC 1989;13:580–584.

130. Berry CR, Gaschen FP, Ackerman N. Radiographic and ultrasonographic features of hypertrophic feline muscular dystrophy in two cats. Vet Radiol Ultrasound 1992;33: 357–364.

131. Brummer DG, Moise NS. Infiltrative cardiomyopathy responsive to combination chemotherapy in a cat with lymphoma. JAVMA 1989;195:1116–1119.

132. Jacobs G, Hutson C, Dougherty J, et al. Congestive heart failure associated with hyperthyroidism in cats. JAVMA 1986;188:52–56.

133. Abinader EG. Two-dimensional and M-mode echocardiographic features of a left ventricular false tendon. J Cardiovasc Ultrasound 1983;2:299–301.

134. Liu S-K, Tilley LP. Excessive moderator bands in the left ventricle of 21 cats. JAVMA 1982;180:1215–1219.

135. Keren A, Billingham ME, Popp RL. Echocardiographic recognition and implications of ventricular hypertrophic trabeculations and aberrant bands. Circulation 1984;70: 836–842.

136. Dec GW, Fuster V. Idiopathic dilated cardiomyopathy. N Engl J Med 1994;331:1564–1575.

137. Cobb MA. Idiopathic dilated cardiomyopathy: advances in aetiology, pathogenesis and management. J Small Anim Pract 1992;33:113–118.

138. Calvert CA. Dilated congestive cardiomyopathy in Doberman Pinschers. Comp Cont Educ 1986;8:417–430.

139. Keene BW, Panciera DP, Atkins CE, et al. Myocardial L-carnitine deficiency in a family of dogs with dilated cardiomyopathy. JAVMA 1991;198:647–650.

140. McEntee K, Clercx C, Snaps F, et al. Clinical, electrocardiographic and echocardiographic improvements after L-carnitine supplementation in a cardiomyopathic labrador. Canine Pract 1995;20:12–15.

141. Panciera DL. An echocardiographic and electrocardiographic study of cardiovascular function in hypothyroid dogs. JAVMA 1994;205:996–1000.

142. Atwell RB, Kelly WR. Canine parvovirus: a cause of chronic myocardial fibrosis and adolescent congestive heart failure. J Small Anim Pract 1980;21:609–620.

143. Ilgen BE, Conroy JD. Fatal cardiomyopathy in an adult dog resembling parvovirus-induced myocarditis: a case report. J Am Anim Hosp Assoc 1982;18:613–617.

144. Higgins RJ, Krakowka D, Metzler AE, et al. Canine distemper virus associated cardiac necrosis in the dog. Vet Path 1981;18:472–486.

145. Keene BW, Atkins CE, Rush JE. Myocarditis in canine dilated cardiomyopathy. J Vet Intern Med 1993;7:118.

146. Novotny MJ, Hogan PM, Flannigan G. Echocardiographic evidence for myocardial failure induced by taurine deficiency in domestic cats. Can J Vet Res 1994;58:6–12.

147. Pion PD, Kittleson MD, Rodgers QR, et al. Myocardial failure in cats associated with low plasma taurine: a reversible cardiomyopathy. Science 1987;237:764–768.

148. Sisson DD, Knight DH, Helinski C, et al. Plasma taurine concentrations and M-mode echocardiographic measures in healthy cats and in cats with dilated cardiomyopathy. J Vet Intern Med 1991;5:232–238.

149. Pion PD, Kittleson MD, Thomas WP, et al. Clinical findings in cats with dilated cardiomyopathy and relationship of findings to taurine deficiency. JAVMA 1992;201: 267–274.

150. Kramer GA, Fox PR. Plasma taurine concentrations in dogs with acquired heart disease. J Vet Intern Med 3:126.

151. Jacobs GJ. Reviewing the various types of primary cardiomyopathy in dogs. Vet Med 1996;91:524–532.

152. Fuentes VL. Feline heart disease: an update. J Small Anim Pract 1992;33:130–137.

153. Lombard CW. Echocardiographic and clinical signs of canine dilated cardiomyopathy. J Small Anim Pract 1984;25:59–70.

154. Darke PGG, Fuentes VL, Champion SR. Doppler echocardiography in canine congestive cardiomyopathy. Proc 11th ACVIM 1993:531–534.

155. Calvert CA, Chapman WL, Toal RL. Congestive cardiomyopathy in Doberman Pinscher dogs. JAVMA 1982;181:598–602.

156. Calvert CA, Brown J. Use of M-mode echocardiography in the diagnosis of congestive cardiomyopathy in Doberman Pinschers. JAVMA 1986;189:293–297.

157. Moise NS, Dietze AE, Mezza LE, et al. Echocardiography, electrocardiography, and radiography of cats with dilation cardiomyopathy, hypertrophic cardiomyopathy, and hyperthyroidism. Am J Vet Res 47:1476–1486.

158. Koch J, Pedersen HD, Jensen AI, et al. M-mode echocardiographic diagnosis of dilated cardiomyopathy in giant breed dogs. J Vet Med A 1996;43:297–304.

159. Keren A, Popp R. Assignment of patients into the classification of cardiomyopathies. Circulation 1992;86:1622–1633.

160. Fox PR. Canine myocardial disease. In: Fox PR, ed. Canine and feline cardiology. New York: Churchill Livingstone, 1988.

161. Freeman LM, Michel KE, Brown DJ, et al. Idiopathic dilated cardiomyopathy in Dalmatians: nine cases (1990–1995). JAVMA 1996;209:1592–1596.

162. Tidholm A, Jönsson L. Dilated cardiomyopathy in the Newfoundland: study of 37 cases (1983–1994). J Am Anim Hosp Assoc 1996;32:465–470.

163. Gaasch WH. Left ventricular radius to wall thickness ratio. Am J Cardiol 1979;43: 1189–1194.

164. Grossman W, Jones D, McLaurin LP. Wall stress and patterns of ventricular hypertrophy in the human left ventricle. J Clin Inves 1975;56:56–64.

165. Atkins CE, Snyder PS, Keene BW, et al. Efficacy of digoxin for treatment of cats with dilated cardiomyopathy. JAVMA 1990;196:1463–1469.

166. Calvert CA, Jacobs GJ, Pickus CW. Bradycardia-associated episodic weakness, syncope, and aborted sudden death in cardiomyopathic Doberman Pinschers. J Vet Intern Med 1996;10:88–93.

167. O'Grady MR, Horne R. Outcome of 103 asymptomatic Doberman Pinschers: incidence of dilated cardiomyopathy in a longitudinal study. J Vet Intern Med 1995;9:199.

168. Gooding JP, Robinson WF, Mews GC. Echocardiographic characterization of dilation cardiomyopathy in the English Cocker Spaniel. Am J Vet Res 1986; 47:1978–1983.

169. Monnet E, Orton EC, Salman M, et al. Idiopathic dilated cardiomyopathy in dogs: survival and prognostic indicators. J Vet Intern Med 1995;9:12–17.

170. Abramson SV, Burke JF, Kelly JJ, et al. Pulmonary hypertension predicts mortality and morbidity in patients with dilated cardiomyopathy. Ann Intern Med 1992;116:888–895.

171. Pion PD, Kittleson MD, Thomas WP, et al. Response of cats with dilated cardiomyopathy to taurine supplementation. JAVMA 1992;201:275–284.

172. Klein I. Thyroid hormone and the cardiovascular system. Am J Med 1990;88:631–637.

173. Bright JM, McEntee M. Isolated right ventricular cardiomyopathy in a dog. JAVMA 1995;207:64–66.

174. Kullo IJ, Edwards WD, Seward JB. Right ventricular dysplasia: the Mayo clinic experience. Mayo Clin Proc 1995;70:541–548.

175. Sabbah HN, Gheorghiade M, Smith ST, et al. Serial evaluation of left ventricular function in congestive heart failure by measurement of peak aortic blood acceleration. Am J Cardiol 1988;61:367–370.

176. Bonagura JD. Echocardiography. JAVMA 204:516–521.

177. Werner GS, Schaefer C, Dirks R, et al. Doppler echocardiographic assessment of left ventricular filling in idiopathic dilated cardiomyopathy during one year follow-up: relation to the clinical course of the disease. Am Heart J 1993;126:1408–1416.

178. Appleton CP, Hatle LK, Popp RL, Relation of transmitral flow velocity patterns to left ventricular diastolic function: new insights from a combined hemodynamic and Doppler echocardiographic study. J Am Coll Cardiol 1988;12:426–440.

179. Nishamura RA, Abel MD, Hatle LK, et al. Assessment of diastolic function of the heart: background and current applications of Doppler echocardiography. Part II: clinical studies. Mayo Clin Proc 1989;64:181–204.

180. Lavine SJ, Arends D. Importance of left ventricular filling pressure on diastolic filling in dilated cardiomyopathy. Am J Cardiol 1989;64:61–65.

181. Nishimura RA, Appleton CP, Redfield MM, et al. Noninvasive Doppler echocardiographic evaluation of left ventricular filling pressures in patients with cardiomyopathies: a simultaneous Doppler echocardiographic and cardiac catheterization study. J Am Coll Cardiol 1996;28:1226–1233.

182. Harpster NK. The cardiovascular system. In: Holzworth J, ed. Diseases of the cat. Vol 1. Philadelphia: WB Saunders, 1986:820.

183. Fox PR. Feline myocardial diseases. Proc 18th Waltham/OSU Symposium 1994:119–128.

184. Lombard CW, Buergelt CD. Endocardial fibroelastosis in four dogs. J Am Anim Hosp Assoc 1984;20:271–278.

185. Cetta F, O'Leary PW, Seward JB, et al. Idiopathic restrictive cardiomyopathy in childhood: diagnostic features and clinical course. Mayo Clin Proc 70:634–640.

186. Atkins CE, Snyder PS. Cardiomyopathy. In: Allen DG, ed. Small animal medicine. JB Lippincott, 1991:284–296.

187. Brunazzi MC, Chirillo F, Pasqualini M, et al. Estimation of left ventricular diastolic

pressures from precordial pulsed-Doppler analysis of pulmonary venous and mitral flow. Am Heart J 1994;128:293–300.

188. Hatle LK, Appleton CP, Popp RL. Differentiation of constrictive pericarditis and restrictive cardiomyopathy by Doppler echocardiography. Circulation 1989;79:357–370.

189. Bossbaly MJ, Buchanan JW, Sammarco C. Aortic body carcinoma and myocardial infarction in a Doberman Pinscher. J Small Anim Pract 1993;34:638–6422.

190. Traill TA. Wall thickness changes considered as regional myocardial in ischemic heart disease. Hertz 1980;5:275–284.

191. Torry RJ, Myers JH, Adler AL, et al. Effects of nonstransmural ischemia on inner and outer wall thickening in the canine left ventricle. Am Heart J 1991;122:1292–1299.

192. Pandian NG, Kieso RA, Kerber RE. Two dimensional echocardiography in experimental coronary stenosis. II. Relationship between systolic wall thinning and regional myocardial perfusion in severe coronary stenosis. Circulation 1982;66:603–611.

193. Guth BD, White FC, Gallagher KP, et al. Decreased systolic wall thickening in myocardium adjacent to ischemic zones in conscious swine during brief coronary artery occlusion. Am Heart J 1984;107:458–464.

194. Traub-Dargatz JL, Schlipf JW, Boon J, et al. Ventricular tachycardia and myocardial dysfunction in a horse. JAVMA 1994;205:1569–1573.

195. Corya BC. Echocardiography in ischemic heart disease. Am J Med 1977;63:10–20.

196. Sabia P. Afrookteh A, Touchstone DA, et al. Value of regional wall motion abnormality in the emergency room diagnosis of acute myocardial infarction. Circulation 1991;84:85–91.

197. Disizian V, Bonow RO. Current diagnostic techniques of assessing myocardial viability in patients with hibernating and stunned myocardium. Circulation 1993;87:1–20.

198. Bolli R. Myocardial stunning in man. Circulation 1992;86:1671–1691.

199. Preuss KC, Gross GJ, Brooks HL, et al. Time course of recovery of stunned myocardium following variable periods of ischemia in conscious and anesthetized dogs. Am Heart J 1987;114:696–703.

200. Lewis SJ, Sawaga SG, Ryan T, et al. Segmental wall motion abnormalities in the absence of clinically documented myocardial infarction: clinical significance and evidence of hibernating myocardium. Am Heart J 1991;121:1088–1094.

201. Pandian NG, Skorton DJ, Doty DB, et al. Immediate diagnosis of acute myocardial contusion by two-dimensional echocardiography: studies in a canine model of blunt chest trauma. J Am Coll Cardiol 1983;2:488–496.

202. Sherman S. Cor pulmonale. Postgrad Med 1992;91:227–236.

203. Lombard CW, Buergelt CD. Echocardiographic and clinical findings in dogs with heartworm-induced cor pulmonale. Comp Cont Ed 1983;5:971–980.

204. Atkins CE, Keene BW, McGuirk SM. Pathophysiologic mechanism of cardiac dysfunction in experimentally induced heartworm caval syndrome in dogs: an echocardiographic study. Am J Vet Res 1988;49:403–410.

205. Badertscher RR, Losonsky JM, Paul AJ, et al. Two-dimensional echocardiography for dirofilariasis in nine dogs. JAVMA 1988;193:843–846.

206. DeMadron E, Bonagura JD, O'Grady MR. Normal and paradoxical ventricular septal motion in the dog. Am J Vet Res 1985;46:1832–1841.

207. Uehara Y. An attempt to estimate the pulmonary artery pressure in dogs by means of pulsed Doppler echocardiography. J Vet Med Sci 1993;55:307–312.

208. Hagio M. Assessment of the pathological condition of congenital heart disease: morphological and functional diagnosis by combined echocardiography. Jpn J Vet Sci 1990;43:119–129.

209. Brecker SJD, Gibbs JSR, Fox KM, et al. Comparison of Doppler derived haemodynamic variables and simultaneous high fidelity pressure measurements in severe pulmonary hypertension. Br Heart J 1994;72:384–389.

210. Snyder PS. Canine hypertensive disease. Comp Cont Ed Pract Vet 1992;14:E17–23.

211. Remillard RL, Ross JN, Eddy JB. Variance of indirect blood pressure measurements and prevalence of hypertension in clinically normal dogs. Am J Vet Res 1991;52:561–565.

212. Dukes J. Hypertension: a review of the mechanisms, manifestations, and management. J Small Anim Pract 1991;33:119–129.

213. Kobayashi DL, Peterson ME, Graves TK, et al. Hypertension in cats with chronic renal failure or hyperthyroidism. J Vet Intern Med 1990;4:58–62.

214. Mahoney LT, Brody MJ. A method for indirect recording of arterial pressure in conscious cats. J Pharm Meth 1978;1:61–66.

215. Klevans LR, Hirkaler G, Kovacs JL. Indirect blood pressure determination by Doppler technique in renal hypertensive cats. Am J Physiol 1979;237:H720–H723.

216. Grandi AM, Venco A, Sessa F, et al. Determinants of left ventricular function before and after regression of myocardial hypertrophy in hypertension. Am J Hypertens 1993;6: 708–712.

217. Karpov RS, Tkachenko OG, Trissvetova EL, et al. Evaluation of cardiac performance in hypertension. Am J Hyper 1992;5:190S–145S.

218. Wicker P, Roudaut R, Haissaguere M, et al. Prevalence and significance of asymmetric septal hypertrophy in hypertension: an echocardiographic and clinical study. Eur Heart J 1983;4(Suppl G):1–5.

219. Morioka S, Simon G. Echocardiographic evidence for early left ventricular hypertrophy in dogs with renal hypertension. Am J Cardiol 1982;49:1890–1895.

220. Lesser M, Fox PR, Bond B. Non-invasive blood pressure evaluation in cats with left ventricular hypertrophic diseases. J Vet Intern Med 1990;4:117.

221. Bovée KC, Douglas PS. Abnormal left ventricular shape and function in hypertensive dogs. J Vet Intern Med 1990;4:117.

222. Devereaux RB, De Simone G, Ganau A, et al. Left ventricular hypertrophy and hypertension. Clin Exper Hyperten 1993;15:1025–1032.

223. Rosenthal J. Systolic and diastolic cardiac function in hypertension. J Cardiovasc Pharm 1992;19:S112–S115.

224. Troy AD, Chakko S, Gash AK, et al. Left ventricular function in systemic hypertension. J Cardiovasc Ultrasound 1983;2:251–257.

225. Hatle L. Doppler echocardiographic evaluation of diastolic function in hypertensive cardiomyopathies. Eur Heart J 1993;14(Suppl J):88–94.

226. Berg RJ, Wingfield W. Pericardial effusion in the dog: a review of 42 cases. J Am Anim Hosp Assoc 1984;20:721–730.

227. Cobb MA, Brownlie SE. Intrapericardial neoplasia in 14 dogs. J Small Anim Pract 1992;33:309–316.

228. Freestone JF, Thomas WP, Carlson GP, et al. Idiopathic effusive pericarditis with tamponade in the horse. Equine Vet J 1987;19:38–42.

229. DeMadron E. Pericarditis with cardiac tamponade secondary to feline infectious peritonitis in a cat. J Am Anim Hosp Assoc 1986;22:65–69.

230. Rush JE, Keene BW, Fox PR. Pericardial disease in the cat: a retrospective evaluation of 66 cases. J Am Anim Hosp Assoc 1990;26:39–46.

231. Vacirca G, Mantelli F, Ferro E, et al. Pericardial effusion with feline infectious peritonitis. Comp Animal Pract—Infect Disease 1989;19:25–27.

232. Bunch SE, Bolton GE, Hornbuckle WE. Pericardial effusion with restrictive pericarditis associated with congestive cardiomyopathy in the cat. J Am Anim Hosp Assoc 1981;17:739–745.

233. Liu S-K. Acquired cardiac lesions leading to congestive heart failure in the cat. Am J Vet Res 1970;31:2071–2088.

234. Berg J. Pericardial disease and cardiac neoplasia. Semin Vet Med Surg: Small Anim 1994;9:185–191.

235. Pipers FS, Hamlin RL. Clinical use of echocardiography in the domestic cat. JAVMA 1981;176:49–56.

236. Bonagura JD, Pipers FS. Echocardiographic features of pericardial effusion in dogs. JAVMA 1981;179:49–56.

237. Berry CR, Lombard CW, Hager DA, et al. Echocardiographic evaluation of cardiac tamponade in dogs before and after pericardiocentesis: four cases (1984–1986). JAVMA 1988;192:1597–1603.

238. DeMadron E, Prymak C, Hendricks J. Idiopathic hemorrhagic pericardial effusion with organized thrombi in a dog. JAVMA 1987;191:324–326.

239. Berg RJ, Wingfield WE, Hoopes PJ. Idiopathic hemorrhagic pericardial effusion in eight dogs. JAVMA 1984;185:988–992.

240. Pories WJ, Gaudain VA. Cardiac tamponade. Surg Clin North Am 1975;55:573–589.

241. Vörös K, Felkai C, Szilagyi Z, et al. Two-dimensional echocardiographically guided pericardiocentesis in a horse with traumatic pericarditis. JAVMA 1991;198:1953–1956.

242. Fuentes VL, Long KJ, Darke PGG, et al. Purulent pericarditis in a puppy. J Small Anim Pract 1991;32:585–588.

243. Shenoy MM, Dhar S, Gittin R, et al. Pulmonary edema following pericardiotomy for cardiac tamponade. Chest 1984;86:647–648.

244. Klopfenstein HS, Schuchard GH, Wann LS, et al. The relative merits of pulsus paradoxes and ventricular diastolic collapse in the early detection of cardiac tamponade: an experimental echocardiographic study. Circulation 1985;71:829–833.

245. Kaplan LM, Epstein SK, Schwartz SL, et al. Clinical, echocardiographic, and hemodynamic evidence of cardiac tamponade caused by large pleural effusions. Am J Respir Crit Care Med 1995;151:904–908.

246. Robinson JA, Marr CM, Reef VB, et al. Idiopathic, aseptic, effusive, fibrinous, nonrestrictive pericarditis with tamponade in a Standardbred filly. JAVMA 1992;201: 1593–1598.

247. Thomas WP, Sisson D, Bauer TG, et al. Detection of cardiac masses in dogs by two-dimensional echocardiography. Vet Radiol 1984;25:65–72.

248. Fruchter AM, Miller CW, O'Grady MR. Echocardiographic results and clinical considerations in dogs with right atrial/auricular masses. Can Vet J 1992;33:171–174.

249. De Madron E. Malignant pericardial effusion in dogs: seven cases. Eur J Companion Anim Pract 1991;1:52–62.

250. Windberger U, Dreier HK, Von Bomhard D, et al. Echocardiographic evaluation of pericardial effusions: a report of 2 cases. Eur J Comp Anim Pract 1993;3:51–55.

251. DiFruscia R, Perrone MA, Bonneau NH, et al. Heart base tumor and pericardial effusion in a dog. Can Vet J 1989;30:150–154.

252. Tillson DM, Fingland RB, Andrews GA. Chemodectoma in a cat. J Am Anim Hosp Assoc 1994;30:586–590.

253. Meurs KM, Miller MW, Mackie JR, et al. Syncope associated with cardiac lymphoma in a cat. J Am Anim Hosp Assoc 1994;30:583–585.

254. Paola JP, Hammer AS, Smeak DD, et al. Aortic body tumor causing pleural effusion in a cat. J Am Anim Hosp Assoc 1994;30:281–285.

255. Keene BW, Rush JE, Cooley AJ, et al. Primary left ventricular hemangiosarcoma diagnosed by endomyocardial biopsy in a dog. JAVMA 1990;197:1501–1503.

256. Atkins CE, Badertscher RR, Greenlee P, et al. Diagnosis of an intracardiac fibrosarcoma using two dimensional echocardiography. J Am Anim Hosp Assoc 1984;20:131–137.

257. Bright JM, Toal RL, Blackford LM. Right ventricular outflow obstruction caused by primary cardiac neoplasia. J Vet Intern Med 1990;4:12–16.

258. Ware WA, Merkley DF, Riedesel DH. Intracardiac thyroid tumor in a dog: diagnosis and surgical removal. J Am Anim Hosp Assoc 1994;30:20–23.

259. Bernard W, Reef VB, Clark S, et al. Pericarditis in horses: six cases (1982–1986). JAVMA 1990;196:468–471.

260. Campbell SL, Forrester SD, Johnston SA, et al. Chylothorax associated with constrictive pericarditis in a dog. JAVMA 1995;206:1561–1564.

261. Thomas WP, Reed JR, Bauer TG. Constrictive pericardial disease in the dog. JAVMA 1984;184:546–553.

262. Mantri RR, Singh M, Radhakrishnan S, et al. Left atrial dilation in constrictive pericarditis: a pre and post-operative echocardiographic study. Intern J Cardiol 1994;45:69–75.

263. Yaphé W, Giovengo S, Moise S. Severe cardiomegaly secondary to anemia in a kitten. JAVMA 1993;202:961–964.

264. Varat MA, Adolph RJ, Fowler NO. Cardiovascular effects of anemia. Am Heart J 1972;83:415–426.

265. Nakajima T, Fujioka S, Tokunaga K, et al. Noninvasive study of left ventricular performance in obese patients: influence of duration of obesity. Circulation 1985;71: 481–486.

266. Chakko S, Mayor M, Allison MD, et al. Abnormal left ventricular diastolic filling in eccentric left ventricular hypertrophy of obesity. Am J Cardiol 1991;68:95–98.

267. Stoddard MF, Tseuda K, Thomas M, et al. The influence of obesity on left ventricular filling and systolic function. Am Heart J 1992;124:694–699.

268. Alpert MA, Hashimi MW. Obesity and the heart. Am J Med Sci 1993;306:117–123.

269. Romano M, Carella G, Cotecchia MR, et al. Abnormal systolic time intervals in obesity. Am Heart J 1986;112:356–360.

270. De Divitiis O, Fazio S, Petitto M, et al. Obesity and cardiac function. Circulation 1981;64:477–482.

271. Gordon T, Kannel WB. Obesity and cardiovascular diseases: the Farmingham study. Clin Endocrinol Metab 1976;5:367–375.

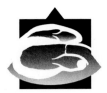

5

Congenital Heart Disease

▼

The echocardiographic evaluation of congenital heart disease is probably the most challenging application of cardiac ultrasound. If the cardiac examination is approached in a logical manner and all aspects of the heart are systematically examined, most defects will be found and accurately diagnosed. Doppler echocardiography helps positively identify some defects. Many congenital heart defects, however, exist in combination with other defects. Use common sense and logic when assessing the changes seen in the heart. Each defect creates predictable changes in cardiac chamber and vessel size even when other concurrent abnormalities are present. Changes not consistent with a visible defect imply the presence of another defect. Following are the descriptions of individual defects.

OBSTRUCTIONS TO FLOW

Outflow obstructions created by aortic or pulmonic stenosis create excessive work for the ventricles and lead to concentric hypertrophy of the respective chamber. The hypertrophy develops to normalize systolic wall stress (1). Pulmonic stenosis causes hypertrophy of both the right ventricular wall and the septum, whereas aortic stenosis causes increased free wall and septal thicknesses. Typically, the chamber size is smaller than normal secondary to the hypertrophy. Mild obstructions to outflow may not result in any visible changes within the heart; therefore, Doppler studies are necessary to confirm the presence of mild stenosis on either side of the heart.

Inflow obstruction secondary to mitral and tricuspid stenosis is much less common. The resistance to filling of the ventricular chambers results in dilated atria. The atrioventricular valves often are incompetent as well.

The varying morphologic manifestations of these stenotic lesions are presented here. Regardless of the appearance of the valves, outflow tracts, or inflow tracts the effects on the ventricular or atrial chambers are similar.

Outflow Obstructions

Aortic Stenosis

Subaortic stenosis is a common defect in large breed dogs. The golden retriever, rottweiler, boxer, German shepherd, pointer, and Newfoundland are among the breeds most susceptible to this congenital defect. Aortic stenosis is rare in cats and cows but features of the disease are similar to those found in dogs and humans (2–10).

FIGURE 5.1 A fibrous band (*arrow*) is seen just below the aortic valve in this dog with subvalvular aortic stenosis. There is visible concentric left ventricular hypertrophy but no apparent muscular obstruction. *Plane*, right parasternal left ventricular outflow view; *RV*, right ventricle; *LV*, left ventricle; *AO*, aorta; *LA*, left atrium.

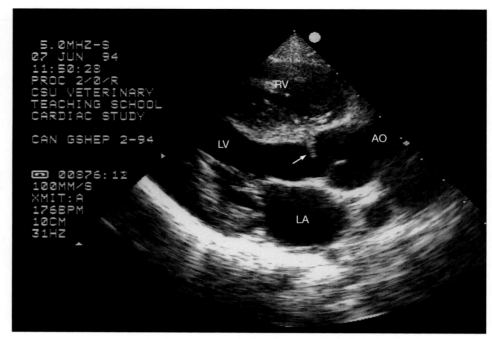

FIGURE 5.2 The discrete fibrous ring (*arrow*) is in close proximity to the aortic valves in this dog with aortic stenosis. There appears to be some impingement of the muscular septum into the outflow tact (*large arrow*). *Plane*, modified right parasternal long-axis left ventricular outflow view; *LV*, left ventricle; *AOV*, aortic valve; *MV*, mitral valve.

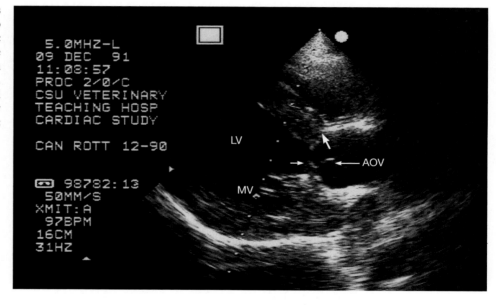

Aortic stenosis may manifest as supravalvular, valvular, or subvalvular. Although supravalvular stenosis is extremely rare in other animals, it frequently is seen in cats (9). Valvular stenosis also rarely is seen as a single entity but does occur in conjunction with the most common form of stenosis, the subvalvular form (11,12). Supravalvular stenosis in the cat often is accompanied by valvular stenosis as well (9). Regardless of the type of stenosis, the effects on the heart are similar. Only the stenotic lesion itself will differ in appearance.

The left ventricular outflow obstruction may be discrete and fixed in that a fibrous ring is present within the left ventricular outflow tract. This band of tissue may be small and may encircle the outflow tract with very little protrusion into the lumen of the tract or it may be extensive, creating a small orifice for blood flow. Fibrous rings may be seen just below the aortic valve on right parasternal left ventricular outflow views (Figs. 5.1 and 5.2). Small fibrous bands may not be visualized. Tilt the transducer back and forth and in and out of the long-axis plane to bring the

Subvalvular Aortic Stenosis

Features of the Obstruction

- Fibrous ring is below aortic valves.
- Ring may pull mitral valve up to outflow tract.
- Small fibrous bands may not be seen.
- If a dynamic component is present, the band usually extends from it.
- Rarely, the anterior mitral valve is stiff and creates a tunnel.
- Rarely, there may be hypoplasia of the annulus.

obstructive band into view. The ring is usually in close proximity to the aortic valve annulus, but it may be seen further down into the outflow tract several millimeters away from the annulus (Fig. 5.3). The band of tissue is reflected onto the mitral annulus, which can be appreciated on real-time images (13). The mitral valve leaflet is pulled up toward the outflow tract before extending into the ventricular chamber instead of normally extending straight out from the posterior aortic wall (Figs. 5.1 and 5.4).

Subaortic stenosis also may manifest as a dynamic obstruction involving hypertrophy or a muscular ridge at the base of the interventricular septum. This is seen best on right parasternal long-axis left ventricular outflow views. The muscle impinges into the outflow tract and the obstruction becomes even greater during contraction (3) (Fig. 5.5). The degree of obstruction can vary from beat to beat depending on loading conditions, heart rate, sympathetic stimulation, etc. Dynamic

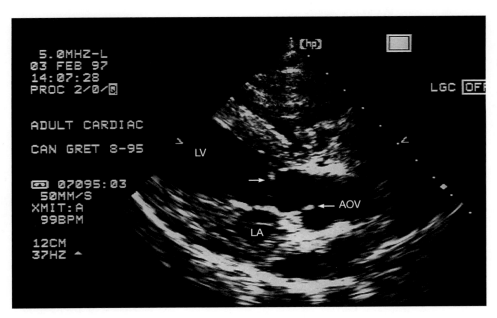

FIGURE 5.3 The fibrous tissue creating outflow obstruction (arrow) is located further down in the left ventricular outflow tract of this dog. No dynamic component is visible. Plane, modified right parasternal long-axis left ventricular outflow view; LV, left ventricle; AOV, aortic valve; LA, left atrium.

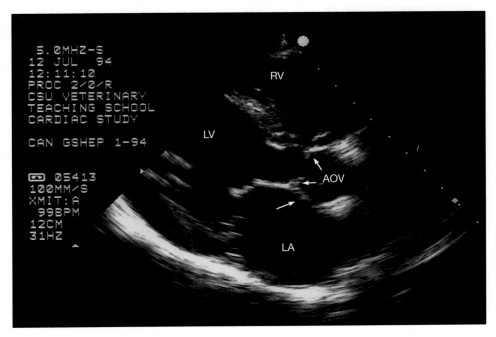

FIGURE 5.4 The mitral valve is pulled up toward the outflow tract (arrow), a sign that a ring is present even when a fibrous band is not visualized. The left atrium and ventricle appear dilated as well as hypertrophied, suggesting that a concurrent problem creating volume overload is present in addition to the obstruction. Plane, right parasternal long-axis left ventricular outflow view; RV, right ventricle; LV, left ventricle; AOV, aortic valve; LA, left atrium.

FIGURE 5.5 Significant concentric hypertrophy is present in this dog with dynamic subvalvular obstruction. The muscle protrudes into the outflow tract (*arrow*). There is no visible ring. *View*, right parasternal long-axis left ventricular outflow view; *RV*, right ventricle; *VS*, ventricular septum; *AO*, aorta; *LA*, left atrium; *LVW*, left ventricular wall.

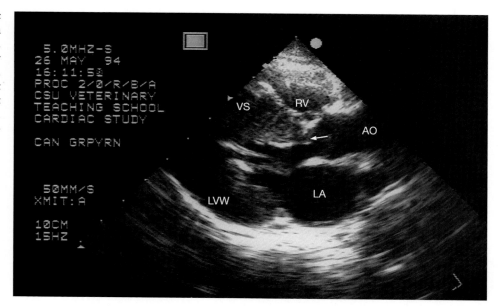

FIGURE 5.6 The fibrous ring extends from the base of the septum at its maximum extension into the outflow tract when both dynamic and discrete obstructions are present (*arrow*). *Plane*, right parasternal long-axis left ventricular outflow view; *LV*, left ventricle; *AO*, aorta; *LA*, left atrium.

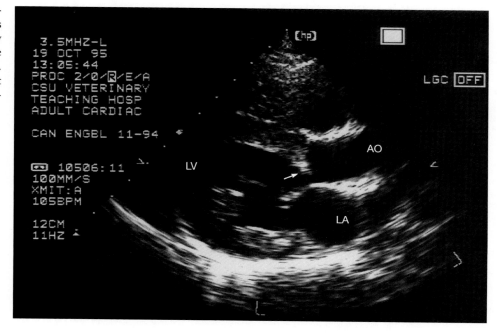

and fixed obstructions may occur together, with the fibrous ring extending from the base of the septum at its maximum extension into the outflow tract (Fig. 5.6).

Sometimes a tunnel type of stenosis is present. The mitral valve is stiff and forms the posterior wall of the obstructive subvalvular tunnel while the septum forms the anterior wall of the tunnel (Fig. 5.7). The mitral valve may be dysplastic. A fibrous band may be present but is often difficult to see in these hearts. The width of the tunnel is much less than the width of the aorta (13).

The annulus of the aorta also may be affected. A small diameter at the level of the leaflets is seen when hypoplasia of the aorta exists (Fig. 5.8). There may or may not be dynamic obstruction or a subvalvular membrane with this type of stenosis. This form of stenosis also has been seen in calves (9).

Partial fusion of the cusps can exist and may be seen on long- or short-axis views of the aortic valves (Fig. 5.9). Asymmetric opening of the cusps is especially easy to see on heart base transverse views. This is difficult to identify on M-mode images because reduced flow through the valves will cause incomplete opening of the valve on M-mode images. Stiff, immobile leaflets without fusion may be seen with any of the manifestations of aortic stenosis especially in boxers and cats (14–16) (Fig. 5.10). Aortic valve dysplasia has been reported in the cow. Thick, malformed cusps caused stenosis and significant insufficiency (8).

The post stenotic dilation observed with aortic stenosis may be seen on right parasternal long-axis left ventricular outflow views of the heart, but it is seen best on left parasternal cranial long-axis images of the left ventricular outflow tract and aorta (Figs. 5.8 and 5.11). The walls of the aorta diverge away from each other, distal to the aortic valves. The sinus of Valsalva often is dilated, and sometimes one or both of the coronary artery ostia may be dilated as well.

Measuring the left ventricular free wall and septum will reveal the presence of hypertrophy (11–13,17). This increase in thickness may be apparent even without

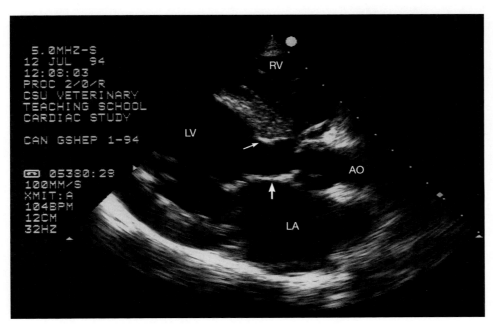

FIGURE 5.7   A stiff anterior mitral valve leaflet helps form a tunnel type of subvalvular stenosis (*arrow*). On real-time images, the mitral valve would show limited motion and may be insufficient. A small muscular ridge is seen in the outflow tract as well (*small arrow*). *Plane*, right parasternal long-axis left ventricular outflow view; *RV*, right ventricle; *LV*, left ventricle; *LA*, left atrium; *AO*, aorta.

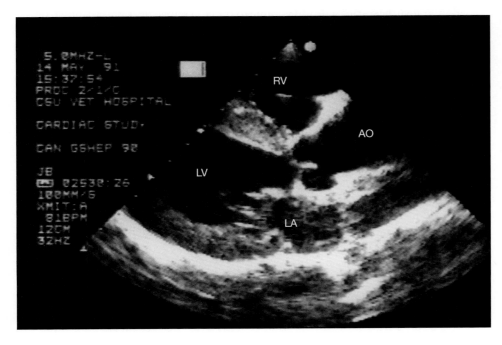

FIGURE 5.8   A small diameter at the level of the aortic valves is seen when aortic annulus hypoplasia creates restriction to flow. A poststenotic dilation is seen. *Plane*, right parasternal long-axis left ventricular outflow view; *RV*, right ventricle; *LV*, left ventricle; *AO*, aorta; *LA*, left atrium.

FIGURE 5.9   The aortic valve cusps do not open symmetrically on this transverse view of the valve, indicating some degree of valvular fusion (*arrow*). *Plane*, right parasternal transverse heart base; *RV*, right ventricle; *RA*, right atrium; *LA*, left atrium.

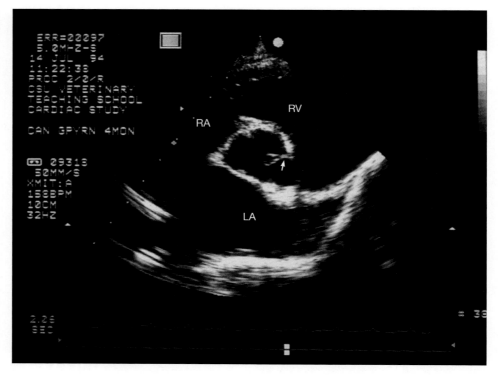

Look for valvular insufficiencies or a shunt if normal or increased LV chamber size is present with moderate to severe aortic stenosis.

quantitative measurements. The degree of hypertrophy correlates well with the severity of the obstruction; however, there are exceptions. Mild hypertrophy sometimes is seen with Doppler-documented moderate to severe obstructions, and conversely, severe gradients sometimes are recorded when little hypertrophy is present. Perhaps the variability, duration, frequency, and severity of dynamic obstruction on a day-to-day basis plays a role in the degree of hypertrophy as is seen in humans with systemic hypertension. The degree of hypertrophy in human patients with hypertension is variable and greatly depends on the duration, frequency, and severity of hypertension during daily activities (18). Some animals have little if any obstruction at rest, but have dramatic gradients when excited as might be expected during some echocardiographic examinations.

Valvular insufficiencies will add volume to the concentrically hypertrophied heart. When quantitative assessment of the left ventricle in a young animal reveals normal left ventricular chamber size, despite hypertrophy of the wall and septum, and a discrete aortic stenosis is clearly apparent, then significant valvular insufficiencies or a shunt of some type is typically present (Fig. 5.12). Myocardial failure in older dogs may affect the ability of the heart to hypertrophy adequately, and a more eccentric pattern of enlargement may be seen in these dogs as well.

Both mitral and aortic insufficiencies are seen with subaortic stenosis (2,13,14). Mitral insufficiency may be secondary to dysplasia but more often is secondary to systolic anterior mitral valve motion (3,13). Aortic insufficiency has been reported in one-half to over three-quarters of dogs with aortic stenosis (13,19) (Fig. 5.13). Infective endocarditis is a complication that may develop as the animal becomes older; it was seen in approximately 5% of dogs in one study (2). Congestive heart failure will develop as a consequence of the significant aortic or mitral insufficiency that develops. Congestive heart failure is otherwise fairly uncommon in dogs with subaortic stenosis (2,14).

Left ventricular systolic function is well preserved in hearts with aortic stenosis. Fractional shortening is high and velocity of circumferential shortening increases in young animals with aortic stenosis (11,17). Ejection time typically is normal (17). The myocardium may start to fail when the stenosis is severe or when the disease has been long standing, creating a large load on the heart. The myocardium often displays areas with increased echogenicity indicative of myocardial fibrosis (Fig. 5.14). This is seen in more severely affected animals; myocardial function may be compromised if the fibrosis is extensive. The papillary muscles and the base of the ventricular septum are common sites for fibrosis (Fig. 5.14). The increased echogenicity is seen easily on transverse and long-axis views (3,12).

Left atrial enlargement sometimes is seen in dogs and cats with aortic stenosis (4,17) (Fig. 5.12). There are several potential causes for atrial dilation with subaortic stenosis. Systolic anterior motion of the mitral valve invariably causes the valve to leak. The mitral valve being involved with the fibrous band of tissue creating the obstruction may be insufficient secondary to structural or functional abnormalities

Subvalvular Aortic Stenosis
─────────────────────────────

Hemodynamic Effects
- Concentric hypertrophy
- Function usually preserved
- Systolic anterior motion seen with dynamic obstruction
- Systolic aortic valve closure possible

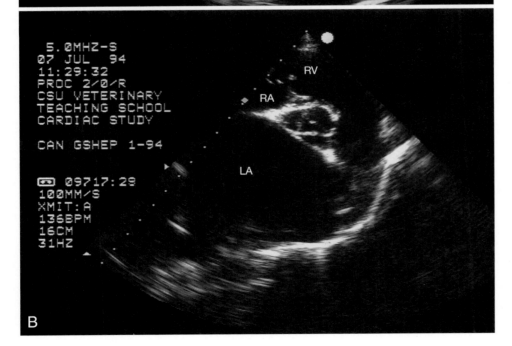

FIGURE 5.10   Stiff, immobile aortic valve cusps without fusion are barely separated at maximal opening (*arrows*). This can be seen on both (**A**) long-axis and (**B**) transverse right parasternal views. *AOV*, aortic valve; *RV*, right ventricle; *LV*, left ventricle; *LA*, left atrium; *RA*, right atrium.

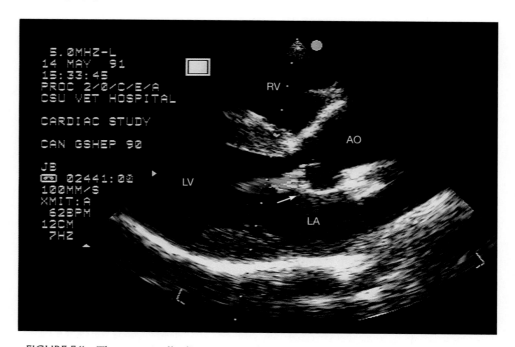

FIGURE 5.11   The aorta walls diverge away from each other in poststenotic dilation of the ascending aorta. The mitral valve is pulled up toward the outflow tract (*arrow*) indicating the presence of a fibrous band even though it is not seen. Very mild aortic insufficiency is present. *Plane,* right parasternal long-axis left ventricular outflow view; *RV,* right ventricle; *LV,* left ventricle; *LA,* left atrium; *AO,* aorta.

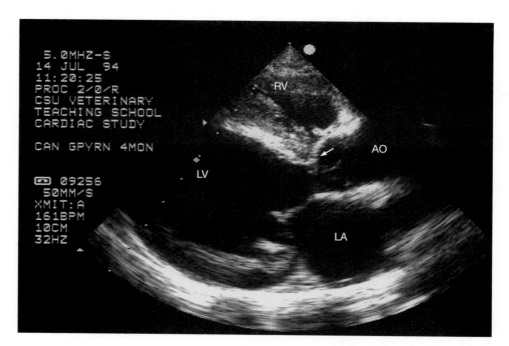

FIGURE 5.12   The infundibular hypertrophy creating outflow obstruction is clearly visible here (*arrow*). Volume overload of the left ventricular and atrial chambers is present. A valvular insufficiency or shunt should be suspected when volume overload exists as well as hypertrophy in young animals with subaortic stenosis. *Plane,* right parasternal long-axis left ventricular outflow view; *RV,* right ventricle; *AO,* aorta; *LV,* left ventricle; *LA,* left atrium.

(Fig. 5.4). Diastolic dysfunction also may be present, leading to a back-up of pressure into the left atrium as the failure progresses (4,10). Some degree of mitral insufficiency is seen in many dogs with aortic stenosis (13,20).

Dynamic outflow obstruction displays the same type of M-mode echocardiographic findings as those seen with obstruction secondary to hypertrophic cardiomyopathy. Systolic anterior motion of the mitral valve confirms the presence of high-velocity flow within the outflow tract. As in hypertrophic obstructive cardiomyopathy, the degree and duration of systolic anterior motion is indicative of the severity of the gradient. Longer apposition to the septum is associated with more severe obstruction (21). Early systolic closure of the aortic valve is seen in almost one-half of dogs with aortic stenosis as flow is interrupted secondary to the obstruction. Systolic closure is seen with both discrete and dynamic aortic stenosis (10–13) (Fig. 5.15).

Color-flow Doppler identifies the turbulent and high-velocity blood flow through the outflow tract and aorta. The aliased color signal helps identify the length and location of a subvalvular obstruction (Figs. 5.16, 5.17, and 5.18). Color-flow Doppler, if available, also should be used to help align the spectral Doppler beam. Although color-flow Doppler is not necessary to evaluate the severity of the stenosis, it helps to identify quickly other complicating factors such as insufficiencies and concurrent shunts.

Left parasternal apical five-chamber views of the heart are used to record spectral Doppler flow through the stenotic region and aorta. Pulsed-wave Doppler can be used to identify the exact location of the obstruction, but otherwise is of little value in assessing the high-velocity flow of aortic stenosis. Move the gate along the outflow tract and into the aorta. An aliased signal will be seen when the high-velocity flow secondary to the obstruction is met. Continuous-wave Doppler will record the high-velocity flow through the stenotic region, and the Bernoulli equation can be applied to calculate a pressure gradient. The Doppler ultrasound beam needs to be as parallel with flow as possible to derive accurate measures of velocity. Deviation from parallel by greater than 15 to 20° will underestimate significantly the severity of the obstruction (22,23). The site of the stenosis does not always line up with the aortic

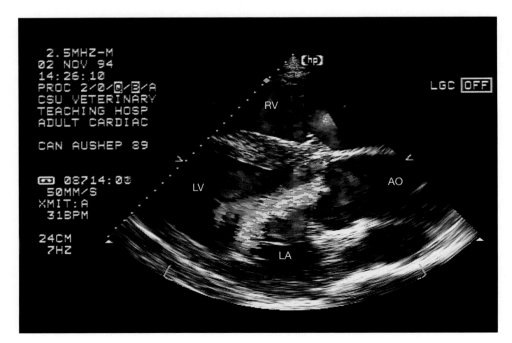

FIGURE 5.13 Aortic insufficiency is present in over three-quarters of dogs with aortic stenosis. The insufficiency here is moderate. *Plane,* right parasternal long-axis left ventricular outflow view; *RV,* right ventricle; *LV,* left ventricle; *AO,* aorta; *LA,* left atrium.

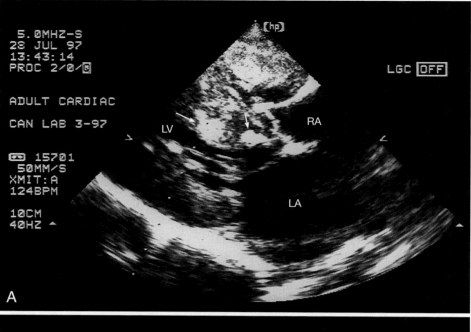

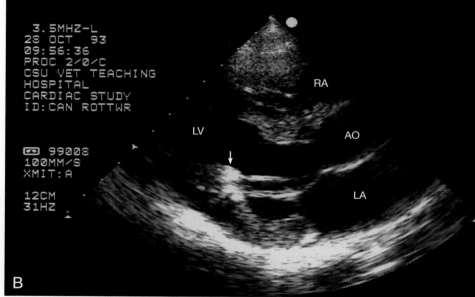

FIGURE 5.14   Areas of increased echogenicity within the myocardium are indicative of myocardial fibrosis. **A.** This interventricular septum contains multiple hyperechoic areas consistent with fibrosis (*arrow*). **B.** Papillary muscles are common sites of fibrosis (*arrow*). Planes: *A*, right parasternal long-axis four chamber; *B*, right parasternal left ventricular outflow view; *LV*, left ventricle; *RA*, right atrium; *LA*, left atrium; *AO*, aorta.

walls, and the beam should not be placed parallel to the aortic walls as they usually are when interrogating the aorta for other reasons. The outflow tract is aligned at an angle toward the mitral valve leaflets in the presence of subvalvular aortic stenosis. All possible angles should be interrogated to determine what the highest velocity truly is (Fig. 5.19).

The flow profile is different than that seen with normal aortic or outflow tract flow. Peak velocity is reached closer to the midpoint of ventricular systole as opposed to within the first third of systole (Figs. 5.20 and 5.21). The flow profile becomes more symmetric as the pressure gradient increases. When dynamic obstruction is present, it may be possible to record the concave dagger shape during acceleration. This is a reflection of the reduction in forward flow as the septum contracts.

One study has shown that the optimal window for recording the flow velocities in aortic stenosis when using a dedicated Doppler probe is the subcostal window (20). Maximal velocities were underestimated by 26% when flow was interrogated

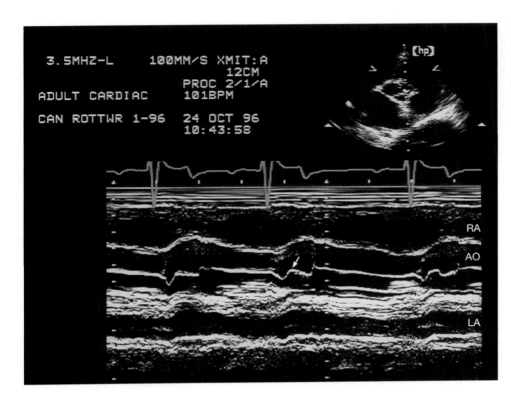

FIGURE 5.15 Early systolic closure of the aortic valve cusps (*arrow*) is seen in almost one-half of dogs with aortic stenosis and may be seen with both discrete and dynamic obstructions to flow. *RA*, right atrium; *AO*, aorta; *LA*, left atrium.

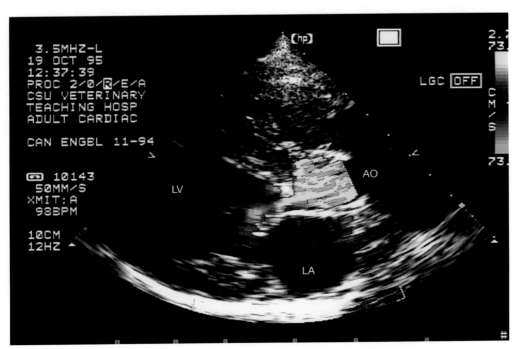

FIGURE 5.16 The aliased color-flow pattern starts at the level of obstruction in this dog with both dynamic and discrete obstruction. *Plane*, right parasternal long-axis left ventricular outflow view; *LV*, left ventricle; *AO*, aorta; *LA*, left atrium.

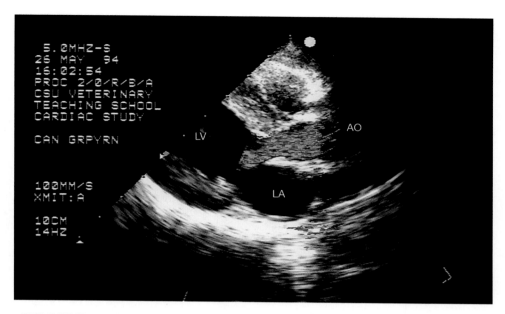

FIGURE 5.17   In this dog with subvalvular dynamic obstruction, the aliased color-flow pattern starts at the point where the infundibular septum has its maximal excursion into the outflow tract. *Plane,* right parasternal long-axis left ventricular outflow view; *LV,* left ventricle; *LA,* left atrium; *AO,* aorta.

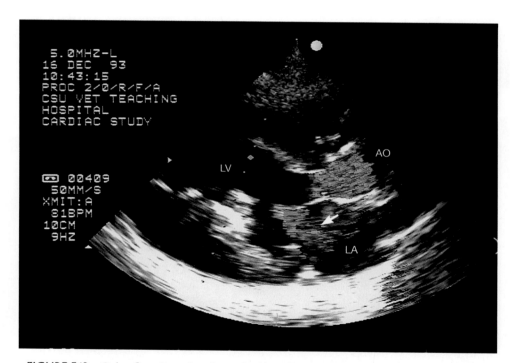

FIGURE 5.18   Color-flow Doppler shows both outflow obstruction and mitral insufficiency (*arrow*) in this dog with dynamic obstruction. The mitral valve is pulled up toward the outflow tract implying the presence of a fibrous ring as well. Fibrosis is present within the papillary muscle. *Plane,* right parasternal long-axis left ventricular outflow view; *LV,* left ventricle; *LA,* left atrium; *AO,* aorta.

on left apical windows as compared to subcostal windows. The animals, however, were sedated, and the pressure needed to use a subcostal window is typically uncomfortable in the awake dog. Experience also plays a role here, and parasternal apical windows are just as valid in the hands of an experienced sonographer. With the exception of examinations in surgical candidates for postoperative gradient comparison or for research studies, a pressure gradient above 90 mm Hg in a parasternal window is adequate to assess the severity and define the prognosis in an animal. Where transducer location and velocity tracings may make a difference is in the identification of mild stenotic lesions. Flow velocities may exceed normal values in a subcostal window and still be normal in a left apical parasternal window.

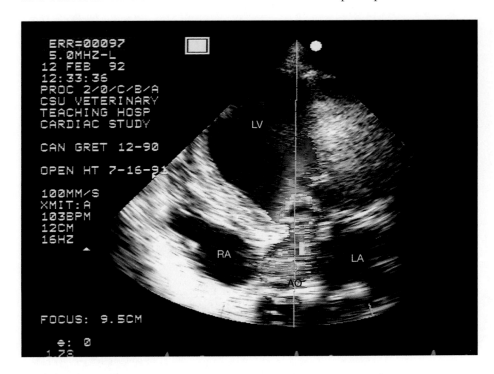

FIGURE 5.19   The outflow tract is not usually in line with the aorta when subvalvular obstruction exists. The Doppler beam should be aligned along the outflow tract if subvalvular stenosis is present as opposed to being parallel to the aorta walls. Color-flow Doppler can identify the direction of high-velocity flow. *Plane*, left parasternal apical five-chamber view; *LV*, left ventricle; *RA*, right atrium; *AO*, aorta.

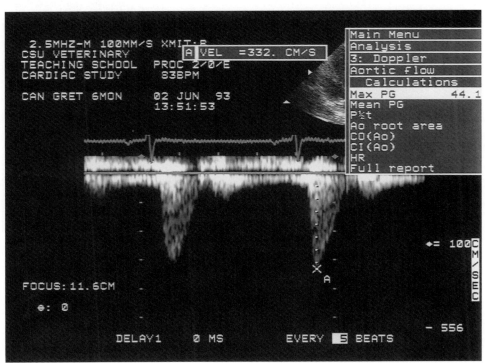

FIGURE 5.20   Mild aortic stenosis is present in this dog with a flow velocity of 332 cm/sec and a pressure gradient of 44 mm Hg. The flow profile remains normal in shape when mild obstruction is present.

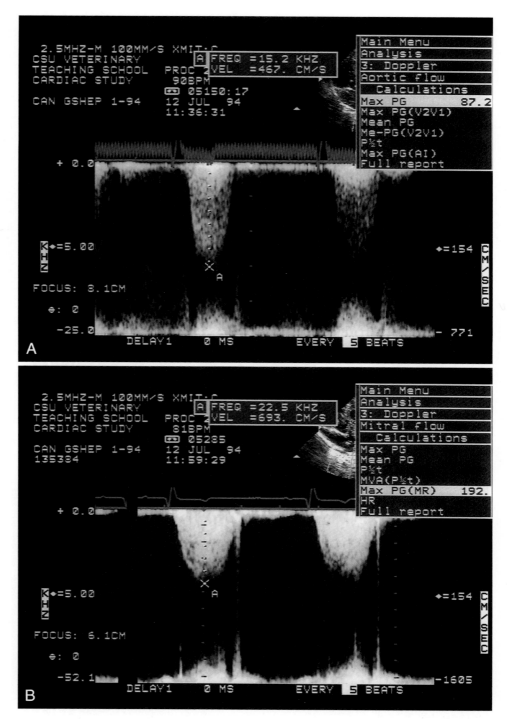

FIGURE 5.21 **A.** As aortic stenosis becomes more severe, the Doppler flow profile changes from its normal shape. Peak velocity is reached closer to mid systole and its shape is more symmetric. The start of ejection coincides with the latter part of the QRS complex. **B.** Mitral insufficiency jets may be recorded by mistake when trying to obtain aortic flow velocities. Mitral regurgitant jets start early in systole near the onset of the QRS and end later than aortic flow, well beyond the T wave.

Real-time images do not show evidence of abnormalities when obstruction is this mild (20).

Take care to record outflow tract and aortic flow and not mitral regurgitant flow when trying to obtain velocities for pressure gradients. Color-flow Doppler helps localize the turbulent jet, but patient movement, respiratory movement, and motion of the heart can complicate matters, and a mitral regurgitant jet inadvertently may be recorded instead of outflow. Mitral regurgitation will start early in the systolic period, and flow is seen near the onset of the QRS complex. Left ventricular outflow and aortic flow will start later in systole coinciding with the latter part of the QRS complex (Fig. 5.21). Mitral regurgitant flow also lasts longer and extends well beyond the T wave, because insufficiencies typically last into the isovolumic relaxation phase of diastole (20,24) (Fig. 5.21). Mistaking a mitral regurgitant jet for aortic flow occurs more often when a nonimaging Doppler probe is used.

> Mitral regurgitation like aortic outflow is also negative and has high velocities, but starts earlier and lasts longer than aortic outflow.

When mitral insufficiency is present, the pressure gradient of the regurgitant jet should be used if possible to confirm the pressure gradient obtained across the stenosis (Fig. 5.21). A gradient across an aortic stenosis of 100 mm Hg indicates left ventricular pressures of at least 200 mm Hg, and the mitral regurgitation velocity should reflect this pressure, measuring approximately 7 m/sec ($4 \times 7^2 = 196$). This assumes that left atrial enlargement is minimal and atrial pressures are estimated at less than 10 mm Hg.

> Use mitral insufficiency pressure gradients to confirm and support the gradient obtained across an aortic stenosis.

Pressure gradients of less than 50 mm Hg are considered mild in severity, and the animal may never show any clinical signs related to the disease. Pressure gradients between 50 and 80 mm Hg represent moderate obstruction to outflow, whereas gradients higher than this imply severe stenosis and carry a poorer prognosis for the animal (2,23).

Controversy still exists as to what velocity must be exceeded before the diagnosis of aortic stenosis can be made (14). Values range from greater than 170 cm/sec to greater than 250 cm/sec. There is agreement that velocities exceeding 250 cm/sec are consistent with the presence of aortic stenosis. Velocities greater than 200 cm/sec are uncommon in dogs but may be seen in athletic animals. When flow velocities fall between 200 and 250 cm/sec, one cannot determine if the animal is free from stenosis. Velocities less than 200 cm/sec are usually considered normal. Subvalvular aortic stenosis is a progressive disease and severity may increase until the animal is full grown. A normal pressure gradient at several weeks of age or a mild pressure gradient at a young age, therefore, does not represent the absence of disease or the presence of insignificant obstruction, because the disease may still progress to the severe stage (6,14,25).

> Doppler Assessment of Aortic Stenosis
> - Use left apical five chamber.
> - Gradients less than 50 = mild stenosis.
> - Gradients from 50 to 80 = moderate stenosis.
> - Gradients greater than 80 = severe obstruction.

The pressure gradient obtained from Doppler echocardiography is affected by cardiac output. Flow through the aorta and the size of the aortic orifice are important (24). Repeat evaluation where gradients are lower may indicate poorer flow through the aorta secondary to myocardial failure or more significant mitral insufficiency. Aortic insufficiency also affects velocity of flow because the regurgitant volume is involved in the aortic flow velocity (Fig. 5.22). Mild insufficiencies probably will not affect the gradient to any great degree, but moderate to severe insufficiencies, which are at times present, will overestimate the severity of the actual physical obstruction. The same applies to any other cardiac defect that adds volume to flow through the aorta. Do not base the diagnosis of aortic stenosis on high-velocity aortic flow alone. Patent ductus arteriosus may be found in conjunction with aortic stenosis and the severity of the stenosis cannot be determined accurately until the ductus has been ligated.

> When a PDA is present as well as AS, an accurate gradient cannot be derived.

Pulmonic Stenosis

Pulmonic stenosis occurs with a higher incidence in the bullmastiff, beagle, bulldog, boxer, spaniel, keeshond, Schnauzer, Chihuahua, and terrier breed (26–29). It has been reported in the cat as well (9,31). Pulmonic stenosis is valvular; however, fixed subvalvular constriction may occur by itself or in conjunction with the valvular stenosis. Subvalvular obstruction as a dynamic component also may develop secondary to compensatory hypertrophy. Supravalvular stenosis rarely occurs (27–31).

Four different views are available to image the pulmonic valves and artery: the right parasternal transverse and oblique views, and the left cranial pulmonary artery and transverse views. The site for the clearest valvular image varies from animal to animal, so all views should be used in evaluating dogs with pulmonic stenosis.

There are two types of valvular pulmonic stenosis. One involves thick immobile dysplastic cusps and the other involves fusion of the peripheral edges of the semilunar

FIGURE 5.22 Aortic insufficiency is present in most dogs with subvalvular aortic stenosis. Here, a Doppler signal indicates the presence of aortic insufficiency (*arrow*). The volume associated with the regurgitation will elevate systolic flow velocities and the calculated pressure gradient.

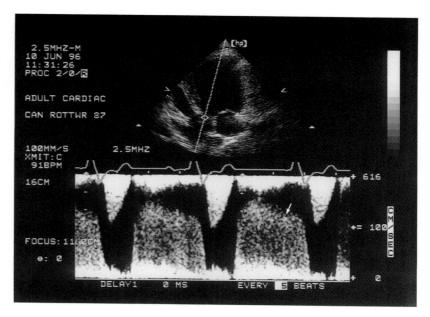

FIGURE 5.23 **A.** Doming of the pulmonic valve cusps (*arrow*) during systole is seen when pulmonic stenosis involves fusion of the leaflets. The body of the leaflet moves to the walls of the artery, but the tips remain pointed toward the center of the vessel. **B.** During diastole the cusps often appear to billow up toward the right ventricle (*arrow*), and the fused valve tips appear bright and thick. *Plane*, right parasternal transverse heart base; *RA*, right atrium; *RVW*, right ventricular wall; *RV*, right ventricle; *AO*, aorta; *PA*, pulmonary artery; *RMPA*, right main pulmonary artery.

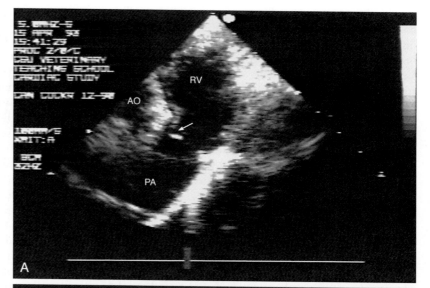

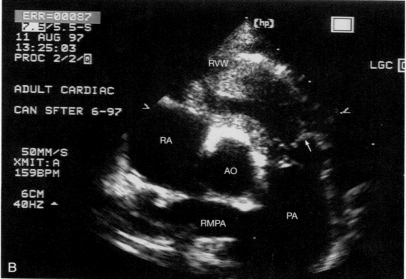

valves (12). When valvular fusion exists, the semilunar cusps are fused toward the tips of the leaflet, resulting in doming of the valves (Fig. 5.23). This means that the body of the leaflets moves toward the walls of the artery while the tips of the cusps remain pointed toward the center of the artery and stay in close proximity to each other throughout systole. Freeze-frame imaging of the leaflets show that the leaflets do not move toward the artery wall as they normally would. The severity of stenosis is related to the degree of fusion. When valvular dysplasia is present, the valve will appear thickened and immobile. There is often no fusion of the cusps, motion is restricted, and the annulus may be narrow and hypoplastic (12,29,30,32–34) (Fig. 5.24).

Infundibular hypertrophy may be part of the congenital lesion or may appear as a secondary change after concentric hypertrophy develops. The majority (96%) of dogs in a study that included 29 dogs had subvalvular hypertrophy (27,30). The muscle can be seen within the right ventricular outflow tract (Fig. 5.25). This is best seen on right parasternal transverse views because inadequate near field resolution sometimes precludes visualization of the hypertrophy on left cranial views. When color-flow Doppler is used, the narrow outflow tract can be defined with greater accuracy (Fig. 5.25).

The poststenotic dilation seen with pulmonic stenosis is seen best on right parasternal transverse views of the pulmonary artery. The pulmonary artery will become wider distal to the valves. This is different than the pulmonary artery dilation seen with pulmonary hypertension, patent ductus arteriosus, or other volume overloading of the artery. The width of the artery at the level of the stenotic pulmonic valves will remain normal, but may be smaller than normal if the annulus is hypoplastic. The dilation occurs beyond the valves (Fig. 5.24). With volume overload or pulmonary hypertension, the artery will be dilated at the level of the valves and remain dilated to the same degree distal to the valve. The dilated pulmonary artery segment may be seen as a prominent circular structure on right parasternal long-axis views below the aorta at the base of the left atrium. The degree of pulmonary artery dilation does not appear to correlate with the severity of the obstruction (29).

The afterload created by the obstruction to flow causes the right ventricular wall and interventricular septum to hypertrophy. Severe septal hypertrophy may contribute to the dynamic outflow obstruction on both the right and left side of the heart. The hypertrophy is concentric and a small ventricular chamber is seen (Fig. 5.26). Increases in chamber size suggest that significant tricuspid or pulmonic insufficiencies are present or possibly a shunt exists in addition to the pulmonic stenosis. When diastolic pressures are elevated paradoxical septal motion may be seen. The paradoxical motion is subtle unless the volume overload is significant (11,27,30).

Right atrial dilation is reported in dogs with pulmonic stenosis (27). This may be secondary to dilation and regurgitation as a result of diastolic or systolic dysfunction, or it may be secondary to tricuspid insufficiency caused by concurrent dysplasia (11,29) (Fig. 5.27). Almost 50% of dogs with pulmonic stenosis have some degree of tricuspid insufficiency. When tricuspid insufficiency is present, the regurgitant jet should be interrogated with a Doppler beam to help confirm the pressure gradient obtained across the pulmonic valve (Fig. 5.28). A tricuspid regurgitant jet also may be used to derive the only pressure gradient if it is difficult to obtain a pulmonary flow profile. A tricuspid regurgitant jet with velocities of 4.33 cm/sec, for instance, signifies that right ventricular systolic pressures are at least 75 mm Hg (4×4.33^2). If pulmonary artery pressures are close to normal at approximately 20 mm Hg, then a pressure gradient of 55 mm Hg can be applied to the pulmonic stenosis (right ventricular pressure is 55 mm Hg higher than the pulmonary artery pressure of 20 mm Hg).

When the pulmonic stenosis is moderate to severe, the left ventricular chamber size will decrease secondary to decreased right ventricular cardiac output. The left ventricular chamber will appear concentrically hypertrophied (Figs. 5.26 and 5.27). Wall and septal thickness will be higher than normal and chamber size will be small. The interventricular septum will bow down toward the left ventricular chamber because right-sided pressure will exceed left-sided pressures and paradoxical septal motion may be present. The left atrium also will be smaller than expected.

Pulmonic Stenosis

Features of the Obstruction
- Usually valvular
- Doming of leaflets indicates fusion.
- Dysplastic cusps are thick and immobile.
- Dynamic obstruction may be primary or secondary.

The diameter of the PA at the level of the valve is usually normal and dilates towards the bifurcation. This differentiates the dilation from that seen with pulmonary hypertension or PDA.

Pulmonic Stenosis

Hemodynamic Effects
- Concentric RV hypertrophy
- Good function
- The VS is involved in the hypertrophy.
- Motion of the VS is paradoxical only if valvular insufficiencies are present.
- The LV is small with moderate to severe pulmonic stenosis.

FIGURE 5.24 **A.** Valvular dysplasia is the cause of pulmonic stenosis in this dog. The valve leaflets are thick, echodense (*arrow*), and have reduced motion during systole. The pulmonic valves in this dog are thick and are obviously stenotic during real-time imaging. The annulus is still of normal size. Poststenotic dilation is present. **C.** Hypoplasia of the pulmonary annulus is present in this animal with pulmonic stenosis. The diameter of the artery is much smaller than the aorta. *Planes,* right parasternal transverse heart base; *RV,* right ventricle; *RA,* right atrium; *AO,* aorta; *RMPA,* right main pulmonary artery; *LMPA,* left main pulmonary artery.

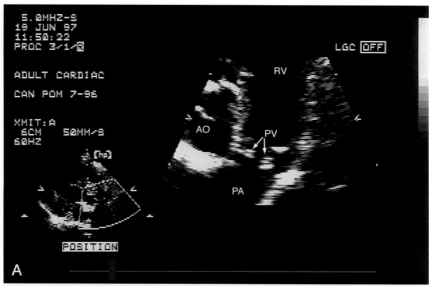

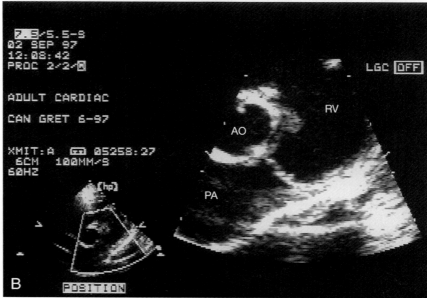

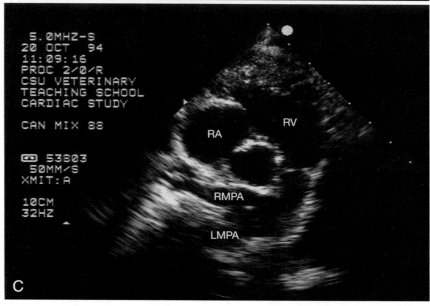

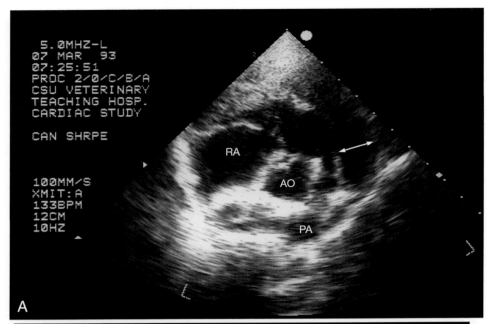

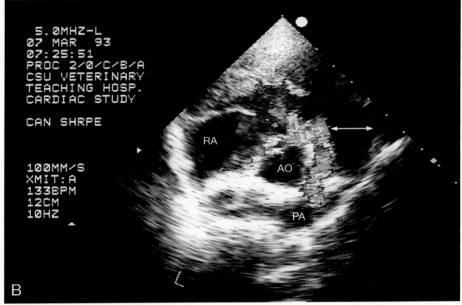

FIGURE 5.25 **A.** The lateral wall of the pulmonary outflow tract is hypertrophied, creating dynamic outflow obstruction in addition to the valvular stenosis. Lateral gain does not fill in the muscle (*arrow*) but color-flow Doppler (**B**) can identify the small outflow tract and narrowing at the level of the valves. *Plane*, right parasternal transverse heart base; *RA*, right atrium; *PA*, pulmonary artery; *AO*, aorta.

Spectral Doppler of the pulmonic stenosis will record high-velocity flow (22,23) (Fig. 5.29). Use a view that provides the highest flow velocities. If real-time images are inconclusive, a pulsed wave gate can be placed within the outflow tract to determine whether any subvalvular obstruction is present.

Normal pulmonary artery flow is typically less than 130 cm/sec but there are reports of normal flow up to 160 cm/sec. The assessment of severity is similar to that used in aortic stenosis. A gradient of less than 50 mm Hg is considered mild. Gradients between 51 and approximately 75 mm Hg are moderate in severity, and higher gradients are associated with severe pulmonic stenosis (23). More severe stenosis has a higher mortality rate (29). When dynamic outflow obstruction exists, a dagger-shaped flow profile will exist similar to that seen in aortic stenosis and hypertrophic cardiomyopathy.

Doppler Assessment of Pulmonic Stenosis

- Try all three views and use the highest velocity.
- Gradients less than 50 = mild stenosis.
- Gradients from 50 to 80 = moderate stenosis.
- Gradients greater than 80 = severe obstruction.

Use tricuspid insufficiency pressure gradients to confirm and support the gradient obtained across the pulmonic stenosis.

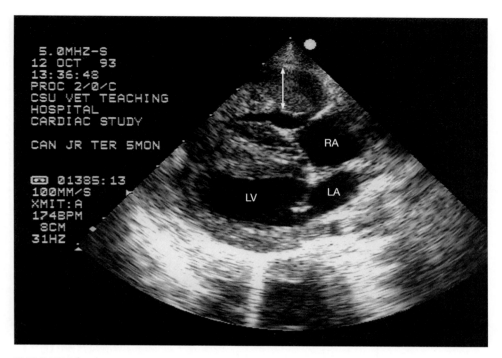

FIGURE 5.26 Concentric right ventricular hypertrophy develops secondary to the increased afterload created by pulmonic stenosis. The right ventricular wall is thick (*arrow*) and the chamber is small. The left ventricular chamber is usually small secondary to decreased preload when stenosis is moderate to severe. *Plane*, right parasternal four-chamber view; *RA*, right atrium; *LV*, left ventricle; *LA*, left atrium.

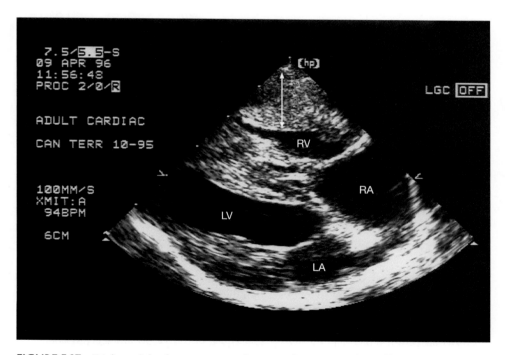

FIGURE 5.27 Right atrial enlargement may be seen when tricuspid insufficiency or ventricular dysfunction is present in hearts with pulmonic stenosis. The right ventricular wall (*arrow*) is severely hypertrophied and the left ventricular chamber appears concentrically hypertrophied as well. *Plane*, right parasternal long-axis four-chamber view; *RV*, right ventricle; *RA*, right atrium; *LV*, left ventricle; *LA*, left atrium.

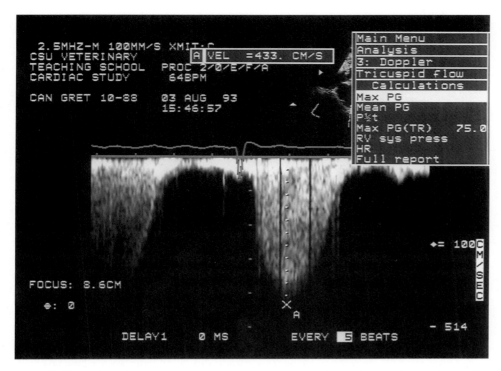

FIGURE 5.28 The velocity of a tricuspid regurgitant jet can be used to confirm or derive the pressure gradient across the pulmonary artery when pulmonic stenosis is present. Here, right ventricular pressures are at least 75 mm Hg based on the tricuspid regurgitant jet velocity. If pulmonary artery pressures are normal at approximately 20 mm Hg the pressure gradient across the stenosis must be close to 55 mm Hg.

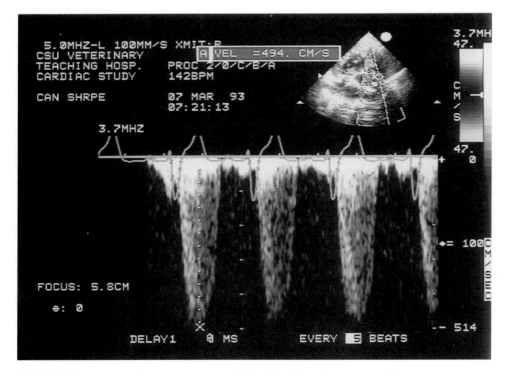

FIGURE 5.29 High-velocity flow is recorded within the pulmonary outflow tract or across the valves when pulmonic stenosis exists. Here, velocities of 494 cm/sec are consistent with a pressure gradient of 97 mm Hg and severe stenosis.

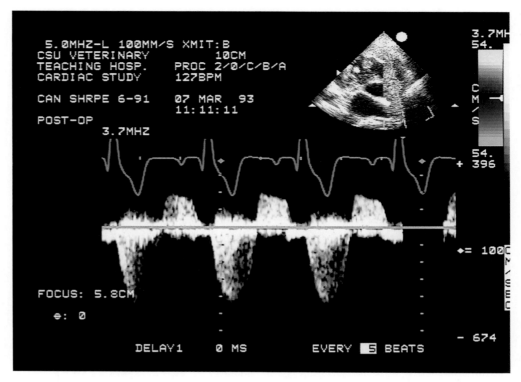

FIGURE 5.30   Pulmonic insufficiency and stenosis are recorded on this Doppler tracing. Significant pulmonic insufficiency will elevate the derived pressure gradient.

Color-flow Doppler helps define the extent of obstruction. The mosaic pattern associated with turbulence and high velocity will start at the level of the valves when valvular obstruction is present. The outflow tract will be defined by the aliased color flow signal when either fixed or dynamic subvalvular obstruction is present. The location and width of the outflow tract and the valvular orifice are well defined with color but usually overestimate the size of the stenotic area. If available, use color-flow Doppler to help align the spectral Doppler beam properly.

As with aortic stenosis, flow through the pulmonary artery affects the derived pressure gradient. Any shunt or significant pulmonic insufficiency that adds volume to the pulmonary flow will increase the pulmonary flow velocity (Fig. 5.30). The pressure gradient will not truly reflect the degree of physical obstruction.

Left-to-right shunts will increase velocities across a valve and will increase the derived pressure gradient.

Inflow Obstructions

Mitral Stenosis

Mitral stenosis is a rare congenital abnormality in dogs and cats that may occur as a single entity or in combination with other defects. In humans, it often is found in conjunction with subaortic stenosis, patent ductus arteriosus, ventricular septal defect, endocardial fibroelastosis, and coarctation of the aorta. Mitral stenosis has been reported in dogs with subaortic stenosis, patent ductus arteriosus, and pulmonic stenosis (35). Mitral stenosis in humans usually is acquired secondary to endocarditis, rheumatic fever, or a variety of other causes; however, its development as an acquired lesion in animals cannot be confirmed (35). In the cat and dog, mitral stenosis may be related to congenital mitral valve dysplasia (35,36).

Mitral stenosis has varying morphologic features, which may include thickened leaflets with hypertrophied papillary muscles; a supravalvular ring; billowing leaflets with abnormal chordae all attached to one papillary muscle, creating a tunnel; and hypoplastic valves (35–37). The diagnosis of mitral stenosis was the first clinical application of ultrasound in the human; the disease has some characteristic echocardiographic findings. M-mode echocardiography shows thick mitral leaflets, parallel motion of the anterior and posterior mitral valve leaflets, reduced mitral valve EF slope, and a dilated left atrium. Two-dimensional findings include a dilated left atrium, doming of the mitral valve leaflets, reduced excursion of the mitral leaflets, thick mitral valve leaflets, and possibly a supravalvular ring (Figs. 5.31, 5.32, and 5.33). Doppler echocardiography will show high pressure gradients, increased pressure half-times, and often, mitral insufficiency (35–37).

Concordant mitral valve motion means the leaflets move in parallel—the posterior and anterior leaflets do not move away from each other as they normally do. The posterior leaflet will move upward toward the septum at the same time as the anterior leaflets. This is seen when there is fusion of the leaflets or commissures, which is easy to document on M-mode images. Two-dimensional images show doming of the mitral valve leaflets when there is fusion of the cusps (Fig. 5.32). The leaflet tips will point downward toward each other at maximal opening. The anterior leaflet body will bow or dome up toward the outflow tact, and sometimes the posterior leaflet domes toward the free wall of the left ventricle.

Mitral leaflet fusion also reduces the anterior and posterior excursion of the leaflets during diastole. To document the reduced excursion of the mitral tips during diastole, look at the leaflet tips and not along the leaflet body where they will billow up toward the outflow tract. To document this on M-mode images, the M-mode cursor must be positioned at the leaflet tips. The mitral valve EF slope also is reduced.

Although the finding of concordant motion is diagnostic of mitral stenosis, the latter two findings, reduced EF slope and reduced excursion, are not specific for the disease. Reduced excursion may be seen in the presence of aortic insufficiency, a common finding in dogs with subaortic stenosis. Almost one-half of dogs with mitral stenosis in one report also had subaortic stenosis (35). Poor flow into the left ventricle for any reason also will reduce mitral valve motion and excursion. Doming of the body of the leaflets will differentiate reduced motion secondary to aortic insufficiency

Mitral Stenosis

Features of the Obstruction
- Thick leaflets
- Doming of leaflets
- Abnormal papillary muscles
- Abnormal chordae
- Tunnel type of inflow
- Supravalvular ring

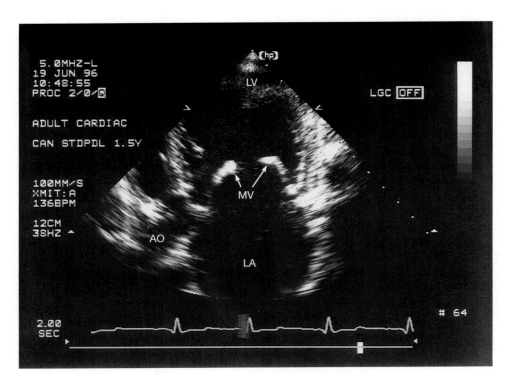

FIGURE 5.31 When the tips of the mitral valves point toward each other (*arrows*) as opposed to pointing toward the left ventricular camber during maximal mitral valve excursion, the leaflets dome, a sign of mitral stenosis. *Plane,* left parasternal apical five chamber; *LV,* left ventricle; *LA,* left atrium; *AO,* aorta; *MV,* mitral valve.

or reduced flow, from poor excursion secondary to mitral stenosis. Reduced ventricular compliance may cause slow early mitral valve closure, which often is seen with heart disease resulting in left ventricular hypertrophy. Reports show mitral stenosis in humans in which concordant mitral valve motion is not present or may not be evident (36–38).

Thick mitral valves are almost always present with mitral stenosis but also may be seen with dysplastic valves, subaortic stenosis, and acquired degenerative or infective lesions. The diagnosis of mitral stenosis, as opposed to these other differentials, can be made when the other features of stenosis are present, including: doming, reduced EF slope, concordant diastolic motion, and reduced pressure half-times (37).

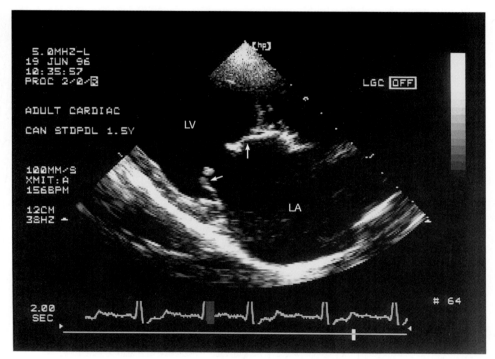

FIGURE 5.32 Doming of the mitral valves may be seen on parasternal long-axis views as well. The leaflet tips point toward each other at maximal excursion implying fusion of the valve leaflets. Both leaflets dome (arrows). The left atrium is dilated secondary to back pressure and possibly insufficiency. Plane, right parasternal long-axis four-chamber view; LV, left ventricle; LA, left atrium.

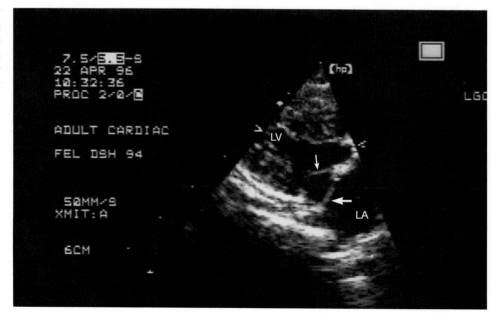

FIGURE 5.33 Mitral stenosis may manifest itself as a supravalvular ring (large arrow). The mitral valves are normal (small arrow). Plane, right parasternal long-axis four-chamber view; LV, left ventricle; LA, left atrium.

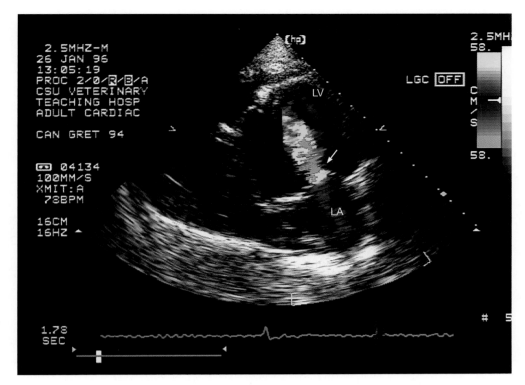

FIGURE 5.34   Color-flow Doppler shows a narrow aliased signal during diastole when mitral stenosis is present (*arrow*). The aliasing starts at the level of the narrow mitral valve orifice. *Plane*, left parasternal apical four chamber; *LV*, left ventricle; *LA*, left atrium.

Restriction to left ventricular filling causes left atrial pressures to increase and the left atrium to dilate (Fig. 5.32). Increases in left atrial pressure are affected by cardiac output. Increased volume flowing through the restricted orifice will elevate the transmitral pressure gradient. Elevations in pressure secondary to increases in output, such as excitement or exercise, may exacerbate the clinical signs associated with mitral stenosis. The development of atrial arrhythmias, especially atrial fibrillation, will decrease flow into the ventricle and elevate atrial pressures. The degree of left atrial dilation is affected not only by the obstruction to left ventricular inflow but also to the degree of mitral insufficiency.

Chronic elevation in left atrial and pulmonary venous pressure will lead to chronic interstitial changes within the pulmonary arterioles and secondary pulmonary hypertension. Pulmonary hypertension will affect the right side of the heart. Echocardiographic evidence of pulmonary hypertension includes right ventricular and pulmonary artery dilation, right ventricular hypertrophy, tricuspid insufficiency, and changes in the pulmonary flow profile. The echocardiographic findings in pulmonary hypertension are discussed in Chapter 4. When hypertension becomes significant, decreases in left ventricular preload may alleviate some of the symptoms of mitral stenosis (39).

The narrow mitral orifice secondary to fusion of the mitral valve commissures creates an aliased color jet flowing into the left ventricle during diastole representative of increased velocity and turbulence (Fig. 5.34). When an aortic valve or outflow tract disorder is also present, be sure to differentiate this mitral jet from diastolic aortic insufficiency within the outflow tract. Systolic aliased signals also may be seen because many of these patients have mitral insufficiency as well (35,37).

Spectral Doppler of mitral inflow shows high-velocity flow profiles with reduced slopes or lack of closure during early diastole. The inflow profile should be recorded from left parasternal apical four- or five-chamber views of the heart. The reduced

Mitral Stenosis
Hemodynamic Effects
- Concordant MV motion
- Dilated left atrium
- Increased pressure half-time
- Possible pulmonary hypertension
- Often, mitral insufficiency

Pressure Half-Time
Affected By
- Irregular heart rates
- Valvular insufficiencies

slope reflects lack of or delayed normal early diastolic closure (Fig. 5.35). Measurement of the slope allows calculation of a pressure half-time. Pressure half-time is the time required for pressure to decrease to one half its peak value. Normal pressure half-times in the dog are 29 ± 8 msec and are reported to be less than 30 msec in the cat. (35–37). Pressure half-times in mitral stenosis usually exceed 90 msec in humans and may be much higher. Reported pressure half-times exceed 80 msec in cats and 100 msec in dogs with mitral stenosis (35–37). The severity of stenosis correlates directly with pressure half-time. The longer the half-time the more severe the stenosis. Pressure half-times are affected by a variety of other factors including the presence of aortic insufficiency and irregular heart rhythms (37,40). The velocity across the stenosis directly depends on left ventricular pressures. In the presence of aortic insufficiency, left ventricular diastolic pressures increase more rapidly secondary to this second source of blood volume, especially if the insufficiency is acute. Pressure half-time will decrease correspondingly despite the presence of possible severe mitral stenosis. When measuring pressure half-times, be sure to trace the actual outline of the E to F slope. If the slope has a curve, follow the curve while tracing the slope. Ignore the A wave if present, use a sweep speed of 100 mm/sec for greater accuracy, and average at least 3 beats. If the animal is in atrial fibrillation or has another irregular rhythm, average the half-times of 5 to 10 beats (41).

Mitral valve area can be calculated using pressure half-times. This information is used to determine the timing of surgical intervention and is of lesser value at this time in animals. Apply the following equation to calculate an orifice area:

$$Area = 220/P\frac{1}{2}$$

where $P\frac{1}{2}$ is measured in msec, and the area is reported as cm^2.

Mitral valve area in humans also is measured directly from transverse images of the mitral valve. Normal mitral valve area in the dog is 3.69 ± 1.42 cm^2. An area greater than 2.5 cm^2 (normal, 4 to 6 cm^2) in humans typically creates only mild symptoms. In humans, a valve area of less than 1 cm^2/m^2 of body surface area represents severe mitral stenosis. This has not been studied in animals. Problems with direct measurement include poor resolution, improper selection of the frame for measurement, and gain settings. When the transverse image is not perpendicular to the mitral valve and an oblique view is used, the size of the mitral orifice may be assessed incorrectly. The tips of the mitral valve leaflets must be seen in cross section, otherwise the orifice size will be overestimated secondary to billowing of the body of the leaflets.

Mitral stenosis creates an obstruction to inflow that results in elevated left atrial pressures. The Bernoulli equation can be applied to peak or mean mitral inflow velocities to determine the pressure gradient. The more restrictive the stenosis, the higher the gradient. Normal dogs should have pressure gradients less than 5 mm Hg between the left atrium and left ventricle during diastole (35). A gradient greater than this suggests the presence of mitral stenosis (Fig. 5.35). Pressure gradients for any given orifice area, however, are influenced by the amount of volume flowing through it. For any given mitral valve area, larger volumes will increase the pressure gradient. Therefore, animals with mitral stenosis and significant mitral insufficiency will have higher pressure gradients than animals with the same valvular area and little or no mitral insufficiency. Likewise, low flow states will underestimate the pressure gradient. Elevations in left ventricular diastolic pressure secondary to aortic insufficiency or poor left ventricular compliance also will reduce the gradient derived for any given stenotic area.

Evidently, any one given feature of mitral stenosis cannot be used to make the diagnosis. A combination of features plus characteristic real-time images consistent with reduced mitral valvular motion, doming, thickened leaflets, abnormal chordae, supravalvular rings, etc., will provide accuracy in diagnosing mitral stenosis correctly, even if the assessment of severity is sometimes not possible.

Normal Pressure Half-Time

Dogs
    29 ± 8 msec
Cats
    < 30 msec

Normal MV Area

3.69 ± 1.42 cm^2
See appendix for correlation to BSA

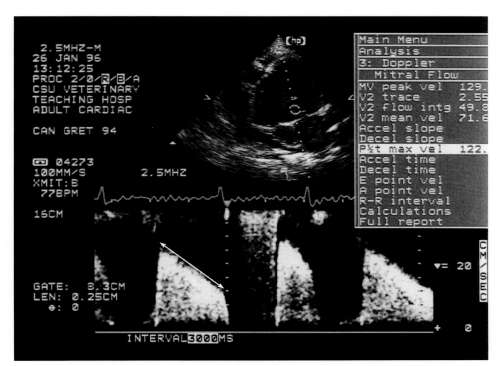

FIGURE 5.35   Spectral Doppler shows a reduced rate of mitral valve closure resulting in a long pressure half-time when mitral stenosis is present. The ultrasound machine will calculate pressure half-time when the closing slope is traced (*arrow*). The half-time here is 122. A pressure gradient also can be calculated from the mitral inflow profile. A mean gradient is more accurate than peak gradient. A gradient greater than 5 mm Hg suggests obstruction.

Tricuspid Stenosis

Congenital tricuspid stenosis is rare and not reported as a single entity in veterinary medicine. This is unrelated to tricuspid dysplasia or atresia. Tricuspid stenosis in conjunction with patent ductus arteriosus and pulmonic stenosis is described in an Arabian foal (42). Figure 5.36 shows an example of tricuspid stenosis in a dog.

The features of tricuspid stenosis are similar to those seen with mitral stenosis. There is doming of the leaflets, reduced excursion of the valve tips, concordant motion of the anterior and septal leaflets, a dilated right atrium, and often, tricuspid insufficiency. Spectral and color-flow Doppler findings also are similar.

CARDIAC SHUNTS

Congenital heart defects may occur by themselves or in combination with other defects. To identify all the defects that may be present in a young animal with congenital heart disease, one must understand what happens to the heart secondary to each abnormality. When considering intracardiac shunts, cardiac enlargement involves only those chambers that are included in the route of the shunting blood through the heart and lungs. A direct correlation exists between the clinical signs related to the cardiac shunt, the size of the defect, and the degree of volume overload in the involved chambers.

The pathway of blood in ventricular septal defect includes the left ventricle, right ventricle, pulmonary artery, left atrium, and back to the left ventricle. Only those chambers and vessels will be volume overloaded. The aorta and right atrium are not involved in the shunt pathway and, therefore, should be normal if no other defects are present.

Atrial septal defects cause shunting blood to flow through the left atrium, right atrium, right ventricle, pulmonary artery, and back to the left atrium. The left ventricle and aorta are not involved in the pathway and should be of normal size.

Patent ductus arteriosus includes the following in its shunt pathway: aorta, pulmonary artery, left atrium, left ventricle, and back to the aorta. The right atrium and ventricle are not part of the pathway and should not be enlarged if there are no other defects or complications.

Tricuspid Stenosis

Features of the Obstruction
- Thick leaflets
- Doming of leaflets
- Abnormal papillary muscles
- Abnormal chordae
- Tunnel type of inflow

Tricuspid Stenosis

Hemodynamic Effects
- Concordant TV motion
- Dilated right atrium
- Increased pressure half-time
- Often tricuspid insufficiency

Always measure pulmonary and aortic flow velocities in congenital heart disease. Increases in pulmonary flow suggest a VSD or ASD in the absence of PS. Increases in aortic flow suggest a PDA if AS is absent. These measures can help identify a defect not visible on real-time images.

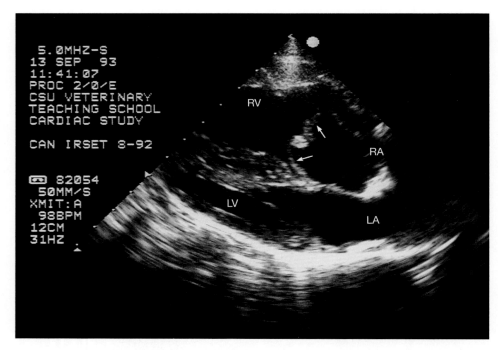

FIGURE 5.36   Doming of thick abnormal tricuspid valves (*arrow*) with fusion of the tips is seen in this dog with tricuspid stenosis. This dog also had an atrial septal defect not seen in this image. *Plane,* right parasternal long-axis four-chamber view; *RV,* right ventricle; *RA,* right atrium; *LV,* left ventricle; *LA,* left atrium.

When one defect has been identified but there is enlargement of a chamber or vessel that is not normally part of the shunt pathway, another defect is most likely present or complications secondary to the shunt may exist. Each shunt will be considered in the following section and complications or possible concurrent problems will be discussed.

Ventricular Septal Defect

A ventricular septal defect (VSD) is a common congenital cardiac defect in the cat and dog and is the most common congenital defect in the horse, llama, and cow (42–46). Most VSDs are easy to identify using echocardiography, but small defects may require Doppler examination to confirm their presence. It is in the assessment of their hemodynamic significance where cardiac ultrasound and especially Doppler ultrasound are useful.

Ventricular septal defects usually are located high in the membranous septum just below the right or noncoronary aortic valve cusp in the left ventricular outflow tract and just under the tricuspid valve in the right side of the heart. Careful examination will allow most defects to be seen on right parasternal long-axis left ventricular outflow views where the muscular ventricular septum joins the anterior aortic wall (Figs. 5.37 and 5.38). Four-chamber views should never be used to identify high membranous defects because these images often have normal echo dropout at the ventricular septum junction and atrioventricular junction. Right parasternal transverse views at the levels of the chordae tendineae and aortic valve also may show the defect (Figs. 5.39 and 5.40). The high membranous hole typically will be seen under the tricuspid valve above the aorta. Occasionally, a VSD will be supracristal, in the area proximal to both the aortic and pulmonic valves as opposed to the tricuspid valve. A supracristal defect will not be seen in long-axis views. Color-flow Doppler may show turbulence within the right side of the heart but a point of origin will not be seen on four-chamber or left ventricular outflow planes. The defect may be seen on transverse views of the heart base on the right side of the image just proximal to

Do not use four-chamber views to diagnose a VSD.

the pulmonic valve within the right ventricular outflow tract (Fig. 5.41). Color-flow Doppler usually is necessary to accurately identify this defect. Ventricular septal defects also may be muscular (22,44,46) (Fig. 5.42). They may be found anywhere along the ventricular septum. If a distinct defect is not seen, a pulsed-wave Doppler gate should interrogate the right side of the septum regardless.

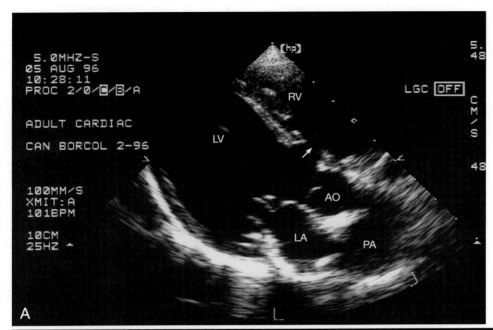

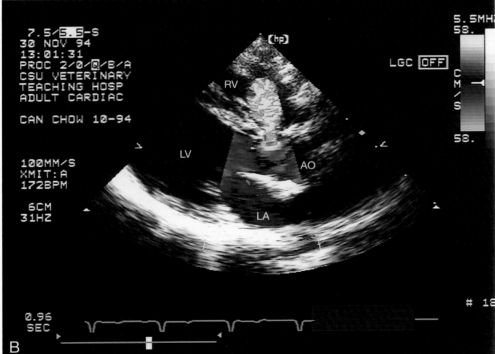

FIGURE 5.37   **A.** A large ventricular septal defect is seen just below the aortic valves (*arrow*). Volume overload of the left ventricular chamber is evident. The pulmonary artery also is dilated secondary to the large volume flowing through the shunt. **B.** Color-flow Doppler documents left-to-right shunting through a high membranous ventricular septal defect. *Planes,* right parasternal long-axis left ventricular outflow view; *RV,* right ventricle; *LV,* left ventricle; *LA,* left atrium; *AO,* aorta; *PA,* pulmonary artery.

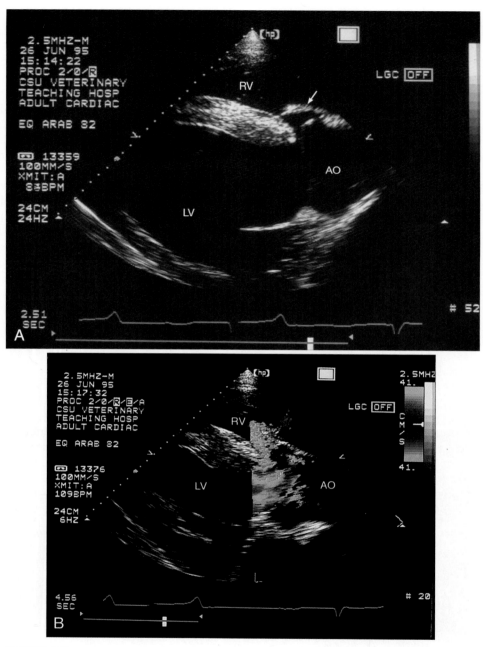

FIGURE 5.38   **A.** A ventricular septal defect is clearly seen under the tricuspid valve (*arrow*) in this horse. **B.** Color-flow Doppler confirms its presence. *Plane,* right parasternal long-axis left ventricular outflow view; *RV,* right ventricle; *LV,* left ventricle; *AO,* aorta.

Small defects at any location may not be visible with two-dimensional echocardiography, and Doppler studies will be necessary to confirm the presence of the VSD (Fig. 5.43). One study showed that only 82% of ventricular septal defects were seen on two-dimensional examinations (17).

Hemodynamically significant VSDs cause the right and left ventricular chambers to dilate (17,46). The left ventricle always sees the volume of blood being shunted because the shunted blood must return to the left heart via the left atrium and ventricle. The location of the defect, however, determines the degree of right ventricular dilation. Because most VSDs are located high in the membranous septum, just proximal to the aortic valve and under the tricuspid valve, the shunted blood will flow through the right ventricular chamber on its way to the pulmonary artery and

VSD—Shunt Pathway

Left ventricle →
Right ventricle →
Pulmonary artery →
Lungs →
Left atrium →
Left ventricle

the RV will dilate. Some defects, however, are within the crista or above (supracristal) and are located more toward the right ventricular outflow tract near the pulmonic valve. In these cases, the volume flows directly into the pulmonary artery and the right ventricle may remain normal in size.

The VSD size is also a factor in how much dilation is present. A small defect may not create any measurable volume overload of the chambers, which helps in deciding how hemodynamically significant the shunt is. Large shunts will create large chambers. Chamber dilation is directly proportional to the volume of blood being shunted. Even without Doppler studies to measure pressures and volume through the vessels, the size of the chambers and vessels tells us whether the volume is significant (22,43). The pulmonary artery usually is dilated in animals with ventricular septal defects regardless of whether there is other right-sided volume overload. The artery sees all of the shunted blood. The vessel will be enlarged along its length from the level of the pulmonic valve cusps and past the bifurcation of the pulmonary artery. No narrowing or increased distension should be seen at any point from the valves on. This differentiates the dilation from that seen in pulmonic stenosis when there is poststenotic dilation and the diameter of the pulmonary artery changes. The pulmonic valves should move normally. Slow motion or frame by frame analysis should show the cusps move completely toward the walls of the pulmonary artery during systole; failure to do so suggests pulmonic stenosis.

An M-mode feature that may help confirm the presence of a small defect when it cannot be seen on two-dimensional examinations and when Doppler is unavailable is systolic tricuspid valve flutter (Fig. 5.44). During systole, shunted blood strikes the septal leaflet after passing through the defect. This was present in 38% of dogs with VSD in one study (17). This finding is only reliable in the absence of tricuspid insufficiency. A large right atrium suggests the presence of tricuspid insufficiency and systolic flutter may be secondary to regurgitant flow as opposed to a shunt.

Aortic insufficiency is commonly seen when high membranous or pericristal defects are present. The aortic valve cusps may prolapse into the ventricular septal

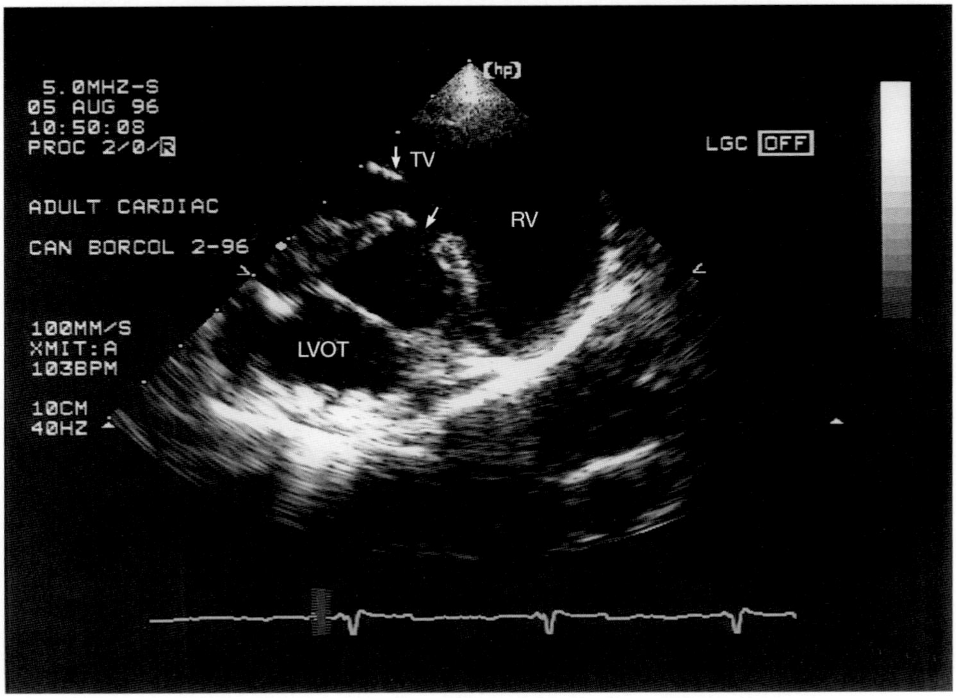

Significant shunts usually = significant volume overloads

FIGURE 5.39   Membranous ventricular septal defects (*arrow*) are seen at the level of the outflow tract on transverse views of the heart base. *RV*, right ventricle; *LVOT*, left ventricular outflow tract; *TV*, tricuspid valve.

defect (17,46,47). The severity of aortic insufficiency should be evaluated with spectral and color-flow Doppler if they are available. Even when a septal defect is hemodynamically insignificant, a significant aortic insufficiency may set the stage for the development of heart failure. Analysis of aortic insufficiency is discussed in chapters 3 and 4.

Pulsed-wave Doppler will identify the presence of a VSD no matter how small the defect. Meticulously moving the Doppler gate along the right ventricular side of the septum and under the tricuspid valve leaflet on right parasternal left ventricular

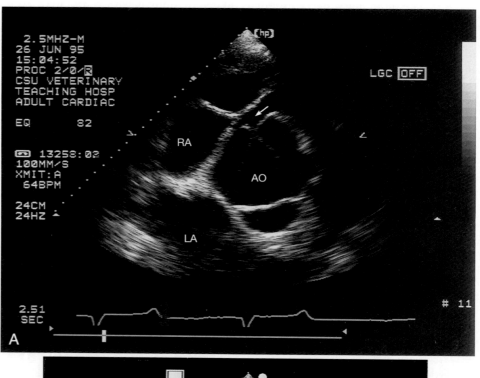

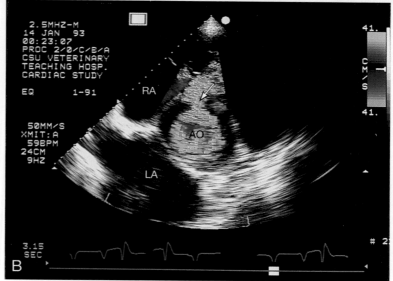

FIGURE 5.40   **A.** The ventricular septal defect is right at the level of the aortic valves in this horse (*arrow*). The tricuspid valve can be seen within the right ventricular chamber above the defect. **B.** Color-flow Doppler shows the left-to-right shunting through the ventricular septal defect on transverse planes also. *Plane,* right parasternal transverse heart base; *RA,* right atrium; *AO,* aorta; *LA,* left atrium.

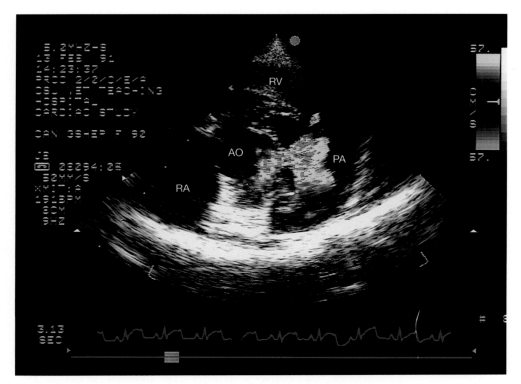

FIGURE 5.41   Supracristal ventricular septal defects are seen adjacent to the aortic and pulmonic valves as opposed to under the tricuspid valves. Here, color-flow Doppler shows the left-to-right shunt crossing the defect just above the level of the pulmonic valves. *Plane,* right parasternal transverse heart base; *RV,* right ventricle; *AO,* aorta; *PA,* pulmonary artery; *RA,* right atrium.

outflow views will identify the location of a shunt. The gate also should be moved from tricuspid valve to pulmonic valve on right parasternal transverse views between the levels of the mitral valve and aortic valve. If a VSD is present, aliased systolic flow is recorded. When the pulsed Doppler gate is placed along the ventricular septum on a tipped left ventricular outflow view, diastolic filling from the tricuspid valve can be recorded. This tricuspid inflow will be positive or upward just as VSD flow. However, tricuspid inflow is not aliased and will be present during diastole.

The velocity of blood flow through a small restrictive VSD should be high, reflecting left ventricular pressures of approximately 120 mm Hg and right ventricular pressures of approximately 20 mm Hg. A pressure gradient of approximately 100 mm Hg is expected, and a velocity close to 5 m/sec should be recorded across the defect (Fig. 5.45). Documenting velocities and pressure gradients consistent with restrictive flow suggests that the effect of the shunt is hemodynamically negligible at the time of the examination (22).

> Restrictive VSDs have high-pressure gradients.

Large unrestrictive VSDs allow the pressures between the right and left ventricles to equilibrate, and smaller pressure gradients will exist. Therefore, the velocity of blood flow across the shunt will be lower (22) (Fig. 5.46). Velocity of blood flow also will be lower secondary to the size of the aperture, allowing the blood to flow through with less turbulence than if the defect was smaller. An analogy would be a river in which the water becomes turbulent and rapids are created as the water courses through narrow areas. Lower gradients, therefore, are indicative of larger defects, higher right ventricular pressures, and hemodynamically significant shunts. Obtaining a systemic blood pressure and subtracting the pressure gradient across the VSD from it will provide a good estimate of right-sided pressure. In the absence of pulmonic stenosis, the right-sided pressure is equal to pulmonary artery systolic pressures and the presence and degree of pulmonary hypertension can be assessed.

> Low pressure gradients =
> • Large defects
>   or
> • Pulmonary hypertension
>   or both

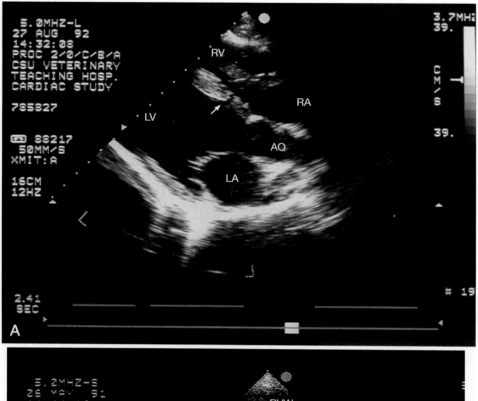

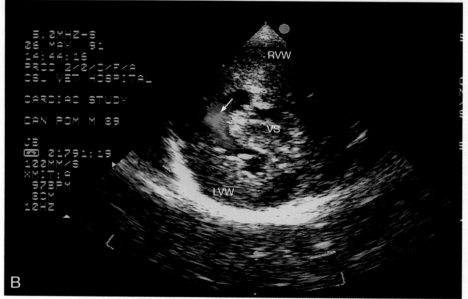

FIGURE 5.42   Muscular ventricular septal defects may be seen anywhere along the septum. **A.** A small defect (*arrow*) is seen within the ventricular septum of this llama. (Used with permission from Boon JA, Knight AP, Moore DH. Llama cardiology. Vet Clin North Am Food Anim Pract. 1994;10[2]:365.) **B.** A large muscular septal defect (*arrow*) is located toward the ventricular apex of this dog. Color-flow Doppler shows very little turbulence associated with this right-to-left shunt. This dog also had pulmonic and aortic stenosis. Severe biventricular hypertrophy is present. *RVW,* right ventricular wall, *LVW,* left ventricular wall; *VS,* ventricular septum; *RV,* right ventricle; *LV,* left ventricle; *LA,* left atrium; *AO,* aorta; *RA,* right atrium.

Pulmonary artery pressures of less than 30 mm Hg would not be of concern. However, pressures between 50 and approximately 80 mm Hg or more suggest the presence of moderate pulmonary hypertension and pressures above 80 or 90 mm Hg indicate servere pulmonary hypertension.

    All of the shunted blood volume must enter the pulmonary artery. The velocity of

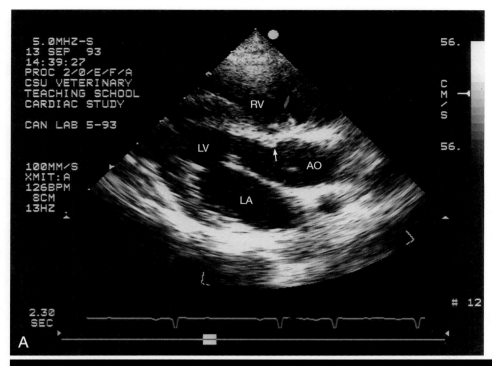

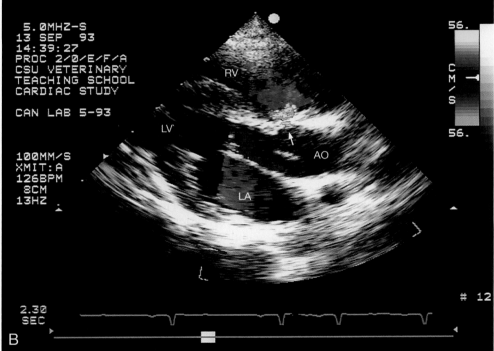

FIGURE 5.43   Very small ventricular septal defects may not be seen on two-dimensional images. They create very little, if any, changes in cardiac size. **A.** The base of the ventricular septum appears mildly abnormal (*arrow*) but no defect is seen in this apparently normal heart. **B.** Color-flow Doppler documents the presence of a small restrictive ventricular septal defect (*arrow*). *Plane*, right parasternal long-axis left ventricular outflow view; *RV*, right ventricle; *LV*, left ventricle; *LA*, left atrium; *AO*, aorta.

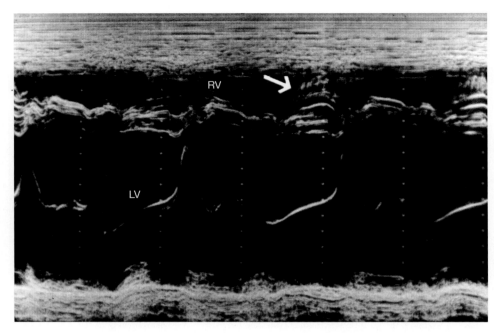

FIGURE 5.44 M-mode images may help in the diagnosis of ventricular septal defect. Tricuspid valve flutter is seen as the shunted blood strikes the leaflet during systole (*arrow*). *RV,* right ventricle; *LV,* left ventricle.

The higher the pulmonary artery velocity, the more significant the volume being shunted in the absence of pulmonic stenosis.

blood flow within the artery will increase in direct proportion to the amount of excess volume flowing through the orifice. Small shunt volumes will not elevate velocities to any great degree, whereas large volumes flowing through the same size vessel must increase in velocity. This reflects the physical law of continuity that dictates that when all other factors are held constant, flow in equals flow out, and velocity must increase between the two areas to maintain this relationship. The larger the VSD, the greater the amount of shunting, and the higher the pulmonary flow velocity. However, as pulmonary hypertension develops, this will no longer hold true because the elevated right-sided pressures will tend to reduce the pressure gradient, which will decrease the velocity of the shunt and the amount of blood being shunted from left to right. As this happens, look for signs of pulmonary hypertension including right ventricular hypertrophy and dilation, a very large pulmonary artery, decreased left ventricular and atrial chamber sizes, and paradoxical septal motion. The changes associated with pulmonary hypertension are described in detail in Chapter 4. All causes of pulmonary hypertension create similar changes. Tricuspid insufficiency, if present, can help determine the right ventricular and pulmonary artery pressures.

A shunt ratio of systemic to pulmonary blood flow may be calculated by obtaining the flow velocity integral of pulmonary flow or mitral flow, both of which will reflect the volume flowing through the pulmonary system, and the flow velocity integral of aortic or systemic flow is calculated. Multiplying these integrals by the cross-sectional area of the interrogated flow will allow volume to be determined and a ratio can be calculated. This is discussed in greater detail in Chapter 3. Accurate planes through the measured areas, good Doppler tracings, and experience will increase the accuracy of calculating volumetric flow and shunt ratios. A ratio of greater than 2.0 is considered to have significant hemodynamic effects on the heart, and a ratio in excess of 2.5 warrants surgical correction of the defect in humans.

Patent Ductus Arteriosus

Patent ductus arteriosus (PDA) is a common defect in young animals. Poodles, keeshonds, cocker spaniels, German shepherds, Pomeranians, collies, and Shetland

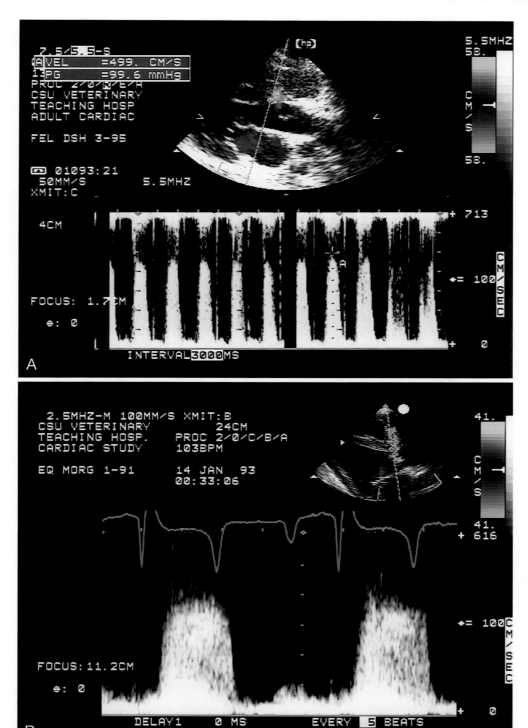

FIGURE 5.45   Both of these Doppler images show high-velocity flow through ventricular septal defects. **A.** A velocity of almost 5 m/sec and a calculated pressure gradient of 100 mm Hg are consistent with a restrictive, hemodynamically insignificant ventricular septal defect. **B.** The velocity of flow across the ventricular septal defect in this horse is approximately 4.5 m/sec, reflecting normal left- and right-sided pressures.

sheepdogs all have an increased risk for maintaining a patent ductus. The defect is also common in calves and cats (9,45); however, PDA is rare in the horse (48). Because the other clinical and radiographic features of PDA are usually very diagnostic and clear cut, echocardiography is not necessary to diagnose PDA. However, echocardiography does confirm the diagnosis (especially if conflicting clinical or physical signs exist) and identifies the presence of other coexisting defects.

Blood flow in PDA involves the pulmonary artery, left atrium, left ventricle, and aorta up to the level of the ductus. Echocardiographic images will show volume overload of all these structures (Fig. 5.47). The larger the shunt, the larger the volume overload will be. Long-axis images will show bowing of the interventricular and atrial septums toward the right side of the heart. Left ventricular outflow views typically show a large left atrium, and the left atrial to aortic root ratio will be large (11,12,17).

A large pulmonary artery will be seen on both right and left parasternal transverse images of the heart base. The dilation includes the artery at the level of the pulmonic valves as well as the right and left main pulmonary artery branches (Fig. 5.48). Differentiation between the dilated pulmonary artery seen with PDA and the artery dilation seen with pulmonary hypertension or pulmonic stenosis is made easily. An artery dilated secondary to hypertension should show the concurrent right ventricular changes of hypertrophy and usually dilation if the pressures are high enough. Pulmonic stenosis rarely causes dilation of the artery at the level of the valves, and the vessel walls will diverge away form each other past the stenosis.

The ductus is angled from the aorta to the pulmonary artery so that flow is directed up toward the pulmonic valve. One or more of the pulmonic valves often prolapse as the ductal flow strikes them. They may prolapse significantly but remain competent.

Despite significant dilation of the left ventricular chamber often inadequate hypertrophy of the wall and septum exists. This, coupled with the fact that the shunt is beyond the ventricular chamber, elevates the systolic wall stress, and the parameters of function in hearts with PDA are often low or within the normal range. Fractional shortening is elevated in volume-overloaded hearts if myocardial function is preserved, but PDA is an exception (Fig. 5.49). Depressed fractional shortening

PDA—Shunt Pathway

Aorta →
Pulmonary artery →
Lungs →
Left atrium →
Left ventricle →
Aorta

Fractional shortening typically is not elevated with PDA, secondary to high afterload.

FIGURE 5.46 A low pressure gradient of 53.9 mm Hg across the ventricular septal defect in this dog is consistent with a large defect that allows right and left ventricular pressures to equilibrate and/or indicates the presence of pulmonary hypertension or stenosis. Right ventricular pressures are approximately 50 to 60 mm Hg.

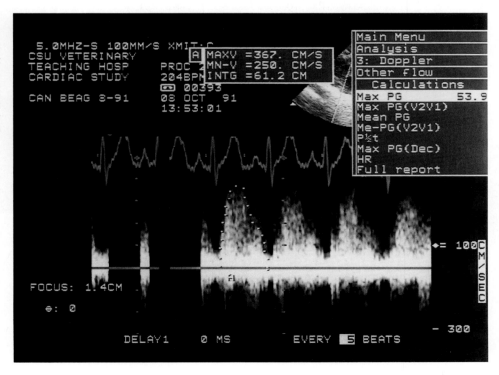

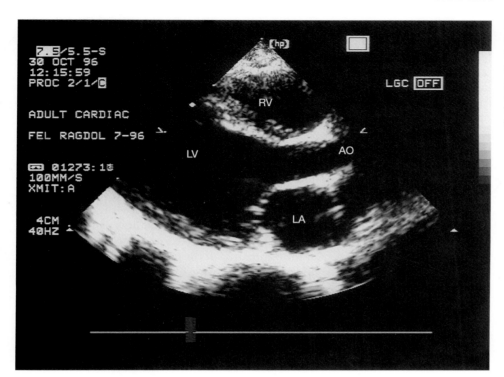

FIGURE 5.47   Patent ductus arteriosus results in left ventricular and left atrial volume overload because these chambers are involved in the shunt pathway. *Plane,* right parasternal long-axis left ventricular outflow view; *RV,* right ventricle; *LV,* left ventricle; *LA,* left atrium; *AO,* aorta.

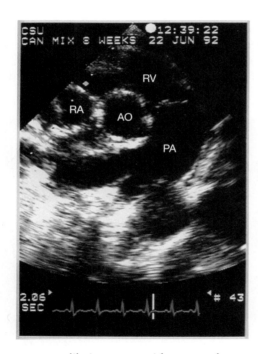

FIGURE 5.48   Pulmonary artery dilation occurs with a patent ductus arteriosus. The dilation involves the entire artery from the valve to and including the bifurcation. *Plane,* right parasternal transverse heart base; *RV,* right ventricle; *AO,* aorta; *PA,* pulmonary artery; *RA,* right atrium.

does not necessarily indicate myocardial failure in young animals with PDA. In older animals, left ventricular function may never return to normal after ligation of the ductus.

The ductus is not visualized on standard views of the heart; only the effects of the volume overload are seen, which are diagnostic for PDA because no other congenital defect by itself creates these types of changes within the heart. Careful examination and manipulation of the transducer on left cranial long-axis planes at the level of the pulmonary artery allows visualization of the ductus in some animals. The pulmonary artery and its bifurcation must be clearly imaged, and the sound beam should be angled cranially and twisted slightly back and forth to see the descending aorta, pulmonary artery, and ductus at the same time (12,22). Color-flow Doppler helps identify the ductus (Fig. 5.50). However, the ductus does not have to be seen to confirm the presence of PDA when the other changes associated with the defect are present.

Color-flow Doppler shows turbulence within the main pulmonary artery when a patent ductus is present. The aliased signal usually will fill the artery and extend from the bifurcation up to the valves (Fig. 5.51). This can be seen on any of the views that show the main pulmonary artery segment. The turbulence in most animals completely fills the artery and no specific jet related to ductal flow can be identified. When small shunts are present, however, a well-defined jet sometimes is seen (Fig. 5.52). The jet will originate near the bifurcation of the pulmonary artery on the right side of the image and will be directed upward toward the pulmonic valves.

Spectral Doppler shows a classic flow pattern that is not seen with any other congenital defect. Using any of the pulmonary artery views place the Doppler beam over the artery with the gate located approximately halfway between the valves and the bifurcation. Continuous positive flow will be seen on the spectral tracing (Fig. 5.53). Negative flow may be either continuous or primarily systolic. In cases where a distinct jet of ductal flow is present, the gate may need to be moved side to side within the artery before the continuous flow pattern is seen (12,22,49). The continuous upward flow is seen regardless of which imaging plane is used and regardless of whether the Doppler cursor is positioned exactly parallel with flow. To obtain a pressure gradient from the pulmonary artery to the aorta, a left cranial long-axis view of the pulmonary artery must be used. This allows the beam to be aligned with the ductal flow and maximal velocities are recorded (Fig. 5.54). Because

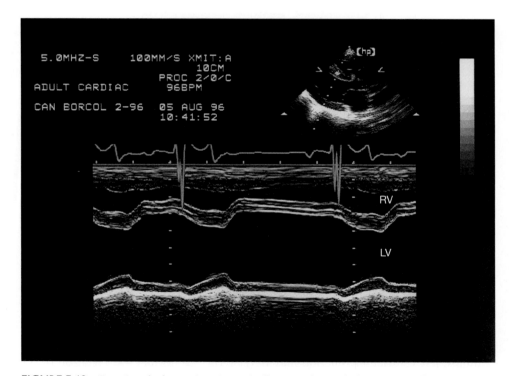

FIGURE 5.49 Fractional shortening is typically not elevated despite significant volume overload in hearts with patent ductus arteriosus. The fractional shortening here is approximately 36% in a significantly dilated left ventricle. *RV*, right ventricle; *LV*, left ventricle.

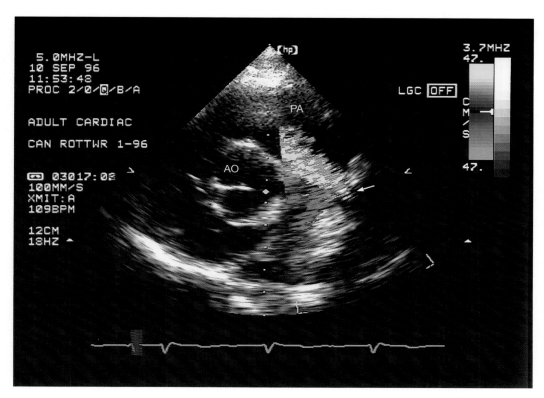

FIGURE 5.50   The patent ductus may sometimes be seen on left cranial views of the pulmonary artery and is easier to identify when color-flow Doppler is used. The aliased color-flow jet is seen flowing from the ductus (*arrow*) into the pulmonary artery in this image. *Plane*, left cranial modified transverse pulmonary artery; *PA*, pulmonary artery; *AO*, aorta.

pulmonary artery pressures should be approximately 20 mm Hg and aortic pressure should be approximately 120 mm Hg, a gradient close to 100 mm Hg is expected. A lower pressure gradient is seen if the ductus is large or if pulmonary hypertension is present. Pressure gradients in congenital heart disease provide information that helps assess hemodynamic significance and prognosis. Because most PDAs are ligated, obtaining a pressure gradient in PDA is not as important as it is with other defects.

Aortic flow velocities always are elevated in animals with PDA (Fig. 5.55). The higher the flow velocity, the greater the amount of shunted blood. This finding can be used to help identify the presence of a shunt in cases in which multiple defects are present. A dog with pulmonic stenosis, for example, should have normal to low aortic flow velocities. High aortic flow velocities suggest the presence of a PDA. Pulmonary to systemic flow ratios can be calculated the same as with other shunts. This is discussed in detail in Chapter 3.

> Aortic flow velocities always are elevated with PDA. The higher the velocity, the more significant the shunt in the absence of AS.

The cardiac changes associated with a reverse patent ductus arteriosus are related to pulmonary hypertension. Both the right ventricle and pulmonary artery will be very large. Both volume overload and hypertrophy of the right ventricular chamber will be present. The right atrium will be normal, unless significant tricuspid insufficiency is present. The left side of the heart will be small secondary to a decrease in preload. One cannot differentiate the cardiac changes associated with hypertension secondary to a reverse shunt from those resulting from other causes such as primary pulmonary hypertension or thromboembolic disease. A bubble study can be used to determine whether the pulmonary hypertension is secondary to a PDA. This procedure is described later in this section.

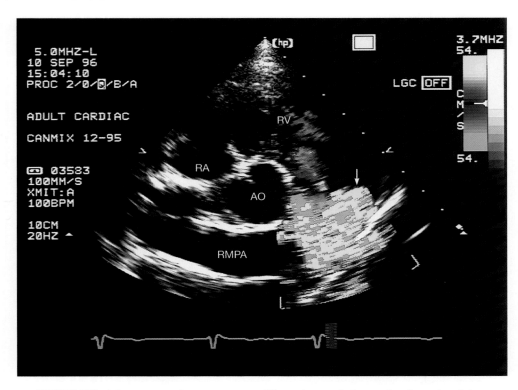

FIGURE 5.51 The entire pulmonary artery fills with a turbulent color-flow signal in most hearts with patent ductus arteriosus. The turbulence stops at the level of the pulmonic valves and extends to the bifurcation. Here, the color-flow signal outlines a prolapsing pulmonic valve (*arrow*) and a small red jet of pulmonic insufficiency is also seen. *Plane,* right parasternal transverse heart base; *RV,* right ventricle; *RMPA,* right main pulmonary artery; *AO,* aorta; *RA,* right atrium.

Atrial Septal Defects

Old English sheepdogs, Samoyeds, and boxers are predisposed to having atrial septal defects. Atrial septal defects also are reported in cats and horses, but this defect overall is uncommon (50–53). Three types of atrial septal defects occur. The most common defect, ostium secundum defect, is located in the middle of the atrial septum. Less common is the ostium primum defect located at the junction of the atrioventricular valves and the atrial septum. The least common atrial septal defect is the sinus venosus type located near the junction of the pulmonary vein and left atrium. Patent foramen ovale may exist in the same area as the ostium secundum but has less hemodynamic significance than a true atrial septal defect; however, if atrial pressures become elevated, that will create a more significant shunt.

> Dropout of the middle portion of the atrial septum often is seen in normal hearts.

The right atrium, right ventricle, pulmonary artery, and left atrium are all involved in the shunt pathway of an atrial septal defect and will all be volume overloaded. The degree of volume overload depends on the defect size of and the pressure difference between the left and right atrium. Large defects will volume overload the chambers and artery significantly and may cause secondary tricuspid and mitral insufficiencies. Small defects may not show any measurable or obvious dilation on real-time images.

Large volume overloads of the right side of the heart will elevate right ventricular diastolic pressures, and paradoxical septal motion is seen when right-sided pressures exceed left ventricular diastolic pressures. The motion is subtle when the difference is minimal, but can become dramatic with larger disparities in pressure. Paradoxical septal motion is the most common echocardiographic hemodynamic change seen in humans with large atrial septal defects (54).

Ostium primum defects have abnormal atrioventricular valves because the

ASD—Shunt Pathway

Left atrium →
Right atrium →
Right ventricle →
Pulmonary artery →
Lungs →
Left atrium

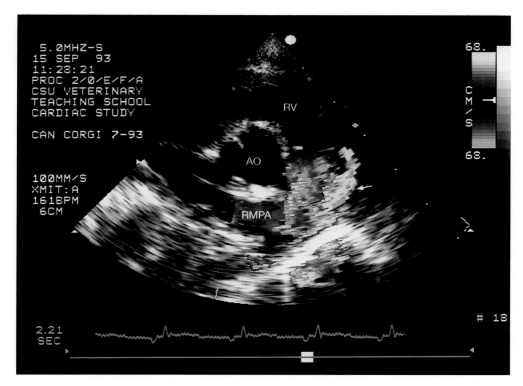

FIGURE 5.52   A well-defined jet representing ductal flow is seen within the pulmonary artery (*arrow*). *Plane*, right parasternal transverse heart base; *RV*, right ventricle; *RMPA*, right main pulmonary artery; *AO*, aorta.

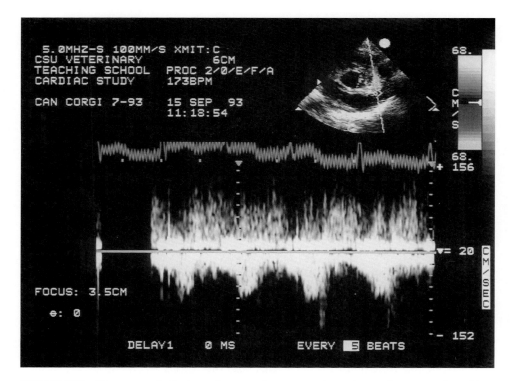

FIGURE 5.53   The spectral display of patent ductus arteriosus is continuous and positive because flow is directed toward the pulmonic valve. Negative diastolic flow will be seen as well as the normal negative systolic pulmonary flow profile.

FIGURE 5.54 Maximal velocities for ductal flow are obtained from left cranial views of the pulmonary artery. A classic flow profile is seen and a maximum gradient of 84 mm Hg is obtained from the pulmonary artery to aorta, reflecting normal aortic and pulmonary pressures.

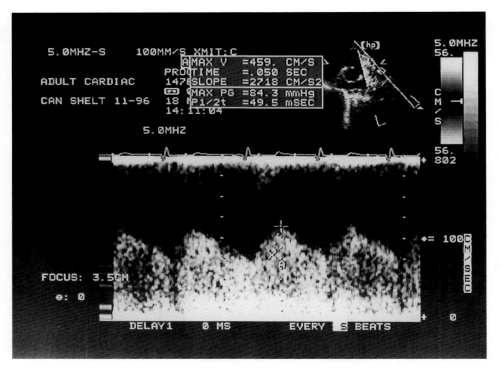

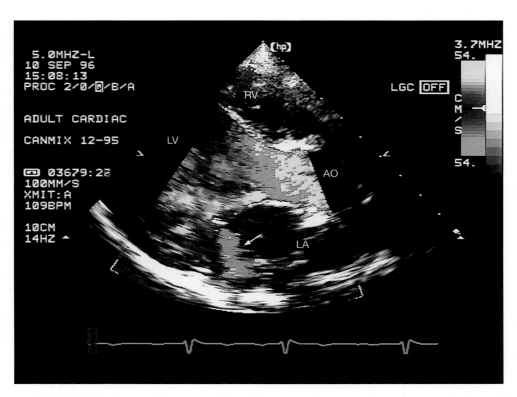

FIGURE 5.55 Aortic velocities are elevated in patent ductus arteriosus because the shunted blood must flow through the ascending aorta. Spectral Doppler will record elevated velocities and color-flow images will show aliasing within the aorta secondary to the increased velocities. A relative stenosis is created. A small jet of mitral insufficiency also is seen (*arrow*). *Plane*, right parasternal long-axis left ventricular outflow view; *LV*, left ventricle; *AO*, aorta; *LA*, left atrium; *RV*, right ventricle.

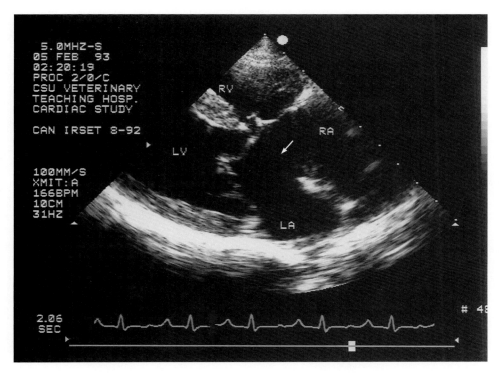

FIGURE 5.56 Ostium primum defects are located at the lower part of the atrial septum just above the mitral and tricuspid valve annuluses (*arrow*). The atrioventricular valves will extend across the defect. Both valves may be dysplastic and insufficient. *Plane*, right parasternal long-axis four-chamber view; *RV*, right ventricle; *RA*, right atrium; *LV*, left ventricle; *LA*, left atrium.

annuluses of these valves are located at the junction of what would normally be the atrial and ventricular septums (Fig. 5.56). Tricuspid dysplasia and atresia may be seen with ostium primum defects (52,53).

Patent foramen ovale is seen in the middle of the atrial septum just as secundum defects are. The membrane that would normally close the foramen on the left side of the atrial septum may be seen on real-time images (Fig. 5.57). This often is seen in neonates.

Spectral and color-flow Doppler can help identify the presence of an atrial septal defect when it is too small to see or when there is doubt as to whether a perceived defect in the atrial septum is real. Place the Doppler gate along the right side of the atrial septum on right parasternal four-chamber views and interrogate along the septum. Almost continuous positive flow will be recorded when an ASD is present. Flow is more prominent during atrial diastole that coincides with the onset of the QRS complex. This first prominent peak may be biphasic. This positive waveform should return almost to baseline when a second lower velocity peak should be seen during atrial systole (50,55) (Fig. 5.58). Vena caval flow, which often is recorded on right parasternal four-chamber views, needs to be differentiated from atrial septal defect flow. Both flows are positive and have two phases to flow. Vena caval flow, however, varies with respiration and has a sharper, more defined positive flow profile with rapid acceleration and deceleration when compared with ASD flow. Vena caval flow also has a much smaller peak coinciding with the P wave (55).

The mean pressure gradient obtained by tracing the shunt flow profile can help differentiate between hemodynamically significant defects and small restrictive ones. Restrictive ASDs will have higher velocities because the pressures between both atria do not equilibrate as they would with large holes. A restrictive ASD will have velocities that reflect 5 to 10 mm of difference in pressure between the two chambers.

Tricuspid flow will be higher than mitral flow when an ASD is present. Pulmonary flow also will be elevated.

Recording tricuspid and mitral flow also helps identify the presence of an ASD. However, this is only valid if no mitral or tricuspid insufficiencies are present. A larger volume of blood will flow past the tricuspid valves than the mitral valve with ASDs. Flow velocities will therefore be greater across the tricuspid valve than the

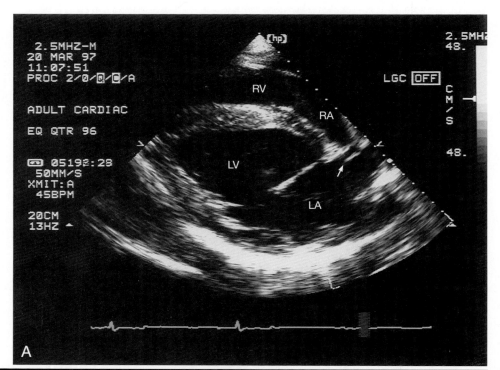

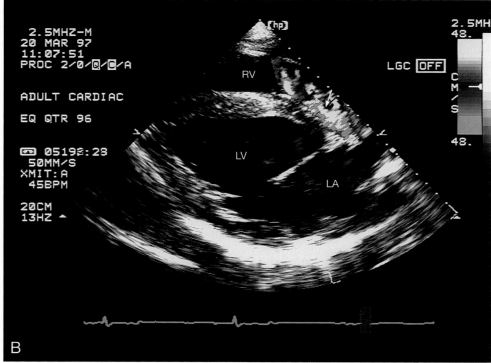

FIGURE 5.57   A patent foramen ovale is located in the middle of the atrial septum. **A.** The membrane that normally would close the defect is seen on the left side of the atrial septum (*arrow*). **B.** Color-flow Doppler may show a mildly aliased signal as blood flows through the defect from left to right (*arrow*). *Planes*, right parasternal long-axis four-chamber view; *RV*, right ventricle; *LV*, left ventricle; *RA*, right atrium; *LA*, left atrium.

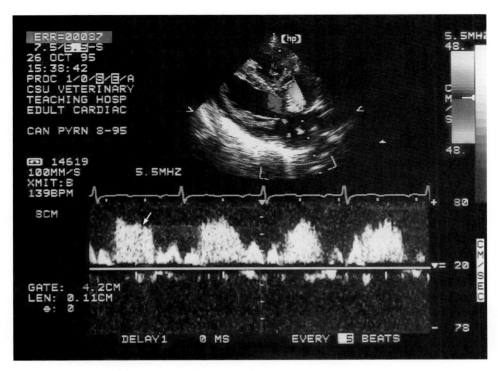

FIGURE 5.58 Spectral Doppler of the flow across an atrial septal defect shows an initial positive peak during early atrial diastole. This peak may be biphasic and is barely discernible in this image (*arrow*). The second peak coincides with atrial contraction and is of lower velocity.

mitral valve when an ASD is present. These flows should be recorded from left parasternal apical and cranial long-axis views of the heart.

The shunted volume of blood must flow past the pulmonary artery and velocity of pulmonary flow will be increased as a result. Although small defects may not increase flow velocities much, a shunt must be suspected when velocities are above the normal range. Pulmonic stenosis should be ruled out first when pulmonary flow velocities are elevated. Comparison of flow velocity integrals of the pulmonary artery and the aorta provides an estimate of the severity of the shunt. The higher the pulmonary flow integral is when compared with aortic flow, the greater the volume of blood that must be flowing through this vessel as compared with the aorta. Pulmonary to systemic flow ratios can be calculated as described in Chapter 3. A ratio of 2:1 or higher signifies a hemodynamically significant shunt. Ratios greater than 2.5 are considered significant enough to warrant surgical intervention.

The flow velocity integral of the pulmonary artery and aorta is more accurate in estimating pulmonary to systemic flow ratios, but when the information cannot be obtained to derive this value, shunt ratios can be estimated from mean transatrial flow velocity. Mean flow velocity of the shunt, derived by tracing the flow profile, has a correlation coefficient of .80 when compared with catheterization-derived flow ratios. The slope of the equation is 10.7, whereas the Y intercept is 14.5 (55). This method has not been confirmed in animals.

Large volume shunts may create pulmonary interstitial changes resulting in pulmonary hypertension. When this occurs, and right atrial pressures begin to exceed left atrial pressures, the shunt will reverse. Reverse atrial septal defects follow a different flow pathway and the left ventricle is now involved. Severe right ventricular hypertrophy as well as a prominent pulmonary artery is seen. Doppler flow will be negative when the shunt is interrogated on right parasternal four-chamber views. Aortic flow velocities will be elevated because the shunt now involves that vessel.

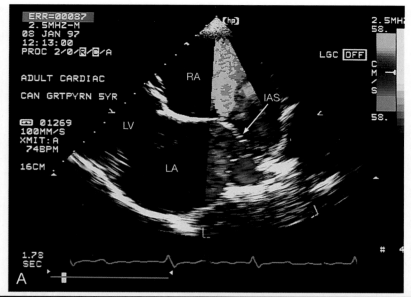

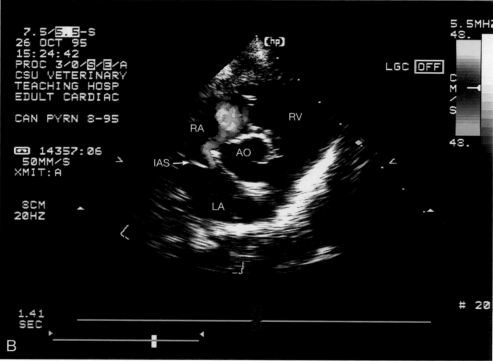

FIGURE 5.59   Flow through an atrial septal defect may not show much, if any, aliasing because pressure gradients are not high. **A.** A prominent aliased signal is seen flowing through the secundum atrial septal on this four-chamber view. **B.** Transverse images of the heart base show low-velocity flow through an atrial septal defect. *RV,* right ventricle; *RA,* right atrium; *IAS,* interatrial septum; *LA,* left atrium; *AO,* aorta.

Color-flow Doppler may show a small turbulent jet crossing the atrial septum (Fig. 5.59). Gradients are small, however, and depending on the transducer and the depth of interrogation, the velocity of shunting blood may not exceed the Nyquist limit. The more restrictive the ASD, the more likely an aliased signal will be seen. Often, a small aliased signal showing a velocity increase proximal to the defect may be seen, but flow through the defect and beyond will be normal.

Endocardial Cushion Defects

When both a large ostium primum atrial septal defect and a large ventricular septal defect are present, the abnormality is called an endocardial cushion defect and also may be referred to as complete atrioventricular canal (12,56).

Two-dimensional echocardiographic images of an endocardial cushion defect are dramatic. The right parasternal four-chamber view shows a large atrial septal defect as well as the ventricular septal defect (Fig. 5.60). The mitral and tricuspid valve originate from the endocardial cushion and are usually dysplastic. Often, just one large atrioventricular valve with an anterior tricuspid leaflet and a large posterior mitral leaflet is seen. When septal mitral and tricuspid leaflets are present, they are usually continuous through the endocardial cushion defect. The right atrium, right ventricle, and left atrium always are dilated, and the left ventricle may be dilated. The valves are usually insufficient and the defects are so large that neither color-flow nor spectral Doppler can help determine the direction of flow.

Truncus Arteriosus

Truncus arteriosus is a rare congenital anomaly that involves the truncus, a single large vessel, leaving the heart opposed to both a pulmonary artery and an aorta. A large ventricular septal defect provides access to the truncus from both the right and left ventricles. The truncus will divide into pulmonary and arterial flow after leaving the heart and cannot be imaged using echocardiography.

Right parasternal or left parasternal long-axis images will show a large ventricular septal defect with one large vessel cranial to the defect (Fig. 5.61). The vessel may appear to override the VSD but also can appear to leave either of the ventricles. A complete examination of the heart is necessary to identify the existence of only one great vessel and to differentiate this defect form tetralogy of Fallot or atresia of either great vessel. Spectral and color-flow Doppler will show the shunting blood and perhaps insufficient valve but are not necessary to diagnose this defect (12,57).

Bubble Studies

Bubble studies help confirm the existence of right-to-left shunting. Normal saline is drawn into a syringe, shaken vigorously, and all large bubbles of air are pushed from the syringe leaving only microbubbles within the solution. Several milliliters of saline are used in larger dogs and less than one milliliter is used in cats and other small animals. The saline is injected into a peripheral vein while the heart is being imaged. A right parasternal four-chamber view is used to detect atrial septal defects and a right parasternal long-axis left ventricular outflow view should be used to detect ventricular septal defects. Dense echoes associated with the air-filled fluid can be seen crossing the atrial or ventricular septums into the left-sided chambers (11,12,58).

Because the shunt in patent ductus arteriosus is extracardiac, and blood flows from the pulmonary artery into the descending aorta, a bubble study using cardiac images will not help determine the existence of a reverse PDA—the abdominal aorta image should be used instead (Fig. 5.62). After a bubble study rules out a reverse VSD or ASD as a cause of hypertension, while looking at right parasternal long-axis images, inject the saline while looking at the abdominal aorta. The dense echoes associated with the microbubbles will show up in the vessel if a reverse PDA exists. It is important to rule out VSD and ASD because these reverse flows also will be seen in the abdominal aorta (58).

Bubble Studies
- Help identify R → L shunts
- Use the abdominal aorta for PDA

MISCELLANEOUS CONGENITAL DEFECTS
Tetralogy of Fallot

The combination of pulmonic stenosis, right ventricular hypertrophy, overriding aorta, and ventricular septal defect creates a congenital anomaly called tetralogy of Fallot. When the pulmonic stenosis is severe enough to elevate right-sided systolic pressures beyond those found within the left ventricle and systemic circulation, the

The VSD and overriding aorta are the same defect on an echo image of tetralogy of Fallot.

FIGURE 5.60 Endocardial cushion defects have a large ostium primum atrial septal defect and a ventricular septal defect. **A.** Long-axis four-chamber images show large portions of both the atrial and ventricular septums missing. Only one tricuspid valve and one mitral valve leaflet is present. (Reprinted with permission from Boon JA, Knight AP, Moore DH. Llama cardiology. Vet Clin North Am Food Anim Pract 1994;10[2]:364.) **B.** Transverse views of the heart base show the large ostium primum defect of this endocardial cushion defect (*arrow*). **C.** Transverse images at the level of the left ventricle show the large ventricular septal defect associated with the endocardial cushion defect (*arrow*). *AO,* aorta; *RA,* right atrium; *LA,* left atrium; *TV,* tricuspid valve; *RV,* right ventricle; *LV,* left ventricle; *IAS,* interatrial septum.

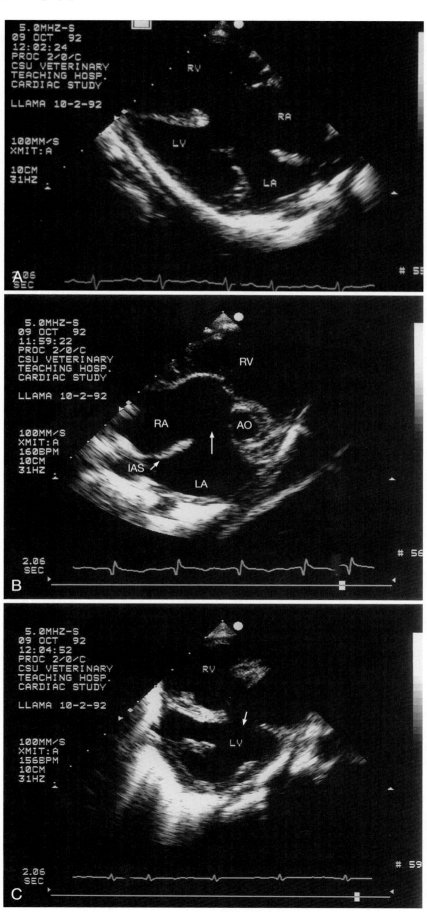

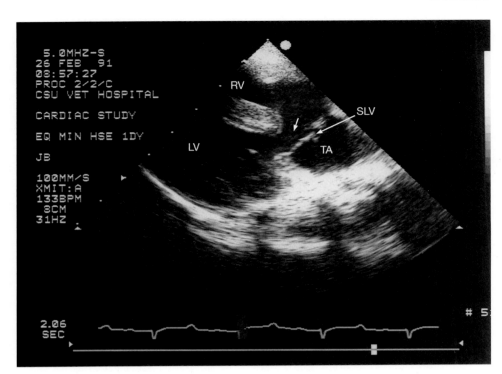

FIGURE 5.61 One large vessel allows blood to leave the ventricular chambers with truncus arteriosus. A large ventricular septal defect (*arrow*) allows both right and left ventricular flow to access the truncus. The pulmonary artery and aorta will not be visible when other aspects of the heart are imaged. *RV*, right ventricle; *LV*, left ventricle; *TA*, truncus arteriosus; *SLV*, semi-lunar valve.

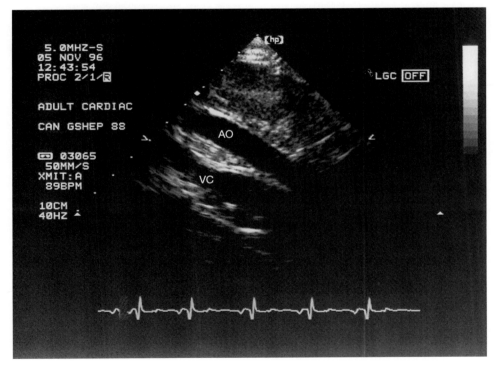

FIGURE 5.62 The abdominal aorta has to be examined for the presence of reverse patent ductus arteriosus when performing a bubble study. Dense echoes associated with reverse flow will fill the aorta if a reverse shunt of any kind is present. A bubble study within the heart will have to rule out reverse atrial or ventricular septal defects. The defects will also cause bubbles to appear in the aorta. *AO*, aorta; *VC*, vena cava.

blood will flow from right to left through the ventricular septal defect. However, not all animals with tetralogy of Fallot have right-to-left shunting, and acyanotic tetralogies can occur. Several canine breeds are predisposed to developing this congenital defect including keeshonds and bulldogs (16,59). Tetralogy of Fallot is also a common complex congenital defect in horses and cats (9,11,42,48,60).

The pulmonic stenosis in animals with tetralogy of Fallot is similar to isolated pulmonic stenosis. The defect may be valvular, subvalvular, or both. The majority of

FIGURE 5.63 The ventricular septal defect of tetralogy of Fallot is usually obvious. **A.** The walls of the aorta (*arrows*) will straddle or override the ventricular septum. Right ventricular hypertrophy is severe. **B.** The ventricular septum is lined up with the center of the aortic valves (*arrow*) in this dog with tetralogy of Fallot. Severe right and left ventricle hypertrophy is present. Septal hypertrophy also is creating obstruction to left ventricular outflow. *Plane,* right parasternal long-axis left ventricular outflow view; *RV,* right ventricle; *LV,* left ventricle; *VS,* ventricular septum; *AO,* aorta; *LA,* left atrium.

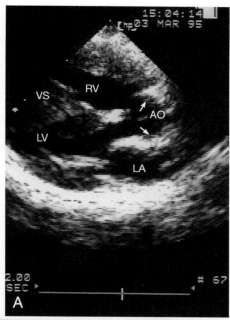

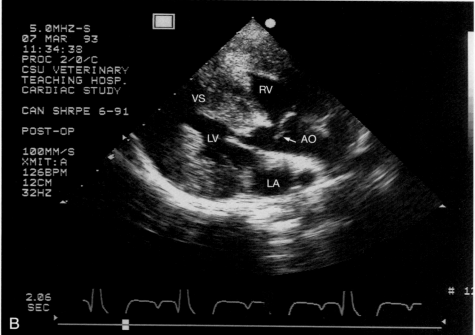

dogs with tetralogy of Fallot appear to have valvular stenosis (61). Hypoplasia of the pulmonary artery beyond the obstruction may be present. A poststenotic dilation is absent in most animals (62).

Spectral Doppler of pulmonary flow can document the degree of obstruction (22). Pressure gradients in excess of 100 mm Hg suggest that right-to-left shunting or bidirectional shunting is present. When severe subvalvular or valvular stenosis is present it is sometimes difficult to obtain an adequate image of the pulmonary outflow tract and valve, and spectral Doppler is often difficult to obtain in these animals. Color-flow Doppler will delineate the boundaries of the outflow tract and may help position the Doppler cursor. Examine all four views for obtaining the pulmonary artery. If pulmonary flow cannot be obtained, check for tricuspid insufficiency as an alternative way to derive right ventricular pressures.

Severe right ventricular hypertrophy is always present as a result of the pressure overload generated by the pulmonic stenosis (17,61). The right ventricular cavity is usually small, unless valvular regurgitations are present. Left ventricular chamber size is also small when tetralogy of Fallot is present, regardless of whether the shunt is right to left or left to right. The left ventricle will appear concentrically hypertrophied. Invasive studies of left ventricular pressures in dogs with tetralogy of Fallot reveal pressures as low as 36 (17,61). A left-to-right shunt would volume overload the left ventricle and sometimes the right ventricle; however, when a moderate to severe pulmonic stenosis is present a decreased volume flows through the pulmonary circulation and into the left side of the heart. Although logically a right-to-left shunt should volume overload the left ventricle, the overriding aorta causes the shunted blood to flow directly into the aorta and the left ventricle never encounters the volume. The severe pulmonic stenosis, which must be present with right-to-left shunts, additionally results in decreased preload within the left ventricular chamber.

The ventricular septal defect is usually obvious and large. The walls of the overriding aorta will straddle the ventricular septum (Fig. 5.63). Only when septal hypertrophy is severe will the defect become less obvious. Manipulating the transducer and sound beam in slightly different directions can help determine whether the septum is intact and whether the aorta is overriding. Color-flow and spectral Doppler will show shunting of blood across the defect no matter how difficult it is to interpret on real-time images. The direction of shunting may be left to right and positive on spectral displays, bidirectional with low velocity flow in both directions, or right to left with negative flow on spectral tracings (Fig. 5.64). Pressure gradients can be derived just as they are for isolated ventricular septal defects.

When a pressure gradient can be obtained from both the pulmonic stenosis and the ventricular septal defect, they should make sense in that the gradient across the septal defect should reflect right-sided pressures and the degree of pulmonic stenosis. A pulmonary stenosis gradient of 130 mm Hg, for instance, should result in right-to-left shunting. A pressure gradient across the septum should be approximately 10 to 20 mm Hg, if systemic systolic pressures are approximately 110 to 120 mm Hg. A gradient of 60 mm Hg across a left-to-right flowing septal defect indicates that right ventricular pressures are approximately 60 mm Hg. The pulmonic stenosis would therefore have a gradient of approximately 40 to 50 mm Hg if pulmonary pressures are assumed to be approximately 10 to 20 mm Hg. Because of the pulmonic stenosis, pulmonary pressure will typically be lower than the 20 to 25 mm Hg present in healthy dogs (61). When multiple defects are present, always cross-check the derived gradients. If, when checking them they don't make sense, then one of the gradients is in error.

Bubble studies can document the presence of a right-to-left shunt across a ventricular septal defect. Inject 1 or 2 mL of vigorously shaken saline into a peripheral vein. The microbubbles will appear echodense on echocardiographic images and will be seen flowing into the left ventricular outflow tract when a reverse shunt is present. When a left-to-right shunt is present, the defect is more difficult to document with bubble studies, unless an area of negative contrast is seen (11,48,61).

Significant septal hypertrophy sometimes creates a secondary obstruction to left ventricular outflow (Fig. 5.63). Look for the M-mode signs of obstruction: systolic anterior mitral valve motion and early systolic aortic valve closure. Spectral and color-flow Doppler will show aliased and high-velocity signals when left-sided obstruction is present. A left-sided obstruction is proximal to the ventricular septal defect, which should be reflected in the analysis of pressure gradients. In other words, systemic pressures are used in assessing the shunt and right ventricular pressures and not the left ventricular pressures as is done with isolated ventricular septal defects.

Cor Triatriatum

Cor triatriatum refers to the division of the right or left atrium into cranial and caudal chambers. The membrane on the right side is a remnant of the embryonic right sinus venosus valve. When the membrane is present within the right atrium, it is referred

Besides RV hypertrophy, the left ventricle appears hypertrophied in tetralogy of Fallot because the shunted volume directly enters the aorta and pulmonic stenosis restricts flow into the left heart.

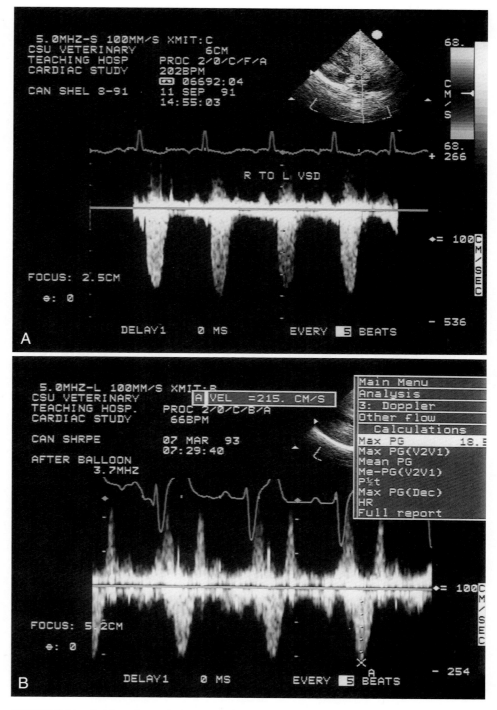

FIGURE 5.64   **A.** Flow through the ventricle septal defect of a tetralogy of Fallot typically is reversed and a negative flow profile is recorded. **B.** Flow may be bidirectional, however, when right and left ventricular pressures are fairly equal.

to as cor triatriatum dexter (63,64). Its presence within the left atrium is referred to as cor triatriatum sinister. Cor triatriatum dexter is found in the dog, whereas cor triatriatum sinister is found primarily in cats. Although it may be the only defect present, cor triatriatum is often associated with tricuspid valve anomalies, pulmonic stenosis, patent ductus arteriosus, and patent foramen ovale in humans (65,66).

Echocardiographic images of the right atrium show a membrane dividing the chamber into two (Fig. 5.65). The membrane also may form a tunnel type of connection between the cranial and caudal chambers as opposed to forming a distinct division into two chambers. The perforation, which allows blood to flow from the cranial to the caudal chamber, is often not apparent without Doppler echocardiography. The membrane may be seen on right parasternal transverse or long-axis views as well as on left apical four- and five- chamber views. Rotate the transducer in several directions in order for the sound beam to interrogate cranial aspects of the right atrium, because sometimes the membrane is located more cranial near the vena cava (63,64).

The membrane varies in its location within the right atrium in humans. The cranial chamber may receive both the caudal and cranial vena cava or only one of the vena cava. The tricuspid valve may be within either chamber depending on the site of the membrane and its angle through the atrium. The majority of dogs have a cranial chamber, which receives the cranial vena cava, and a caudal chamber, which receives the caudal vena cava and the coronary sinus. The tricuspid valve is located within the cranial chamber and may or may not be normal (63,64,67–69). Ebstein's anomaly has been reported in the dog as a concurrent defect (64). Tricuspid regurgitation may or may not be present. Atypical angles and planes through the right atrium are sometimes necessary to visualize the membrane.

The membrane may create an obstruction to flow from the cranial to caudal chamber. Spectral or color-flow Doppler can confirm the presence of obstruction. A pressure gradient between the two chambers will be recorded and turbulent flow can be documented. A diffuse membrane with many fenestrations, called the Chiari network, is a variant of cor triatriatum, and in most cases the Chiari network is not hemodynamically significant.

The cranial chamber and vena cava will dilate if a significant obstruction to flow into the right side of the heart exists. The rest of the heart may appear perfectly normal. Any young animal with signs of right side heart failure should be examined thoroughly for cor triatriatum dexter. As an isolated defect no murmur will be auscultated.

Cor triatriatum sinister shows the same features as triatriatum dexter except the membrane divides the left atrium into cranial and caudal chambers (Fig. 5.66). This membrane should be differentiated from supravalvular mitral stenosis. The fibrous ring associated with mitral stenosis is always distal to the fossa ovalis and closer to the valve. The membrane of cor triatriatum sinister is located proximal to the fossa ovalis near the base of the atrium. Abnormalities within the heart may not be apparent unless the cranial aspects of the atrium are examined. An obstruction to flow may exist and Doppler can confirm the presence of a pressure gradient. Significant gradients may cause left heart failure and pulmonary hypertension.

Atrioventricular Valve Dysplasia

Dysplasia of the atrioventricular valves result in valvular insufficiencies. The degree of dysplasia and regurgitation is variable. The cardiac changes associated with these defects are similar to those seen when the valvular insufficiencies are secondary to acquired valvular lesions. Cardiac changes associated with mitral dysplasia include eccentric left ventricular hypertrophy, elevated parameters of left ventricular function, left atrial dilation, and excessive wall and septal motion (12). Right-sided changes associated with tricuspid dysplasia include right ventricular volume overload, possible paradoxical septal motion, and right atrial dilation (12). For further descriptions of these changes, refer to Chapter 4 and the discussions on acquired mitral and tricuspid valve disease. Descriptions of the two-dimensional appearance of the dysplastic atrioventricular valves follow.

The appearance of the valvular apparatus varies and any combination of abnormally shaped leaflets and papillary muscle may be seen. The leaflets may be

Valvular Dysplasias
_____

May Affect
• Leaflets
• Chordae
• Papillary muscles

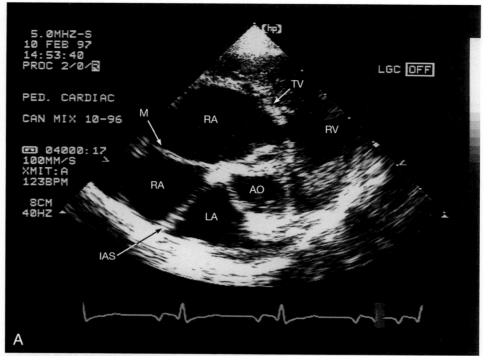

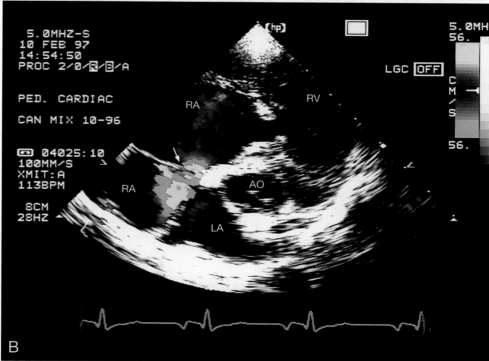

FIGURE 5.65 **A.** A membrane divides the right atrial chamber into cranial and caudal chambers when cor triatriatum dexter exists. **B.** The connection (*arrow*) between the two parts of the right atrium may not be obvious without color-flow Doppler. *Plane,* right parasternal transverse heart base; *RA,* right atrium; *TV,* tricuspid valve; *RV,* right ventricle; *LA,* left atrium; *IAS,* interatrial septum; *AO,* aorta; *M,* membrane.

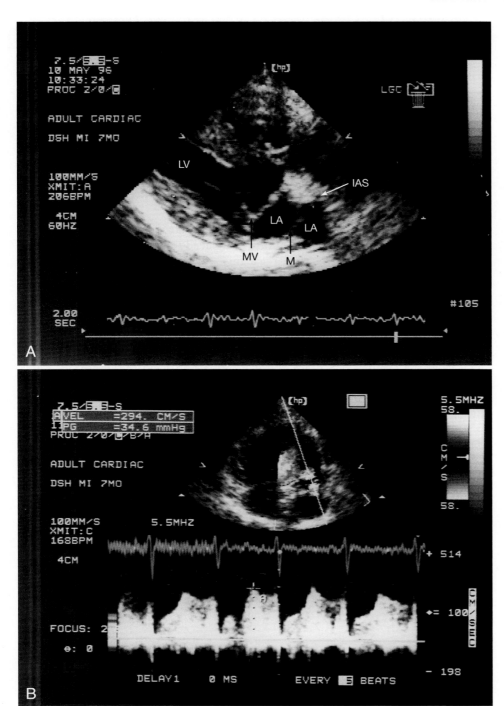

FIGURE 5.66   **A.** A membrane separates the left atrial chamber in cranial and caudal sections with cor triatriatum sinister. **B.** Spectral Doppler reveals a pressure gradient of 35 mm Hg between the left atrium cranial and caudal chambers. *Plane A*, right parasternal four-chamber view; *Plane B*, left parasternal apical four-chamber view; *LV,* left ventricle; *LA,* left atrium; *IAS,* interatrial septum; *M,* membrane; *MV,* mitral valve.

thick, long, short, contain clefts, or have some degree of commissural fusion. The papillary muscles may be abnormally shaped, elongated, or large (9,11,16).

Tricuspid Dysplasia

This defect of the tricuspid valve is particularly common in Labrador retrievers; however, other large breed dogs are predisposed to the defect (11). The septal leaflet is tethered to the right side of the septum. Short chordae may be visible as the leaflet tries to move toward its normal closed position during systole (Fig. 5.67). The middle of the leaflet often buckles away from the septum while the tips remain closely apposed to the septum. The anterior leaflet is typically elongated and may come close to achieving closure of the tricuspid valves during systole (Fig. 5.68). Sometimes it is difficult to define where the anterior leaflet of the tricuspid valve is and where the chordae tendineae start (17).

An unusual variation of tricuspid dysplasia is Ebstein's anomaly. In this type of tricuspid dysplasia, the tricuspid annulus is displaced toward the apex of the right ventricle. The right atrial chamber is large in this defect and is referred to as atrialized. The annulus can be identified on right parasternal long-axis four-chamber views of the heart. In normal hearts, the mitral annulus and tricuspid annulus should be aligned almost directly across from each other. The tricuspid valve is typically 1 to 2 mm further toward the apex of the heart than the mitral annulus. With Ebstein's anomaly, the tricuspid annulus is clearly displaced toward the apex. Be sure to examine the septal cusp carefully because a severely tethered leaflet may only move away from the septum at a more apical location and yield the appearance of a displaced annulus. However, in this instance, the valve is dysplastic (17).

Even though the right atrium is enlarged because the leaflets close in a more apical

Be sure to see restricted motion and tethered leaflets in more than one view. TV often appear to have restricted motion on parasternal four-chamber views when the RV is very dilated.

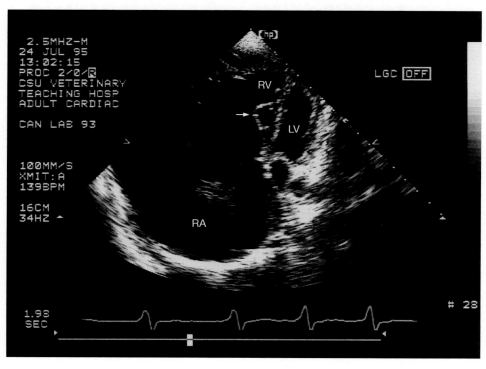

FIGURE 5.67 Tricuspid dysplasia may involve any aspect of the tricuspid apparatus; however, typically the septal leaflet of the valve is tethered to the interventricular septum by short chordae. The leaflet can be seen buckling as it tries to move away from the septum (*arrow*). The tip of the leaflet remains in close apposition to the septum. Severe dilation secondary to severe insufficiency is present. *Plane*, left parasternal apical four-chamber view; *RV*, right ventricle; *RA*, right atrium; *LV*, left ventricle.

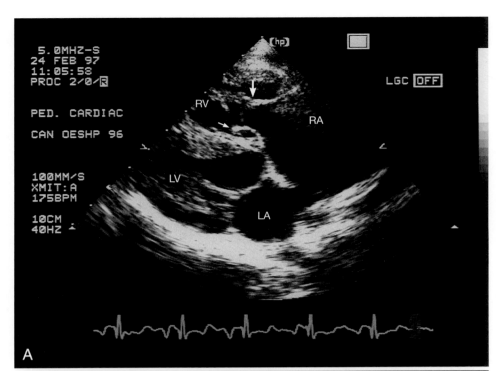

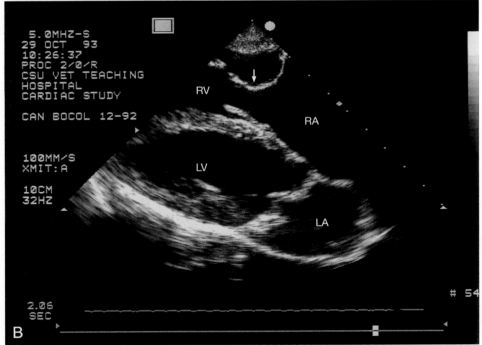

FIGURE 5.68 **A.** Right parasternal long-axis images also may show the tricuspid valve septal leaflet tightly adhered to the ventricular septum (*small arrow*). Often, the anterior tricuspid valve leaflet is elongated and there is abnormal attachment to papillary muscles (*large arrow*). **B.** An elongated anterior leaflet and a long tethered septal leaflet is seen in this heart with tricuspid dysplasia. The right atrium is dilated and the leaflets close in a more apical location. *Planes,* right parasternal long-axis views; *RA,* right atrium; *RV,* right ventricle; *LV,* left ventricle; *LA,* left atrium.

location than normally, tricuspid insufficiency is not always severe. Often, valves with abnormal architecture on echocardiographic images are only mildly to moderately incompetent.

Mitral Dysplasia

Mitral dysplasia is particularly common in cats (9). As with tricuspid dysplasia, the leaflets may be short and thick or elongated, which may be associated with abnormally shaped, elongated or large papillary muscles. The septal leaflet is not usually tethered to the septum as with tricuspid dysplasia, but tethering does occur

FIGURE 5.69 Herniated abdominal contents are visible within the pericardial sac of this dog (*arrows*) on right parasternal long-axis views (**A**) and transverse views (**B**) of the heart. When loops of bowel are present, clear images of the heart may be impossible to obtain. This dog had compressed bowel within its pericardial sac with little air. *RA*, right atrium; *RV*, right ventricle; *LV*, left ventricle; *LA*, left atrium; *P*, pericardium.

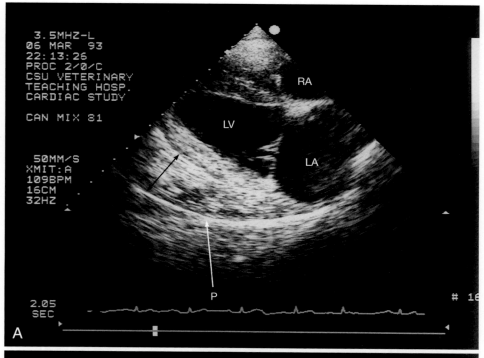

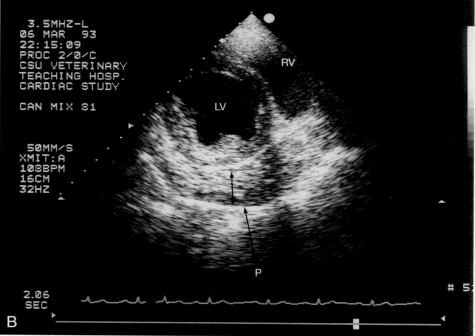

on occasion. The valves may display increased echogenicity and abnormal motion secondary to malformation of the mitral apparatus. There may be prolapse and some degree of restriction to inflow (11,16).

Pericardial Diaphragmatic Hernia

The echocardiographic features of pericardioperitoneal diaphragmatic hernias have been only briefly described (12). Real-time images will show tissue within the pericardial sac, which is visible on multiple views. The pericardial sac will diverge away from the walls of the ventricles, and the herniated tissue will be seen between the sac and the ventricular walls (Fig. 5.69). Pericardial effusion, if present, is usually trivial to mild. When the liver or spleen are involved in the hernia, imaging is fairly easy and the organs can be visualized within the sac. When bowel is involved in the hernia, so much air present may be present that a diagnostic image of the heart is not possible. The pericardial sac should be identified as a bright, echodense line extending from the left and right atrial walls.

REFERENCES

1. Grossman W, Jones D, McLaurin LP. Wall stress and patterns of hypertrophy. J Clin Invest 1975;56:56–64.
2. Kienle RD, Thomas WP, Pion PD. The natural clinical history of canine congenital subaortic stenosis. J Vet Int Med 1994;8:423–431.
3. Buoscio DA, Sisson D, Zachary JF, et al. Clinical and pathological characterization of an unusual form of subvalvular aortic stenosis in four golden retriever puppies. J Am Anim Hosp Assoc 1994;30:100–110.
4. Stepien RL, Bonagura JD. Aortic stenosis: clinical findings in six cats. J Small Anim Pract 1991;32:341–350.
5. O'Grady MR, Holmberg DL, Miller CW, et al. Canine congenital aortic stenosis: a review of the literature and commentary. Can Vet J 1989;30:811–815.
6. Pyle RL, Patterson DF, Chacko S. The genetics and pathology of discrete subaortic stenosis in the Newfoundland dog. Am Heart J 1976;92:324–334.
7. Buchanan JW. Causes and prevalence of cardiovascular disease. In: Kirk RW, Bonagura JD, eds. Current Vet Therapy XI. Philadelphia: WB Saunders, 1992;647–655.
8. Watson TDG, Marr CM, McCandlish IAP. Aortic valve dysplasia in a calf. Vet Rec 1991;129:380–382.
9. Bolton GR, Liu SK. Congenital heart diseases of the cat. Vet Clin North Am 1977;7:341–353.
10. Wingfield WE, Boon JA, Miller CW. Echocardiographic assessment of congenital aortic stenosis in dogs. JAVMA 1983;183:673–676.
11. Bonagura JD, Herring DS. Echocardiography: congenital heart disease. Vet Clin North Am: Small Anim Pract 1985;15:1195–1208.
12. Kaplan P M. Congenital heart disease. Probl Vet Med 1991;3:500–519.
13. Monnet E, Orton EC, Gaynor JS, et al. Open resection for subvalvular aortic stenosis in dogs. JAVMA 1996;209:1255–1261.
14. Fuentes VL. Aortic stenosis in Boxers. Vet Annu 1993;33:220–229.
15. Bonagura JD. Contemporary issues in small animal practice: cardiology. New York: Churchill Livingstone, 1987.
16. Darke PGG. Congenital heart disease in dogs and cats. J Small Anim Pract 1989;30:599–607.
17. Wingfield WE, Boon JA. Echocardiography for the diagnosis of congenital heart defects in the dog. Vet Clin North Am: Small Anim Pract 1987;17:735–753.
18. Devereaux RB, De Simone G, Ganau A, et al. Left ventricular hypertrophy and hypertension. Clin Exper Hypertens 1993;15:1025–1032.
19. O'Grady MR. The incidence of aortic valve insufficiency in congenital canine aortic stenosis: a Doppler echocardiographic study. J Vet Int Med 1990;4:129.
20. Lehmkuhl LB, Bonagura JD. Comparison of transducer placement sites for Doppler echocardiography in dogs with subaortic stenosis. Am J Vet Res 1994;55:192–198.
21. Pollick C, Morgan CD, Gilbert BW, et al. Muscular subaortic stenosis: the temporal relationship between systolic anterior motion of the anterior mitral leaflet and the pressure gradient. Circulation 1982;66:1087–1094.
22. Moise NS. Doppler echocardiographic evaluation of congenital cardiac disease. J Vet Int Med 1989;3:195–207.
23. Thomas WP. Doppler echocardiographic estimation of pressure gradients in dogs with congenital pulmonic and subaortic stenosis. Proc 8th ACVIM 1990:867–869.
24. Richards KL. Assessment of aortic and pulmonic stenosis by echocardiography. Circulation 1991;84:I182–I187.
25. Patterson DF. Congenital defects of the cardiovascular system of dogs: studies in comparative cardiology. Adv Vet Sci Comp Med 1976;20:1–37.
26. Eyster GE. Pulmonic stenosis. In: Bojrab MJ, ed. Current Techniques in Small Animal Surgery. 2nd ed. Philadelphia: WB Saunders, 1983:462–469.

27. Malik R, Church DB, Hunt GB. Valvular pulmonic stenosis in bullmastiffs. J Small Anim Pract 1993;34:288–292.

28. Patterson DF, Haskins ME, Schnarr WR. Hereditary dysplasia of the pulmonary valve in beagle dogs. Am J Cardiol 1981;47:631–641.

29. Bonagura JD. Congenital heart disease. In: SJ Ettinger, ed. Textbook of Veterinary Medicine, 3rd ed. Philadelphia: WB Saunders, 1989:1000–1005.

30. Fingland RB, Bonagura JD, Myer CW. Pulmonic stenosis in the dog: 29 cases (1975–1984). JAVMA 1986;189:218–226.

31. Hawe RS. Pulmonic stenosis in a cat. J Am Anim Hosp Assoc 1981;17:777–782.

32. Emmanouilides GC, Baylen BG. Pulmonary stenosis. In: Adam FH, Emmanouilides GC, eds. Moss' Heart Disease in Infants, Children, and Adolescents, 3rd ed. Baltimore: Williams and Wilkins, 1993:308–323.

33. Hurst JW, Schlant RC. The pathology of normal physiology, clinical recognition and medical and surgical treatment of congenital heart disease. In: The Heart. New York: McGraw-Hill, 1990:726–730.

34. Martin MWS, Godman M, Fuentes LV, et al. Assessment of balloon pulmonary valvuloplasty in six dogs. J Small Anim Pract 1992;33:443–449.

35. Lehmkuhl LB, Ware WA, Bonagura JD. Mitral stenosis in 15 dogs. J Vet Int Med 1994;8:2–17.

36. Stamoulis ME, Fox PR. Mitral valve stenosis in three cats. J Small Anim Pract 1993;34:452–456.

37. Fox PR, Miller MW, Liu S. Clinical, echocardiographic, and Doppler imaging characteristics of mitral valve stenosis in two dogs. JAVMA 1992;201:1575–1579.

38. Shiu MF, Jenkins BS, Webb-Peploe MM. Echocardiographic analysis of posterior mitral leaflet movement in mitral stenosis. Br Heart J 1978;40:372–376.

39. Feldman T. Rheumatic mitral stenosis. Postgrad Med 1993;93:93–104.

40. Hatle L. Doppler evaluation of mitral stenosis. Cardiol Clin 1990;8:233–247.

41. Labovitz AJ, Williams GA. Doppler echocardiography: the quantitative approach. Malvern, PA: Lea and Febiger, 1992.

42. Bayly WM, Reed SM, Leathers CW, et al. Multiple congenital heart anomalies in five Arabian foals. JAVMA 1982;181:684–689.

43. Lombard CW, Scarratt WK, Buergelt CD. Ventricular septal defects in the horse. JAVMA 1983;183:562–565.

44. Boon JA, Knight AP, Moore DH. Llama cardiology. Vet Clin North Am Food Anim Pract 1994;10:353–370.

45. Gopal T, Leipold HW, Dennis SM. Congenital cardiac defects in calves. Am J Vet Res 1986;47:1120–1121.

46. Reef VB. Evaluation of ventricular septal defects in horses using two dimensional and Doppler echocardiography. Equine Vet J 1995;19(Suppl):86–96.

47. Sisson D, Luethy M, Thomas WP. Ventricular septal defect accompanied by aortic regurgitation in five dogs. J Am Anim Hosp Assoc 1991;27:441–448.

48. Reef VB. Echocardiographic findings in horses with congenital cardiac disease. Comp 1991;13:109–117.

49. O'Grady MR, Cockshutt JR, Khanna A, et al. Patent ductus arteriosus in a Holstein calf: a two-dimensional and Doppler echocardiographic study of the ductus arteriosus and validation. Can Vet J 1991;32:303–304.

50. Kirberger RM, Berry WL. Atrial septal defect in a dog: the value of Doppler echocardiography. J S Afr Vet Assoc 1992;63:43–48.

51. Olivier NB. Congenital heart disease in dogs. In Fox PR, ed. Canine and Feline Cardiology. New York: Churchill Livingstone, 1988:357–389.

52. Taylor FG, Wotton PR, Hillyer MH, et al. Atrial septal defect and atrial fibrillation in a foal. Vet Rec 1991;128:80–81.

53. Church DB, Allan GS. Atrial septal defect and Eisenmenger's syndrome in a mature cat. Aus Vet J 1990;67:380.

54. McCann WD, Harbold NB, Giuliani BR. The echocardiogram in right ventricular volume overload. JAMA 1972;221:1243–1245.

55. Marx GR, Allen HD, Goldberg SJ, et al. Transatrial septal velocity measurement by Doppler echocardiography in atrial septal defect: correlation with Qp:Qs ratio. Am J Cardiol 1985;55:1162–167.

56. Ecke P, Malik R, Kannegieter NJ. Common atrioventricular canal in a foal. NZ Vet J 1991;39:97–98.

57. Steyn PF, Holland P, Hoffman J. An angiocardiographic diagnosis of persistent truncus arteriosus. J S Afr Vet Assoc 1989;60:106–108.

58. Goodwin JK, Holland M. Contrast echoaortography as an aid in the diagnosis of right-to-left shunting patent ductus arteriosus. Vet Radiol Ultrasound 1995;36:157–159.

59. Patterson DF. Epidemiologic and genetic studies of congenital heart disease in the dog. Circ Res 1968;23:171–202.

60. Reef VB. Cardiovascular disease in the equine neonate. Vet Clin North Am: Equine Pract 1985;1:117–129.

61. Ringwald RJ, Bonagura JD. Tetralogy of Fallot in the dog: clinical findings in 13 cases. J Am Anim Hosp Assoc 1988; 24:33–43.

62. Patterson DF, Pyle RL, Van Mierop L, et al. Hereditary defects of the conotruncal septum in keeshond dogs: pathologic and genetic studies. Am J Cardiol 1979;34:187–205.

63. Brayley KA, Lunney J, Ettinger SJ. Cor triatriatum dexter in a dog. J Am Anim Hosp Assoc 1994;30:153–156.

64. Tobias AH, Thomas WP, Kittleson MD, et al. Cor triatriatum dexter in two dogs. JAVMA 1993;202:285–290.

65. Hansing CE, Young WP, Rowe GG. Cor triatriatum dexter: persistent right sinus venosus valve. Am J Cardiol 1972;30:559–563.

66. Mazzucco A, Bortolotti U, Stellin G, et al. Anomalies of the systemic venous return: a review. J Cardiac Surg 1990;5:122–133.

67. Miller MW, Bonagura JD, DiBartoli SP, et al. Budd-Chiari-like syndrome in two dogs. J Am Anim Hosp Assoc 1989;25:177–283.

68. Stern A, Fallon RK, Aronson E, et al. Cor triatriatum dexter in a dog. Comp Continu Educ 1986;8:401–413.

69. Linde-Sipman JS, Stokhof AA. Triple atria in a pup. JAVMA 1974;165:539–541.

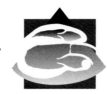

Appendix I

EFFECT OF ANGLE OF INCIDENCE (Θ) ON DOPPLER-DERIVED VELOCITY

Velocity (V) of blood flow is derived using the Doppler equation:

$$V = \frac{c \times f_d}{2(f_o) \times \cos \theta} \qquad \text{(Eq. 1.3)}$$

where C = speed of sound in soft tissue, f_d = Doppler frequency shift, f_o = transducer frequency, and θ = angle of interrogation with respect to blood flow. When the Doppler equation is changed to calculate the frequency shift, you can see that the cosine of the intercept angle directly affects the frequency shift and velocity.

$$f_d = \frac{V \times (2\,f_o) \times \cos \theta}{C} \qquad \text{(Eq. 1.4)}$$

The following examples using a 5-MHz transducer show how increasing angles decrease the derived velocity dramatically.

a) With a true blood flow velocity of 5 m/sec toward the transducer, and a transducer frequency of 5.0 MHz, the frequency shift will be 32,468 cycles per second when the sound beam is perfectly parallel with flow.

$$f_d = \frac{5 \times 2(5,000,000) \times \cos (0°)}{1540}$$

$$f_d = 32,468$$

Inserting this frequency shift into the velocity equation results in the true velocity of 5 m/sec.

$$V = \frac{1540 \text{ m/sec} \times 32,468 \text{ cycles/sec}}{2(5,000,000 \text{ cycles/sec})} = \frac{50,000,720}{10,000,000} = 5.0 \text{ m/sec}$$

b) As the interrogation angle increases, calculated velocities are less than actual velocities because the cosine is no longer equal to 1, and the calculated frequency shift is underestimated. The cosine of 10° is 0.98.

$$f_d = \frac{5 \times 2(5,000,000) \times \cos(10°)}{1540}$$

$$f_d = 31,818$$

The calculated velocity at this angle of incidence is:

$$V = \frac{1540 \text{ m/sec} \times 31{,}818 \text{ cycles/sec}}{2(5{,}000{,}000 \text{ cycles/sec})} = \frac{48{,}999{,}720}{10{,}000{,}000} = 4.9 \text{ m/sec}$$

c) The cosine of 20° is 0.94:

$$f_d = \frac{5 \times 2(5{,}000{,}000) \times \cos(20°)}{1540}$$

$$f_d = 30{,}128$$

The calculated velocity at this angle of incidence is:

$$V = \frac{1540 \text{ m/sec} \times 30{,}128 \text{ cycles/sec}}{2(5{,}000{,}000 \text{ cycles/sec})} = \frac{46{,}397{,}120}{10{,}000{,}000} = 4.6 \text{ m/sec}$$

d) The cosine of 30° is 0.87:

$$f_d = \frac{5 \times 2(5{,}000{,}000) \times \cos(30°)}{1540}$$

$$f_d = 28{,}247$$

The calculated velocity at this angle of incidence is:

$$V = \frac{1540 \text{ m/sec} \times 28{,}247 \text{ cycles/sec}}{2(5{,}000{,}000 \text{ cycles/sec})} = \frac{43{,}500{,}380}{10{,}000{,}000} = 4.4 \text{ m/sec}$$

e) The cosine of 40° is 0.77:

$$f_d = \frac{5 \times 2(5{,}000{,}000) \times \cos(40°)}{1540}$$

$$f_d = 25{,}000$$

The calculated velocity at this angle of incidence is:

$$V = \frac{1540 \text{ m/sec} \times 25{,}000 \text{ cycles/sec}}{2(5{,}000{,}000 \text{ cycles/sec})} = \frac{38{,}500{,}000}{10{,}000{,}000} = 3.9 \text{ m/sec}$$

This information is graphically illustrated in Figure 1.23.

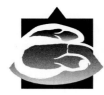

Appendix II

EFFECT OF TRANSDUCER FREQUENCY ON THE NYQUIST LIMIT

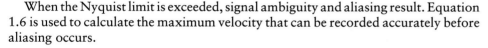

When the Nyquist limit is exceeded, signal ambiguity and aliasing result. Equation 1.6 is used to calculate the maximum velocity that can be recorded accurately before aliasing occurs.

$$Vmax = \frac{(1540 \text{ m/sec})^2}{8(f_o) \times D}$$

(Eq. 1.6)

The equation shows that the maximal velocity (Vmax) that can be recorded at any given depth (D) with no ambiguity is inversely proportional to transducer frequency (f_o). The following examples all use the same gate depth but vary in transducer frequency. You can see that higher velocities can be recorded before the Nyquist limit is reached by using lower-frequency transducers.

a) Using a 5.0-MHz transducer to sample an area at 7 cm:

$$Vmax = \frac{1540^2}{8(5 \times 10^6) \times 0.07} = 0.85 \text{ m/sec}$$

b) Using a 3.5-MHz transducer at the same depth:

$$Vmax = \frac{1540^2}{8(3.5 \times 10^6) \times 0.07} = 1.21 \text{ m/sec}$$

c) Using a 2.5-MHz transducer at the same depth.

$$Vmax = \frac{1540^2}{8(2.5 \times 10^6) \times 0.07} = 1.7 \text{ m/sec}$$

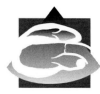

Appendix III

EFFECT OF SAMPLE DEPTH ON THE NYQUIST LIMIT

When the Nyquist limit is exceeded, signal ambiguity and aliasing result. Equation 1.6 is used to calculate the maximum velocity that can be recorded accurately before aliasing occurs.

$$\text{Vmax} = \frac{(1540 \text{ m/sec})^2}{8(f_o) \times D}$$
(Eq. 1.6)

The equation shows that the maximal velocity (Vmax) that can be recorded without aliasing is inversely proportional to gate depth (D) for any given transducer frequency (f_o). The following examples all use the same transducer frequency but vary in sampling depth. You can see that the Nyquist limit is reached at lower velocities as gate depth increases.

a) Using a 5-MHz transducer at a sample depth of 7 cm:

$$\text{Vmax} = \frac{1540^2}{8(5 \times 10^6) \times 0.07} = 0.85 \text{ m/sec}$$

b) Using a 5-MHz transducer at a sample depth of 12 cm:

$$\text{Vmax} = \frac{1540^2}{8(5 \times 10^6) \times 0.14} = 0.49 \text{ m/sec}$$

c) Using a 5-MHz transducer at a depth of 20 cm:

$$\text{Vmax} = \frac{1540^2}{8(5 \times 10^6) \times 0.21} = 0.30 \text{ m/sec}$$

From these examples it becomes clear that as sampling depth increases, you must use lower-frequency transducers to record higher velocities without aliasing.

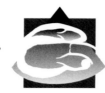

Appendix IV

ECHOCARDIOGRAPHIC REFERENCE VALUES

Reference values for dogs, cats, horses, cows, pigs, sheep, and llamas are included in this appendix. Reference tables for cats, horses, cows, pigs, and llamas may be used without regard for body weight because no significant correlations exist between weight and cardiac size in these animals. Cardiac size in the dog, growing calves, and foals increases with increasing body size. Tables of regression equations are included in which body weight or body surface area may be inserted into the appropriate equations to determine the expected cardiac dimension. The equations are especially useful when they are programmed into a computer and used to generate reports.

For convenience, also included are tables of expected values in dogs for each cardiac parameter of size at specific weights. These tables may be used for all canine breeds. The general reference tables only list expected values for up to 150-lb dogs. Instructions for generating normal ranges in dogs larger than 150 lbs are outlined after the tables. Specific values that have been generated for some canine breeds are listed.

Parameters of function are not significantly correlated to body size, and although various physiologic influences affect the parameters, they may be applied without regard for body weight or surface area in all animals. Most parameters of function are listed within the individual species reference tables along with the cardiac dimension reference ranges.

HOW TO MAKE M-MODE ECHOCARDIOGRAPHIC MEASUREMENTS

Instructions for measuring the most common parameters of size and function are described in the following section. Function typically is measured by calculation packages within the ultrasound equipment; however, an understanding of how they are measured is important.

If all possible M-mode measurements described here are made, three different views are used. The number next to the description has a corresponding number on the echocardiographic diagram. See the text in Chapter 3 for details on how to interpret and apply the numbers once they have been derived from the echocardiograms.

Diastolic measurements are made at the end of diastole and should correspond to the beginning of the QRS complex on the ECG tracing. Systolic measurements are made at the smallest left ventricular measurements at peak downward septal motion or at the end of the T wave on the ECG.

MEASUREMENT OF THE AORTA AND LEFT ATRIUM (Fig. Ap-1)

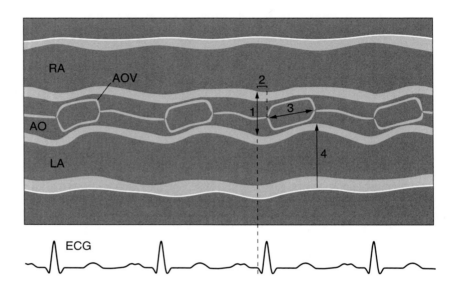

1. AORTIC ROOT (AO):
   Measured from the top of the anterior (top) wall to the top of the posterior (bottom) wall at end-diastole
2. PRE-EJECTION PERIOD (PEP):
   Measured from the onset of the QRS complex to the opening of the aortic valve
3. LEFT VENTRICULAR EJECTION TIME (LVET):
   Measured from the opening of the aortic valve to the closing
4. LEFT ATRIUM (LA):
   Measured from the top of the posterior aortic wall straight down to the pericardium at the end of ventricular systole (point of maximum aortic upward movement)

MEASUREMENT OF THE MITRAL VALVE (Fig. Ap-2)

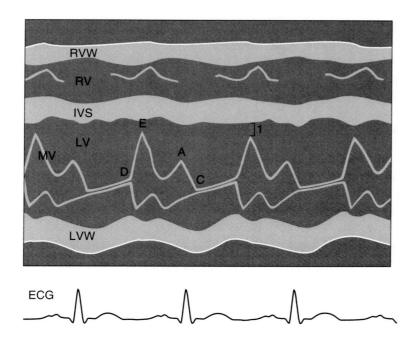

1. E POINT TO SEPTAL SEPARATION (EPSS):
   Measured from the E point straight up to the left ventricular side of the septum

MEASUREMENT OF THE LEFT VENTRICLE (Fig. Ap-3)

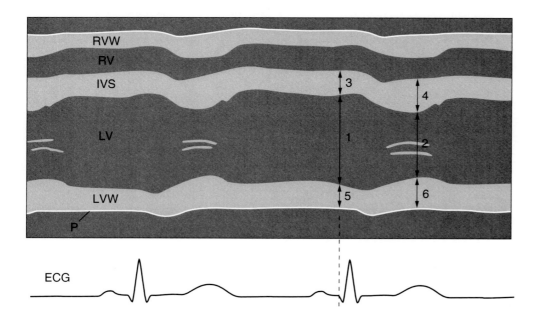

1. END-DIASTOLIC DIMENSION (LVd):
   Measured at the level of the chordae tendineae, from the bottom of the ventricular
   septum to the top of the left ventricular wall at diastole

2. END-SYSTOLIC DIMENSION (LVs):
   Measured at the level of the chordae at peak downward septal motion if septal motion is normal; or measured at the peak upward motion of the left ventricular wall if septal motion is abnormal

3. SEPTAL DIASTOLIC THICKNESS (VSd):
   Measured from the top of the right side of the septum to the bottom of the left side of the septum at the beginning of the QRS complex

4. SEPTAL SYSTOLIC THICKNESS (VSs):
   Measured from the top of the right side of the septum to the bottom of the left side of the septum at the same point the LV systolic dimension was measured

5. LEFT VENTRICULAR WALL DIASTOLIC THICKNESS (LVWd):
   Measured at end-diastole from the top of the ventricular wall to the top of the pericardium

6. LEFT VENTRICULAR WALL SYSTOLIC THICKNESS (LVWs):
   Measured at end-systole from the top of the ventricular wall to the top of the pericardium at the same point systolic chamber size was measured

CALCULATIONS FOR LEFT VENTRICULAR FUNCTION

1. LEFT VENTRICULAR FRACTIONAL SHORTENING (%FS):

$$((LVd - LVs) / LVd) \times 100$$

M-MODE REFERENCE VALUES IN NONANESTHETIZED CATS

Parameter	Jacobs[a] Range	Pipers[b] Range	Sisson[c] Range	Moise[d] $\bar{x} \pm SD$
RVd (cm)	0.00–0.70	—	0.0–0.83	—
RVs (cm)	0.27–0.94	—	—	—
RVWs (cm)	0.23–0.43	—	—	—
LVd (cm)	1.20–1.98	1.12–2.18	1.08–2.14	1.51 ± 0.21
LVs (cm)	0.52–1.08	0.64–1.68	0.40–1.12	0.69 ± 0.22
% FS	39.0–61.0	23–56	40.0–66.7	55 ± 10.2
LVET (sec)	0.10–0.18	0.11–0.19	—	—
Vcf (cm/sec)	2.35–4.95	1.27–4.55	—	—
VSd (cm)	0.22–0.40	0.28–0.60	0.30–0.60	0.50 ± 0.07
VSs (cm)	0.47–0.70	—	0.40–0.90	0.76 ± 0.12
VS% Δ	—	—	—	33.5 ± 8.2
LVWd (cm)	0.22–0.44	0.32–0.56	0.25–0.60	0.46 ± 0.05
LVWs (cm)	0.54–0.81	—	0.43–0.98	0.78 ± 0.10
LVW% Δ	—	—	—	39.5 ± 7.6
AO (cm)	0.72–1.19	0.40–1.18	0.60–1.21	0.95 ± 0.15
LA (cm)	0.93–1.51	0.45–1.12	0.70–1.70	1.21 ± 0.18
LA/AO	0.95–1.65	—	0.88–1.79	1.29 ± 0.23
EPSS (cm)	0.00–0.21	—	0.00–0.20	0.04 ± 0.07
HR	147–242	120–240	120–240	182 ± 22
Kg	1.96–6.26	2.3–6.8	2.7–8.2	4.3 ± 0.5
N	30	25	79	11

[a]Jacobs G, Knight DH. M-mode echocardiographic measurements in nonanesthetized healthy cats: Effects of body weight, heart rate, and other variables. Am J Vet Res 1985;46:1705–1711.

[b]Pipers FS, Reef V, Hamlin RL. Echocardiography in the domestic cat. Am J Vet Res 1979;40:882–886.

[c]Sisson DD, Knight DH, Helinski C, et al. Plasma taurine concentrations and m-mode echocardiographic measures in healthy cats and in cats with dilated cardiomyopathy. J Vet Intern Med 1991;5:232–238.

[d]Moise NS, Dietz AE, Mezza LE, et al. Echocardiography, electrocardiography, and radiography of cats with dilation cardiomyopathy, hypertropic cardiomyopathy, and hyperthyroidism. Am J Vet Res 1986;47:1476–1486.

2. VELOCITY OF CIRCUMFERENTIAL FIBER SHORTENING (Vcf):

$$((LVd - LVs) / (LVET \times LVd))$$

Dimensions in this equation must be in centimeters and ejection time must be in seconds

3. LEFT VENTRICULAR WALL SYSTOLIC THICKENING (LVW % △):

$$((LVWs - LVWd) / LVWd) \times 100$$

4. SEPTAL SYSTOLIC THICKENING (VS % △):

$$((VSs - VSd) / VSd) \times 100$$

M-MODE REFERENCE VALUES IN ANESTHETIZED OR SEDATED CATS

Parameter	Allen[a] x̄ ± SD	Fox[b] Range	Allen[c] x̄ ± SD
RVd (cm)	—	0.12–0.75	—
RVs (cm)	—	—	—
LVd (cm)	1.30 ± 0.12	1.07–1.73	1.29 ± 0.09
LVs (cm)	0.86 ± 0.16	0.49–1.16	0.88 ± 0.08
%FS	34.5 ± 2.51	30.0–60.0	31.1 ± 4.67
LVET (sec)	0.17 ± 0.02	0.100–0.132	0.16 ± 0.02
PEP (sec)	—	0.024–0.058	—
PEP/LVET	—	0.228–0.513	—
Vcf (cm/sec)	2.05 ± 0.48	2.44–5.00	2.02 ± 0.45
VSd (cm)	0.40 ± 0.03	0.22–0.49	—
VSs (cm)	—	—	—
LVWd (cm)	0.40 ± 0.4	0.21–0.45	—
LVWs (cm)	—	—	—
VS/LVW	—	0.69–1.42	—
AO (cm)	0.90 ± 0.07	0.71–1.15	—
LA (cm)	1.00 ± 0.07	0.72–1.33	—
LA/AO	—	0.73–1.64	—
EPSS (cm)	—	—	—
HR	175 ± 20	160–300	163 ± 13
Kg	3.64 ± 0.66	2.05–6.80	3.50 ± 0.41
N	10	30	8
Drug	Sodium pentobarbital	Ketamine hydrochloride	Xylazine-sodium pentobarbital

[a]Allen, DG. Echocardiographic study of the anesthetized cat. Can J Comp Med 1982;46:115–122.

[b]Fox PR, Bond BR, Peterson ME. Echocardiographic reference values in healthy cats sedated with ketamine hydrochloride. Am J Vet Res 1985;46:1479–1484.

[c]Allen, DG, Downey RS. Echocardiographic assessment of cats anesthetized with xylazine-sodium pentobarbital. Can J Comp Med 1983;47:281–283.

REFERENCE VALUES FOR TWO-DIMENSIONAL MEASUREMENTS IN CATS

Parameter/View	Mean	SD
Short-axis views		
AO area	0.7	0.15
LVd	13.5	1.38
LVs	8.4	1.46
VSd	3.9	0.83
VSs	5.9	0.82
LVWd	3.5	0.71
LVWs	5.5	0.83
Long-axis views		
LVd	12.6	1.04
LVs	8.0	1.49
VSd	3.6	0.52
VSs	5.8	0.58
LVWd	3.7	0.49
LVWs	6.1	0.55

Weight = 3.6 ± 1.05; N = 13 (7 awake, 6 sedated).

Data from DeMadron E, Bonagura JD, Herring DS. Two dimensional echocardiography in the normal cat. Vet Radiol 1985;26:149–158.

M-MODE REFERENCE VALUES IN SPECIFIC CANINE BREEDS

Parameter	Greyhound[a] Range	Greyhound[a] Range	Greyhound[b] Range	English Pointer[c] x̄ ± SD
AO (mm)	—	—	—	24.1 ± 1.7
LA (mm)	—	—	—	22.6 ± 2.0
LA/AO	—	—	—	0.94 ± 0.07
LVd (mm)	36.0–49.0	40.0–49.0	40–50	39.2 ± 2.4
LVs (mm)	27.0–37.0	29.0–38.0	28–36	25.3 ± 2.4
%FS	16.0–32.0	17.0–35.0	24–37	35.5 ± 4.0
%EF	31.0–60.0	35.0–64.0	—	—
LVET (msec)	—	—	153–209	—
LVETI	—	—	216–253	—
PEP/LVET	—	—	0.32–0.54	—
Vcf (circ/sec)	—	—	1.2–2.2	—
PEP (msec)	—	—	55–82	—
VSd (mm)	9.0–14.0	8.0–14.0	10–16	6.9 ± 1.1
VSs (mm)	11.0–16.0	10.0–17.0	—	10.6 ± 1.0
LVWd (mm)	10.0–15.0	9.0–14.0	8–13	7.1 ± 0.7
LVWs (mm)	13.0–18.0	12.0–18.0	—	11.5 ± 1.3
Kg	20.7–32.5	20.7–32.5	25.0–36.3	19.2 ± 2.8
N	16	16	11	16
HR	—	—	66–131	107 ± 17
Drugs	Acepromazine & pethidine	No	No	No

[a]Page A, Edmunds G, Atwell RB. Echocardiographic values in the greyhound. Aus Vet J 1993;70:361–364.

[b]Snyder PS, Sato T, Atkins CE. A comparison of echocardiographic indices of the nonracing, healthy greyhound to reference values from other breeds. Vet Radiol Ultrasound 1995;36:387–392.

[c]Sisson D, Schaeffer D. Changes in linear dimensions of the heart, relative to body weight as measured by m-mode echocardiography in growing dogs. Am J Vet Res 1991;52:1591–1596.

M-MODE REFERENCE VALUES IN SPECIFIC CANINE BREEDS

Parameter	Beagle[a] Range	Miniature Poodle[b] Range	Corgi[b] Range	Afghan[b] Range	Golden Retriever[b] Range
AO (cm)	—	0.8–1.3	1.5–2.2	2.0–3.4	1.4–2.7
LA (cm)	—	0.8–1.8	1.2–2.4	1.8–3.5	1.6–3.2
LVd (cm)	1.80–3.30	1.6–2.8	2.8–4.0	3.3–5.2	3.7–5.1
LVs (cm)	0.80–2.70	0.8–1.6	1.2–2.3	2.0–3.7	1.8–3.5
%FS	20–70	35–57	33–57	24–48	27–55
%EF	40–100	—	—	—	—
EPSS (cm)	—	0–0.2	0–0.5	0–1.0	0.1–1.0
VSd (cm)	0.50–1.10	0.4–0.6	0.6–0.9	0.8–1.2	0.8–1.3
VSs (cm)	0.60–1.20	0.6–1.0	1.0–1.4	0.8–1.8	1.0–1.7
LVWd (cm)	0.60–1.30	0.4–0.6	0.6–1.0	0.7–1.1	0.8–1.2
LVWs (cm)	0.70–1.70	0.6–1.0	0.8–1.3	0.9–1.8	1.0–1.9
Kg	5.5–12.0	1.4–9.0	8–19	17–36	23–41
N	50	20	20	20	20

[a]Crippa L, Ferro E, Melloni E, et al. Echocardiographic parameters and indices in the normal Beagle dog. Lab Animals 1992;26:190–195.

[b]Morrison SA, Moise NS, Scarlett J, et al. Effect of breed and body weight on echocardiographic values in four breeds of dogs of differing somatotype. J Vet Intern Med 1992;6:220–224.

M-MODE REFERENCE VALUES IN SPECIFIC CANINE BREEDS

Parameter	Cocker Spaniel[a] x̄ ± SD	Newfoundland[b] 90% CI	Wolfhound[b] 90% CI	Great Dane[b] 90% CI	Spanish Mastiff[c] x̄ ± SD
AO (cm)	—	2.6–3.3	2.9–3.1	2.8–3.4	2.86 ± 0.07
AOexc (cm)	—	0.5–1.3	0.8–1.3	0.6–1.3	—
LA (cm)	—	2.4–3.3	2.2–3.5	2.8–4.6	2.85 ± 0.09
LA/AO	—	0.8–1.25	0.75–1.15	0.9–1.5	0.97 ± 0.02
LVd (cm)	3.38 ± 0.33	4.4–6.0	4.6–5.9	4.4–5.9	4.77 ± 0.14
LVs (cm)	2.22 ± 0.28	2.9–4.4	3.3–4.5	3.4–4.5	2.90 ± 0.11
%FS	34.3 ± 4.5	22–37	20–34	18–36	39 ± 1.6
%EF	—	44–66	38–61	33–65	—
LVET (sec)	—	0.14–0.20	0.14–0.19	0.12–0.18	—
Vcf (cir/sec)	—	1.1–2.5	1.0–2.2	1.0–2.3	—
EPSS (cm)	—	0.3–1.4	0.1–1.0	0.5–1.2	—
VSd (cm)	0.82 ± 0.13	0.7–1.5	0.9–1.45	1.2–1.6	0.98 ± 0.04
VSs (cm)	—	1.1–2.0	1.1–1.7	1.4–1.9	1.56 ± 0.05
VS%Δ	—	0–45	0–32	6–32	61.2 ± 2.4
VSexc (cm)	—	0.4–1.0	0.5–1.0	0.2–0.8	—
LVWd (cm)	0.79–0.11	0.8–1.3	0.9–1.3	1.0–1.6	0.97 ± 0.04
LVWs (cm)	—	1.1–1.6	1.1–1.7	1.1–1.9	1.52 ± 0.04
LVW%Δ	—	11–40	10–38	–9–29	56.8 ± 2.5
LVWexc (cm)	—	0.8–1.7	0.8–1.3	0.9–1.5	—
HR	—	70–120	70–120	100–130	107 ± 5
Kg	12.2 ± 2.3	47–70	50–80	52–75	52.4 ± 3.3
N	12	27	20	15	12

CI, confidence interval.

[a]Gooding JP, Robinson WF, Mews GC. Echocardiographic assessment of left ventricular dimensions in clinically normal English Cocker Spaniels. Am J Vet Res 1986;47:296–300.

[b]Koch J, Pedersen HD, Jensen AL, et al. M-mode echocardiographic diagnosis of dilated cardiomyopathy in giant breed dogs. J Vet Med A 1996;43:297–304.

[c]Bayón A, Fernández del Palacio MJ, Montes AM, et al. M-mode echocardiography study in growing Spanish mastiffs. J Small Anim Pract 1994;35:473–479.

NORMAL SYSTOLIC TIME INTERVALS IN THE DOG[a]

Parameter	Atkins[b] x̄ ± SD	Pipers[c] Unanesthetized Regression Equation	r	Pipers[c] Anesthetized Regression Equation	r
LVET (msec)	159 ± 15				
LVETI (msec)	227 ± 15	Y = 222 − 0.55 (HR)	0.93	Y = 290 − 0.70 (HR)	0.95
PEP (msec)	54 ± 7				
PEP/LVET	0.24 ± 0.05	Y = 0.15 + 0.0025 (HR)	0.73	Y = 0.17 + 0.0013 (HR)	0.71
Vcf (cir/sec)	2.48 ± 0.50				
QAVC (msec)	214 ± 18	Y = 282 − 0.51 (HR)	0.93	Y = 346 − 0.75 (HR)	0.88
HR	124 + 23				

Y, measurement of the parameter; r, correlation coefficient.

[a]Independent upon body weight.

[b]Atkins CE, Snyder PS. Systolic time intervals and their derivatives for evaluation of cardiac function. J Vet Intern Med 1992;6:55–63.

[c]Pipers FS, Andrysco RM, Hamlin RL. A totally noninvasive method for obtaining systolic time intervals in the dog. Am J Vet Res 1978;39:1822–1826.

M-MODE REFERENCE VALUES IN GROWING PUPPIES

Parameter/Breed	1 Month x̄ ± SD	2 Months x̄ ± SD	3 Months x̄ ± SD
Kg			
Spanish mastiffs[a]	3.37 ± 0.08	9.08 ± 0.47	15.35 ± 0.75
English pointers[b]	1.47 ± 0.26	3.84 ± 1.04	7.68 ± 1.46
HR			
Spanish mastiffs	199 ± 7.7	160 ± 3.6	139 ± 4.9
English pointers	177 ± 24.0	181 ± 31.7	144 ± 11.5
LVd (mm)			
Spanish mastiffs	16.60 ± 0.27	24.82 ± 0.71	28.29 ± 0.73
English pointers	14.5 ± 1.7	20.3 ± 1.8	26.1 ± 2.0
LVs (mm)			
Spanish mastiffs	8.65 ± 0.29	15.00 ± 0.37	18.67 ± 0.58
English pointers	8.9 ± 1.5	12.2 ± 1.6	16.6 ± 1.6
LVWd (mm)			
Spanish mastiffs	4.73 ± 0.16	5.76 ± 0.14	7.02 ± 0.25
English pointers	3.0 ± 0.3	4.0 ± 0.6	4.7 ± 0.8
LVWs (mm)			
Spanish mastiffs	7.61 ± 0.21	9.24 ± 0.20	10.69 ± 0.39
English pointers	5.0 ± 0.6	6.9 ± 0.7	8.3 ± 0.8
VSd (mm)			
Spanish mastiffs	4.92 ± 0.15	5.97 ± 0.15	7.04 ± 0.22
English pointers	3.2 ± 0.6	4.0 ± 0.6	4.8 ± 0.7
VSs (mm)			
Spanish mastiffs	7.81 ± 0.19	9.41 ± 0.24	10.88 ± 0.38
English pointers	4.8 ± 0.5	6.4 ± 0.8	7.7 ± 0.6
LA (mm)			
Spanish mastiffs	10.94 ± 0.27	15.78 ± 0.40	18.64 ± 0.35
English pointers	8.5 ± 0.9	12.0 ± 1.1	15.6 ± 1.7
AO (mm)			
Spanish mastiffs	9.77 ± 0.26	15.00 ± 0.40	18.63 ± 0.39
English pointers	8.5 ± 0.6	12.5 ± 1.2	16.2 ± 1.3
LA/AO			
Spanish mastiffs	0.90 ± 0.03	0.95 ± 0.02	1.00 ± 0.02
English pointers	1.01 ± 0.16	0.97 ± 0.06	0.96 ± 0.08
%FS			
Spanish mastiffs	47.84 ± 1.51	39.27 ± 0.99	34.02 ± 1.05
English pointers	38.4 ± 5.4	40.0 ± 4.8	36.3 ± 3.4

Spanish mastiffs, N = 66; English pointers, N = 16.

[a]Bayon A, Fernández del Palacio MJ, Montes AM, et al. M-mode echocardiography study in growing Spanish mastiffs. J Small Anim Pract 1994;35:473–479.

[b]Sisson D, Schaeffer D. Changes in linear dimensions of the heart, relative to body weight, as measured by m-mode echocardiography in growing dogs. Am J Vet Res 1991;52:1591–1596.

GENERAL M-MODE REFERENCE VALUES FOR ADULT DOGS[a]

Parameter (mm)/ Reference		Regression Equation	$S\hat{Y}_{xo}$	CI $(t_{0.025})$
AO	1	$\hat{Y}_o = 12.83 + (12.17)x_0$	$\sqrt{0.21 + 12.64(x_o - 0.73)^2}$	$\hat{Y}_o \pm (2.101)(S\hat{Y}_{xo})$
	2	$\hat{Y}_o = 14 + (0.353)x_0$		
LA	1	$\hat{Y}_o = 12.63 + (12.05)x_0$	$\sqrt{0.32 + 19.27(x_o - 0.73)^2}$	$\hat{Y}_o \pm (2.101)(S\hat{Y}_{xo})$
	2	$\hat{Y}_o = 13 + (0.380)x_0$		
LVd	1	$\hat{Y}_o = 15.63 + (31.25)x_0$	$\sqrt{0.72 + 43.64(x_o - 0.73)^2}$	$\hat{Y}_o \pm (2.101)(S\hat{Y}_{xo})$
	2	$\hat{Y}_o = 22 + (0.733)x_0$		
LVs	1	$\hat{Y}_o = 9.00 + (21.18)x_0$	$\sqrt{0.37 + 22.67(x_o - 0.73)^2}$	$\hat{Y}_o \pm (2.101)(S\hat{Y}_{xo})$
	2	$\hat{Y}_o = 12 + (0.515)x_0$		
LVWd	1	$\hat{Y}_o = 4.05 + (4.08)x_0$	$\sqrt{0.04 + 2.61(x_o - 0.73)^2}$	$\hat{Y}_o \pm (2.101)(S\hat{Y}_{xo})$
	2	$\hat{Y}_o = 5 + (0.158)x_0$		
LVWs	1	$\hat{Y}_o = 6.67 + (6.35)x_0$	$\sqrt{0.10 + 5.79(x_o - 0.73)^2}$	$\hat{Y}_o \pm (2.101)(S\hat{Y}_{xo})$
VSd	1	$\hat{Y}_o = 4.59 + (6.33)x_0$	$\sqrt{0.16 + 2.80(x_o - 0.72)^2}$	$\hat{Y}_o \pm (2.145)(S\hat{Y}_{xo})$
	2	$\hat{Y}_o = 6 + (0.133)x_0$		
VSs	1	$\hat{Y}_o = 7.92 + (8.46)x_0$	$\sqrt{0.34 + 6.09(x_o - 0.72)^2}$	$\hat{Y}_o \pm (2.145)(S\hat{Y}_{xo})$

1. Boon J, Wingfield WE, Miller CW. Echocardiographic indices in the normal dog. Vet Radiol 1983;5:214–221.

2. Lombard CW. Normal values of the canine m-mode echocardiogram. Am J Vet Res 1984;45:2015–2018.

$\hat{Y}_o$, estimate of the mean measurement at a given body surface area or weight; x_0, body surface area of the dog for reference 1 and weight for reference 2; $S\hat{Y}_{xo}$, variance of the estimate about the regression line. CI, 95% confidence interval about the regression line.

[a]Dependent upon body weight.

GENERAL TWO-DIMENSIONAL REFERENCE VALUES FOR ADULT DOGS[a]

Parameter (mm) View/Figure	Regression Equation	$S^2_{y.x}$	95% CI
LVd length RP (Fig. 3.19)	$y = 37.73 + 1.29(x_i)$	$(2.46 + 0.0509(X_i - 18.05)^2)$	$y \pm 2.16(s_{y.x})$
LVd length RP (Fig. 3.20)	$y = 37.21 + 1.17(x_i)$	$(3.82 + 0.0931(X_i - 17.89)^2)$	$y \pm 2.14(s_{y.x})$
LVd length LP (Fig. 3.21)	$y = 28.39 + 1.26(x_i)$	$(2.05 + 0.0456(X_i - 18.52)^2)$	$y \pm 2.13(s_{y.x})$
LVs length LP (Fig. 3.21)	$y = 20.63 + 1.03(x_i)$	$(1.79 + 0.0399(X_i - 18.52)^2)$	$y \pm 2.13(s_{y.x})$
LVd long axis (Fig. 3.17)	$y = 21.99 + 0.64(x_i)$	$(0.68 + 0.0152(X_i - 18.52)^2)$	$y \pm 2.13(s_{y.x})$
LVs long axis (Fig. 3.17)	$y = 15.10 + 0.51(x_i)$	$(0.64 + 0.0143(X_i - 18.52)^2)$	$y \pm 2.13(s_{y.x})$
LVd short axis (Fig. 3.18)	$y = 23.97 + 0.57(x_i)$	$(0.99 + 0.0220(X_i - 18.52)^2)$	$y \pm 2.13(s_{y.x})$
LVs short axis (Fig. 3.18)	$y = 17.03 + 0.48(x_i)$	$(0.55 + 0.0123(X_i - 18.52)^2)$	$y \pm 2.13(s_{y.x})$
LVd int area sax (Fig. 3.47)	$y = 3.86 + 0.29(x_i)$	$(0.20 + 0.045(X_i - 18.52)^2)$	$y \pm 2.13(s_{y.x})$
VSd long axis (Fig. 3.17)	$y = 3.65 + 0.18(x_i)$	$(0.08 + 0.0017(X_i - 18.52)^2)$	$y \pm 2.13(s_{y.x})$
VSs long axis (Fig. 3.17)	$y = 4.71 + 0.29(x_i)$	$(0.12 + 0.0026(X_i - 18.52)^2)$	$y \pm 2.13(s_{y.x})$
VSd short axis (Fig. 3.18)	$y = 3.97 + 0.23(x_i)$	$(0.08 + 0.0019(X_i - 18.52)^2)$	$y \pm 2.13(s_{y.x})$
VSs short axis (Fig. 3.18)	$y = 5.90 + 0.23(x_i)$	$(0.13 + 0.0029(X_i - 18.52)^2)$	$y \pm 2.13(s_{y.x})$
LVWd long axis (Fig. 3.17)	$y = 3.41 + 0.24(x_i)$	$(0.12 + 0.0026(X_i - 18.52)^2)$	$y \pm 2.13(s_{y.x})$
LVWs long axis (Fig. 3.17)	$y = 5.82 + 0.27(x_i)$	$(0.10 + 0.0021(X_i - 18.52)^2)$	$y \pm 2.13(s_{y.x})$
LVWd short axis (Fig. 3.18)	$y = 3.00 + 0.27(x_i)$	$(0.12 + 0.0026(X_i - 18.52)^2)$	$y \pm 2.13(s_{y.x})$
LVWs short axis (Fig. 3.18)	$y = 4.59 + 0.31(x_i)$	$(0.19 + 0.0043(X_i - 18.52)^2)$	$y \pm 2.13(s_{y.x})$
LA r–1 lax RP (Fig. 3.19)	$y = 20.65 + 0.63(x_i)$	$(0.83 + 0.0185(X_i - 18.52)^2)$	$y \pm 2.13(s_{y.x})$
LA b–a lax RP (Fig. 3.19)	$y = 17.20 + 0.58(x_i)$	$(0.56 + 0.0124(X_i - 18.52)^2)$	$y \pm 2.13(s_{y.x})$
LA area lax RP (Fig. 3.22)	$y = 2.64 + 0.38(x_i)$	$(0.18 + 0.0040(X_i - 18.52)^2)$	$y \pm 2.13(s_{y.x})$
LA area lax LP (Fig. 3.21)	$y = 1.23 + 0.40(x_i)$	$(0.30 + 0.0073(X_i - 17.82)^2)$	$y \pm 2.18(s_{y.x})$
AO valve RP (Fig. 3.23)	$y = 9.55 + 0.22(x_i)$	$(0.16 + 0.0035(X_i - 18.52)^2)$	$y \pm 2.13(s_{y.x})$
AO sinus RP (Fig. 3.23)	$y = 11.87 + 0.40(x_i)$	$(0.25 + 0.0056(X_i - 18.52)^2)$	$y \pm 2.13(s_{y.x})$
AO valve LP (Fig. 3.24)	$y = 9.07 + 0.29(x_i)$	$(0.24 + 0.0058(X_i - 19.37)^2)$	$y \pm 2.20(s_{y.x})$
AO sinus LP (Fig. 3.24)	$y = 13.46 + 0.38(x_i)$	$(0.20 + 0.0053(X_i - 19.01)^2)$	$y \pm 2.18(s_{y.x})$
AO asc LP (Fig. 3.24)	$y = 8.38 + 0.31(x_i)$	$(0.05 + 0.0012(X_i - 19.58)^2)$	$y \pm 2.23(s_{y.x})$
AO area sax RP (Fig. 3.25)	$y = 0.72 + 0.11(x_i)$	$(0.01 + 0.0003(X_i - 18.52)^2)$	$y \pm 2.13(s_{y.x})$

Y, measurement for the parameter; X_i, body weight; $S^2_{y.x}$, standard deviation about the regression line; CI, confidence interval; RP, right parasternal; LP, left parasternal; int, internal; sax, short axis; lax, long axis; asc, ascending; r–l, right to left dimension; b–a, base apex dimension.

Data adapted from O'Grady MR, Bonagura JD, Powers JD, et al. Quantitative cross-sectional echocardiography in the normal dog. Vet Radiol 1986;27:34–49.

[a]Dependent upon body weight.

CANINE REFERENCE VALUES FOR PARAMETERS OF FUNCTION[a]

Parameter	N	Mean	STD DEV	95% CI
LVET (msec)	37	177.84	16.90	160.90-194.70
PEP (msec)	34	56.77	18.20	19.75-93.79
PEP/LVET	33	0.32	0.11	0.10-0.54
LA/AO	59	0.98	0.15	0.83-1.13
EPSS (mm)	58	3.70	2.00	0.30-7.70
FS (%)	64	39.63	6.26	33.70-45.90
Vcf (circ/sec)	36	2.21	0.40	1.40-3.02
VS%Δ	63	53.59	19.60	34.00-73.20
LVW%Δ	63	60.76	15.10	45.70-75.90
VSd/LVWd	62	1.26	0.22	1.04-1.48
VSd/LVd	63	0.28	0.06	0.22-0.34
HR (beats/min)	66	97.60	24.30	49.00-146.00

Data from Boon J, Wingfield W, Miller C. Echocardiographic indices in the normal dog. Vet Radiol 1983;24:214–221. Additional data courtesy of June Boon, Colorado State University, Veterinary Teaching Hospital.

[a]Independent of body weight.

DETERMINING REFERENCE VALUES FOR DOGS WEIGHING MORE THAN 150 POUNDS

Normal ranges for dogs larger than 150 lb may be determined by applying the following calculations. These are based on the fact that a linear correlation exists between the cardiac parameter and the body surface area. The regression equation slope can then be used to adjust the value of the dog's echocardiographic parameter down to 1 m^2.

To adjust your echocardiographic measurements to 1 m^2, use the following table and instructions:

Parameter (mm)	Slope	95% CI for 1 m^2
AO	17.44	25.6-27.3
AO exc	4.74	8.1-9.1
LA	15.35	24.2-26.4
LVd	27.82	40.9-44.4
LVs	19.05	25.4-27.9
VSd	5.60	10.3-11.5
VSs	8.75	15.6-16.9
VS exc	4.09	7.0-7.8
LVWd	4.61	8.3-9.3
LVWs	7.07	13.4-14.6
LVW exc	6.48	10.8-12.2

Data from Boon J, Wingfield W, Miller C. Echocardiographic indices in the normal dog. Vet Radiol 1983;24:214–221. Additional data courtesy of June Boon, Colorado State University, Veterinary Teaching Hospital.

exc, excursion.

1. Subtract the body surface area (BSA) of your patient from 1. The result will be negative if the BSA of your patient is greater than 1 m^2. (See the table correlating weight with BSA.)

2. Multiply the above result by the slope of the regression equation for the parameter in question.

3. Add to that the echocardiographic measurement from your scan.

Example: For a dog that is 1.2 m^2 and has a left ventricular end-diastolic measurement of 47.4 mm on your echocardiogram, the calculation is as follows:

$$((1-1.2) \times 27.82) + 47.4 = 41.8$$

A measurement of 41.8 would be normal because the normal range for left ventricular end-diastolic dimension at 1 m^2 is 40.9–44.4.

BODY SURFACE AREA FOR DOGS

LBS	KG	BSA		LBS	KG	BSA
151	68.6	1.68		177	80.5	1.87
152	69.1	1.69		178	80.9	1.88
153	69.5	1.70		179	81.4	1.88
154	70.0	1.70		180	81.8	1.89
155	70.5	1.71		181	82.3	1.90
156	70.9	1.72		182	82.7	1.90
157	71.4	1.72		183	83.2	1.91
158	71.8	1.73		184	83.6	1.92
159	72.3	1.74		185	84.1	1.92
160	72.7	1.75		186	84.5	1.93
161	73.2	1.75		187	85.0	1.94
162	73.6	1.76		188	85.5	1.94
163	74.1	1.77		189	85.9	1.95
164	74.5	1.78		190	86.4	1.96
165	75.0	1.78		191	86.8	1.97
166	75.5	1.79		192	87.3	1.97
167	75.9	1.80		193	87.7	1.98
168	76.4	1.80		194	88.2	1.99
169	76.8	1.81		195	88.6	1.99
170	77.3	1.82		196	89.1	2.00
171	77.7	1.83		197	89.5	2.01
172	78.2	1.83		198	90.0	2.01
173	78.6	1.84		199	90.5	2.02
174	79.1	1.85		200	90.9	2.03
175	79.5	1.85		201	91.4	2.03
176	80.0	1.86				

M-MODE REFERENCE VALUES IN GROWING FOALS (6 PONIES, 10 THOROUGHBREDS)

Parameter	24 Hours Mean	SD	7 Days Mean	SD	4 Weeks Mean	SD	2 Months Mean	SD	3 Months Mean	SD
RVd (cm)	2.37	0.40	2.61	0.27	2.64	0.34	2.90	0.09	2.74	0.23
LVd (cm)	5.81	0.53	6.50	0.53	7.40	0.65	7.45	0.71	7.76	0.65
LVs (cm)	4.67	0.56	5.50	0.41	6.52	0.11	6.86	0.18	6.92	0.88
%FS	21.3	2.93	20.1	5.01	16.3	1.77	18.2	4.51	21.1	1.4
LVET (msec)	303	69.8	260	47.1	250	55.6	364	79.8	344	90.4
PEP (msec)	48.5	6.24	51.9	8.61	52.1	15.0	69.3	12.3	65.8	10.1
PEP/LVET	0.16	0.02	0.20	0.04	0.21	0.05	0.19	0.04	0.19	0.05
Vcf (cir/sec)	1.00	0.37	0.83	0.15	0.54	0.12	0.58	0.08	0.59	0.10
VSd (cm)	1.27	0.25	1.35	0.23	1.38	0.20	1.42	0.31	1.46	0.09
VS%Δ	48.8	19.5	43.1	12.0	36.1	13.7	41.1	12.9	50.0	12.5
LVWd (cm)	0.55	0.04	0.70	0.08	1.28	0.14	1.48	0.19	1.58	0.16
LVW/VS	0.43	0.06	0.52	0.07	0.93	0.11	0.93	0.11	1.08	0.12
AO (cm)	3.70	0.25	3.61	0.29	4.19	0.21	3.95	0.16	4.34	0.32
LA (cm)	3.01	0.70	3.23	0.50	3.52	0.92	3.48	0.75	3.82	0.60
LA/AO	0.81	0.15	0.90	0.15	0.84	0.14	0.88	0.14	0.88	0.33
HR	91	15	93	22	76	17	70	13	69	13
Kg	46.96	8.98	56.89	10.05	80.66	13.67	96.48	12.96	111.83	16.08
N	16		16		16		16		16	

Adapted from Stewart JH, Rose RJ, Barko AM. Echocardiography in foals from birth to three months old. Equine Vet J 1984;16:332–341.

M-MODE REFERENCE VALUES IN PONY FOALS (12 PONY FOALS)

Parameter	Mean	SD	Range	Regression Equation	r
%FS	34	8	24–50		
VSd (mm)	11	2	7–14		
LVWd (mm)	9	2	6–13		
LA/AO	0.82	0.1	0.55–1.08		
RVd (mm)			8–20	y = 0.16x + 9	0.55
LVd (mm)			26–63	y = 0.47x + 26	0.74
LVs (mm)			15–47	y = 0.38x + 15	0.65
AO (mm)			21–38	y = 0.21x + 22	0.63
LA (mm)			16–34	y = 0.23x + 16	0.62
Kg	27	10	14–57		

Adapted from Lombard CW, Evans M, Martin L, et al. Blood pressure, electrocardiogram and echocardiogram measurements in the growing pony foal. Equine Vet J 1984;16:342–347.

y, measurement for the parameter; x, body weight; r, correlation coefficient.

M-MODE REFERENCE VALUES IN ADULT HORSES

Parameter	Dressage[a] Mean	SD	Show-Jumping[a] Mean	SD	Untrained[a] Mean	SD	Endurance[b] Mean	SD	Unconditioned[b] Mean	SD	THB and THB Crosses[c] Mean	SD
RVd (mm)	39	8	41	5	42	8	—	—	—	—	3.83	0.91
RVs (mm)	35	6	38	5	38	6	—	—	—	—	2.71	1.00
LVd (mm)	116	7	121	10	115	7	101	2	95	3	11.9	0.71
LVs (mm)	82	6	86	8	82	7	60	2	52	3	7.35	0.72
%FS	29	5	29	5	28	5	42	1	46	2	38.76	4.59
LVET (sec)	—	—	—	—	—	—	0.44	0.01	0.40	0.02	—	—
PEP (sec)	—	—	—	—	—	—	0.08	0.01	0.50	0.01	—	—
Vcf (cir/sec)	—	—	—	—	—	—	0.91	0.05	1.16	0.07	—	—
VSd (mm)	35	4	30	3	33	5	28	1	27	1	3.02	0.39
VSs (mm)	43	7	40	5	40	6	45	1	44	1	4.55	0.55
VSexc (mm)	—	—	—	—	—	—	20	1	19	1	—	—
VS%Δ	—	—	—	—	—	—	59	3	66	4	—	—
LVWd (mm)	30	3	26	4	27	6	24	1	18	1	—	—
LVWs (mm)	36	5	32	5	32	6	36	1	33	1	3.96	0.63
LVWexc (mm)	—	—	—	—	—	—	24	1	26	1	—	—
LVW%Δ	—	—	—	—	—	—	53	5.4	86	7	—	—
VS/LVW	—	—	—	—	—	—	1.22	0.1	1.57	0.07	—	—
AO (mm)	78	6	74	9	75	6	64	1	58	1	8.50	0.51
LA (mm)	56	5	60	4	58	8	43	1	41	1	—	—
LA/AO	—	—	—	—	—	—	0.68	0.02	0.71	0.02	—	—
EPSS (mm)	—	—	—	—	—	—	15	1	10	1	—	—
Age (yr)	10.1	1.8	8.8	1.7	8.3	2.9	6–208[d]		1–25[d]		2–17[d]	
Kg	602	38	587	40	549	44	329–523[d]		186–636[d]		432–648[d]	
N	15		15		15		53		32		26	

[a]Stadler P, Rewel A, Deegen E. M-mode echocardiography in dressage- and show-jumping horses of class "S" and in untrained horses. J Vet Med A 1993;40:292–306.

[b]Paull KS, Wingfield WE, Bertone JJ, et al. Echocardiographic changes with endurance training. In: Gillespie JR, NE Robinson, eds. Equine exercise physiology 2. Davis: ICEEP Publications, 1987.

[c]Long, KJ, Bonagura JD, Darke PGG. Standardized imaging technique for guided m-mode and Doppler echocardiography in the horse. Equine Vet J 1992;24:226–235.

[d]Range.

REFERENCE VALUES FOR MEASUREMENTS FROM TWO-DIMENSIONAL IMAGES IN THE ADULT HORSE

Parameter	Mean	SD	Range
RVd (cm)	5.9	0.61	4.4–6.8
RVs (cm)	4.7	0.61	3.0–5.6
LVd (cm)	11.3	1.37	8.0–14.0
LVs (cm)	7.3	0.76	5.9–9.1
%FS	35.3	3.9	26.3–43.5
VSd (cm)	3.8	0.27	3.4–4.4
VSs (cm)	4.7	0.48	3.9–5.7
AO (cm)	7.8	0.4	7.3–8.4
LA (cm)	12.6	1.26	10.8–15.7
LA/AO	1.4	0.1	1.2–1.7

N = 18; weight = 482 kg (range = 411–551 kg).

Adapted from Voros K, Holmes JR, Gibbs, et al. Measurement of cardiac dimensions with two dimensional echocardiography in the living horse. Equine Vet J 1991;23:461.

M-MODE REFERENCE VALUES IN THE ADULT COW

Parameter	Mean	SD
RVd (cm)	3.04	0.56
LVd (cm)	7.54	0.80
LVs (cm)	3.97	1.16
%FS	43.5	5.80
LVET (msec)	408	13.8
QAVC (msec)	59.4	7.9
PEP (msec)	55.1	17.8
Vcf (cir/sec)	0.87	0.14
VSd (cm)	2.24	0.26
LVWd (cm)	2.00	0.19
AO (cm)	6.00	0.40
LA (cm)	4.80	0.57
HR	47.8	5.90

N = 15; weight = ~300 kg.

Adapted from Pipers FS, Reef V, Hamlin RL, et al. Echocardiography in the bovine animal. Bov Pract 1978;13:114–118.

ECHOCARDIOGRAPHIC REFERENCE VALUES FOR FRIESIAN AND BELGIAN WHITE AND BLUE CALVES

Parameter	Long Axis M-mode Mean	SE	Short Axis M-mode Mean	SE	Two-Dimensional Measurements Mean	SE
LVd (mm)	51.3	1.5	50.2	1.1	48.2	1.1
LVs (mm)	29.1	1.2	28.7	1.2	30.9	1.2
%FS	43.1	2.0	42.8	2.1	37.0	2.3
VSd (mm)	12.4	0.4	11.8	0.3	11.8	0.3
VSs (mm)	19.9	0.8	19.2	0.7	18.3	0.6
VS%Δ	60.4	3.6	63.1	2.4	57.4	2.8
LVWd (mm)	11.9	0.4	10.9	0.4	11.1	0.3
LVWs (mm)	20.5	0.6	19.6	1.0	17.7	0.7
LVW%Δ	76.1	2.7	76.5	3.6	62.9	3.7
VS/LVW	1.03	0.03	1.07	0.03	1.05	0.02
AO (mm)	31.5	0.9	—		—	
LA (mm)	25.9	0.5	—		—	
LA/AO	0.83	0.02	—		—	

N = 18; weight 84.9 ± 5 kg; age = 81.8 ± 3.7 days.

Adapted from Amory H, Jakovljevic S, Lekeux P. Quantitative m-mode and two dimensional echocardiography in calves. Vet Rec 1991;128:25–31.

M-MODE REFERENCE VALUES IN GROWING FRIESIAN CALVES

Parameter	18 Days Mean	SE	1 Month Mean	SE	2 Months Mean	SE	3 Months Mean	SE	4 Months Mean	SE
RVd (mm)	13.4	0.5	15.7	0.9	—	—	20.8	0.5	18.6	0.4
RVs (mm)	7.5	0.6	9.9	0.9	—	—	10.8	0.8	8.6	0.4
LVd (mm)	41.5	1.2	44.6	2.1	52.2	2.1	49.8	1.3	57.9	0.9
LVs (mm)	26.1	0.6	27.3	1.7	30.6	2.0	25.4	1.9	30.4	3.1
%FS	36.9	1.6	39.1	1.8	41.5	2.7	49.1	2.8	47.5	5.1
VSd (mm)	9.2	0.3	11.6	0.3	11.3	0.6	13.3	0.4	14.8	0.3
VSs (mm)	14.6	0.5	16.7	0.4	18.7	0.7	20.9	0.8	26.0	1.5
VS%Δ	58.4	4.5	43.2	2.9	66.9	5.5	57.1	3.0	75.6	10.7
LVWd (mm)	9.0	0.5	12.0	0.9	10.9	0.5	16.6	1.5	14.0	0.2
LVWs (mm)	14.8	0.4	18.1	0.7	18.9	0.7	25.0	1.4	24.0	0.5
LVW%Δ	65.8	4.8	55.4	7.4	73.9	4.8	53.2	7.4	71.3	1.9
VS/LVW	1.03	0.04	1.01	0.05	1.03	0.02	0.83	0.07	1.06	0.01
AO (mm)	26.5	0.8	28.9	0.6	28.9	0.7	34.3	1.1	37.2	0.9
LA (mm)	21.2	0.5	22.9	0.3	25.3	0.8	27.3	0.9	29.7	1.9
LA/AO	0.81	0.03	0.80	0.02	0.87	0.01	0.80	0.04	0.80	0.07
Kg	33.9	1.7	45.4	0.8	67.7	4.5	95.4	1.1	119.4	1.9
Age (days)	18.18	2.5	30.6	5.3	68.3	6.5	93.8	6.2	121.2	3.3
N	11		10		6		5		5	

Adapted from Amory H, Lekeux P. Effects of growth on functional and morphological echocardiographic variables in Friesian calves. Vet Rec 1991;128:349–354.

REGRESSION EQUATIONS CORRELATING CARDIAC DIMENSIONS WITH BODY WEIGHT IN FRIESIAN AND BELGIAN BLUE AND WHITE CALVES

Parameter	Friesian Calves	Belgian White and Blue
LVd (mm)		
M-mode from long axis	$Y = -2.5 + 30.8 \log BW$	$Y = 7.9 + 22.1 \log BW$
M-mode from short axis	$Y = 1.4 + 26.3 \log BW$	$Y = 11.3 + 20.0 \log BW$
Measurements from 2D short axis	$Y = 6.3 + 23.0 \log BW$	$Y = 3.8 + 22.9 \log BW$
LVs (mm)		
M-mode from long axis	$Y = 20.2 + 6.1 \log BW$	$Y = 16.0 + 7.9 \log BW$
M-mode from short axis	$Y = 14.8 + 7.4 \log BW$	$Y = 18.0 + 6.6 \log BW$
Measurements from 2D short axis	$Y = 20.5 + 4.7 \log BW$	$Y = 27.2 + 1.9 \log BW$
VSd (mm)		
M-mode from long axis	$Y = 0.01 + 6.9 \log BW$	$Y = -5.3 + 9.3 \log BW$
M-mode from short axis	$Y = -0.3 + 6.4 \log BW$	$Y = -6.3 + 9.5 \log BW$
Measurements from 2D short axis	$Y = -0.9 + 6.5 \log BW$	$Y = -6.2 + 9.4 \log BW$
VSs (mm)		
M-mode from long axis	$Y = -13.3 + 18.0 \log BW$	$Y = -17.2 + 18.8 \log BW$
M-mode from short axis	$Y = -8.7 + 14.9 \log BW$	$Y = -16.3 + 18.0 \log BW$
Measurements from 2D short axis	$Y = -7.3 + 13.5 \log BW$	$Y = -21.9 + 21.0 \log BW$
LVWd (mm)		
M-mode from long axis	$Y = 1.3 + 5.4 \log BW$	$Y = -8.9 + 10.5 \log BW$
M-mode from short axis	$Y = 1.1 + 4.8 \log BW$	$Y = -12.3 + 11.8 \log BW$
Measurements from 2D short axis	$Y = -1.9 + 7.2 \log BW$	$Y = -8.3 + 9.8 \log BW$
LVWs (mm)		
M-mode from long axis	$Y = -9.9 + 16.3 \log BW$	$Y = -22.4 + 21.7 \log BW$
M-mode from short axis	$Y = -8.4 + 15.2 \log BW$	$Y = -26.9 + 23.5 \log BW$
Measurements from 2D short axis	$Y = -9.3 + 14.2 \log BW$	$Y = -30.7 + 25.3 \log BW$
AO (mm)		
M-mode from long axis	$Y = -1.0 + 18.0 \log BW$	$Y = 1.6 + 14.3 \log BW$
LA (mm)		
M-mode from long axis	$Y = 1.4 + 13.9 \log BW$	$Y = -8.2 + 17.8 \log BW$
N	17	8

Adapted from Amory H, Kafidi N, Lekeux P. Echocardiographic evaluation of cardiac morphologic and functional variables in double-muscled calves. Am J Vet Res 1992;53:1540–1547.

Y, M-mode variable; *BW*, body weight in kg.

PARAMETERS OF FUNCTION OBTAINED FROM LONG-AXIS M-MODE IMAGES IN FRIESIAN AND BELGIAN WHITE AND BLUE CALVES

Parameter	Friesian		Belgian White and Blue	
	Mean	SE	Mean	SE
%FS	43.2	0.7	40.0	1.0
VS%Δ	63.6	2.2	44.7	3.1
LVW%Δ	71.3	2.6	44.8	3.7
VS/LVW	1.01	0.02	0.94	0.03
LA/AO	0.82	0.01	0.92	0.01

N = 17 Friesian; 8 Belgian white and blue (BWB).

Adapted from Amory H, Kafidi N, Lekeux P. Echocardiographic evaluation of cardiac morphologic and functional variables in double-muscled calves. Am J Vet Res 1992;53:1540–1547.

REFERENCE ECHOCARDIOGRAPHIC M-MODE VALUES FOR SHEEP

Parameter	Mean	SD	Range
RVd (mm)	20.3	5.6	12.6–33.5
RVs (mm)	13.6	5.3	6.6–27.3
RVWd (mm)	5.1	1.1	3.4–8.2
RVWs (mm)	9.4	2.2	6.0–13.1
LVd (mm)	51.7	7.4	37.3–63.3
LVs (mm)	32.3	4.6	24.8–40.5
VSd (mm)	9.4	1.7	6.2–13.6
VSs (mm)	14.1	2.2	10.2–18.6
LVWd (mm)	8.9	2.0	6.2–13.9
LVWs (mm)	15.3	3.3	11.4–27.3
AO (mm)	32.9	3.3	28.3–39.7
LA (mm)	30.2	3.5	22.6–36.3
LA/AO	0.92	0.10	0.79–1.13
%FS	37.2	5.7	27.3–49.0
LVW%Δ	75.1	28.5	30.2–133.9
VS%Δ	52.4	27.7	20.4–150.0
VSd/LVWd	1.07	0.18	0.7–1.43
LVET (msec)	252	35	200–320
Vcf (cir/sec)	1.52	0.28	1.12–2.04

Age = 2–5 years; weight = 55–95 kg.

Data from Moses BL, Ross JN. M-mode echocardiographic values in sheep. Am J Vet Res 1987;48:1313–1318.

M-MODE REFERENCE VALUES FOR MATURE PIGS

Parameter	Mean	SD	Range
LVd (mm)	3.32	0.45	2.7–3.8
LVs (cm)	1.87	0.34	1.4–2.5
LVWd (cm)	0.61	0.12	0.4–0.8
VSd (cm)	0.71	0.13	0.5–0.9
LA (cm)	1.60	0.22	1.4–2.0
AO (cm)	1.9	0.30	1.6–2.5
LVET (msec)	220	90	160–270
PEP (msec)	80	50	50–120
%FS	44.8	8.7	34–59
Vcf (cir/sec)	1.12	0.49	0.7–1.4
HR	94	6	72–110

Age = 1 year; weight = ~ 30 kg.

Data from Pipers FS, Muir WW, Hamlin RL. Echocardiography in swine. Am J Vet Res 1978;39:707–710.

M-MODE REFERENCE VALUES FOR GROWING PIGS

Parameter	Age		
	63 Days	90 Days	112 Days
LVd (mm)	35.7 ± 5.1	39.9 ± 4.0	38.5 ± 3.5
LVs (mm)	23.3 ± 5.0	25.3 ± 3.5	24.5 ± 2.1
%FS	36.3 ± 5.4	36.9 ± 3.7	36.5 ± .07
LA (mm)	11.9 ± 2.6	16.0 ± 3.0	17.5 ± 3.5
AO (mm)	18.8 ± 2.1	21.9 ± 2.6	21.5 ± 2.1
HR	165 ± 16	130 ± 7	160 ± 40
Kg	18.0 + 4.7	27.9 + 5.5	32.7 + 6.4

Data from Gwathmey JK, Nakao S, Come PC, et al. Echocardiographic assessment of cardiac chamber size and functional performance in swine. Am J Vet Res 1989;50:192–197.

M-MODE REFERENCE VALUES IN ADULT LLAMAS

Parameter	Mean	SD	Range
LVd (mm)	62.01	6.57	48.97–74.53
LVs (mm)	37.15	6.81	20.64–53.52
%FS	40.03	9.42	25.90–62.42
LVWd (mm)	11.60	2.52	7.96–18.97
LVWs (mm)	20.82	4.28	14.42–30.11
LVWexc (mm)	14.74	4.87	8.63–28.13
LVW%Δ	81.93	29.80	33.04–159.80
VSd (mm)	12.35	1.80	9.75–16.79
VSs (mm)	21.17	3.27	15.19–27.73
VSexc (mm)	12.29	3.78	6.50–22.70
VS%Δ	72.60	22.93	39.66–117.80
VSd/LVd	0.20	0.04	0.15–0.27
VSd/LVWd	1.10	0.21	0.68–1.52
HR	61.70	13.70	45.00–93.00

Data from Boon JA, Knight AP, Moore DH. Llama cardiology. Vet Clin North Am Food Anim Pract 1994;10:353–370.

CANINE
REFERENCE VALUES FOR AORTIC DOPPLER FLOW VARIABLES

	Vmax Range (cm/sec)	Vmax $\bar{x} \pm$ (SD) (cm/sec)	FT $\bar{x} \pm$ (SD) msec	PEP $\bar{x} \pm$ (SD) msec	PEP/ET $\bar{x} \pm$ (SD)	TTP $\bar{x} \pm$ (SD) msec	TTP/FT $\bar{x} \pm$ (SD)	Acc $\bar{x} \pm$ (SD) cm/sec^2	FVI $\bar{x} \pm$ (SD) m
Yuill (CW)(1)	104–138	118.1 (10.8)	—	—	—	—	—	—	—
Gaber (PW)(2)	—	118.9 (17.8)	—	—	—	—	—	—	—
Brown (PW)[a](3)	65–137	106 (21)	205 (15)	—	—	—	—	—	0.146 (0.029)
Kirberger (PW)(4)	106–229	157 (33)	182 (29)	58 (12)	—	55 (15)	0.30 (0.07)	32 (14)	—
Kirberger (CW)(4)	99–210	149 (27)	—	—	—	—	—	—	—
Bonagura (PW)(5)	≤170	$\bar{x} = 120$	—	—	—	—	—	—	—
Darke (6)	—	119 (24)	—	—	0.22 (0.06)	50 (10)	—	34 (16)	—

[a]Sedation used.

CANINE
REFERENCE VALUES FOR PULMONARY DOPPLER FLOW VARIABLES

	Vmax Range (cm/sec)	Vmax $\bar{x} \pm$ (SD) (cm/sec)	FT $\bar{x} \pm$ (SD) msec	PEP $\bar{x} \pm$ (SD) msec	PEP/ET $\bar{x} \pm$ (SD)	TTP $\bar{x} \pm$ (SD) msec	TTP/FT $\bar{x} \pm$ (SD)	Acc $\bar{x} \pm$ (SD) cm/sec^2	FVI $\bar{x} \pm$ (SD) m
Yuill (CW)(1)	76–122	98.1 (9.4)	—	—	—	—	—	—	—
Gaber (PW)(2)	—	99.8 (15.3)	—	—	—	—	—	—	—
Brown (PW)[a](3)	34–129	84 (17)	219 (18)	—	—	—	—	—	0.131 (0.028)
Kirberger (PW)(4)	88–161	120 (20)	184 (28)	51 (10)	—	79 (17)	0.43 (0.07)	16 (5)	—
Kirberger (CW)(4)	60–191	125 (26)	—	—	—	—	—	—	—
Bonagura (PW)(5)	≤130	$\bar{x} = 107$	—	—	—	—	—	—	—
Darke (6)	—	99 (22)	—	—	0.14 (0.03)	70 (20)	—	21 (11)	—

[a]Sedation used.

CANINE
REFERENCE VALUES FOR MITRAL DOPPLER FLOW VARIABLES

| | Peak E Velocity | | Peak A Velocity | | | | |
	Range cm/sec	$\bar{x} \pm$ (SD) cm/sec	Range cm/sec	$\bar{x} \pm$ (SD) cm/sec	E:A Range	E:A $\bar{x} \pm$ (SD)	FVI $\bar{x} \pm$ (SD) cm
Yuill (CW)(1)	70–108	86.2 (9.5)	—	—	—	—	—
Gaber (PW)(2)	—	75.0 (11.8)	—	—	—	—	—
Kirberger (PW)(4)	59–118	91 (15)	33–93	63 (13)	1.04–2.42	1.48 (0.31)	—
Bonagura (PW)(5)	≤100	$\bar{x} = 76$	<75	$\bar{x} = 49$	—	—	—
Yamamoto (PW)[a](7)	—	56 (18)	—	44 (11)	—	1.3 (0.3)	9.4 (3.2)
Darke (6)	—	65 (18)	—	43 (13)	—	1.55 (0.36)	—

[a]Anesthetized.

CANINE
REFERENCE VALUES FOR TRICUSPID DOPPLER FLOW VARIABLES

| | Peak E Velocity | | Peak A Velocity | | | |
	Range cm/sec	$\bar{x} \pm$ (SD) cm/sec	Range cm/sec	$\bar{x} \pm$ (SD) cm/sec	E:A Range	E:A $\bar{x} \pm$ (SD)
Yuill (CW)(1)	52–92	68.9 (8.4)	—	—	—	—
Gaber (PW)(2)	—	56.2 (16.1)	—	—	—	—
Kirberger (PW)(4)	49–131	86 (20)	33–94	58 (16)	0.69–3.08	1.60 (0.56)
Bonagura (PW)(5)	≤80	$\bar{x} = 60$	<60	$\bar{x} = 48$	—	—
Darke (6)	—	57 (15)	—	37 (15)	—	1.62 (0.36)

EQUINE
REFERENCE VALUES FOR AORTIC DOPPLER FLOW VARIABLES

	Vmax Range (cm/sec)	Vmax $\bar{x} \pm$ (SD) (cm/sec)	Acc $\bar{x} \pm$ (SD) m/sec²	TTP $\bar{x} \pm$ (SD) msec	PEP $\bar{x} \pm$ (SD) msec	ET $\bar{x} \pm$ (SD) msec	VTI $\bar{x} \pm$ (SD) cm
Reef (8)	60–170	101 (29)	—	—	—	—	—
Blissitt (9)	78–115	94 (9)	8 (1.4)	122 (21)	75 (18)	467 (31)	25.4 (3.2)
Stadler (10)	—	81 (21)	5.0 (1.8)	—	—	—	23.3 (7.4)

EQUINE
REFERENCE VALUES FOR PULMONARY DOPPLER FLOW VARIABLES

	Vmax Range (cm/sec)	Vmax $\bar{x} \pm$ (SD) (cm/sec)	Acc $\bar{x} \pm$ (SD) cm/sec²	TTP $\bar{x} \pm$ (SD) msec	PEP $\bar{x} \pm$ (SD) msec	ET $\bar{x} \pm$ (SD) msec	VTI $\bar{x} \pm$ (SD) cm
Reef (8)	50–190	109 (42)	—	—	—	—	—
Blissitt (9)	78–104	91 (8)	4.4 (0.7)	208 (27)	61 (17)	501 (30)	25.7 (3.1)
Stadler (10)	—	97 (12)	3.7 (1.0)	—	—	—	32.0 (5.2)

EQUINE
REFERENCE VALUES FOR MITRAL DOPPLER FLOW VARIABLES

| | Peak E Velocity | | Peak A Velocity | | | | |
	Range cm/sec	x̄ ± (SD) cm/sec	Range cm/sec	x̄ ± (SD) cm/sec	E:A Range	E:A x̄ ± (SD)	Dec Time x̄ ± (SD) sec
Reef (8)	20–150	70 (24)	11–130	31 (10)	—	—	—
Blissett (9)	41–112	70 (14)	24–63	42 (1)	0.95–3.6	1.8 (0.6)	0.22 (0.03)

EQUINE
REFERENCE VALUES FOR TRICUSPID DOPPLER FLOW VARIABLES

| | Peak E Velocity | | Peak A Velocity | | | | |
	Range cm/sec	x̄ ± (SD) cm/sec	Range cm/sec	x̄ ± (SD) cm/sec	E:A Range	E:A x̄ ± (SD)	Dec Time x̄ ± (SD) sec
Reef (8)	20–90	49 (17)	10–90	39 (18)	—	—	—
Blissitt (9)	77–105	90 (10)	48–107	69 (14)	0.87–2.0	1.3 (0.3)	0.24 (0.04)

SHEEP
REFERENCE VALUES FOR PEAK DOPPLER FLOW VELOCITIES[11]

	Range (cm/sec)	x̄ ± SD (cm/sec)
Aorta	70–140	99.1 ± 16.2
Pulmonary	68–116	92.7 ± 13.9
Mitral E	48–83	63.8 ± 9.2
Mitral A	47–90	68.4 ± 12.7
Tricuspid E	30–78	51.9 ± 12.7
Tricuspid A	30–81	44.8 ± 14.6

SHEEP
REFERENCE VALUES FOR DOPPLER-DERIVED SYSTOLIC TIME INTERVALS[11]

	Aorta	Pulmonary
Acc time (msec)	9.6–80	6.1–19.2
TTP (msec)	20–90	50–170
LVET (msec)	190–270	190–280
TTP/LVET	0.11–0.38	0.23–0.68
PEP (msec)	40–70	40–90
PEP/TTP	0.48–3.50	0.39–0.93
PEP/LVET	0.18–0.37	0.17–0.42

REFERENCES

1. Yuill C, O'Grady M. Doppler-derived velocity of blood flow across the cardiac valves in the normal dog. Can J Vet Res 1991;55:185–192.
2. Gaber C. Normal pulsed Doppler flow velocities in adult dogs. Proc 5th ACVIM 1987:923.
3. Brown D, Knight D, King R. Use of pulse-wave Doppler echocardiography to determine aortic and pulmonary velocity and flow variables in clinically normal dogs. Am J Vet Res 1991;52:543–550.
4. Kirberger RM, Bland-Van Den Berg P, Darazs B. Doppler echocardiography in the normal dog: Part II — factors influencing flow velocities and a comparison between left and right heart blood flow. Vet Radiol and Ultrasound 1992;33:380–386.
5. Bonagura JD, Miller MW. Veterinary echocardiography. Am J Cardiovasc Ultrasound & Allied Tech 1989;6:229–264.
6. Darke PGG, Fuentes VL, Champion SR. Doppler echocardiography in canine congestive cardiomyopathy. Proc 11th ACVIM 1993:531–534.
7. Yamamoto K. Masuyama T, Tanouchi J, et al. Effects of heart rate on left ventricular filling dynamics: assessment from simultaneous recordings of pulsed Doppler transmitral flow velocity pattern and haemodynamic variables. Cardiovasc Res 1993;27:935–941.
8. Reef V, Lalezari K, De Boo J, et al. Pulsed-wave Doppler evaluation of intracardiac blood flow in 30 clinically normal standard bred horses. Am J Vet Res 1989;50:75–90.
9. Blissitt KJ, Bonagura JD. Pulsed wave Doppler echocardiography in normal horses. Equine Vet J Suppl 1995;19:38–46.
10. Stadler P, Kinkel N, Deegen E. Evaluation of systolic heart function on the horse with PW Doppler echocardiography compared with thermodilution. Dtsch Tierärztl Wschr 1994;101:312–315.
11. Kirberger RM. Pulsed wave Doppler echocardiographic evaluation of intracardiac blood flow in normal sheep. Res Vet Sci 1993;55:189–194.

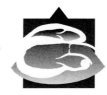

Index

Italic page numbers indicate figures; page numbers followed by t indicate tables.

Abscesses, pericardial sac, 370
Acoustic impedance, 5–6, 6t
Aliasing, 23
American College of Veterinary Internal Medicine, Echocardiography Committee of The Specialty of Cardiology, 46
American Society of Echocardiography (ASE), recommendations for M-mode images, 169
Anemia, effects on the heart, 371–372
Angle correction, spectral Doppler, 115
Angle of incidence, effect on Doppler-derived velocity, 447–448
Angle of interrogation, Doppler equation, 18, *19, 19t, 20*
Aorta
  left parasternal short-axis images, 69, *70–71*, 91, *94*
  long-axis view, *48*
  measurement, 163–165, *167*, 454
  M-mode measurement, 177–179, *179*
Aortic flow
  color-flow Doppler, 137, *144–146*
  spectral Doppler, 119–120, *119–121*, 182–183
Aortic insufficiency, 286–297
  color-flow Doppler, 290–296, *293*
  left ventricular size and function, 290–293
  spectral Doppler, 293, *296–297*
  valve appearance and motion, 286–290, *287–292*
Aortic root
  measurement, 454
  M-mode imaging, 111, *115–116*
Aortic stenosis, 214–215, 383–397, *384–398*
  color-flow Doppler, 391
  Doppler assessment, 397, *400–404*
  subvalvular, 384–388
Aortic valve
  aortic insufficiency effects, 286
  motion, on M-mode images, 225, *226–227*
Artifacts, 27–32
  mirror-image on Doppler display, 32, *33*
  patient movement and breathing, 27, *30*
  reverberation, 30–32, *31*
  side-lobe, 27–30, *31*
Atrial contraction, 205, *205*
Atrial septal defects, 424–431, *425–433*
  color-flow Doppler, 427
  spectral Doppler, 427
Atrioventricular valve dysplasia, 437
Atrium
  left, 163–165, *167*
    measurement, 454
  left parasternal short-axis images, 69, *70–71*
  right and left pressures, 221–223, *223–224*
Attenuation, 7
Axial resolution, 12, *13*

Baseline
  color-flow Doppler, 134, *134*
  spectral Doppler, 116, *117*
Blood flow. *see also* Flow
  laminar, 23
  turbulent, 23
Body surface area, dogs, 462t
Body weight, correlation with cardiac dimensions, Friesian and Belgian Blue and White calves, 467t
Bubble studies, 431

Cardiac catheterization, noninvasive, Doppler echocardiography, 210
Cardiac dimensions, correlation with body weight, Friesian and Belgian Blue and White calves, 467t
Cardiac effusions, 1
Cardiac masses, 1
Cardiac shunts, 409–431
Cardiac size, quantitative assessment, two-dimensional imaging, 160
Cardiac tamponade, 358–359, *359*
Cardiomyopathy
  dilated, 320–332, *325–332*
  hypertrophic, 304–320, *304–323*
    complications, 317–319, *318–319*
    hemodynamic and functional information, 308–317, *310–318*
    left ventricular false tendons, 320, *322–323*
    left ventricular size, 304–308, *304–308*
  restrictive, 332–337, *334–336*
  right ventricular, 328, *331*
Cats, positioning, 38, *38*
Chordae tendineae, ruptured, 267, *268–271*
Circumferential fiber shortening, velocity of, 457
Color-flow Doppler. *see* Doppler ultrasound
Color-flow processing, color-flow Doppler, 132
Color map, color-flow Doppler, 132
Color position, color-flow Doppler, *135*, 136
Color sector width, color-flow Doppler, 134–136, *135*
Committee on Standards for Veterinary Echocardiography, 45
Compress, two-dimensional echocardiography, 41
Constrictive pericarditis, 371, *372*
Continuous-wave Doppler. *see* Doppler ultrasound
Cor triatriatum, 435–437, *438–439*
Cows, positioning, 40
Cursor
  M-mode imaging technique, 104, *105–107*
  spectral Doppler, 114, *116*
Cycles, 2, *4*

Deceleration time, measure of diastolic function, 204–205, *205*
Depth
  color-flow Doppler, 132, *133*
  sample, effect on Nyquist limit, 451
Depth controls, two-dimensional echocardiography, 41, *42*

Diastolic function, 203–209
    Doppler assessment, 204–205, *204–205*
    Doppler evaluation, 206–207, *206–211*
Diastolic pressure, right and left ventricle, 220–221, *221–222*
Diastolic pulmonary pressures, 218, *219*
Diastolic systemic pressures, 217–218, *218*
Dogs, positioning, 38, *38*
Doppler, Christian Johann, 14–16
Doppler-derived systolic time intervals, sheep, 472t
Doppler-derived velocity, angle of incidence effects, 447–448
Doppler equation, 17–18
Doppler flow
    peak velocities, sheep, 472t
    profiles, normal, 118–119
    variables
        aortic
            canine, 470t
            equine, 471t
        mitral
            canine, 471t
            equine, 472t
        pulmonary
            canine, 470t
            equine, 471t
        tricuspid
            canine, 471t
            equine, 472t
Doppler gain, 117
Doppler physics, 13–26
Doppler shift, 14–16, *15*
Doppler tracing, 16, *16*
Doppler ultrasound, 1
    color-flow, 14, 23–26, *25–28*, 128–147
        aortic insufficiency, *290–296, 293*
        aortic stenosis, 391
        atrial septal defects, 427
        controls, 129–136
        evaluation, 184–186, *184–187*
        mitral insufficiency, 276–284, *279–283*
        mitral stenosis, 407, *407*
        patent ductus arteriosus, 422
        Tetralogy of Fallot, 434
    continuous-wave, 14, 17, *18*
    flow velocities, 1, *3*
    pulsed-wave, 14, 17, *17*
        presence of ventricular septal defect, 414
        spectral broadening of, 23, *24*
    spectral. *see* Spectral Doppler
Drop, transducer, 72

Echocardiography
    Doppler, pressure determination, 210
    examination, 35–150
    M-mode, 103–112, *105–107*
        controls, 104
        hemodynamic information, 223–236, *225–235*
        measurement and application, 169–179
        measurements, 453–454
    patient positioning, 27, 37–40, *38*
    patient preparation, 36, *36–37*
    reference values, 453–473
        Friesian and Belgian White and Blue calves, 466t
    two-dimensional, 41–103
        controls, 41–42
        evaluation of size and flow profiles, 151–186
    uses of, 1
End-diastolic dimension, 455
Endocardial cushion defects, 431
Endocardial fibroelastosis, 337
Endocardiosis, 261
Endocarditis, 301–304, *302–303*
End-systolic dimension, 456

Far field, 9–12, *10, 11*
Fibrinous pericarditis, *370, 370–371*

Five chamber, 88, *89*
    large animal, 63, *69, 101, 101–102, 104*
    long-axis image, *55, 62*
Flow velocity
    Doppler-derived, effect of angle of incidence, 447–448
    Doppler ultrasound, 1, *3*
Flow velocity integral, 199
    spectral Doppler, 180, *181*
Four chamber, 49–50, *51–53, 57, 64*, 88, *89*
    large animal, 63, *68, 95, 97, 100*, 100–101
    right parasternal long-axis, 157–159, *158–159*
    small animal, 80, *83*
Fractional shortening, left ventricular, 188–189, *189–190*, 203
Frame rate, 25, *28*
Frequency, sound waves, 3, *4*

Gain, color-flow Doppler, 129, *133*
Gain controls, two-dimensional echocardiography, 41, *43*
Gate, spectral Doppler, 114
Gate depth, velocity measurement and, 23, 23t, *24*
Gate size, spectral Doppler, 114

Heart
    long-axis left ventricular outflow view, *47–50*
    long-axis view, 45, *45*
    miscellaneous conditions, 371–373
    short-axis view, 46, *46*
Heart base
    aorta, 53, *58–59*, 86, 100
    pulmonary artery, 53, *60–61*, 86, 100, 101, *103*
    right parasternal transverse, 159, *160–162*
    right ventricle, 101, *103*
    tumors, 360–361, *362–364*
Heart disease
    acquired, 261–382
    congenital, 383–445
Heartworms, pulmonary hypertension and, 350–351
Hemangiosarcoma, 361–367, *365–367*
Horses, positioning, 39, *39*
Hypertension. *see* specific type

Idiopathic dilated cardiomyopathy. *see* Cardiomyopathy, dilated
Imaging technique. *see also* specific type
    M-mode, 104–112
    terms, 72
    two-dimensional, 72, *73–75*
Interventricular septum, on M-mode images, 227–229, *233–236*
Intracardiac neoplasia, 367–370, *369*
Isovolumic relaxation time, measure of diastolic function, 204, *204*

Lateral resolution, 12–13, *14*
Left atrium, M-mode measurement, 177–179, *179*
Left parasternal apical images, 55, 88–90, *89–90*, 102
Left ventricle
    calculation of function, 456–462
    chamber, wall, and septum, measurement, 160–163, *163–166*
    diastolic pressure, 220–221, *221–222*
    function, 186–188
    left parasternal long-axis images, 101, *102*
    left parasternal short-axis images, 69, *72*
    measurement, 455
    M-mode imaging, 104–105, *108–110*
    M-mode measurement, 170–176, *171–176*
    with papillary muscle and chordae tendineae, 50, *54–55, 84–85, 87*
    with pulmonary artery, 55, *61*, 86, *88*
    right parasternal short-axis images, 98, *98–99*
    right parasternal transverse, 159, *160*
    size and function
        in aortic insufficiency, 290–293
        in mitral insufficiency, 267–276, *271–278*
    systolic pressures, 215, *216*
Left ventricular ejection time, measurement, 454
Left ventricular false tendons, 320, *322–323*
Left ventricular fractional shortening, 456

Left ventricular outflow, 46, 47, 75, 90, 92
    large animal, 92–95, 95
    right parasternal long-axis, 151–157, 152–157
    small animal, 57, 63, 65
Left ventricular outflow tract, spectral Doppler, 120
Left ventricular wall, on M-mode images, 227
Left ventricular wall diastolic thickness, 456
Left ventricular wall systolic thickness, 456, 457
Lift, transducer, 72
Llamas, positioning, 40, 40
Long-axis, 45, 45
    left parasternal, 57, 90, 100, 100–103
    right parasternal, 75–88, 76–87, 92–95, 94–95

Mitral and tricuspid flow, color-flow Doppler, 136–137,
    140–143
Mitral dysplasia, 441–442
Mitral inflow, spectral Doppler, 124–127, 126–127
Mitral insufficiency, 216, 261–286
    color-flow Doppler, 276–284, 279–283
    diastolic, 286
    left ventricular size and function, 267–276, 271–278
    spectral Doppler, 284–285, 284–286
    valvular appearance and motion, 261–267, 262–271
Mitral stenosis, 215, 215, 404–409, 404–409
    Doppler assessment, 407
    spectral Doppler, 407
Mitral valve, 53, 56, 85
    aortic insufficiency effects, 286
    degenerative lesions, 261–263, 262–264
    measurement, 455
    M-mode imaging, 110–112, 112–114
    M-mode measurement, 176–177, 178
    right parasternal short-axis images, 98–99, 99–100
    spectral Doppler, 183
Mitral valve motion, on M-mode images, 225, 230
Mitral valve prolapse, 263–267, 265–267
M-mode imaging, 1. see also Echocardiography, M-mode
    how to make measurements, 453–454
    long-axis, Friesian and Belgian White and Blue calves, 468t
    reference values
        adult cow, 466t
        adult dogs, 461t
        adult horses, 465t
        adult llamas, 468t
        anesthetized or sedated cats, 457t
        growing foals, 464t
        growing puppies, 460t
        growth Friesian calves, 467t
        nonanesthetized cats, 456t
        pigs, 468t
        pony foals, 464t
        sheep, 468t
        specific canine breeds, 458t, 459t
Motion-mode imaging. see Echocardiography, M-mode; M-mode
    imaging
Myocardial infarction, 337–341, 337–342
Myocardium, abnormalities, 1

Near field, 9–12, 10, 11
Nyquist limit, 21, 21–22, 22
    effect of sample depth, 451
    effect of transducer frequency on, 449

Obesity, effects on the heart, 372–373
Ostium primum defects, 424–425, 427
Outflow obstructions, 383–404, 404–409

Packet size, 26, 29
Parameters of function, reference values, canine, 462t
Patent ductus arteriosus, 418–423, 421–424
    color-flow Doppler, 422
    spectral Doppler, 422
Peak and mean velocity, spectral Doppler, 180, 181
Pericardial diaphragmatic hernia, 442, 442
Pericardial diseases, 370–371

Pericardial effusion, 356–370, 357–358
    cardiac function with, 359–360, 360
    neoplasia as a cause of, 360
    pericardial diseases as cause of, 370–371
Pericardial tumors, 370
Pericarditis
    constrictive, 371, 372
    fibrinous, 370, 370–371
Persistence
    color-flow Doppler, 136
    two-dimensional echocardiography, 42
Point, transducer, 72
Positioning
    large animal, 39, 39–40, 40
    small animal, 37, 37–39, 38
Pre-ejection period, measurement, 454
Pressure gradients, Doppler measurement, 210, 211
Pulmonary artery, left parasternal short-axis images, 69, 70–71, 91, 94
Pulmonary flow
    color-flow Doppler, 137, 146–147
    spectral Doppler, 120–121, 122–124, 183
Pulmonary hypertension, 342–352, 342–352
    heartworms in, 350–351
Pulmonic stenosis, 214–215, 397–404
    Doppler assessment, 401
    spectral Doppler, 401, 403
Pulsed-wave Doppler. see Doppler ultrasound
Pulse repetition frequency, 8–9, 9, 10, 19

Reference values, dogs weighing more than 150 pounds, 462t
Reflection, 6–7, 7
Refraction, 6–7, 7
Regurgitant fractions, 218–220
Resolution, transducers and, 8–13
Respiratory motion, M-mode abnormalities, 172, 173
Right atrium, left parasternal short-axis images, 91, 94
Right atrium and auricle, small animal, 63, 66, 91
Right ventricle
    diastolic pressure, 220–221, 221–222
    systolic pressures, 216, 217
Right ventricular outflow, 91
    small animal, 63, 67–68
    spectral Doppler, 124
Rotate, transducer, 72

Scale, spectral Doppler, 117
Scanning table, small animal positioning, 37, 38
Scattering, 6–7, 7, 8
Sector width, two-dimensional echocardiography, 42, 44
Septal and wall boundaries, M-mode abnormalities, 172, 174
Septal diastolic thickness, 456
Septal systolic thickness, 456, 457
Shaving, preparation for echocardiography, 36, 36–37
Short-axis, 45–46, 46
    left parasternal, 69, 70, 91, 94
    right parasternal, 50, 53, 81–84, 86, 95–100
Shunt ratios, 1, 220
Sound
    attenuation, 7
    reflection, refraction, and scattering, 6–7, 7, 8
Sound beams, 1, 2
    generated by transducers, 9–12, 10, 11
Sound waves, 1, 2, 3
    frequency, 3, 4
    velocity, 4, 4–5, 5
Spectral Doppler, 112–128
    aortic insufficiency, 290–296, 293
    atrial septal defect, 427
    controls, 114–118
    dilated cardiomyopathy, 328, 332
    measurement and assessment, 179–184, 180–183
    mitral inflow, 407
    mitral insufficiency, 284–285, 284–286
    patent ductus arteriosus, 422
    pulmonary hypertension, 348–350, 348–351
    pulmonic stenosis, 401, 403

Spectral Doppler—*Continued*
  systemic hypertension, 355
  Tetralogy of Fallot, 434
Spectral tracings, 16, *16*
Speed of sound, *4*, 4–5, 5t
Stenotic lesions, 1
Stroke volume, 199
Subcostal images, 72
Sweep speed
  M-mode imaging technique, 104
  spectral Doppler, 118
Systemic hypertension, 352–355, *353–355*
Systolic function
  Doppler evaluation, 199–204, *200–202*
  M-mode evaluation, 188–193
  two-dimensional measurement, 193–199, *194–198*
Systolic time intervals
  left ventricular, 191–193
  normal, dog, 460t
  spectral Doppler, 180–182, *181*

Temporal resolution, 12–13
Tetralogy of Fallot, 431–432, *434, 436*
Time-gain compensation, two-dimensional echocardiography, 41, *43*
Tissues
  half-power distances of, 7, 8t
  speed of sound, *4*, 4–5, *5*
Transducers, 3
  face, 72
  frequency, effect on Nyquist limit, 449
  frequency, effects of, 19, *19*
  mechanical, 10
  phased-array, 10–12, *12*

reference marks, 72, *73–75*
resolution and, 8–13
selection, 40–41
variable focal zones in, 9
Tricuspid and pulmonic insufficiencies, 298–301, *299–301*
Tricuspid dysplasia, *440*, 440–441
Tricuspid flow, spectral Doppler, 127–128, *128–132*
Tricuspid insufficiency, 216
Tricuspid stenosis, 409, *410*
Tricuspid valve, spectral Doppler, 183–184
Truncus arteriosus, 431
Two-dimensional images, 1, *2*
Two-dimensional measurement, reference values
  adult dogs, 461t
  adult horse, 466t
  cats, 458t

Ultrasound
  cardiac. *see* Echocardiography
  physics of, 1–34
  pulsed, 8–9, *9, 10*

Valvular disease, degenerative, 261
Valvular lesions, 1
Variance maps, ultrasound, 25, *27*
Ventricular filling
  rapid, measure of diastolic function, 204, *205*
  restriction to, diastolic function, 206, *207*
Ventricular septal defect, 410–418, *411–420*

Wall filters, spectral Doppler, 118, *118*
Wavelengths, 2, *4*
  at commonly used frequencies, 4t